Hip Surgery: A Patient's Guide to Hip Replacement, Resurfacing and Arthroplasty

Editor: Marlow Coffey

FOSTER ACADEMICS

www.fosteracademics.com

www.fosteracademics.com

FOSTER ACADEMICS

Cataloging-in-Publication Data

Hip surgery : a patient's guide to hip replacement, resurfacing and arthroplasty / edited by Marlow Coffey.
p. cm.
Includes bibliographical references and index.
ISBN 978-1-63242-549-2
1. Hip joint--Surgery. 2. Total hip replacement. 3. Artificial hip joints. I. Coffey, Marlow.
RD549 .H57 2018
617.581 059 2--dc23

Foster Academics,
118-35 Queens Blvd., Suite 400,
Forest Hills, NY 11375, USA

ISBN 978-1-63242-549-2 (Hardback)

Printed and bound in China.

Contents

Preface

The procedure of placing a prosthetic implant in place of a hip joint is called a hip surgery. In severe cases, the only treatment for a hip dysfunction is a surgery. Some of the techniques used while performing the surgery are posterior approach, antero-lateral approach, lateral approach and minimally invasive approach. The various studies that are constantly contributing towards advancing technologies and evolution of this field are examined in detail. A number of latest researches have been included to keep the readers up-to-date with the global concepts in this area of study.

This book is a comprehensive compilation of works of different researchers from varied parts of the world. It includes valuable experiences of the researchers with the sole objective of providing the readers (learners) with a proper knowledge of the concerned field. This book will be beneficial in evoking inspiration and enhancing the knowledge of the interested readers.

In the end, I would like to extend my heartiest thanks to the authors who worked with great determination on their chapters. I also appreciate the publisher's support in the course of the book. I would also like to deeply acknowledge my family who stood by me as a source of inspiration during the project.

Editor

1

SSRIs Increase Risk of Blood Transfusion in Patients Admitted for Hip Surgery

Hermien Janneke Schutte[1], Sofie Jansen[1], Matthias U. Schafroth[2], J. Carel Goslings[3], Nathalie van der Velde[1], Sophia E. J. A. de Rooij[1]*

1 Section of Geriatric Medicine, Department of Medicine, Academic Medical Center, Amsterdam, The Netherlands, **2** Department of Orthopedic Surgery, Academic Medical Center, Amsterdam, The Netherlands, **3** Trauma Unit, Department of Surgery, Academic Medical Center, Amsterdam, The Netherlands

Abstract

Background: Recent studies have shown that an increased bleeding tendency can be caused by Selective Serotonin Reuptake Inhibitors (SSRI) use. We aimed to investigate the occurrence and risk of blood transfusion in SSRI users compared to non-SSRI users in a cohort of patients admitted for hip-surgery.

Methods: We conducted a retrospective cohort study of patients who underwent planned or emergency hip surgery from 1996 to 2011 in the Academic Medical Center in Amsterdam. Primary outcome measure was risk of blood transfusion. Secondary outcome measures were pre- and postoperative hemoglobin level. Multivariate logistic regression was used to adjust for potential confounders.

Results: One-hundred and fourteen SSRI users were compared to 1773 non-SSRI users. Risk of blood transfusion during admission was increased for SSRI users in multivariate analyses (OR 1.7 [95% CI 1.1–2.5]). Also, pre-operative hemoglobin levels were lower in SSRI users (7.8±1.0 mmol/L) compared to non-SSRI users (8.0±1.0 mmol/L) ($p = 0.042$)), as were postoperative hemoglobin levels (6.2±1.0 mmol/L vs. 6.4±1.0 mmol/L respectively) ($p = 0.017$)).

Conclusions: SSRI users undergoing hip surgery have an increased risk for blood transfusion during admission, potentially explained by a lower hemoglobin level before surgery. SSRI use should be considered as a potential risk indicator for increased blood loss in patients admitted for hip surgery. These results need to be confirmed in a prospective study.

Editor: Halvard Boenig, German Red Cross Blood Service Frankfurt, Germany

Funding: These authors have no support or funding to report.

Competing Interests: The authors have declared that no competing interests exist.

* E-mail: s.e.derooij@amc.uva.nl

Introduction

Peri-operative blood transfusions increase the relative risk of postoperative infections and are associated with considerable morbidity and mortality [1,2]. An important indication for blood transfusions is major peri-operative blood loss [3]. The amount of peri-operative blood loss can be negatively influenced by the use of drugs that increase bleeding tendency, such as anti-thrombotic drugs [4]. However, increased bleeding tendency is also associated with the use of Selective Serotonin Reuptake Inhibitors (SSRIs) [5–8]. In a recent large cohort study, peri-operative use of SSRIs was even directly associated with a higher risk of adverse events, such as in-hospital mortality and hospital readmission within 30 days [9].

In the Netherlands, the use of SSRIs is widely spread with over 500,000 prescribed patients in 2011 [10]. The most common indications for SSRI prescription in general practice are depression (53.5%) and anxiety (18.7%) [11].

Several studies have shown that use of SSRIs is associated with an increased risk of gastrointestinal bleeding. Within studies, associations varied from modest to strong [5–8,12]. Despite these outcomes, only a few studies have addressed the association between SSRI use and peri-operative blood loss. These reference studies showed ambiguous result [13,14]. Consequently, the association between SSRI use and increased risk of peri-operative bleeding remains unclear. As hip surgery is known to be the leading indication for blood transfusion in orthopedic patients [15], we aimed to study whether SSRIs increase risk of blood transfusion during admission in a cohort of patients undergoing hip surgery.

Methods

Setting and population

The current study was performed within a large cohort of hip surgery patients that consisted of all consecutive patients admitted for either planned or emergency hip surgery from 1996 to 2011 in an academic hospital. This cohort was gathered for a study in which the occurrence of ECG abnormalities was studied in patients undergoing hip surgery [16]. Inclusion criteria were age ≥ 50 years, pre-operative ECG present in hospital records. Exclusion criteria were previous hip fracture, hip fracture due to High Energy Trauma (HET) and pathological fracture due to malignancy or other diseases. Hip surgeries included all proximal femur fracture surgeries, including osteosynthesis and (hemi-) arthroplasty. This study was conducted according to the principles expressed in the Declaration of Helsinki. The medical ethics committee of the Academic Medical Center (Amsterdam) approved the conduction of this study and waived the necessity to obtain informed consent from participants because of the observational design.

Covariate information

The following covariates were collected: age at the time of surgery (years), gender, Charlson Comorbidity Index (CCI) [17], home situation at time of admission, type of surgery, date of surgery, estimated glomerular filtration rate (eGFR) by the Modification of Diet in Renal Decease (MDRD) equation [18], previously diagnosed clinical depression and all drug use. Home situation was defined as community dwelling (living at home or in assisted living) or living in an institution (nursing home, home for elderly or other hospital). Type of surgery was defined as either emergency hip surgery (all proximal femur fractures with subsequent surgery) or planned hip surgery (treatment for osteoarthritis or avascular necrosis through total hip replacement). Date of surgery was categorized as before 2004 or from 2004 and onwards, corresponding the change in blood transfusion guidelines. All data were retrieved from patients' medical records.

Markers for increased bleeding tendency

Primary outcome measure was the occurrence of blood transfusion during hospital stay (pre-, peri- and postoperative). In 1998, local guidelines advised pre-operative blood transfusion from a hemoglobin level of 4.5–5.0 mmol/L and a postoperative blood transfusion from 4.5–5.5 mmol/L. In 2004, new national guidelines for blood transfusion introduced the prevailing '4-5-6 rule', which combined age, American Society of Anesthesiologists (ASA) score and hemoglobin level [19,20].

Secondary outcome variables were the amount of packed cells administered and pre- and postoperative serum hemoglobin levels (mmol/L). To investigate peri-operative loss of hemoblobin, a delta-hemoglobin level was defined (pre-operative hemoglobin level subtracted from the postoperative hemoglobin level). Pre-operative serum hemoglobin was defined as most recent hemoglobin level before surgery within 72 hours. Postoperative hemoglobin level was obtained from the first postoperative blood samples within 72 hours.

SSRI and other drug use

Medication use at time of admission was verified through hospital charts, pharmacy notes and/or referral letters. Drugs were listed and grouped according to ATC codes. SSRI use included all types of SSRIs registered and prescribed at the time of surgery. All anti-thrombotic agents, (heparin, vitamin K antagonists and platelet aggregation inhibitors), were also registered. Furthermore, non-steroidal anti-inflammatory drugs (NSAIDs) and anti-rheumatic drugs were registered.

Health care consumption

Other variables that were possibly related to increased bleeding tendency in the setting of major surgery were explored. Duration of surgery was defined as the actual duration of surgery, excluding duration of pre- and postoperative care in the operating room and recovery. Duration of hospital admission (days) and hospital readmission within 30 days after admission (all causes included) were also gathered.

Statistical analysis

Baseline characteristics and outcome variables were calculated either as the mean and SD or as frequency and percentage of occurrence. Independent samples T-tests were used for continuous variables and Chi-square test for dichotomous variables. Histograms of continuous variables were analyzed to affirm normal distribution. In non-normally distributed data, we used Mann-Whitney U and Kruskal-Wallis non-parametric tests. A p-value $\leq$ 0.05 was considered statistically significant. To assess for potential confounders, multivariate logistic regression analyses were performed. Variables were considered confounders when they altered the coefficient of the main variable by more than ten percent [21]. In the multivariate logistic regression analyses, multiple imputation was used for variables that had more than ten percent missing values [22]. As it is known that patients undergoing emergency hip-surgery are usually frailer than patients undergoing planned hip-surgery, potentially influencing our results, we repeated our analyses in patients undergoing emergency hip-surgery exclusively.

Finally, potential influence by change in guidelines was analyzed by testing for potential interaction (interaction term between date of blood transfusion categorized as before 2004, or from 2004 and onwards and SSRI use).

Statistical analyses were performed with SPSS (IBM SPSS Statistics version 19.0).

Results

In total, 1887 hip surgery patients were included, of whom 114 were SSRI users. Table 1 represents the baseline characteristics of SSRI users and non-users. Age and gender were equally distributed between both groups. On average, SSRI users had more comorbidity, more often underwent emergency hip surgery and more often lived in institutions compared to non-SSRI users. Date of surgery, estimated GFR and use of anti-thrombotic and non-steroidal anti-inflammatory drugs (NSAIDS) were equal in both groups.

Table 2 represents the association of SSRI use with different markers for increased bleeding tendency. Forty-eight percent of SSRI users underwent blood transfusion during admission, compared to 38% of non-SSRI users ($p = 0.021$). Pre-operative hemoglobin levels were lower in SSRI users than non-SSRI users ($p = 0.042$), as were postoperative hemoglobin levels ($p = 0.017$). Delta-hemoglobin level showed no difference between SSRI users and non-users. Length of hospital stay, duration of surgery and readmission rate within thirty days were equal in both groups.

Table 3 shows associations between blood transfusion during hospitalization and use of SSRIs, anti-thrombotic drugs and NSAIDs. Model 1 represents the odds ratios adjusted for age and gender and model 2 the odds ratios adjusted for age, gender, established depressive disorder and the estimated glomerular filtration rate (variables that changed the regression coefficient by more than 10%). After adjustment in the second model, SSRI users had an increased risk of blood transfusion (OR 1.7 [95% CI 1.1–2.5]). Odds ratios for blood transfusion were also increased for anti-thrombotic drug use (OR 1.3 [1.1–1.6]) and NSAIDs/anti-rheumatic drug use (OR 1.4 [1.0–1.8]). After further adjustment for pre-operative hemoglobin levels (model 3), odds ratios for blood transfusion for all three drug types remained increased. However, the association between SSRI use and blood transfusion lost statistical significance.

Repeating the multivariate logistic regression in emergency hip-surgery patients exclusively ($n = 1312$), SSRI use remained positively associated with an increased risk of blood transfusion (OR 1.7 [95% CI 1.1–2.6]).

Table 1. Baseline Characteristics of SSRI users and non-SSRI users.

Variable	SSRI users (n = 114) Mean (±)/n (%)	non- SSRI users (n = 1773) Mean (±)/n (%)	p
Age at the time of surgery (years)	78.1 (±11.7)	77.0 (±11.4)	0.317
Gender			
Female	85 (74.6%)	1269 (71.0%)	0.492
Type of surgery			
Acute	99 (86.8%)	1213 (68.4%)	<0.001
Date of surgery			
In 2004 and onwards	55 (48.2%)	755 (42.6%)	0.236
Home situation at admission (n = 1739)			
Communitiy dwelling	55 (48.2%)	1326 (74.8%)	<0.001
Charlson Comorbidity Index	1.5 (±1.5)	1.2 (±1.5)	0,029
eGFR (n = 1822)	85.5 (±34.1)	83.1 (±30.0)	0,463
Clinical Depression	24 (32.0%)	90 (5.0%)	<0.001
Anti-thrombotic drug use	41 (36.0%)	595 (33.6%)	0.598
NSAIDs/anti- rheumatic drug use	15 (13.2%)	271 (15.3%)	0.539

SSRI = Selective Serotonin Reuptake Inhibitor;
eGFR = estimated Glomerular Filtration Rate;
NSAIDs = Non-Steroidal Anti Inflammatory Drugs;
± = standard deviation.

Finally, the interaction term between date of blood transfusion (categorized as before 2004, or from 2004 and onwards) and SSRI use in the regression models was not significant ($p = 0.278$).

Because of >10% missing values, for the latter analyses imputation of pre-operative hemoglobin levels and estimated glomerular filtration rate was performed.

Discussion

The results of our study show that patients who used SSRIs at the time of hip surgery had an increased risk of blood transfusion during hospitalization. A lower pre-operative hemoglobin level in SSRI users potentially causes this greater risk.

The results of our study correspond to a study by Movig et al. In this study, risk of blood transfusion was quadrupled among SSRI users [14]. Their study participants were younger patients undergoing planned spine, knee and hip surgery, whereas our

Table 2. Markers for increased bleeding tendency and health care consumption.

	SSRI users (n = 114) Mean (±)/n (%)	non-SSRI users (n = 1773) Mean (±)/n (%)	p
Blood transfusion during admission	55 (48.2%)	663 (37.7%)	0.021
Amount of packed cells administered during admission (n = 718) †	2.9 (±1.9)	3.1 (±3.1)	0.631
Pre-operative hemoglobin level (n = 1499) (mmol/L) ‡	7.8 (±1.0)	8.0 (±1.0)	0.042
Postoperative hemoglobin level (n = 1743) (mmol/L) ‡	6.2 (±1.0)	6.4 (±1.0)	0.017
Delta hemoglobin level (n = 1323) (mmol/L) §	1.7 (±0.8)	1.7 (±0.9)	0.624
Readmission within 30 days	9 (7.9%)	92 (5.2%)	0.213
Duration of surgery (n = 1884) (minutes)	91.0 (43.4%)	93.9 (38.7%)	0.449
Length of hospital stay (days)	13.9 (±11.8)	15.5 (±15.5)	0.288

† = only transfused patients included;
‡ = pre-operative hemoglobin level: <72 hours before surgery, postoperative hemoglobin level: <72 hours after surgery;
§ = (postoperative hemoglobin - pre-operative hemoglobin);
SSRI = Selective Serotonin Reuptake Inhibitor;
± = standard deviation.

Table 3. Odds Ratios (OR) for blood transfusion during admission (n = 1887).

	Model 1		Model 2		Model 3	
	OR	**95% CI**	**OR**	**95% CI**	**OR**	**95% CI**
SSRI	1.5	(1.0–2.2)	1.7	(1.1–2.5)	1.4	(0.9–2.2)
Anti-thrombotic	1.4	(1.2–1.7)	1.3	(1.1–1.6)	1.3	(1.0–1.6)
NSAIDs/anti-rheumatic drugs	1.4	(1.0–1.8)	1.4	(1.0–1.8)	1.3	(1.0–1.8)

Model 1 = adjusted for age and gender;
Model 2 = adjusted for age, gender, eGFR, depression;
Model 3 = adjusted for age, gender, eGFR, depression, pre-operative hemoglobin level (<72 hours after surgery), Missing variables for pre-operative hemoglobin level and eGFR were imputed through multiple imputation;
CI = Confidence Interval;
OR = Odds Ratio;
aOR = adjusted Odds Ratio;
SSRI = Selective Serotonin Reuptake Inhibitor;
eGFR = estimated Glomerular Filtration Rate;
NSAIDs = Non-steroidal Anti Inflammatory Drugs.

study exclusively included older patients undergoing hip surgery. Hip surgery is known to be the leading indication for blood transfusion in orthopedic patients [15]. In our cohort this may have caused more events in both SSRI users and non-SSRI users, possibly overshadowing the effects of SSRIs on bleeding tendency alone. Another study by van Haelst et al. reported an increase in peri-operative blood loss in SSRI users compared to non-SSRI users in a cohort of patients undergoing elective hip surgery [13]. However, this did not result in a significant increase in blood transfusions in SSRI users. Van Haelst et al. exclusively included elective hip surgery patients who differ from patients undergoing emergency hip surgery regarding comorbidity and drug use, which might explain the differences with our findings. The differences between our results and the mentioned studies could also be explained by the fact that hospitals employ different triggers or criteria for blood transfusion [23].

The results of our study also show that SSRI users had lower pre- and postoperative hemoglobin levels compared to non-SSRI users. As delta-hemoglobin level was equal in both groups, the lower post-operative hemoglobin level in SSRI users is most likely explained by the lower pre-operative hb levels in SSRI users. These results are comparable to both reference studies, in which lower pre-operative hemoglobin levels were also found in SSRI users, however not significant [13,14]. Since it is unclear whether reference studies used hemoglobin levels measured within 72 hours peri-operatively, it is difficult to compare these results with ours.

Adjustment for pre-operative hemoglobin level altered the ORs for blood transfusion according to SSRI use, confirming the influence of pre-operative hemoglobin level on risk of blood transfusion. We considered pre-operative hemoglobin as an intermediate, since extra pre-operative blood loss would be a trigger for blood transfusion.

In this study's frail population, reasons for lower starting hemoglobin levels could be manifold. Our theory is that SSRI users have lower starting hemoglobin level due to increased bleeding in the hip-fracture, caused by a lower anti-platelet aggregation function. Although SSRI users more often underwent emergency hip-surgery, were more often institutionalized and had more comorbidity, the adjustment for these potential confounders did not influence our results. Also, repeating our analysis in emergency hip-surgery patients exclusively did not lead to different results.

The underlying mechanism of the increased bleeding tendency is currently attributed to the known ability of SSRIs to block the 5-HTT transporter in neurons. 5-HTT transporters in neurons have the same structure as those in platelets and can therefore cause a low serotonin level in platelets, which has a decreasing effect on the platelet aggregation function [24]. This theory is currently accepted; however recently a new theory suggests that SSRIs cause additional damage to the gastrointestinal mucosa, which might lead to gastrointestinal bleeding [25]. Potentially, SSRI users had more (occult) gastro-intestinal blood loss. In this retrospective study however, potential mucosal defects and gastro-intestinal blood loss could not be objectivized and therefore we can only speculate on this potential pathway.

Literature also suggests that a clinical depression is associated with increased or decreased platelet aggregation [26,27]. However, not all study participants who used SSRIs had a diagnosis of clinical depression. In our analysis, we therefore regarded clinical depression as a potential confounder. Correcting for depression in our analyses did however not change the significance of our results, indicating that SSRIs were not acting just as a mediator for clinical depression.

Our study has several strengths. First of all, the size of this study cohort is considerably larger than two other studies. Furthermore, considering the mean age, comorbidity and type of surgery of the study subjects, our cohort probably represents the population that is mostly troubled by adverse effects of SSRI use [28].

However, due to the retrospective design of the study, interpretation of our findings is to some extent limited. The registration of SSRIs relied on the registrations in surgical charts. Detailed information on medication use (such as dose and duration) was inconsistent due to the routine registration diversity among physicians. SSRI use was therefore potentially underreported, which might have led to a dilution of the actual effect size. Furthermore, the indication for blood transfusion in hospitals is currently customarily based on the ASA score and hemoglobin level, therefore it does not depend solely on the amount of blood loss [3]. As we have no reason to assume that this was differential for both groups, we do not consider confounding by indication.

The hospital's criteria for blood transfusion changed during the study period [3]. However, analysis showed no interaction between date of blood transfusion (categorized as before 2004, or from 2004 and onwards) and SSR use. Therefore, change in guidelines was not considered as a moderator.

Finally, it is possible that the prescription of certain anticoagulant drugs was stopped a few days before surgery. Therefore the association between use of these drugs and blood transfusion could be underestimated. However, it is unlikely that this has affected our main results. But to fully compare SSRIs with these other drugs, more information regarding actual drug use would be needed.

This study showed that SSRI users have an increased risk of blood transfusion during hospitalization compared to non-SSRI users (OR1.7 [95%CI 1.1–2.5]). A lower pre-operative hemoglobin level in SSRI users most likely caused this increased risk of blood transfusion. The increased risk has implications for clinical practice, especially for the peri-operative care of frail older patients who are at increased risk of peri-operative complications per sé. Use of SSRIs around surgery is momentarily not mentioned as a potential risk indicator for increased bleeding tendency in orthopedic and anesthetic guidelines. However, our findings need to be validated in a prospective cohort study.

Acknowledgments

The authors would like to thank Ms. Janet MacNeil-Vroomen for her help with multiple imputation, and Sanquin Blood Supply Foundation for providing information on Blood Transfusion protocols and procedures.

Author Contributions

Conceived and designed the experiments: SEJAR SJ NV HJS. Performed the experiments: SJ HJS. Analyzed the data: SJ HJS. Contributed reagents/materials/analysis tools: JCG MUS. Wrote the paper: SJ HJS.

References

1. Rogers MA, Blumberg N, Heal JM, Hicks GL Jr. (2007) Increased risk of infection and mortality in women after cardiac surgery related to allogeneic blood transfusion. J Womens Health (Larchmt) 16: 1412–1420.
2. Shander A, Spence RK, Adams D, Shore-Lesserson L, Walawander CA (2009) Timing and incidence of postoperative infections associated with blood transfusion: analysis of 1,489 orthopedic and cardiac surgery patients. Surg Infect (Larchmt) 10: 277–283.
3. Centraal Begeleidings Orgaan (2011) Blood Transfusion Guideline.
4. Radovanovic I, Queally J, Bahari S, Sproule J, McElwain J (2012) Anticoagulant use and its effect on bleeding and complications in total knee arthroplasty. Acta Orthop Belg 78: 187–191.
5. de Abajo FJ, Garcia-Rodriguez LA (2008) Risk of upper gastrointestinal tract bleeding associated with selective serotonin reuptake inhibitors and venlafaxine therapy: interaction with nonsteroidal anti-inflammatory drugs and effect of acid-suppressing agents. Arch Gen Psychiatry 65: 795–803.
6. Carvajal A, Ortega S, Del OL, Vidal X, Aguirre C, et al. (2011) Selective serotonin reuptake inhibitors and gastrointestinal bleeding: a case-control study. PLoS One 6: e19819.
7. Andrade C, Sandarsh S, Chethan KB, Nagesh KS (2010) Serotonin reuptake inhibitor antidepressants and abnormal bleeding: a review for clinicians and a reconsideration of mechanisms. J Clin Psychiatry 71: 1565–1575.
8. Vidal X, Ibanez L, Vendrell L, Conforti A, Laporte JR (2008) Risk of upper gastrointestinal bleeding and the degree of serotonin reuptake inhibition by antidepressants: a case-control study. Drug Saf 31: 159–168.
9. Auerbach AD, Vittinghoff E, Maselli J, Pekow PS, Young JQ, et al. (2013) Perioperative use of selective serotonin reuptake inhibitors and risks for adverse outcomes of surgery. JAMA Intern Med 173: 1075–1081.
10. College van zorgverzekeringen (2012) Aantal gebruikers 2007–2011 voor ATC-subgroep N06AB: Selectieve serotonine-heropnameremmers.
11. Gardarsdottir H, Heerdink ER, van Dijk L, Egberts AC (2007) Indications for antidepressant drug prescribing in general practice in the Netherlands. J Affect Disord 98: 109–115.
12. Targownik LE, Bolton JM, Metge CJ, Leung S, Sareen J (2009) Selective serotonin reuptake inhibitors are associated with a modest increase in the risk of upper gastrointestinal bleeding. Am J Gastroenterol 104: 1475–1482.
13. van Haelst IM, Egberts TC, Doodeman HJ, Traast HS, Burger BJ, et al. (2010) Use of serotonergic antidepressants and bleeding risk in orthopedic patients. Anesthesiology 112: 631–636.
14. Movig KL, Janssen MW, de Waal MJ, Kabel PJ, Leufkens HG, et al. (2003) Relationship of serotonergic antidepressants and need for blood transfusion in orthopedic surgical patients. Arch Intern Med 163: 2354–2358.
15. Cobain TJ, Vamvakas EC, Wells A, Titlestad K (2007) A survey of the demographics of blood use. Transfus Med 17: 1–15.
16. Jansen S (2012) ECG abnormalities as a predictor for hip fractures. European Geriatric Medicine 3: S2–S3.
17. Charlson ME, Pompei P, Ales KL, MacKenzie CR (1987) A new method of classifying prognostic comorbidity in longitudinal studies: development and validation. J Chronic Dis 40: 373–383.
18. Levey AS, Bosch JP, Lewis JB, Greene T, Rogers N, et al. (1999) A more accurate method to estimate glomerular filtration rate from serum creatinine: a new prediction equation. Modification of Diet in Renal Disease Study Group. Ann Intern Med 130: 461–470.
19. Centraal Begeleidings Orgaan (2004) Blood Transfusion Guideline.
20. Owens WD, Felts JA, Spitznagel EL Jr. (1978) ASA physical status classifications: a study of consistency of ratings. Anesthesiology 49: 239–243.
21. Rothman KJ, Greenland S. (2008) Modern Epidemiology. Lippincot Williams & Wilkins.
22. White IR, Royston P, Wood AM (2011) Multiple imputation using chained equations: Issues and guidance for practice. Stat Med 30: 377–399.
23. Wu WC, Trivedi A, Friedmann PD, Henderson WG, Smith TS, et al. (2012) Association between hospital intraoperative blood transfusion practices for surgical blood loss and hospital surgical mortality rates. Ann Surg 255: 708–714.
24. Cook EH Jr, Fletcher KE, Wainwright M, Marks N, Yan SY, et al. (1994) Primary structure of the human platelet serotonin 5-HT2A receptor: identify with frontal cortex serotonin 5-HT2A receptor. J Neurochem 63: 465–469.
25. Takeuchi K, Tanaka A, Nukui K, Kojo A, Gyenge M, et al. (2011) Aggravation by paroxetine, a selective serotonin reuptake inhibitor, of antral lesions generated by nonsteroidal anti-inflammatory drugs in rats. J Pharmacol Exp Ther 338: 850–859.
26. Ziegelstein RC, Parakh K, Sakhuja A, Bhat U (2009) Platelet function in patients with major depression. Intern Med J 39: 38–43.
27. Morel-Kopp MC, McLean L, Chen Q, Tofler GH, Tennant C, et al. (2009) The association of depression with platelet activation: evidence for a treatment effect. J Thromb Haemost 7: 573–581.
28. Naranjo CA, Herrmann N, Mittmann N, Bremner KE (1995) Recent advances in geriatric psychopharmacology. Drugs Aging 7: 184–202.

2

Troublesome Heterotopic Ossification after Central Nervous System Damage: A Survey of 570 Surgeries

François Genêt[1]*, Claire Jourdan[1], Alexis Schnitzler[1], Christine Lautridou[2], Didier Guillemot[3], Thierry Judet[2], Serge Poiraudeau[4], Philippe Denormandie[2]

1 Service de Médecine Physique et de Réadaptation, Hôpital Raymond Poincaré, Garches, France, **2** Service de Chirurgie Orthopédique et Traumatologique, Hôpital Raymond Poincaré, Garches, France, **3** Unité Fonctionnelle de Santé Publique, Hôpital Raymond Poincaré, Garches, France, **4** Service de Médecine Physique et de Réadaptation, Hôpital Cochin, Paris, France

Abstract

Background: Heterotopic ossification (HO) is a frequent complication after central nervous system (CNS) damage but has seldom been studied. We aimed to investigate features of HO for the first time in a large sample and the rate of early recurrence of HO in terms of the time of surgery.

Methodology/Principal Findings: We retrospectively analyzed data from an anonymous prospective survey of patients undergoing surgery between May 1993 and November 2009 in our institution for troublesome HO related to acquired neurological disease. Demographic and HO characteristics and neurological etiologies were recorded. For 357 consecutive patients, we collected data on 539 first surgeries for HO (129 surgeries for multiple sites). During the follow-up, recurrences requiring another surgery appeared in 31 cases (5.8% [31/539]; 95% confidence interval [CI]: 3.8%–7.8%; 27 patients). Most HO requiring surgery occurred after traumatic brain injury (199 patients [55.7%]), then spinal cord injury (86 [24.0%]), stroke (42 [11.8%]) and cerebral anoxia (30 [8.6%]). The hip was the primary site of HO (328 [60.9%]), then the elbow (115 [21.3%]), knee (77 [14.3%]) and shoulder (19 [3.5%]). For all patients, 181 of the surgeries were performed within the first year after the CNS damage, without recurrence of HO. Recurrence was not associated with etiology ($p = 0.46$), sex ($p = 1.00$), age at CNS damage ($p = 0.2$), multisite localization ($p = 0.34$), or delay to surgery ($p = 0.7$).

Conclusions/Significance: In patients with CNS damage, troublesome HO and recurrence occurs most frequently after traumatic brain injury and appears frequently in the hip and elbow. Early surgery for HO is not a factor of recurrence.

Editor: Mel Feany, Brigham and Women's Hospital, Harvard Medical School, United States of America

Funding: These authors have no support or funding to report.

Competing Interests: The authors have declared that no competing interests exist.

* E-mail: francois.genet@rpc.aphp.fr

Introduction

Heterotopic ossification (HO) is defined as the formation within the soft tissues of abnormal, ectopic lamellar bone containing bone marrow [1,2,3,4]. It has 3 etiologies: 1) trauma (fractures, dislocations, post-surgery, burns), 2) genetic (fibrodysplasia ossificans progressiva (FOP), progressive osseous heteroplasia and Albright hereditary osteodystrophy), and 3) neurologic (mainly spinal cord injury [SCI] and traumatic brain injury [TBI]) [1,5,6].

In patients with central nervous system (CNS) damage, HO is a frequent complication, ranging from 11% to 76% of cases depending on the etiology and the study because of varied diagnostic criteria [7,8,9]. Symptomatic HO develops in approximately 10% of patients with TBI [10,11,12]. In SCI, the HO frequency varies from 5% to 60% depending on the study and whether the diagnosis is based on clinical symptoms or standard radiography results [13,14,15,16].

The etiopathogenesis of HO is poorly understood [2]. CNS damage is believed to activate local factors such as bone morphogenic protein or systemic factors such as prostaglandin E2, or both [1,4,6]. These factors could induce bone-forming mesenchymal cells to differentiate to osteoblasts in the periphery of the muscle and stimulate the formation of bone[1,4,12,17]. Another potential mechanism is the disruption of joint proprioception after neurologic damage, thus changing the relationship among the different peri-articular tissues [18]. For patients with TBI, osteogenic blood factors have been suggested[12,17].

For patients with CNS damage, HO causes pain, inflammation and loss of range of motion (ROM) as the joint gradually becomes ankylosed [4,5,12,19,20]. The condition may have major repercussions on function, with, in many cases, loss of independence [2,6]. Currently, the only effective treatment is surgery [4,5,19,20,21]. Indications for surgery have changed recently [4]. Until recently, surgery was delayed until the HO was fully formed [4,21,22,23,24], and studies of small samples of patients (analyzed by reviews) have suggested that the rate of recurrence is not affected by HO maturity [4,25,26]. Indications for surgery relate to vascular or neurological involvement, effect on function, hygiene (e.g., access to the perineum) and pain [5,20,26]. Surgery can be performed as soon as co-morbidity factors are under control, even in patients with major neurologic damage due to the original abnormality (e.g., TBI) [2,26,27,28].

Only a few studies have investigated the epidemiological features of HO (incidence, recurrence, localization) in adult patients with CNS lesions [25]. Furthermore, these studies included few patients [2,10,13,26,29]. The most important series was published by Garland et al., in 1980; the incidence of HO was 11% in a cohort of 496 patients with TBI in a physical medicine and rehabilitation unit [10]. In 2005, Fuller et al. reported on 17 patients with 22 knee HO in a retrospective analysis [19], Simonsen et al. in 2007, reported on 13 patients with HO in 21 locations in a prospective cohort of 114 patients with TBI [29], and Melamed et al. reported on 12 excisions for HO in 9 patients with TBI [26].

We aimed to investigate a neuro-orthopedic complication — HO requiring surgery – in a large cohort of patients with CNS damage admitted to an orthopedic and trauma hospital ward. This unit is part of a tertiary-care teaching hospital specialized in medical treatment, surgery and rehabilitation for motor handicap. We also investigated the rate of recurrence of HO in terms of time to surgery. Results from this large survey might help establish recommendations for treating HO after CNS damage.

Methods

Objectives

The objectives are to investigate features of HO for the first time in a large sample of patients and notably to assess if the time of surgery is associated with the risk of early recurrence of HO.

Participants

This prospective data survey involved consecutive patients undergoing surgery between May 1993 and November 2009 for HO of a joint after CNS injury. Patients with previous removal of HO (before their inclusion in the study) who presented recurrence or could not be followed up by the surgeon or the physical medicine and rehabilitation physician for a minimum of 6 months were excluded, as were those without an initial neurologic aetiology.

Description of Procedures or Investigations undertaken

Patients were referred for a specialized neuro-orthopedic consultation for troublesome HO. Indications for surgery were loss of ROM with functional repercussion, ankylosed joint, and nerve or vessel compression. The surgery and immediate post-operative assessment were performed by the same surgeon.

The following data were collected during consultation by questionnaire and medical records : sex; etiology of the CNS damage (ischemia or hemorrhage for stroke; tetraplegia or paraplegia for SCI, with lesion level; brain-associated lesion [TBI or cerebral anoxia (CA)] and American Spinal Injury Association [ASIA] score [30]); age at CNS damage and at surgery; delay from neurologic trauma to surgery; affected joints; type of HO for the surgical approach of Garland (for incision) [7] (from radiography and computed tomography [CT] scanning: anterior, posterior, internal [anterior and posterior], external [anterior and posterior], and encircling); area of residence (Paris area [Ile de France], near Ile de France, between 200 and 400 km from Ile de France, more than 400 km from Ile de France, and foreign countries and French overseas departments and territories); and follow-up (last consultation, months). Finally, data were collected on complications, especially sepsis and HO recurrence. Several patients had received prophylactic treatment for HO, such as a nonsteroidal anti-inflammatory drug (for pain) into their upstream structure. Radiation therapy was rarely used by the upstream units.

A standardised surgical approach was used for each location of the HO. The surgical goal was resection of the necessary amount of bone to allow for restoration of motion in all planes. Postoperatively, gentle mobilization was started on the second day, and progressed as tolerated. A non-steroidal anti-inflammatory agent, ketoprofene, was given for 10 days after surgery. Neither radiation therapy (RT) nor indomethacin was used after surgery. RT was never carried out after surgery mainly because the post-operative management of such a treatment is too complicated for these kinds of patients. RT was sometimes administered before surgery but only when recurrence occurred (14/31 cases). The main reason was that we are not aware of any evidence demonstrating the efficacy of RT for HO after central nervous system damage. The recurrence rate was very low and well distributed across the 16 years of this study. As there are no recommendations for patients with neurological lesions, we used the same RT protocol as for hip arthroplasty in the patients who received pre-operative RT (4 hours before surgery, 7 to 10 Gy) [31].

Patients were followed up in the rehabilitation unit of the same institution for surgery if they lived locally or by medical consultation if they lived far away. Each patient underwent regular clinical and radiography examinations; they were hospitalized in a surgical care unit for about 1 week, then received regular consultations in rehabilitation units (inpatient care followed by outpatient care for a minimum of 1 year). All patients received intravenous peri-operative antibiotic prophylaxis and anticoagulation medication.

Ethics

The study was approved by the local institutional review board. It was a non-interventional study with usual procedures and without additional procedures (diagnosis or medical supervision). In France, patient consent is not needed for such an anonymous retrospective data analysis. We confirm that the named institutional review board specifically waived the need for consent for this study [Comité de Protection des Personnes Ile de France XI Pavillon Jacques Courtois - 2ème étage 20, rue Armagis 78105 Saint Germain en Laye Cedex. tél : 01.39.27.42.58 - fax : 01.39.27.49.01 mail : cppidf11@chi-poissy-st-germain.fr"]

Statistical methods

Statistical analysis involved use of SAS® v9.1 (SAS Inst., Cary, NC). Data are reported as median, interquartile ranges (IQRs) and numbers and percentages. The chi-square test was used to compare normally distributed qualitative variables and the Fisher test for no normally distributed data. ANOVA was used for analysis of continuous variables, and if significant, the Student t test was used to compare groups with the nearest values. All p values were two tailed, and a $p<0.05$ was considered statistically significant.

Results

Demographic data (Table 1)

Of 402 consecutive patients undergoing surgery for HO between May 1993 and November 2009, 363 with neurologic damage met our inclusion criteria (Fig. 1). Data for the few patients with cerebral palsy (4 patients), multiple sclerosis (1 patient) and Guillain-Barré syndrome (1 patient) were excluded from the analysis. Thus, we analyzed the data for 357 patients (70 females) who underwent 570 surgeries: 539 (94.2%) were first surgeries (multiple sites for 129 patients: 2 surgeries for 97 patients, 3 for 18; 4 for 9, 5 for 3 and 6 for 2) and 31 were for recurrences

Table 1. Demographic Data for Patients Undergoing Surgery for Heterotopic Ossification After Central Nervous System (CNS) Damage.

Patient parameters	TBI n = 199 (55.7)	Stroke n = 42 (11.8)	SCI n = 86 (24.1)	CA n = 30 (8.4)	Total n = 357 (100)
Male (%)	159 (79.9)	26 (61.9)	81 (94.2)	21 (70.0)	287 (80.4)
Age at time of CNS damage (yr) median interquartile range	30.6 23.6–38.8	45.7 37.9–51.5	27.1 21.3–34.7	44.9 32.2–48.3	32.4 24.6–43.3
Age at time of surgery (yr) Median interquartile range	32.2 26.2–41.2	49.7 40.5–54.3	34.7 27.1–42.7	46.5 34.3–49.3	35.4 27.6–46.7
Delay from CNS damage to first surgery (months) Median interquartile range	13.1 8.3–29.0	15.2 9.5–34.7	24.1 13.4–72.4	12.7 9.5–21.0	15.7 9.2–37.5

HO: Heterotopic Ossification; TBI: traumatic Brain Injury; SCI: Spinal Cord Injury; CA: Cerebral Anoxia; CNS: Central Nervous System.

for a rate of recurrence of 5.8% (95% confidence interval [CI]: 3.8–7.8%).

The median delay from neurological trauma to the first surgery was 15.7 months (IQR 9.2 to 37.5 months) (Table 1), and the median delay with multi-site HO was 16.7 months (IQR 9.9 to 40.0 months). Most cases of HO were related to TBI (199 patients [55.7%], 304 surgeries [56.4%]), then SCI (86 patients [24.1%]; 56 paraplegia and 30 tetraplegia; 129 surgeries [23.9%]), stroke (42 patients [11.8%], 10 ischemia and 32 hemorrhage; 55 surgeries [10.2%]) and CA (30 patients [8.6%]; 51 surgeries [9.5%]). The median follow-up by the surgeon was 6.9 months (IQR 5.7 to 19.4 months).

The presence of multiple sites of HO occurred more frequently in patients with CA (16/30; 14 patients with 2 locations, 1 patient with 3 locations and 1 patient with 6 locations) and TBI (74/199; 53 patients with 2 locations, 14 with 3 locations, 4 with 4 locations and 3 with 5 locations) than with SCI (29/86; 14/56 with paraplegia, 15/30 with tetraplegia; 22 with 2 locations, 2 with 3 locations, 4 with 4 locations and 1 patient with 6 locations) and

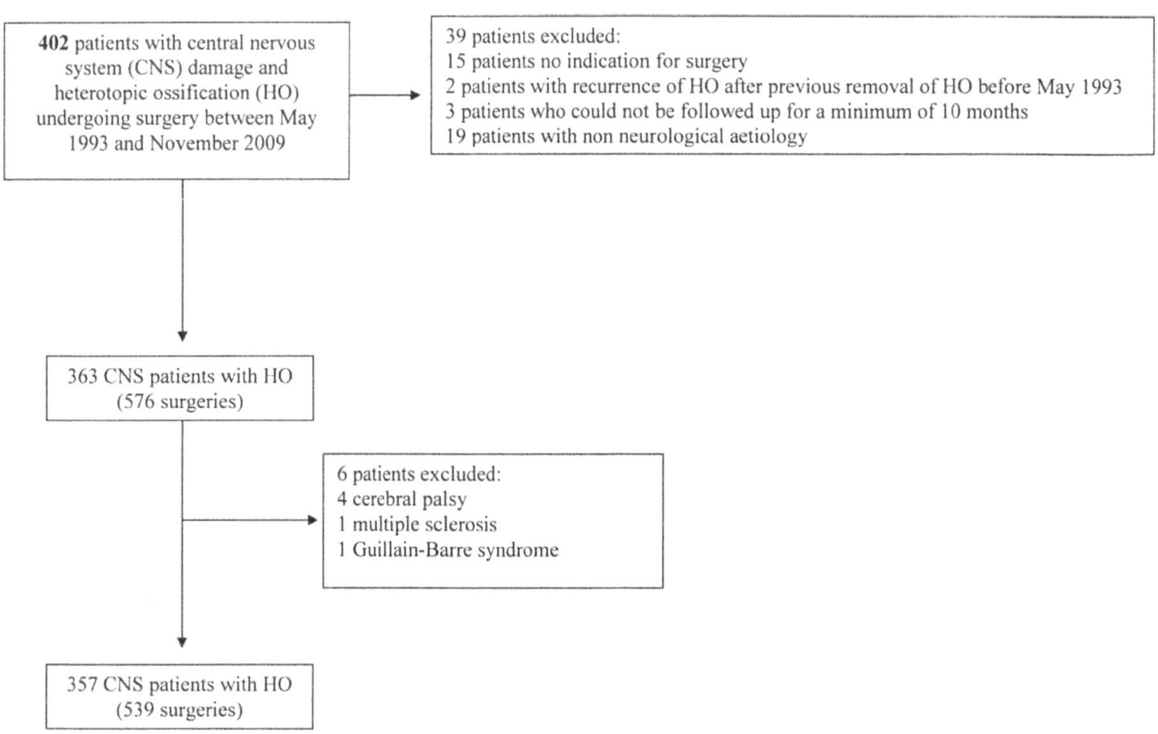

Figure 1. Flow chart of the patients' selected files.

stroke (10/42; 8 patients with 2 locations, 1 patient with 3 locations and 1 patient with 4 locations).

HO surgery side effects

The main side effects were sepsis (16; 3.0%) and HO recurrence (31; 5.8%). All patients with sepsis underwent secondary surgery. Sepsis occurred mainly after SCI (12), then TBI (3) and stroke (1). All patients with HO recurrence underwent secondary surgery. Recurrences occurred after TBI (16), stroke (2), SCI (10), and CA (3). In total, 27 patients (15 with multisite HO) had 1 recurrence and 4 patients (all with multisite HO) had 2 recurrences on 2 different joints. HO recurrence concerned only the hip (25 recurrences) and the elbow (6). Recurrence was more frequent for patients with multisite HO (15/27; 55.6%) than for all patients (127/357; 35.6%). For the 15 patients with multisite HO, recurrence never appeared after the first surgery but after a later surgery on a different site. For 181 surgeries performed within the first year after the CNS damage, no recurrence was reported at 6-month follow-up.

HO sites (Table 2)

For all first surgeries (all etiologies combined), the primary site for HO was the hip joint (328/539; 60.9%). Hip HO occurred most frequently with SCI (96/129; 74.4%) and stroke (40/55; 72.7%). Elbow HO was the next most affected joint (115/539, 21.3%), then the knee (77/539; 14.3%) and shoulder (19/539; 3.5%). Elbow HO occurred most frequently in patients with TBI (85/304; 28.0%) and CA (12/51; 23.5%). Knee HO occurred most frequently in patients with SCI (19/129; 14.7%; 7 for paraplegia, 2 bilateral; and 6 for tetraplegia, 4 bilateral), stroke (8/55; 14.1%) and TBI (43/304; 14.1%). The ratio of knee to hip HO (81.0%) and shoulder to elbow HO (85.8%) was similar for all etiologies.

Lower-limb HO sites (Table 3)

HO in the anterior and internal hip represented 60.0% of the total sites. This incidence was highest for patients with stroke (74.4%), then SCI (70.7%), TBI (51.9%) and CA (50.0%). The principle site of knee HO was internal (77.3%). This incidence was highest for patients with stroke (87.5%), then SCI (84.1%), TBI (75.5%) and CA (57.1%).

Table 2. Sites of Heterotopic Ossification (HO) in Patients Undergoing Surgery After Central Nervous System Damage.

Location of HO	TBI n = 304	Stroke n = 55	SCI n = 129	CA n = 51	Total n = 539
Hip – no. (%)	163 (53.6)	40 (72.7)	96 (74.4)	29 (56.9)	328 (60.9)
Knee – no. (%)	43 (14.1)	8 (14.6)	19 (14.7)	7 (13.7)	77 (14.3)
Shoulder – no. (%)	13 (4.3)	1 (1.8)	2 (1.6)	3 (5.9)	19 (3.5)
Elbow – no. (%)	85 (28.0)	6 (10.9)	12 (9.3)	12 (23.5)	115 (21.3)
Total – no. (%)	304 (56.4)	55 (10.2)	129 (23.9)	51 (9.5)	539 (100)

Data are for Number of First Surgeries Performed.
TBI: traumatic brain injury; SCI: spinal cord injury; CA: cerebral anoxia; CNS: central nervous system.

Upper-limb HO sites (Table 3)

The main site of elbow HO was posterior and internal (82.7%). Similar to hip HO, this incidence was highest for patients with SCI (100.0%; all tetraplegia and 1 paraplegia with associated elbow fracture) and stroke (100.0%), then TBI (81.2%) and CA (66.7%). Only 5 patients with paraplegia exhibited HO in the upper limbs: 4 had an associated brain injury (2 with HO in shoulders and 2 elbows) and one a medical SCI with HO after elbow fracture. Only 19 occurrences of HO (3.5%) were in the shoulder joint, and the main sites were internal (41.2%), posterior (23.5%) and encircling (23.5%).

Univariate analysis of data for patients (Tables 4)

When analyzing data for patients (n = 357), we found a significant association between etiology and delay until first surgery ($F = 11.5$; $p < 0.01$). The shortest delay was observed for CA (12.7 months; IQR 9.5 to 21.0 months), then stroke, TBI and SCI. We found a significant difference between delay until first surgery for SCI (the longest delay) and for stroke (the nearest from SCI) ($F = 7.38$; $p < 0.01$). We suggest that differences between SCI and the other 2 etiologies (TBI and CA) are significant also. We did not find an association of etiology and multiple-site HO ($p = 0.1$). Recurrence was not associated with etiology ($p = 0.46$), sex ($p = 1.00$), or multisite HO ($p = 0.34$).

Univariate analysis of time from CNS damage related to HO recurrence (Table 5)

When analyzing data for patients (n = 357), recurrence was not associated with age at CNS damage ($F = 1.65$; $p = 0.20$) or delay from CNS damage to first surgery (months) ($F = 0.13$; $p = 0.7$). For all surgeries, (including multisite HO), recurrence was not associated with delay from CNS damage to surgery (months) ($F = 2.35$; $p = 0.13$).

Discussion

HO is a frequent complication after CNS damage. This survey of a large sample of patients with CNS damage revealed that most HO requiring surgery occurred after TBI, then SCI, stroke and CA. Multi-site HO was most frequently due to CA and TBI. For all patients, the hip was the primary site of damage, then the elbow, knee and shoulder. The median time from CNS damage to surgery for all etiologies was 15.7 months (IQR 9.2 to 37.5 months), which was shorter than that for SCI (24.1 months; IQR 13.4 to 72.4 months). For all patients, 181 of the surgeries were performed within the first year after the CNS damage, without recurrence at 6-month follow-up. Recurrence was not associated with etiology, sex, age at CNS damage, multisite HO, or delay from CNS damage to surgery, whether analyzing data for patients or surgeries. No association was found between etiology and multisite HO or articulation location of HO. These results suggest that surgery could be proposed as soon as HO becomes troublesome.

In our survey, HO was mainly observed in 4 etiologies and very rarely in other disorders such as multiple sclerosis (1), cerebral palsy (4), or Guillain-Barré syndrome (1). Our observations are unlikely due to recruitment bias because our institution, in charge of the National Adult CP Network, is the main site for HO management in France. This is suggested by our geographical recruitment [Ile de France 220 (63.9%); near Ile de France 41 (11.9%); between 200 and 400 km from Ile de France 22 (6.4%); more than 400 km from Ile de France 23 (6.7%); and foreign countries or French overseas departments and territories 38 (11.1%)]. Better risk factors for HO have been reported to be

Table 3. Sites of Heterotopic Ossification of Patients Undergoing Surgery for Central Nervous System Damage. Data are for Number of First Surgeries Performed.

Site	Hip					*Knee*				
	TBI n = 304	**Stroke n = 55**	**SCI n = 129**	**CA n = 51**	**Total n = 539**	**TBI n = 304**	**Stroke n = 55**	**SCI n = 129**	**CA n = 51**	**Total n = 539**
Anterior – no. (%)	27 (16.9)	9 (23.1)	46 (50.0)	6 (23.1)	88 (27.8)	2 (4.9)	0 (0.0)	1 (5.3)	0 (0.0)	3 (4.0)
Posterior – no. (%)	29 (18.1)	1 (2.6)	12 (13.0)	7 (26.9)	49 (15.5)	4 (9.8)	0 (0.0)	0 (0.0)	0 (0,0)	4 (5.3)
Internal – no. (%)	56 (35.0)	20 (51.3)	19 (20.7)	7 (26.9)	102 (32.2)	31 (75.5)	7 (87.5)	16 (84.1)	4 (57.1)	58 (77.3)
External – no. (%)	28 (17.5)	7 (17.9)	3 (3.3)	2 (7.7)	40 (12.6)	2 (4.9)	1 (12.5)	1 (5.3)	1 (14.3)	5 (6.7)
Encircling – no. (%)	20 (12.5)	2 (5.1)	12 (13.0)	4 (15.4)	38 (11.9)	2 (4.9)	0 (0.0)	1 (5.3)	2 (28.6)	5 (6.7)
Total	160 (50.5)	39 (12.3)	92 (29.0)	26 (8.2)	317 (100)	41 (54.7)	8 (10.7)	19 (25.3)	7 (9.3)	75(100)
Site	**Shoulder**					*Elbow*				
	TBI n = 304	**Stroke n = 55**	**SCI n = 129**	**CA n = 51**	**Total n = 539**	**TBI n = 304**	**Stroke n = 55**	**SCI n = 129**	**CA n = 51**	**Total n = 539**
Anterior – no. (%)	0 (0.0)	0 (0.0)	2 (100.0)	0 (0.0)	2 (11.8)	3 (3.8)	0 (0.0)	0 (0.0)	2 (16.7)	5 (4.6)
Posterior – no. (%)	4 (40.0)	0 (0.0)	0 (0.0)	0 (0.0)	4 (23.5)	22 (27.5)	0 (0.0)	3 (25.0)	3 (25.0)	28 (25.4)
Internal – no. (%)	4 (40.0)	1 (100.0)	0 (0.0)	1 (33.3)	6 (41.2)	43 (53.7)	6 (100.0)	9 (75.0)	5 (41.7)	63 (57.3)
External – no. (%)	0 (0.0)	0 (0.0)	0 (0.0)	0 (0.0)	0 (0.0)	12 (15.0)	0 (0.0)	0 (0.0)	0 (0.0)	12 (10.9)
Encircling – no. (%)	2 (20.0)	0 (0.0)	0 (0.0)	2 (66.7)	4 (23.5)	0 (0.0)	0 (0.0)	0 (0.0)	2 (16.7)	2 (1.8)
Total	10 (62.5)	1 (6.3)	2 (12.5)	3 (18.7)	17 (100.0)	80 (72.7)	6 (5.5)	12 (10.9)	12 (10.9)	110 (100.0)

related to coma severity, coma length, presence of diffuse axonal lesions, spasticity, systemic infection, and overall dysautonomia, which is a high predictive factor of HO [11,25]. These risk factors may explain why HO was observed mainly for patients with CA, TBI, SCI and stroke. Furthermore, notably after TBI, neurological repercussions affect the whole organism and probably also bone hormonal control [32].

As suggested by Garland et al., we found that the main site of HO was the hip (60.9%), then the elbow (21.3%), knee (14.3%) and shoulder (3.5%) [10]. The high incidence in the hip may be linked to HO in this joint having large repercussions on function (e.g., ability to sit, lie or stand). The high incidence in the elbow may be linked to the frequency of ulnar nerve compression, which is a strong indication for surgery. Furthermore, HO often occurred below the level of the CNS lesion in patients with SCI, which may explain the high incidence of lower-limb HO in this group. For the hip, the sites of HO seem to depend on the abnormality: the most frequent site for SCI was anterior (51.1%) but antero-medial for stroke (43.6%). This finding could reflect joint-related constraints, which differ according to muscle control. However, this hypothesis needs to be confirmed with further studies. For all etiologies, the most frequently affected site was medial for the knee (54.7%) and medial, antero- and postero-medial for the elbow (57.3%). These results could be explained by these particular locations having the worse repercussions (e.g., functional, compressive) and therefore needing surgery.

Table 4. Univariate Analysis of Data for Patients (n = 357).

Variables	*p (F statistic)*	*p*
Etiology		
Delay until first surgery	<0.01* (11.46)	
Delay until first surgery for SCI and stroke	<0.01* (7.38)	
Multisite HO		0.1
Recurrence		
Multisite HO		0.34
Sex		1.00
Etiology		0.46
SCI = spinal cord injury; HO = heterotopic ossification		

HO: heterotopic ossification; TBI: traumatic brain injury; SCI: spinal cord injury; CA: cerebral anoxia; CNS: central nervous system.

Currently, the only effective treatment for HO is surgery [4,5,6,21]. Indications for surgery have changed recently [4]. In our experience, surgery is indicated when HO causes loss of function, when pain is difficult to manage medically or with risk of nerve or, more rarely, vessel involvement. In our study, the median time from CNS damage to surgery was 15.7 months (range 9.2 to 37.5 months). This delay was significantly shorter than that for patients with SCI (24.1 months, range 13.4–72.4 months). Discomfort is likely to be a problem earlier in conditions other than SCI because of the typical loss of sensation in SCI and the different functional prognosis.

Some studies, with a small sample of patients with HO, have suggested that early surgery does not increase the rate of recurrence [4,21,25]. In our survey, recurrence was not associated with delay from CNS damage to surgery, whether considering patients or surgeries. None of the 181 patients who underwent surgery within a year of the CNS damage experienced HO recurrence during follow-up. In addition, 4 patients with recurrence had previously benefitted from surgery for troublesome HO on another location without recurrence. The minimum follow-up by the surgeon in our study was 3 months. In our experience, recurrences requiring surgery appear sooner than 3

Table 5. Univariate Analysis of Time from Central Nervous System Damage Related to Heterotropic Ossification Recurrence.

Variables	*P (F statistic)*	With recurrence	Without recurrence
Data for Patients (n = 357)			
Delay from CNS damage to surgery – mo.	0.7 (0.13)	21.5 (9.0; 34.1)	15.6 (9.2; 37.5)
Age at CNS damage – years	0.2 (1.65)	30.0 (21.9; 36.6)	32.5 (24.7; 43.4)
Data for Surgeries (n = 539)			
Delay from CNS damage to surgery – mo.	0.13 (2.35)	28.7 (12.0; 59.1)	16.4 (9.9; 37.9)

Data are median (interquartile range) CNS = central nervous system

months. Furthermore, most patients who underwent surgery for HO came from units in close contact with our institution, and, in cases of recurrence, the surgeon is contacted quickly. Likewise, after 6 months, patients were followed up by a physical and medical rehabilitation physician. Therefore, recurrences were unlikely to be undiagnosed and unreported.

Several other groups have assessed the effect of delayed surgery on HO. Lazarus et al. studied 24 patients who underwent surgery for elbow HO and found that a long delay before surgery was a negative predictor of recovery of ROM [33]. This finding is reinforced by the new approaches in neuro-rehabilitation involving limited ROM. Limited ROM may induce plastic cerebral changes, such as atrophy of motor areas with time, and therefore reduce recovery capacity after ROM has been restored [34]. However, several studies suggested that the more limited the ROM in the pre-operative joint, the better the surgical outcome[33,35]. The sooner the troublesome HO is treated by surgery, the better the functional outcome. Moreover, in a previous study we found that a long delay before surgery can be deleterious, especially for the ankylosis state: often considerable bone loss of articular structure (i.e., femoral head) and high risk of peri-operative fracture [20]. Because of our large sample size, our results demonstrate that delay is not a criterion to decide surgery, as was suggested by our previous work [20], systematic reviews and other previous studies with limited sample size [4,6,25,26]. Almost half of the patients experiencing recurrence (15 of 31) had multisite HO, so this after-effect might occur more in patients with a global increase of bone activity. However, recurrence was not associated with etiology, sex or age at CNS damage.

According to Garland et al. [36], after SCI, there is a significant relationship between hip HO volume and recurrence risk. Garland proposed a "subjective" radiological grading system in a spinal cord injured group of patients (19 patients with 24 HO). There were 5 grades (from minimal to ankylosis), only for the hip. Previously, Brooker et al. (1973) proposed a radiological scale for post operative patients (after total hip arthroplasty) [37]. There were 4 classes (from "Island of bone within the soft tissues about the hip" to "apparent bone ankylosis of the hip") and again only for the hip. Stover et al. (1991) proposed to extend this classification for other articulations and aetiologies and mainly after neurological diseases [16]. Finally, Stover suggested (without carrying out a statistic analysis) that the higher the Brooker status, the higher the recurrence risk [16,37]. Unlike the results of these studies, in our series, the pre-operative extent of HO does not seem to influence the recurrence risk. However, our database is quite varied, containing many aetiologies (4), articulations (4) and surgical indications (functional disabilities, pain, nerve and vessel compressions, hygienic access…) making it difficult to draw reliable conclusions regarding the implication of the volume of preoperative HO in the recurrence risk. Further studies should be carried out on sub-populations of this database (i.e. after TBI and Hip HO). Furthermore, we specify that, in our series, all patients undergoing symptomatic HO were classified as Brooker level 3 or 4 for the hip. As we stated above, we believe the most pertinent risk factors are clinical such as aetiology (SCI), an infectious context (bacteriuria, slough, post operative or post traumatic sepsis such as open fracture), spasticity and the severity of the neurological initial damage.

Our results can be generalized only to patients with HO requiring surgical intervention, not those with HO in general. The prevalence of HO risk is probably underestimated slightly because non-symptomatic cases remain undiagnosed. As well, our study was monocentric, which may influence the generalizability of results. However, our center is a national reference center of rehabilitation, and our large sample size and our patients admitted from a large geographical area should limit questions of recruitment bias.

In conclusion, we performed a large-sample study of HO, a frequent complication after CNS damage but rarely studied, to illuminate features of HO associated with etiology and other factors. In patients with CNS damage, troublesome HO and recurrence occurred most frequently in those with TBI and appeared frequently in the hip and elbow. Early surgery for HO is not a factor of recurrence. Therefore, troublesome HO is the main factor indicating surgery.

Author Contributions

Conceived and designed the experiments: FG SP PD. Performed the experiments: CL PD TJ. Analyzed the data: FG CJ DG. Contributed reagents/materials/analysis tools: FG AS. Wrote the paper: FG SP.

References

1. Balboni TA, Gobezie R, Mamon HJ (2006) Heterotopic ossification: Pathophysiology, clinical features, and the role of radiotherapy for prophylaxis. Int J Radiat Oncol Biol Phys 65: 1289–1299.
2. Cullen N, Bayley M, Bayona N, Hilditch M, Aubut J (2007) Management of heterotopic ossification and venous thromboembolism following acquired brain injury. Brain Inj 21: 215–230.
3. Haran M, Bhuta T, Lee B (2004) Pharmacological interventions for treating acute heterotopic ossification. Cochrane Database Syst Rev. CD003321.
4. Vanden Bossche L, Vanderstraeten G (2005) Heterotopic ossification: a review. J Rehabil Med 37: 129–136.
5. Cipriano CA, Pill SG, Keenan MA (2009) Heterotopic ossification following traumatic brain injury and spinal cord injury. J Am Acad Orthop Surg 17: 689–697.
6. Shehab D, Elgazzar AH, Collier BD (2002) Heterotopic ossification. J Nucl Med 43: 346–353.
7. Garland DE (1991) A clinical perspective on common forms of acquired heterotopic ossification. Clin Orthop Relat Res. pp 13–29.

8. Rogers RC (1988) Heterotopic calcification in severe head injury: a preventive programme. Brain Inj 2: 169–173.
9. Sazbon L, Najenson T, Tartakovsky M, Becker E, Grosswasser Z (1981) Widespread periarticular new-bone formation in long-term comatose patients. J Bone Joint Surg Br 63-B: 120–125.
10. Garland DE, Blum CE, Waters RL (1980) Periarticular heterotopic ossification in head-injured adults. Incidence and location. J Bone Joint Surg Am 62: 1143–1146.
11. Hendricks HT, Geurts AC, van Ginneken BC, Heeren AJ, Vos PE (2007) Brain injury severity and autonomic dysregulation accurately predict heterotopic ossification in patients with traumatic brain injury. Clin Rehabil 21: 545–553.
12. Cadosch D, Toffoli AM, Gautschi OP, Frey SP, Zellweger R, et al. (2010) Serum after traumatic brain injury increases proliferation and supports expression of osteoblast markers in muscle cells. J Bone Joint Surg Am 92: 645–653.
13. Bravo-Payno P, Esclarin A, Arzoz T, Arroyo O, Labarta C (1992) Incidence and risk factors in the appearance of heterotopic ossification in spinal cord injury. Paraplegia 30: 740–745.
14. Riklin C, Baumberger M, Wick L, Michel D, Sauter B, et al. (2003) Deep vein thrombosis and heterotopic ossification in spinal cord injury: a 3 year experience at the Swiss Paraplegic Centre Nottwil. Spinal Cord 41: 192–198.
15. Silver JR (1969) Heterotopic ossification. A clinical study of its possible relationship to trauma. Paraplegia 7: 220–230.
16. Stover SL, Niemann KM, Tulloss JR (1991) Experience with surgical resection of heterotopic bone in spinal cord injury patients. Clin Orthop Relat Res. pp 71–77.
17. Toffoli AM, Gautschi OP, Frey SP, Filgueira L, Zellweger R (2008) From brain to bone: evidence for the release of osteogenic humoral factors after traumatic brain injury. Brain Inj 22: 511–518.
18. da Paz AC, Carod Artal FJ, Kalil RK (2007) The function of proprioceptors in bone organization: a possible explanation for neurogenic heterotopic ossification in patients with neurological damage. Med Hypotheses 68: 67–73.
19. Fuller DA, Mark A, Keenan MA (2005) Excision of heterotopic ossification from the knee: a functional outcome study. Clin Orthop Relat Res 438: 197–203.
20. Genet F, Marmorat JL, Lautridou C, Schnitzler A, Mailhan L, et al. (2009) Impact of late surgical intervention on heterotopic ossification of the hip after traumatic neurological injury. J Bone Joint Surg Br 91: 1493–1498.
21. Pelissier J, Petiot S, Benaim C, Asencio G (2002) [Treatment of neurogenic heterotopic ossifications (NHO) in brain injured patients: review of literature]. Ann Readapt Med Phys 45: 188–197.
22. Beingessner DM, Patterson SD, King GJ (2000) Early excision of heterotopic bone in the forearm. J Hand Surg Am 25: 483–488.
23. Moore TJ (1993) Functional outcome following surgical excision of heterotopic ossification in patients with traumatic brain injury. J Orthop Trauma 7: 11–14.
24. Garland DE, Hanscom DA, Keenan MA, Smith C, Moore T (1985) Resection of heterotopic ossification in the adult with head trauma. J Bone Joint Surg Am 67: 1261–1269.
25. Chalidis B, Stengel D, Giannoudis PV (2007) Early excision and late excision of heterotopic ossification after traumatic brain injury are equivalent: a systematic review of the literature. J Neurotrauma 24: 1675–1686.
26. Melamed E, Robinson D, Halperin N, Wallach N, Keren O, et al. (2002) Brain injury-related heterotopic bone formation: treatment strategy and results. Am J Phys Med Rehabil 81: 670–674.
27. Denys P, Azouvi P, Denormandie P, Samuel C, Patel A, et al. (1996) Late cognitive and behavioural improvement following treatment of disabling orthopaedic complications of a severe closed head injury. Brain Inj 10: 149–153.
28. Charnley G, Judet T, Garreau de Loubresse C, Mollaret O (1996) Excision of heterotopic ossification around the knee following brain injury. Injury 27: 125–128.
29. Simonsen LL, Sonne-Holm S, Krasheninnikoff M, Engberg AW (2007) Symptomatic heterotopic ossification after very severe traumatic brain injury in 114 patients: incidence and risk factors. Injury 38: 1146–1150.
30. Ditunno JF, Jr., Young W, Donovan WH, Creasey G (1994) The international standards booklet for neurological and functional classification of spinal cord injury. American Spinal Injury Association. Paraplegia 32: 70–80.
31. Cipriano C, Pill SG, Rosenstock J, Keenan MA (2009) Radiation therapy for preventing recurrence of neurogenic heterotopic ossification. Orthopedics 32.
32. Cadosch D, Gautschi OP, Thyer M, Song S, Skirving AP, et al. (2009) Humoral factors enhance fracture-healing and callus formation in patients with traumatic brain injury. J Bone Joint Surg Am 91: 282–288.
33. Lazarus M, Guttmann D, Rich C, Keenan M (1999) Heterotopic ossification resection about the elbow. Neurorehabilitation 12: 145–153.
34. Taub E, Miller NE, Novack TA, Cook 3rd EW, Fleming WC, et al. (1993) Technique to improve chronic motor deficit after stroke. Arch Phys Med Rehabil 74: 347–354.
35. de Palma L, Rapali S, Paladini P, Ventura A (2002) Elbow heterotopic ossification in head-trauma patients: diagnosis and treatment. Orthopedics 25: 665–668.
36. Garland DE, Orwin JF (1989) Resection of heterotopic ossification in patients with spinal cord injuries. Clin Orthop Relat Res. pp 169–176.
37. Brooker AF, Bowerman JW, Robinson RA, RileyJr LH (1973) Ectopic ossification following total hip replacement. Incidence and a method of classification. J Bone Joint Surg Am 55: 1629–1632.

3

C-Reactive Protein, Erythrocyte Sedimentation Rate and Orthopedic Implant Infection

Kerryl E. Piper[1], Marta Fernandez-Sampedro[1], Kathryn E. Steckelberg[1], Jayawant N. Mandrekar[2], Melissa J. Karau[1], James M. Steckelberg[1], Elie F. Berbari[1], Douglas R. Osmon[1], Arlen D. Hanssen[4], David G. Lewallen[4], Robert H. Cofield[4], John W. Sperling[4], Joaquin Sanchez-Sotelo[4], Paul M. Huddleston[4], Mark B. Dekutoski[4], Michael Yaszemski[4], Bradford Currier[4], Robin Patel[1,3]*

1 Division of Infectious Diseases, Department of Medicine, Mayo Clinic College of Medicine, Rochester, Minnesota, United States of America, **2** Division of Biomedical Statistics and Informatics, Department of Health Sciences Research, Mayo Clinic College of Medicine, Rochester, Minnesota, United States of America, **3** Division of Clinical Microbiology, Department of Laboratory Medicine and Pathology, Mayo Clinic College of Medicine, Rochester, Minnesota, United States of America, **4** Department of Orthopedic Surgery, Mayo Clinic College of Medicine, Rochester, Minnesota, United States of America

Abstract

Background: C-reactive protein (CRP) and erythrocyte sedimentation rate (ESR) have been shown to be useful for diagnosis of prosthetic hip and knee infection. Little information is available on CRP and ESR in patients undergoing revision or resection of shoulder arthroplasties or spine implants.

Methods/Results: We analyzed preoperative CRP and ESR in 636 subjects who underwent knee (n = 297), hip (n = 221) or shoulder (n = 64) arthroplasty, or spine implant (n = 54) removal. A standardized definition of orthopedic implant-associated infection was applied. Receiver operating curve analysis was used to determine ideal cutoff values for differentiating infected from non-infected cases. ESR was significantly different in subjects with aseptic failure infection of knee (median 11 and 53.5 mm/h, respectively, p = <0.0001) and hip (median 11 and 30 mm/h, respectively, p = <0.0001) arthroplasties and spine implants (median 10 and 48.5 mm/h, respectively, p = 0.0033), but not shoulder arthroplasties (median 10 and 9 mm/h, respectively, p = 0.9883). Optimized ESR cutoffs for knee, hip and shoulder arthroplasties and spine implants were 19, 13, 26, and 45 mm/h, respectively. Using these cutoffs, sensitivity and specificity to detect infection were 89 and 74% for knee, 82 and 60% for hip, and 32 and 93% for shoulder arthroplasties, and 57 and 90% for spine implants. CRP was significantly different in subjects with aseptic failure and infection of knee (median 4 and 51 mg/l, respectively, p<0.0001), hip (median 3 and 18 mg/l, respectively, p<0.0001), and shoulder (median 3 and 10 mg/l, respectively, p = 0.01) arthroplasties, and spine implants (median 3 and 20 mg/l, respectively, p = 0.0011). Optimized CRP cutoffs for knee, hip, and shoulder arthroplasties, and spine implants were 14.5, 10.3, 7, and 4.6 mg/l, respectively. Using these cutoffs, sensitivity and specificity to detect infection were 79 and 88% for knee, 74 and 79% for hip, and 63 and 73% for shoulder arthroplasties, and 79 and 68% for spine implants.

Conclusion: CRP and ESR have poor sensitivity for the diagnosis of shoulder implant infection. A CRP of 4.6 mg/l had a sensitivity of 79 and a specificity of 68% to detect infection of spine implants.

Editor: Stefan Bereswill, Charité-Universitätsmedizin Berlin, Germany

Funding: There was no external funding source.

Competing Interests: The authors have declared that no competing interests exist.

* E-mail: patel.robin@mayo.edu

Introduction

C-reactive protein (CRP), and erythrocyte sedimentation rate (ESR) are inexpensive, non-invasive tests that are often obtained in subjects with orthopedic implants prior to implant removal to assess for implant-associated infection. CRP and, to a lesser extent, ESR, have been shown to be useful in the diagnosis of prosthetic hip and knee infection, especially if validated cut-off values are applied (Table 1). Little information is available, however, on CRP and ESR in patients undergoing revision or resection of shoulder arthroplasties or spine implants.

ESR and CRP have poor sensitivity to detect prosthetic shoulder infection when cutoffs of 30 mm/h or 10 mg/l, respectively, are applied [1]. This may relate to the frequent implication of the low virulence organism, *Propionibacterium acnes*, in shoulder arthroplasty infection [1,2], or to failure to use optimized cutoff values for shoulder arthroplasty infection. There is little data available on the performance of CRP and ESR in the diagnosis of spine implant-associated infection, although Hahn et al. reported that normal CRP and ESR do not rule out late infection associated with spinal instrumentation [3].

We analyzed preoperative CRP and ESR in subjects prior to implant removal at our institution, using a standardized definition of orthopedic implant-associated infection, to determine the sensitivity and specificity of CRP and ESR, using receiver operating curve analysis-optimized cutoffs, for the diagnosis of hip, knee, and shoulder arthroplasty and spine implant-associated infection.

Table 1. Results of studies examining preoperative ESR and CRP for diagnosis of prosthetic joint infection.

	First author	Implant type	Number of arthroplasties	Cutoff (ESR, mm/h; CRP, mg/l)	Sensitivity (%)	Specificity (%)	Positive predictive value (%)	Negative predictive value (%)
ESR	Greidenaus [8]*, ****	Knee	145	≥22.5	93	83	71	96
	Spangehl [19].**	Hip	171	>30	82	85	58	95
	Austin [20]*****	Knee	296	>30	82	85	58	95
	Schinsky [21]***	Hip	235	>30	97	39	42	96
	Baré [22]	Knee	295	>30	63	55	39	77
	Bernard [23]	Hip/knee	171	≥30	87	47	94	26
	Levitsky [24]	Hip/knee	72	>30	60	65	25	90
	Feldman et al. [25]	Hip/knee	33	>50	79	78	Not reported	Not reported
CRP	Greidenaus [8]*, ****	Knee	145	≥13.5	91	86	74	95
	Bottner [26]*	Hip/knee	78	>32	95	96	91	98
	Spangehl [19]**	Hip	142	>10	96	92	74	99
	Austin [20]*****	Knee	296	>10	96	92	74	99
	Schinsky [21]***	Hip	235	>100	94	71	59	96
	Baré [22]	Knee	295	>10	60	63	45	76
	Bernard [23]	Hip/knee	228	≥10	97	81	98	71
	Fink [27]	Knee	145	> 13.5	73	81	59	89
	Müller [28]	Hip	50	>5	95	62	88	80
	Virolainen [29]	Hip/knee	68	>10	79	68	Not reported	Not reported

*Diagnostic cutoff level determined using receiver operating characteristic curve analysis.
**Patients with connective-tissue disorders were excluded from analysis.
***Patients with a preoperative diagnosis of inflammatory arthritis were excluded from analysis.
****Patients with a systemic disease or a condition that could result in an abnormal ESR or CRP, such as rheumatoid arthritis or other inflammatory arthritides, were excluded from analysis.
*****Patients with a confounding factors that can elevate inflammatory markers (inflammatory disorders, collagen vascular disease, urinary tract infection, hepatitis, demyelinating neuropathy or malignancy), were excluded from analysis.

Methods

Study Population

Patients who underwent prosthetic knee, hip, or shoulder arthroplasty or spine implant removal between July 2001 and June 2008 at Mayo Clinic Rochester, Minnesota, were studied. CRP (mg/l) and ESR (mm/h) within one month before the index surgery were analyzed. (If more than one measurement was available, the measurement closest to surgery was studied.) Some patients reported herein have been previously described [1,4,5]. Patients without both CRP and ESR performed within one month before the index surgery were excluded. Patients with underlying inflammatory arthritides were excluded. This study was reviewed and approved by the Mayo Clinic Institutional Review Board. Waivers of informed consent and HIPAA authorization were approved. For subjects residing in Minnesota, only those who had authorized use of their medical record in research (Minnesota Statute 144.335) were included.

Patient Classification

Patients were classified as having orthopedic implant-associated infection if at least one of the following was present: (1) Visible purulence surrounding the implant; (2) acute inflammation on histopathologic examination of permanent tissue sections (as determined by the clinical pathologist); (3) a sinus tract communicating with the implant; or (4) positive periprosthetic tissue culture and positive sonicate fluid culture for the same microorganism [6]. Aseptic failure was defined as implant failure not meeting these criteria.

Specimen Collection

Venous blood was collected in a 3.5 ml serum separator tube for CRP and in a 2.4 ml sodium citrate (0.6 ml) tube for ESR. Intraoperative tissue samples with the most obvious inflammatory changes were collected for histopathologic evaluation and conventional microbiologic culture. Removed implants were placed in an autoclaved (132°C, 27 psi for 15 minutes) 1 liter polypropylene wide mouth container (Nalgene, Lima, Ohio). Specimens were cultured within six hours.

Peri-Implant Tissue Culture

Peri-implant tissue cultures were performed in the Mayo Clinic Clinical Microbiology Laboratory. Tissue specimens were homogenized in 3 ml brain heart infusion broth for 1 minute. The homogenate was inoculated onto aerobic blood, chocolate, and anaerobic blood agar and into thioglycollate broth (BD Diagnostic Systems, Sparks, MD). Aerobic and anaerobic agar plates were incubated at 35–37°C in 5–7% CO_2 aerobically and anaerobically for 2–4 and 7 days, respectively. Thioglycollate broth was incubated anaerobically at 35–37°C for 7 days; turbid broth was subcultured. Microorganisms were identified using routine microbiologic techniques. Peri-implant tissue culture positivity was defined as isolation of the same organism from at least two tissue specimens from the index surgery.

Sonicate Fluid Culture

Sterile Ringer's solution (400 ml) was added to each implant-containing container. The container was vortexed for 30 seconds

(Vortex Genie, Scientific Industries Inc., Bohemia, NY), followed by bath sonication (frequency 40±2 kHz, power density 0.22±0.04 watts/cm^2) in an Aquasonic Model 750T ultrasound bath (VWR Scientific, Weschester, PA) for 5 minutes, and then vortexed again for 30 seconds.

For subjects studied before December 14, 2005, 0.5 ml of sonicate fluid was directly plated onto aerobic and anaerobic sheep blood agar plates which were incubated at 35–37°C in 5–7% CO_2 aerobically and anaerobically for 5 and 7 days, respectively. For subjects studied after December 14, 2005, a concentration step and an extended period of anaerobic incubation were added. Sonicate fluid was placed into conical centrifuge tubes which were centrifuged at 3,150×g for 5 minutes. The supernatant was aspirated (for a one hundred fold concentration) and 0.1 ml of the sediment was plated onto aerobic and anaerobic sheep blood agar plates which were incubated at 35–37°C in 5–7% CO_2 aerobically and anaerobically for 2–4 and 14 days, respectively. Microorganisms were enumerated and identified using routine microbiologic techniques. Sonicate fluid cultures were considered positive based on the following criteria. A cutoff value of at least 5 colony forming units (cfu) per plate was applied to the subjects studied before December 14, 2005. A cutoff value of at least 20 cfu per plate was applied to the subjects enrolled after December 14, 2005. The higher cutoff for subjects after December 14, 2005 was used due to the addition of a concentration step to the sonicate fluid culture procedure yielding higher numbers of microorganisms [1].

C-Reactive Protein

CRP measurements were performed using the Roche/Hitachi Modular System. Briefly, the anti-CRP antibodies coupled to latex microparticles react with antigen to form antigen-antibody complexes. After agglutination, the complex formation was measured turbidimetrically. The linear range of detection was 3 to 200 mg/l.

Erythrocyte Sedimentation Rate

The ESR was determined using the Westergren method. The rate of sedimentation of erythrocytes is measured in a 1:5 dilution of 3.2% sodium citrate solution to whole blood. Blood is drawn up in a column and allowed to sit undisturbed for one hour. The sedimentation is read as the millimeter distance from the top of the column to the meniscus of the erythrocyte sediment.

Statistical Analysis

Descriptive summaries were reported as median values (due to the non Gaussian distribution of the data). ESR and CRP levels between the aseptic failure and the infection groups at the various anatomic locations (knees, hips, shoulders, spine) were compared using the Wilcoxon rank sum test. All tests were two sided; a p-value of less than 0.05 was considered as statistically significant. Analysis was performed using Statistical Analysis Software (SAS) version 9.0. Receiver operating characteristic curves for ESR and CRP were established for knee, hip, and shoulder arthroplasty and spine implant patients, with the optimal cut-off values chosen as those in the upper left corner of the curve, representing the point at which the greatest sensitivity and specificity are achieved.

Funding Source

There was no external funding source.

Results and Discussion

636 subjects who underwent knee (n = 297), hip (n = 221) or shoulder (n = 64) arthroplasty, or spine implant (n = 54) removal were analyzed. 487 subjects with knee (n = 215), hip (n = 187), or shoulder (n = 45) arthroplasties and spine implants (n = 40) removed met the preoperative definition of aseptic failure. 149 subjects who underwent removal of knee (n = 82), hip (n = 34), or shoulder (n = 19) arthroplasties or spine implants (n = 14) met the preoperative definition of orthopedic implant-associated infection.

CRP was significantly different in subjects with aseptic failure and infection of knee (median 4 and 51 mg/l, respectively, $p<0.0001$), hip (median 3 and 18 mg/l, respectively, $p<0.0001$), and shoulder (median 3 and 10 mg/l, respectively, $p = 0.01$) arthroplasties, and spine implants (median 3 and 20 mg/l, respectively, $p = 0.0011$). ESR was significantly different in subjects with aseptic failure and infection of knee (median 11 and 53.5 mm/h, respectively, $p<0.0001$) and hip (median 11 and 30 mm/h, respectively, $p<0.0001$) arthroplasties, and spine implants (median 10 and 48.5 mm/h, respectively, $p = 0.0033$), but not shoulder arthroplasties (median 10 and 9 mm/h, respectively, $p = 0.9883$) (Table 2).

The sensitivities, specificities, positive and negative predictive values, and the p-value from logistic regression of CRP >10 mg/l, ESR >30 mm/h, and CRP >10 mg/l or ESR >30 mm/h to detect infection of knee, hip, and shoulder arthroplasties, and spinal implants are shown in Table 3. The combination of normal

Table 2. Descriptive summary and comparison of aseptic failure versus orthopedic implant-associated infection subjects. Median (range) values are shown.

Knee arthroplasty (n = 297)	**Aseptic failure (n = 215)**	**Orthopedic implant-associated infection (n = 82)**	**P-value**
ESR, mm/h	11 (0–68)	53.5 (6–128)	<0.0001
CRP, mg/l	4 (0.1–174)	51 (3–444)	<0.0001
Hip arthroplasty (n = 221)	**Aseptic failure (n = 187)**	**Orthopedic implant-associated infection (n = 34)**	
ESR, mm/h	11 (0–94)	30 (3–137)	<0.0001
CRP, mg/l	3 (0.3–141)	18 (3–288)	<0.0001
Shoulder arthroplasty (n = 64)	**Aseptic failure (n = 45)**	**Orthopedic implant-associated infection (n = 19)**	
ESR, mm/h	10 (0–32)	9 (1–71)	0.9883
CRP, mg/l	3 (3–26)	10 (3–40)	0.01
Spine implant (n = 54)	**Aseptic failure (n = 40)**	**Orthopedic implant-associated infection (n = 14)**	
ESR, mm/h	10 (0–74)	48.5 (1–83)	0.0033
CRP, mg/l	3 (0.5–183)	20 (3–205)	0.0011

Table 3. Sensitivity and specificity of CRP (>10 mg/l) and/or ESR (>30 mm/h) for the detection of infected knee, hip and shoulder arthroplasty and spinal instrumentation.

	Sensitivity	Specificity	PPV	NPV	Area Under the ROC Curve	p-value from Logistic Regression
Knee ESR >30 mm/h	71 (58/82)	89 (191/215)	71 (58/82)	89 (191/215)	0.80	<0.0001
Knee CRP >10 mg/d	83 (68/82)	79 (170/215)	60 (68/113)	92 (170/184)	0.81	<0.0001
Knee ESR >30 mm/h or CRP >10 mg/l	87 (71/82)	75 (161/215)	57 (71/125)	94 (161/172)	0.81	<0.0001
Hip ESR >30 mm/h	47 (16/34)	84 (158/187)	36 (16/45)	90 (158/176)	0.66	<0.0001
Hip CRP >10 mg/l	74 (25/34)	78 (146/187)	38 (25/66)	94 (146/155)	0.76	<0.0001
Hip ESR >30 mm/h or CRP >10 mg/l	76 (26/34)	71 (132/187)	32 (26/81)	94 (132/140)	0.74	<0.0001
Shoulder ESR >30 mm/h	16 (3/19)	98 (44/45)	75 (3/4)	73 (44/60)	0.57	0.0764
Shoulder CRP >10 mg/l	42 (8/19)	84 (38/45)	53 (8/15)	78 (38/49)	0.63	0.0269
Shoulder ESR >30 mm/h or CRP >10 mg/l	42 (8/19)	82 (37/45)	50 (8/16)	77 (37/48)	0.62	0.0455
Spine ESR >30 mm/h	64 (9/14)	83 (33/40)	56 (9/16)	87 (33/38)	0.73	0.0021
Spine CRP >10 mg/l	57 (8/14)	85 (34/40)	57 (8/14)	85 (34/40)	0.71	0.0038
Spine ESR >30 mm/h or CRP >10 mg/l	79 (11/14)	75 (30/40)	52 (11/21)	91 (30/33)	0.77	0.0013

ESR (≤30 mm/h) and CRP (≤10 mg/l) predicted the absence of infection in 94, 94 and 91% of subjects undergoing knee or hip arthroplasty or spine implant removal, respectively, but only 77% of those subjects undergoing shoulder arthroplasty removal.

Optimized ESR cutoffs for knee, hip and shoulder arthroplasties and spine implants were 19, 13, 26, and 45 mm/h, respectively. Using these cutoffs, sensitivity and specificity to detect infection were 89 and 74% for knee, 82 and 60% for hip, and 32 and 93% for shoulder arthroplasties, and 57 and 90% for spine implants (Table 4).

Optimized CRP cutoffs for knee, hip, and shoulder arthroplasties, and spine implants were 14.5, 10.3, 7, and 4.6 mg/l, respectively. Using these cutoffs, sensitivity and specificity to detect infection were for 79 and 88% knee, 74 and 79% for hip, and 63 and 73% for shoulder arthroplasties, and 79 and 68% for spine implants (Table 4).

Our study is a comprehensive analysis of CRP and ESR in subjects undergoing orthopedic implant removal with and without infection. In patients satisfying the definition for orthopedic implant-associated infection, CRP and ESR values were higher in knee arthroplasty and spine implant patients than in hip arthroplasty patients. Previous investigations have reported higherCRP and ESR values in knee than hip arthroplasty patients with infection [7].

We used receiver operating curve analysis to optimize CRP and ESR cutoffs. The optimized CRP cutoff value for hip arthroplasty infection was similar to the standard cutoff of CRP >10 mg/l often used in clinical practice. Optimized CRP and ESR cutoff

Table 4. Sensitivity and specificity of optimized CRP and ESR for the detection of infected knee, hip and shoulder arthroplasty and spinal instrumentation.

	Sensitivity	Specificity	PPV	NPV	Area Under the ROC Curve	p-value from Logistic Regression
Knee ESR >19 mm/h	89 (73/82)	74 (159/215)	57 (73/129)	95 (159/168)	0.82	<0.0001
Knee CRP >14.5 mg/l	79 (65/82)	88 (189/215)	71 (65/91)	92 (189/206)	0.84	<0.0001
Knee ESR >19 mm/h or CRP >14.5 mg/l	94 (77/82)	69 (149/215)	54 (77/143)	97 (149/154)	0.82	<0.0001
Hip ESR >13 mm/h	82 (28/34)	60 (113/187)	27 (28/102)	95 (113/119)	0.71	<0.0001
Hip CRP >10.3 mg/l	74 (25/34)	79 (147/187)	38 (25/65)	94 (147/156)	0.76	<0.0001
Hip ESR >13 mm/h or CRP >10.3 mg/l	88 (30/34)	55 (103/187)	26 (30/114)	96 (103/107)	0.72	<0.0001
Shoulder ESR >26 mm/h	32 (6/19)	93 (42/45)	67 (6/9)	76 (42/55)	0.63	0.02
Shoulder CRP >7 mg/dl	63 (12/19)	73 (33/45)	50 (12/24)	83 (33/40)	0.68	0.01
Shoulder ESR >26 mm/h or CRP >7 mg/dl	63 (12/19)	73 (33/45)	50 (12/24)	83 (33/40)	0.68	0.01
Spine ESR >45 mm/h	57 (8/14)	90 (36/40)	67 (8/12)	86 (36/42)	0.74	0.001
Spine CRP >4.6 mg/dl	79 (11/14)	68 (27/40)	46 (11/24)	90 (27/30)	0.73	0.01
Spine ESR >45 mm/h or CRP 4.6 mg/dl	79 (11/14)	67 (27/40)	46 (11/24)	90 (27/30)	0.73	0.01

values for knee arthroplasty in our study were >14.5 mg/l and >19 mm/h, similar to the ≥13.5 mg/l and ≥22.5 mm/h values derived by Greidenaus et al. using a similar approach [8].

Overall, CRP and ESR showed the lowest sensitivity for diagnosis of shoulder arthroplasty infection, even applying cutoffs optimized using receiving operating curve analysis. This may relate to the predominance of *P. acnes* in shoulder arthroplasty infection [1,2].

Several investigators have examined the natural history of postoperative ESR and CRP after uncomplicated arthroplasty. CRP levels change more rapidly than ESR levels, and return to normal more rapidly following primary total knee or hip arthroplasty [7,9]. CRP levels usually peak on the second or third day following total hip or knee arthroplasty [10,11,12,13], thereafter dropping to preoperative levels by the third week in total hip arthroplasty patients and by the end of the second month in total knee arthroplasty patients [7,14,15]. CRP levels rise to a higher level postoperatively in total knee than hip arthroplasty patients [11]. A similar rise and fall of CRP is noted postoperatively in total hip or knee arthroplasty patients with underlying rheumatoid arthritis [16]. One study demonstrated that, after uncomplicated arthroplasty, ESR peaks on the fifth postoperative day [13], dropping close to preoperative levels at the end of the third month in total hip arthroplasty patients, and at the end of the ninth month in total knee arthroplasty patients [7]. Other studies suggest, however, that the ESR, although usually normal by six months postoperatively, may be elevated for as long as one year after uncomplicated total hip arthroplasty [14,15].

For patients undergoing uncomplicated spinal surgery, investigators have described ESR peaking earlier than described above, on the fourth day, and normalizing within a two week period in the majority of patients [17]. Additionally, levels in patients undergoing fusion surgery were higher than in those patients undergoing herniated disc removal [17]. In patients with known vertebral osteomyelitis the ESR may be elevated for a prolonged period of time, even in the face of appropriate non-operative treatment [18]. In the referenced series, many patients went on to a successful clinical outcome in spite of the elevated ESR, illustrating the poor specificity of the test when used alone to predict treatment failure [18]. The current study differs in that the ESR was used in a predictive fashion preoperatively, in conjunction with the CRP, and a consistent definition of infection was applied.

In a series of 202 revision total hip arthroplasties, all subjects with infection had an elevated ESR (>30 mm/h) or CRP (>10 mg/l) [19]. In our study, this was not the case.

There are several limitations of our study. ESR and CRP are nonspecific markers of inflammation and may be elevated by chronic inflammatory conditions (e.g., rheumatoid arthritis), surgical intervention, or systemic illness. Patients with underlying inflammatory arthritides were excluded from our study, but we did not assess for recent surgeries or systemic illnesses not involving the joint. We assessed ESR and CRP within the month prior to surgery, at a time when the study subjects had symptoms related to implant failure. Ideally, the timing of ESR and CRP measurement should be standardized (e.g., 24 hours prior to surgery). A final limitation is the lack of a Gold standard definition for prosthetic shoulder and spine implant infection.

In conclusion, CRP and ESR values are higher in knee arthroplasty and spine implant patients than in hip arthroplasty patients with infection, and show the lowest sensitivity for diagnosis of shoulder arthroplasty infection, even applying cutoffs optimized using receiving operating curve analysis.

Presented in part at the Musculoskeletal Infection Society Annual Meeting and 19th Open Scientific Meeting, Aug 7–8, 2009, San Diego, California and at the 29th Annual Interscience Conference on Antimicrobial Agents and Chemotherapy/Infectious Diseases Society of America 46th Annual Meeting, October 25–28, 2008.

Acknowledgments

The authors gratefully acknowledge Andrej Trampuz and Paloma Anguita-Alonso for assistance with data collection.

Author Contributions

Conceived and designed the experiments: KEP MFS MJK JMS RP. Performed the experiments: KEP MFS KES JNM MJK JMS RP. Analyzed the data: KEP MFS KES JNM MJK JMS EFB DRO ADH RHC JWS JSS PMH MBD MJY BC RP. Contributed reagents/materials/analysis tools: EFB DRO ADH DGL RHC JWS JSS PMH MBD MJY BC. Wrote the paper: KEP MFS KES JNM MJK JMS EFB DRO ADH DGL RHC JWS JSS PMH MBD MJY BC RP.

References

1. Piper KE, Jacobson MJ, Cofield RH, Sperling JW, Sanchez-Sotelo J, et al. (2009) Microbiologic diagnosis of prosthetic shoulder infection by use of implant sonication. J Clin Microbiol 47: 1878–1884.
2. Kanafani ZA, Sexton DJ, Pien BC, Varkey J, Basmania C, et al. (2009) Postoperative joint infections due to *Propionibacterium* species: A case-control study. Clin Infect Dis 49: 1083–1085.
3. Hahn F, Zbinden R, Min K (2005) Late implant infections caused by *Propionibacterium acnes* in scoliosis surgery. Eur Spine J 14: 783–788.
4. Trampuz A, Piper KE, Jacobson MJ, Hanssen AD, Unni KK, et al. (2007) Sonication of removed hip and knee prostheses for diagnosis of infection. N Engl J Med 357: 654–663.
5. Fernandez Sampedro M, Huddleston PM, Piper KE, Karua MJ, Dekutoski MB, et al. (In Press) A biofilm approach to detect bacteria on removed spinal implants. Spine.
6. Del Pozo JL, Patel R (2009) Infection associated with prosthetic joints. New England Journal of Medicine 361: 43–50.
7. Bilgen O, Atici T, Durak K, Karaeminogullari, Bilgen MS (2001) C-reactive protein values and erythrocyte sedimentation rates after total hip and total knee arthroplasty. J Int Med Res 29: 7–12.
8. Greidanus NV, Masri BA, Garbuz DS, Wilson SD, McAlinden MG, et al. (2007) Use of erythrocyte sedimentation rate and C-reactive protein level to diagnose infection before revision total knee arthroplasty. A prospective evaluation. J Bone Joint Surg Am 89: 1409–1416.
9. Moreschini O, Greggi G, Giordano MC, Nocente M, Margheritini F (2001) Postoperative physiopathological analysis of inflammatory parameters in patients undergoing hip or knee arthroplasty. Int J Tissue React 23: 151–154.
10. Niskanen RO, Korkala O, Pammo H (1996) Serum C-reactive protein levels after total hip and knee arthroplasty. J Bone Joint Surg Br 78: 431–433.
11. White J, Kelly M, Dunsmuir R (1998) C-reactive protein level after total hip and total knee replacement. J Bone Joint Surg Br 80: 909–911.
12. Choudhry RR, Rice RP, Triffitt PD, Harper WM, Gregg PJ (1992) Plasma viscosity and C-reactive protein after total hip and knee arthroplasty. J Bone Joint Surg Br 74: 523–524.
13. Larsson S, Thelander U, Friberg S (1992) C-reactive protein (CRP) levels after elective orthopedic surgery. Clin Orthop Relat Res. pp 237–242.
14. Shih LY, Wu JJ, Yang DJ (1987) Erythrocyte sedimentation rate and C-reactive protein values in patients with total hip arthroplasty. Clin Orthop Relat Res. pp 238–246.
15. Aalto K, Osterman K, Peltola H, Rasanen J (1984) Changes in erythrocyte sedimentation rate and C-reactive protein after total hip arthroplasty. Clin Orthop Relat Res. pp 118–120.
16. Laiho K, Maenpaa H, Kautiainen H, Kauppi M, Kaarela K, et al. (2001) Rise in serum C reactive protein after hip and knee arthroplasties in patients with rheumatoid arthritis. Ann Rheum Dis 60: 275–277.
17. Jonsson B, Soderholm R, Stromqvist B (1991) Erythrocyte sedimentation rate after lumbar spine surgery. Spine (Phila Pa 1976) 16: 1049–1050.
18. Kowalski TJ, Layton KF, Berbari EF, Steckelberg JM, Huddleston PM, et al. (2007) Follow-up MR imaging in patients with pyogenic spine infections: lack of correlation with clinical features. AJNR Am J Neuroradiol 28: 693–699.
19. Spangehl M, Masri B, O'Connell J, Duncan C (1999) Prospective analysis of preoperative and intraoperative investigations for the diagnosis of infection at the sites of 202 revision total hip arthroplasties. Journal of Bone and Joint Surgery (American) 81: 672–683.

20. Austin MS, Ghanem E, Joshi A, Lindsay A, Parvizi J (2008) A simple, cost-effective screening protocol to rule out periprosthetic infection. J Arthroplasty 23: 65–68.
21. Schinsky MF, Della Valle CJ, Sporer SM, Paprosky WG (2008) Perioperative testing for joint infection in patients undergoing revision total hip arthroplasty. J Bone Joint Surg Am 90: 1869–1875.
22. Baré J, MacDonald SJ, Bourne RB (2006) Preoperative evaluations in revision total knee arthroplasty. Clin Orthop Relat Res 446: 40–44.
23. Bernard L, Lubbeke A, Stern R, Bru JP, Feron JM, et al. (2004) Value of preoperative investigations in diagnosing prosthetic joint infection: retrospective cohort study and literature review. Scand J Infect Dis 36: 410–416.
24. Levitsky KA, Hozack WJ, Balderston RA, Rothman RH, Gluckman SJ, et al. (1991) Evaluation of the painful prosthetic joint. Relative value of bone scan, sedimentation rate, and joint aspiration. J Arthroplasty 6: 237–244.
25. Feldman DS, Lonner JH, Desai P, Zuckerman JD (1995) The role of intraoperative frozen sections in revision total joint arthroplasty. J Bone Joint Surg Am 77: 1807–1813.
26. Bottner F, Wegner A, Winkelmann W, Becker K, Erren M, et al. (2007) Interleukin-6, procalcitonin and TNF-alpha: markers of peri-prosthetic infection following total joint replacement. J Bone Joint Surg Br 89: 94–99.
27. Fink B, Makowiak C, Fuerst M, Berger I, Schafer P, et al. (2008) The value of synovial biopsy, joint aspiration and C-reactive protein in the diagnosis of late peri-prosthetic infection of total knee replacements. J Bone Joint Surg Br 90: 874–878.
28. Müller M, Morawietz L, Hasart O, Strube P, Perka C, et al. (2008) Diagnosis of periprosthetic infection following total hip arthroplasty - evaluation of the diagnostic values of pre- and intraoperative parameters and the associated strategy to preoperatively select patients with a high probability of joint infection. J Orthop Surg 3: 31.
29. Virolainen P, Lahteenmaki H, Hiltunen A, Sipola E, Meurman O, et al. (2002) The reliability of diagnosis of infection during revision arthroplasties. Scand J Surg 91: 178–181.

4

Genetic Evaluation of Hip Score in UK Labrador Retrievers

Thomas W. Lewis[1]*, Sarah C. Blott[1], John A. Woolliams[2]

1 Kennel Club Genetics Centre at the Animal Health Trust, Animal Health Trust, Newmarket, United Kingdom, **2** The Roslin Institute and Royal (Dick) School of Veterinary Studies, University of Edinburgh, Roslin, United Kingdom

Abstract

Hip dysplasia is an important and complex genetic disease in dogs with both genetic and environmental influences. Since the osteoarthritis that develops is irreversible the only way to improve welfare, through reducing the prevalence, is through genetic selection. This study aimed to evaluate the progress of selection against hip dysplasia, to quantify potential improvements in the response to selection via use of genetic information and increases in selection intensity, and to prepare for public provision of estimated breeding values (EBV) for hip dysplasia in the UK. Data consisted of 25,243 single records of hip scores of Labrador Retrievers between one and four years old, from radiographs evaluated between 2000 and 2007 as part of the British Veterinary Association (BVA) hip score scheme. A natural logarithm transformation was applied to improve normality and linear mixed models were evaluated using ASREML. Genetic correlations between left and right scores, and total hip scores at one, two and three years of age were found to be close to one, endorsing analysis of total hip score in dogs aged one to three as an appropriate approach. A heritability of 0.35 ± 0.016 and small but significant litter effect (0.07 ± 0.009) were estimated. The observed trends in both mean hip score and mean EBV over year of birth indicate that a small genetic improvement has been taking place, approximately equivalent to avoiding those dogs with the worst 15% of scores. Deterministic analysis supported by simulations showed that a 19% greater response could be achieved using EBV compared to phenotype through increases in accuracy alone. This study establishes that consistent but slow genetic improvement in the hip score of UK Labrador Retrievers has been achieved over the previous decade, and demonstrates that progress may be easily enhanced through the use of EBVs and more intense selection.

Editor: Amanda Ewart Toland, Ohio State University Medical Center, United States of America

Funding: This work was funded by the Kennel Club Charitable Trust. JAW is grateful to BBSRC for funding through an ISPG. The funders had no role in study design, data analysis, decision to publish, or preparation of the manuscript. Hip score and pedigree data was collated and provided by the UK Kennel Club.

Competing Interests: Hip score and pedigree data was collated and provided by the UK Kennel Club.

* E-mail: tom.lewis@aht.org.uk

Introduction

It has been argued that tackling the spread of heritable diseases in managed populations of animals is an obligation for animal breeding, both for farm and for companion animals [1]. Among companion animals the extent of inherited disease in pedigree dog breeds has recently come under scrutiny [2,3] and it has been reiterated that the appropriate use of genetic selection schemes could be used to tackle such diseases [4]. Thus, researchers have a responsibility to make the best use of the data available to provide the tools that will enable breeders to reduce the disease burden across pedigree dog breeds through effective and efficient genetic selection.

Hip dysplasia is an important and complex genetic disease in dogs, and is one of the most prevalent diseases among larger breeds [5]. It has both genetic and environmental influences [6,7,8] with evidence of gene effects at multiple loci [9] confirming complex underlying genetics. It is a developmental orthopaedic disorder characterised by the formation of a loose, ill-fitting coxofemoral (hip) joint [10], and over time, the malformation leads to abnormal wearing of bone surfaces and the appearance of the osteoarthiritic signs of degenerative joint disease (DJD) [11]. Since the osteoarthritis that develops is irreversible, hip dysplasia is often impossible to treat and so the only way to improve dog welfare, through reducing the prevalence, is through genetic selection.

Various international recording schemes for hip dysplasia have been in existence for several years with a view to providing information to breeders. One of the larger and longer running schemes is the British Veterinary Association (BVA) / Kennel Club (KC) hip scoring scheme, which was established in its current form in 1984 [12] and is used in the UK, Ireland, Australia and New Zealand. Under this scheme, a radiograph of the pelvic area is taken by a general practice vet according to standardised protocols, submitted to the BVA and evaluated by three members of a panel of certified radiologists or small animal surgeons [13]. Nine features of each hip are scored according to the degree of dysplasia observed (0 = no signs) and scores from each feature are summed to give a total from 0–53 for each hip, and 0–106 in total. Although voluntary, the rate of participation in the UK is good; for example, 8–10% of all annually registered Labrador Retrievers (the most popular breed in the UK, with between 33, 398 registrations in 1999 and 45,779 registrations in 2005) are scored per year, equating to 50–60% of all dogs used for breeding. There are other international evaluation schemes of note, operated by the Orthopedic Foundation for Animals (OFA) in the USA and Canada; the Fédération Cynologique Internationale (FCI), an umbrella organisation of more than 80 national kennel authorities in most of Europe, Russia, South America and parts of Asia, [13]; and the PennHIP scheme based at the University of Pennsylvania, USA. There are clear philosophical differences between these global recording schemes in the best way to assess hip dysplasia, particularly over categorical classification of the disease and whether an assessment is made on the condition of both hips or on the worst hip alone.

Reports on the response to selection against the disease are mixed. In the UK, it was reported that there were no discernable improvements in 5 breeds between 1987 and 1995 [14], despite the availability of hip score phenotypes to breeders. There have been reported reductions in the prevalence of disease in some Finnish registered breeds but an increase in others, even when an enforced threshold of hip score was applied to registrations [15]. An improving genetic trend with respect to disease was detected in two Swedish registered breeds [16] and in a retrospective study of data on American Labradors over almost 40 years [17], via calculation of estimated breeding values (EBV). These inconsistencies lead to the impression that progress in breeding away from the disease is currently sub-optimal given the amount of information being generated.

The complex nature of hip dysplasia, the abundance of phenotypic data and the availability of pedigree records are favourable for the calculation of EBV for the scored features indicative of this disease. EBV are the estimates of genetic liabilities obtained after removing as far as possible the environmental influences. The calculation of an EBV combines an individual's phenotypic data with that of its relatives using weights derived from the pedigree, resulting in a more accurate estimate than is possible from using only the individual's own phenotype. EBV have been widely used in the improvement of production traits and traits indicative of health in livestock [18,19], and have more recently been calculated for complex inherited diseases in dogs [16,20,21].

Given the mixed reports of the response to selection against hip dysplasia and the suitability for selection using EBV, this study aimed to assess one of the largest cohorts of data on a single breed (Labrador Retrievers) within the BVA/KC scheme. The objectives were to: 1) evaluate the current effectiveness of the scheme in enabling demonstrable and genetic improvement towards reducing prevalence; 2) quantify the potential benefits from providing better genetic information such as EBV to breeders; 3) prepare the path for routine provision of EBV with the BVA/KC data. These objectives were carried out using both mixed model analysis of the accumulated data of BVA/KC and simulation.

Results

Data distribution

The distribution of hip scores (H) from radiographs taken and evaluated from 2000–2007 (Figure 1) had a mean of 13.22, (mode = 8, median = 10), a standard deviation of 12.29, CV = 0.93, and was highly skewed with coefficient of skewness of 3.39. Evaluation of radiographs taken of dogs aged 1, 2 and 3 years old comprised 90.6% of the scores. Given the progressive nature of the disease it would be expected that parameters would change over a lifetime and so the 'full' dataset used in the analyses described was limited to include only those dogs that were 1, 2 or 3 years (365–1459 days) old at the time of evaluation. This dataset (n = 25,243) had a mean of 13.00 (mode = 8, median = 10), standard deviation of 11.82, CV = 0.91, and coefficient of skewness of 3.44. There were 5,116 sires with a mean of 4.93

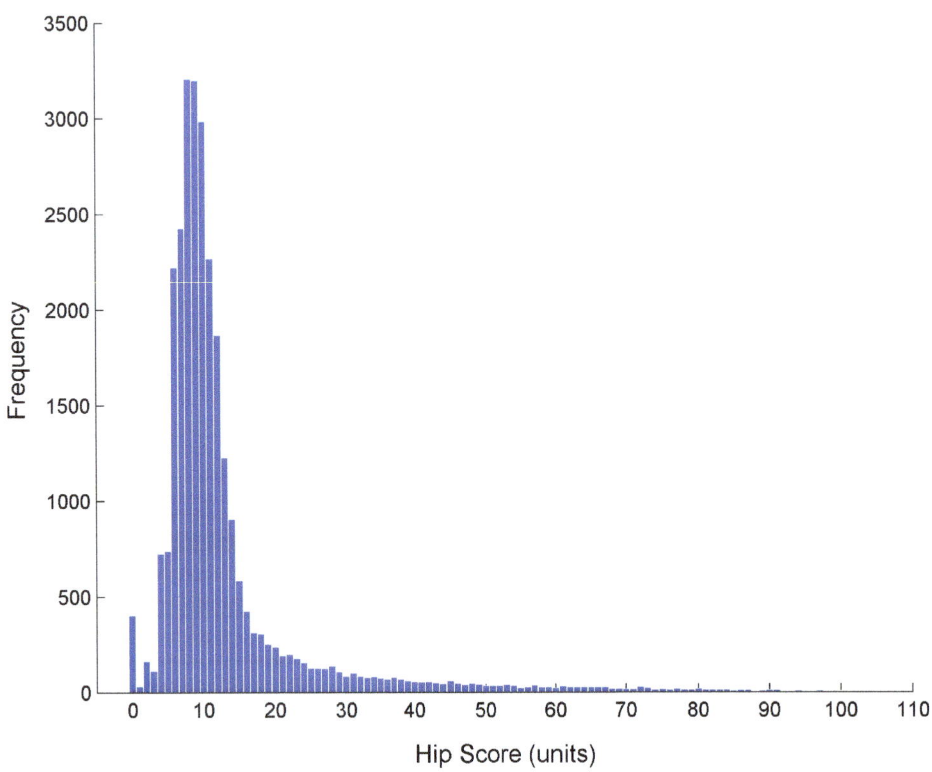

Figure 1. Distribution of hip score from all UK registered Labrador Retrievers. Dogs radiographed from 2000–2007 inclusive (where age at radiograph was above the stipulated 1 year old, recorded sex and coat colour were from the permitted classes male and female, and black, chocolate and yellow respectively, and scores within the defined boundaries of 0 to 106).

scored offspring per sire, and 12,719 dams with a mean of 1.98 scored offspring per dam, and 16,922 litters with a mean of 1.49 scored animals per litter. Generation interval (L) was calculated as 4.3 years. The mean coefficient of inbreeding (calculated over 5 generations of pedigree) was 0.041 (S.D. = 0.039), with 95% of the population <0.125 (the value for progeny of mating between two half-sibs that are otherwise unrelated).

Lateral symmetry of gene expression

Under the BVA/KC scheme, left and right hips are scored separately and summed. The utility of analysis of the total score compared to a bivariate analysis of left and right scores (H_L and H_R) depends upon the phenotypic and additive genetic variances, and the genetic correlation between left and right scores. The preliminary analysis of transformations as described in the Materials and Methods indicated that for individual left and right hip scores natural logarithm transformations of $1+H_L$ and $1+H_R$ were optimal. Very similar estimates of phenotypic variance (0.386±0.0074 and 0.366±0.0070) and heritability (0.30±0.036 and 0.27±0.035) were obtained for transformed left and right hip scores from two year old dogs. The genetic correlation between transformed left and right hip score was estimated with only small error but still could not be distinguished from 1, with a 95% confidence interval of [0.99,1.00]. In contrast, the environmental correlation between left and right hip score was 0.57 (±0.025). Given the similarity of estimates of heritability and phenotypic variances and the near perfect genetic correlation it was considered reasonable to simplify further analyses by using the transformed total score ($\log_e(1+H)$, where $H = H_L+H_R$), since the benefit of bivariate analyses resulting in two EBVs for use in selection, or a differentially weighted sum would be negligible.

Age related expression

To explore any need to model genetic parameters separately for H at different ages, a series of bivariate analyses were conducted for scores of 1, 2 and 3 year old dogs. Preliminary analysis of transformations of total score determined that within each year age group $\log_e(1+H)$ was again the optimum. Models tested the hypothesis of genetic equivalence of transformed hip scores of 1, 2 and 3 year olds. Heritabilities (h^2) and phenotypic variances (σ^2_P) were similar at all three ages ($h^2 = 0.33$–0.34, $\sigma^2_P = 0.34$–0.43) and genetic correlations between total scores at each age were not significantly different to 0.999 indicating the hypothesis of genetic equivalence of scores over this age range is reasonable. In contrast, a comparable bivariate analysis using an identical protocol suggested more dissimilar phenotypic variances and heritability estimates of dogs scored at one and five years old (1825–2189 days, $h^2 = 0.19$, $\sigma^2_P = 0.50$) although the genetic correlation of hip scores at the two ages remained high (0.95, and not significantly different from 1).

Litter and dam effect on hip score

There are reports that hip score may be subject to litter and maternal effects [22] and so litter and dam random effects were first singly and then jointly added to a simple animal model to determine significance, and the results are shown in Table 1. Separate inclusion of either 'litter' or 'dam' as random effects in addition to 'animal' improves the fit compared to the 'animal' only model. However, inclusion of both 'litter' and 'dam' together in addition to 'animal' makes no significant improvement to fit compared to the addition of 'litter' alone. These results indicate that the data analysed contains insufficient records from repeated litters from dams to establish separate effects, or that the dam effects are small. An 'animal'+'litter' model was used in subsequent analyses since it had a greater likelihood compared to 'animal'+'dam'.

Table 1. Model Log likelihoods.

Model	Effects	Log likelihood	Test statistic	P
1.	animal	898.77		
2.	animal+litter	928.00	58.46 c.f. Model 1	<0.001
3.	animal+dam	911.42	25.30 c.f. Model 1	<0.001
4.	animal+dam+litter	928.39	0.78 c.f. Model 2	>0.05
			33.94 c.f. Model 3	<0.001

Log likelihoods of a sequence of models fitting combinations of 'animal', 'litter' and 'dam' terms to $\log_e(1+H)$, together with the test statistic for the likelihood ratio tests. The significance value, P, is obtained from comparison with χ^2_1.

Genetic parameters and trends for total hip score (H)

Using the 'full' dataset described the heritability estimate of $\log_e(1+H)$ was 0.35±0.016. The variation due to litter explained a fraction of 0.07±0.009 of the total variation, much smaller than the genetic. The total phenotypic variation was 0.375±0.0040. For comparison, when untransformed hip score was analysed using the same model the heritability and litter variance fraction were estimated at 0.50±0.018 and 0.06±0.009, and phenotypic variance was 153.1±1.8 (see later).

Figure 2 shows the distribution of EBV, when evaluated on the log scale, of dogs with hip scores H≤4, = 8, = 10, = 13, and ≥37 corresponding to the lower and upper 5% tails of the phenotypic values, the quartiles and the median. The overlapping of the distributions shows the large range of EBV that can occur within a single phenotypic hip score, for example a median score can be associated with EBV either in the best or worst 5%. This refinement of the genetic breeding value is one potential advantage of EBV over phenotype for providing predictions of risk in a breeding program to reduce hip dysplasia.

The mean and standard deviation for EBV of $\log_e(1+H)$ and the observed hip score (H) according to year of birth are displayed in Table 2. Both mean EBV and mean H decrease with year of birth indicating that there is moderate progress against hip dysplasia, and that this is partially mediated by genetic improvement. The decline in H from 1996 to 2006 is 2.69 untransformed units, and regression of H on date of birth equivalent to a fall of 0.376 (±0.031) untransformed units per annum. For the same period EBV declined by a total of 0.155 transformed units, and regression on date of birth was equivalent to a decline of 1.36×10^{-2} (±0.0007) transformed units p.a. This trend in EBV between 1996 and 2006 is equivalent to a 1.4% decline in (1+H) year on year. Translating this estimated decline to observed H shows genetic progress has reduced hip scores by 13% from 1996 to 2006 birth years. This can be compared to the 20% decline observed phenotypically, which includes non genetic factors such as changes in nutrition and exercise regimes, and indicates that genetics has been the dominant factor in improvement. The estimate of total gain achieved in this period of 1996 to 2006 birth years of 0.155 transformed units is equivalent to 0.43 genetic standard deviations. The standard deviation of phenotypic hip score declines over progressive years of birth, consistent with a near constant CV of 0.9, and is indicative of a contraction of the 'tail'.

Accuracy of selection

The accuracy of an EBV in predicting the true breeding value, or genetic liability, at the time of selection is directly proportional to the rate of progress. However, the accuracy of an EBV will change over time as more phenotypic information becomes

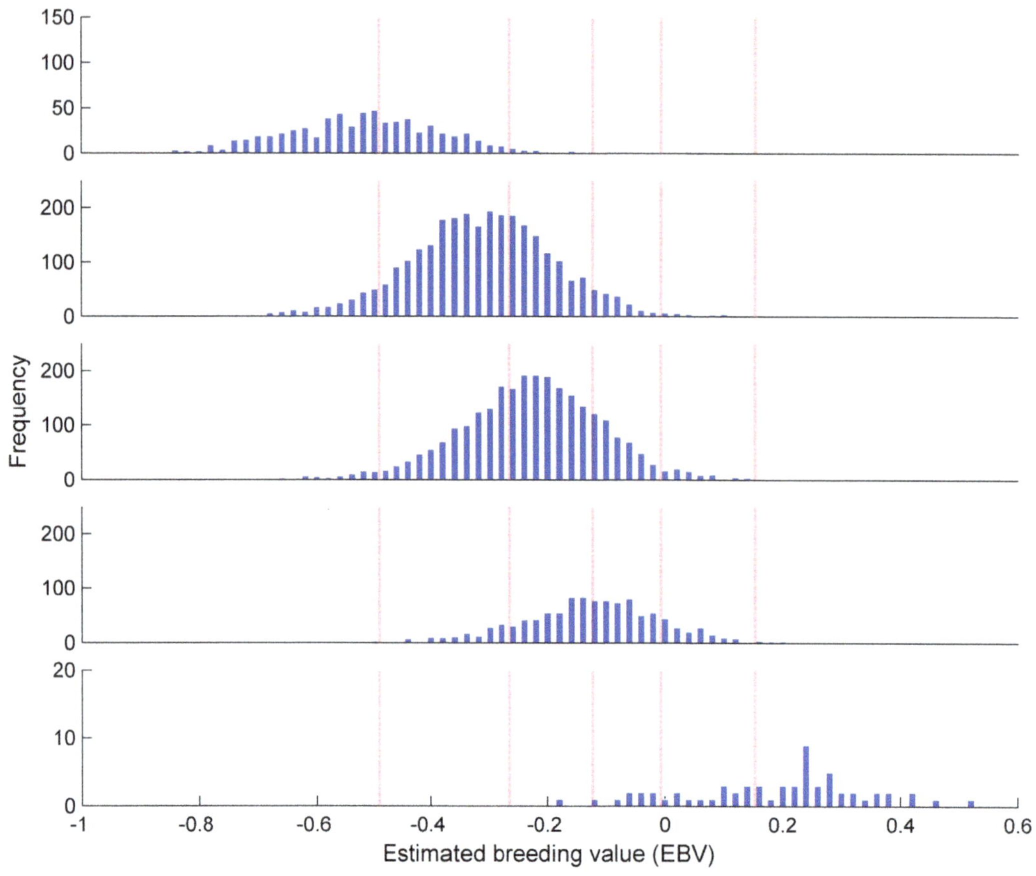

Figure 2. Distribution of EBV over phenotypic scores. Subsets defined by phenotypic scores H≤4, H = 8, H = 10, H = 13 and H≥37 respectively. These subsets represent the lowest (best) 5% (top), individuals with phenotypic values equal to the lower quartile, the median and the upper quartile, and the highest (worst) 5% (bottom). Vertical dashed lines indicate the 5th, 25th, 50th, 75th and 95th percentile for the EBV. EBV are obtained from analysis of $\log_e(1+H)$.

available on the individual or relatives, and so the lifetime profile of EBV accuracy against age will influence the overall utility of EBV and recommendations on how to use them. This profile was examined by comparing results obtained with the full data set to those obtained from a reduced dataset, where the data of the final cohort (779 dogs born in 2006) was set as missing. Estimates from analysis of the reduced data mimic the 'nascent' EBV for the 779 dogs born in 2006 which would have been predicted at birth as $\frac{1}{2}EBV_{sire}+\frac{1}{2}EBV_{dam}$, i.e. prior to scoring and so without individual phenotypic records. The mean accuracy of nascent EBV for the 779 dogs born in 2006, equivalent to EBV for a 'newborn' dog, was 0.55 (S.D. = 0.061). The mean EBV accuracy of the 779 dogs born in 2006 calculated with their scores included in the data was 0.70 (S.D. = 0.023). The different distributions indicate a 1.27-fold improvement in EBV accuracy obtained from the presence of an individual phenotypic record. Mean accuracies of EBV for sires and dams of the 779 dogs born in 2006 using the reduced dataset were 0.78 (S.D. = 0.121) and 0.70 (S.D. = 0.095) respectively, approximating the accuracy of sire and dam EBV at the time of breeding within the current system. Therefore whilst a typical sire has a 1.1-fold higher accuracy than that expected after simply being scored itself, most likely due to information from previous offspring, the accuracy of a typical dam is not supplemented by additional information. Using the full dataset, the mean accuracy of sire and dam EBV was 0.80 (S.D. = 0.103) and 0.72 (S.D. = 0.077) revealing a relatively minor incremental improvement in accuracy of estimate from this additional litter, in the current system.

Table 2. Hip score (H) statistics over year of birth.

Year of birth	n records	EBV		H	
		Mean	s.d.	mean	s.d.
1996	169	−0.160	0.232	14.04	12.40
1997	665	−0.167	0.249	14.59	13.78
1998	1576	−0.174	0.245	14.20	12.53
1999	2703	−0.195	0.239	13.40	11.55
2000	2967	−0.183	0.242	13.89	12.62
2001	3160	−0.201	0.247	13.70	12.76
2002	3465	−0.221	0.236	13.03	11.81
2003	3827	−0.240	0.241	12.88	11.91
2004	3443	−0.245	0.235	12.03	10.99
2005	2489	−0.267	0.234	11.41	9.92
2006	779	−0.315	0.246	11.35	9.87

Mean and standard deviation of EBV and phenotypic hip scores (H) according to year of birth for all records of dogs scored at ≥1 and <4 years old and between 2000 and 2007. EBV are obtained from analysis of $\log_e(1+H)$.

In the absence of EBV, any selection must be based upon the phenotypic score of the individual. In this case the accuracy of selection when selecting on the phenotypic scores of candidates is 0.59 (equal to h). This compares to the accuracy of 0.70 when using the EBV after scoring, indicating a potential 1.19-fold increase in progress – even if selection intensity were not to increase when the EBV was available (see Discussion). Choosing parents on the average of their phenotypic scores produces an accuracy for the new born of 0.42 (calculated as $\sqrt{½}$ h, which is optimistic since it *ignores all potential biases* from fixed effects in such a procedure!). Therefore the accuracy of the nascent EBV for a newborn of 0.55, calculated above, represents 1.31-fold increase in accuracy.

Assessment of historical selection intensity applied

The results reported above may be used to calculate selection intensity (i) that has been applied against hip dysplasia since breeders will only have had access to a phenotype, and so rate of progress, ΔG, is given by $i\ h^2\ \sigma_P\ /\ L$. Substitution with the estimates for $\log_e(1+H)$ of $\sigma_P = 0.61$, $L = 4.3$, $h^2 = 0.35$, and $\Delta G = 1.36 \times 10^{-2}$, gives $i = 0.27$; this is equivalent to only breeding from dogs and bitches in the top 85% of the distribution, assuming a Normal distribution of values.

These calculations were tested using simulation of selection of dogs born in 2005 (n = 2489, 756 males, 1733 females). Figure 3 shows that whenever selection was practiced, i.e. $p < 1.0$, the simulated response to selection indicated a greater response using EBV than phenotypic hip scores for every selection proportion, with the increment becoming larger as selection became more intense. The predicted responses in Figure 3 were used to provide a further estimate of the equivalent selection proportion being applied against hip dysplasia in the UK Labrador Retriever population. For the purpose of this comparison, the responses in Figure 3 need to be corrected for the 1.1-fold higher accuracy of a typical sire: since ΔG is directly related to accuracy but sires only contribute ½ the genes, the responses in Figure 3 need to be increased 1.05-fold. Furthermore responses in Figure 3 may be viewed as being equivalent to progress in a whole generation (with generation interval, L, of 4.3 years). The progress made in a single generation over the period 1996–2006 is $4.3 \times (1.36 \times 10^{-2}/1.05) \sim 0.056$ transformed units. Having corrected for these two factors, the observed response can be seen to be equivalent to a selection proportion of ~0.87 – in good agreement with the calculation above.

Fixed effects on hip score

Analysis of the full data set indicated that males had a lower score compared to females of -0.042 ± 0.0085 ($P < 0.05$) on the transformed scale which is equivalent to approximately half a point when compared to females with a score of 10 (the median) and otherwise similar fixed and random factors. There was a small but detrimental trend ($P < 0.1$) in hip score associated with the coefficient of inbreeding, equivalent to a quarter point increase for a median score of 10 (or 1.3 points for a score of 50) when comparing a coefficient of inbreeding of 0.125 to 0 (values obtained for offspring of half-sib and unrelated matings respectively). However, breeding from such close relatives is rare with less than 5% of animals resulting from a mating equivalent or closer than a

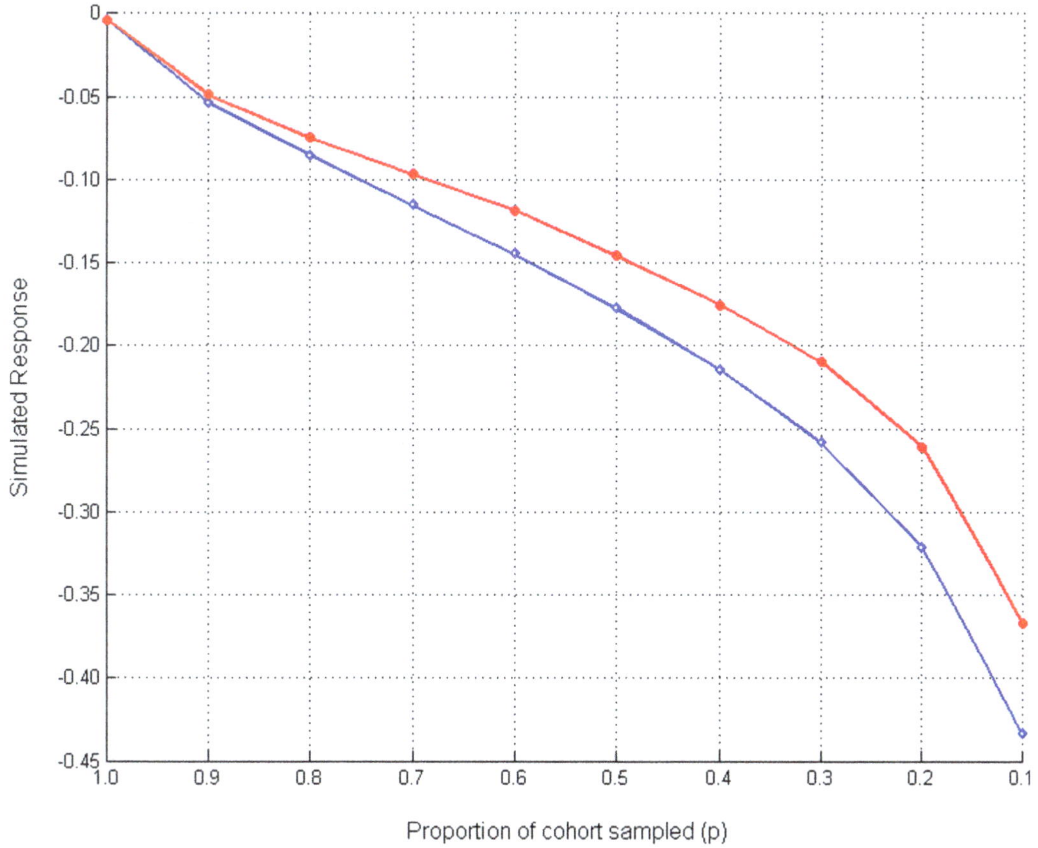

Figure 3. The simulated response to selection. Calculated as the difference in simulated generation mean EBV from parental generation mean EBV, due to selection from sampling within a cohort of dogs with the lowest p proportion phenotypic hip score (red line, closed circles) or EBV (blue line, open diamonds). Response is negative since lower EBVs indicate lower disease liability.

half sib mating. Therefore avoidance of mating close relatives *per se* will have minimal impact upon the distribution of population scores.

Whilst the pedigree accounted for genetic trend, the fitting of a smoothing spline for day of birth protected against any confounding that might have been present. Predicted values of hip score over smoothed splines of absolute day born show a definite cyclical pattern (figure 4) with scores elevated in winter and reduced in summer. This seasonal effect on hip score appears to have peaks and troughs varying between one and two points on the observed scale. The scale and timing of the seasonal effect on hip score is consistent with that reported previously in Labrador Retrievers [23].

The effect of age on hip score is detrimental with a predicted increase of just over a point from 12.8 at one year old to a plateau at 14.0 at about 2 ¼ years. However these differences are not large compared to the standard errors ranging from 0.5 to 0.8 on the untransformed grades. A trend in year of evaluation reflects either procedural change, including personnel, or changes in risk factors, since pedigree inclusion has accounted for any genetic trend in the data. There was no clear and consistent trend in the effect of year of evaluation over 2000–2007.

Comparison of genetic evaluation of transformed and untransformed score

Given the relatively stable temporal trends in evaluation of hip dysplasia it was feasible to compare the relationship of scored offspring with the mean score of the parents, for both H and $\log_e(1+H)$. For the transformed score the slope of the regression of offspring/mid-parent regression of transformed scores was consistent with the heritability estimate reported ($b = 0.32 \pm 0.025$) and yielded a reasonable fit over the distribution apart from the lower 5% (Figure 5). For the untransformed data the slope of the regression was 0.33, lower than the estimated heritability of 0.50 obtained from REML, with major deviations in the upper 5% of the tail. The relevance of this is discussed later.

Genetic association of hip score with coat colour

To explore a possible genetic association of coat colour with hip score, coat colour was fitted as an additional fixed effect in the models described in the Materials and Methods. However there was no significant effect of colour on mean hip score ($P>0.05$) and the magnitude of the estimated genetic variance after adjustment for coat colour was only negligibly different from before adjustment. In conclusion there was no evidence of any genetic association between coat colour and hip dysplasia.

Discussion

This study has shown that despite the large quantity of screening data provided by the BVA/KC hip scoring scheme, progress against hip dysplasia appears minimal; equivalent to that projected from avoiding only the worst 15% of animals for

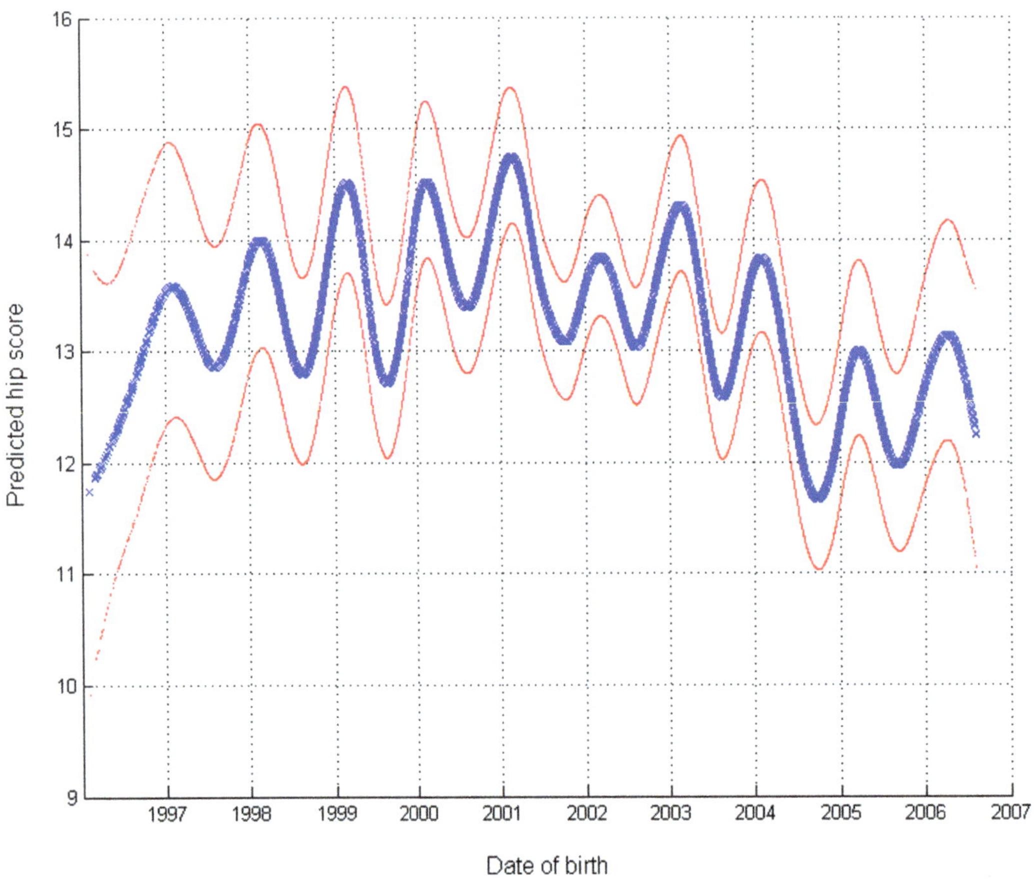

Figure 4. Predicted hip score over date of birth. Undulations within year indicate the seasonal effect on hip score. The blue line is the predicted value and the red lines indicate ±1 standard error. Values shown were obtained from the fitted values for $\log_e(1+H)$ by transforming back to the observed scale. The standard error curves were obtained by first adding ± s.e. to the fitted value on the transformed scale and then transforming back to the observed scale.

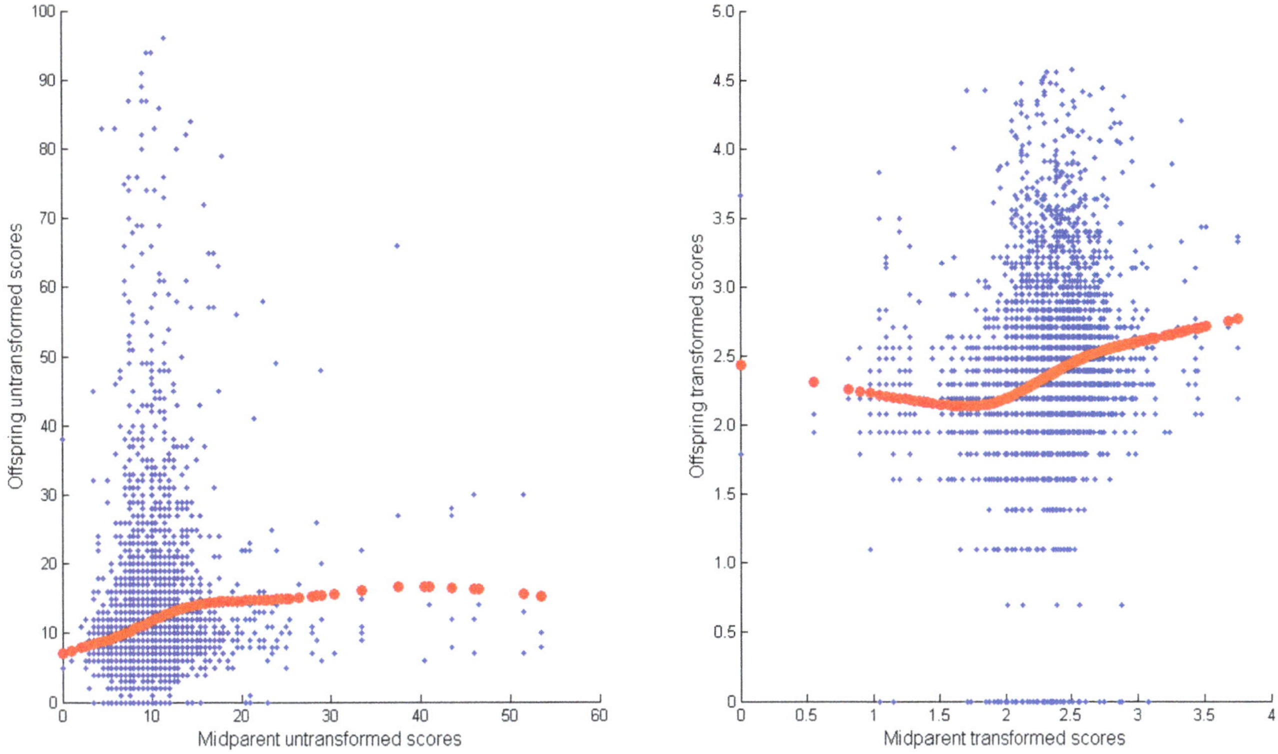

Figure 5. Relationship of offspring to midparent. Hip dysplasia scores (H) untransformed (left) and after transformation of individual scores to $\log_e(1+H)$ (right). The points displayed are for the subset of 5115 records for which score data was available on the individual and both parents. The fitted values from regression on mid-parent are also shown using smoothing splines with 4 d.f. for smoothing the fitted curves (Genstat).

breeding. The introduction of EBV alone would be projected to increase the rate of progress by 19% through additional accuracy of selection even if selection intensity remained unchanged. Barring costly and painful surgery, hip dysplasia is incurable due to the development of osteoarthritis as a consequence of malformation, so genetic selection presents the only effective method of reducing the prevalence. Therefore, as hip dysplasia is one of the most serious diseases in larger breeds of dog, the need for the most efficient and effective genetic selection is clear.

The presented results have demonstrated that the availability of EBV through routine evaluations of the hip score data would hasten progress in alleviating the problem of hip dysplasia via increases in selective accuracy compared to selection based on phenotype alone. However the benefits of EBV extend beyond the simple comparisons of accuracy for a recently scored dog: (i) the EBV for an individual, unlike its phenotypic score, will further increase in accuracy over time by utilising all the available information and being updated as additional information becomes available e.g. from offspring or siblings; (ii) the EBV will provide predictors for those animals that do not have a phenotypic record hence increasing selection opportunities and intensity, which again enhances rate of improvement; (iii) the EBV will be available from the moment of birth for selection (although newborn littermates will have identical EBV) and, in this case, the accuracy (and hence rate of improvement) from using EBV increases by 31% compared to the parental average phenotype; (iv) the EBV will have been corrected for other fixed effects such as sex and age which bias phenotype as a predictor of genetic merit; and (v) it may be argued that taking account of a sustainable rate of inbreeding as well as disease prevalence would restrict the selection pressure that can be applied, however this only serves to place a greater emphasis on the accuracy of the selection that does take place.

Finally with the availability of sequence [24] and dense canine SNP chips, the development of a genomic EBV (an EBV informed by additional information from dense SNP genotypes [25]) would help to distinguish littermates and further increase accuracy, increasing the potential rate of improvement, and might also lead subsequently to scientific benefits through identifying the major QTL. The intention is to make public the EBV for hip score for all KC registered Labrador Retrievers so that all these benefits may be realised.

The analyses of transformations for calculation indicated consistently that a logarithmic transformation was more suitable for the data, despite the observation of a higher estimate of heritability for H untransformed. Two important reasons argue for the use of the transformation. Firstly the Box-Cox analysis optimises transformation on the basis of implicit assumptions with the model; namely normality, lack of heterogeneity in subclass variance, and additivity of model terms, and whilst the procedure has been used here in the context of mixed models rather than a fixed model in which it was developed the underlying principles behind the optimisation may be assumed to hold. These implicit assumptions underpin substantial parts of quantitative genetic theory and therefore it seems a wise precaution to use the transformed scale. A second justification may be found in a more detailed examination of the additivity in a genetic context where similarity between offspring and parent is fundamental, and where in selection theory linearity in regression of offspring on mid-parent an important tenet. This examination was possible because of the relatively stable temporal trends for evaluation of hip score, which testifies to good quality control by the BVA. The implication is that focussing on the upper tail of the distribution alone is unlikely to have the benefit that may be anticipated in reducing the population mean, and that genetic progress needs to be generated by influencing selection within the wider population that is less extreme. Transformation alone does not alter this – the transformation is monotonic and so does not change ranking. However the more linear relationship between offspring and mid-parent will underpin a more predictable response to selection. The lack of linearity and monotonicity in the lower tail of the relationship for $\log_e(1+H)$ is not influential as it affects only the lower 5% of the distribution and that part of the distribution which will always be selected. A possible explanation for the results concerning the lower tail may be lower precision of evaluation, for which there may be some support from the apparent excess of zero individual scores (see Figure 1).

A further caveat of the BVA/KC scheme arises from the possible under-reporting of extremely poor hip scores, since submission of the radiograph to the BVA is voluntary. In such cases, it would be hoped that a prospective hip score severe enough to warrant saving the cost of evaluation by the BVA panellists would dissuade the owner from using the dog in question for breeding. Directed removal of data from one end of the scale is expected to under-estimate heritability and consequently bias estimates of EBV; in particular sires with the poorer breeding values since they are expected to have more offspring with missing (and bad) records. However, selection progress from the existing data will still be expected, and potentially faster than predicted here as a result of the underestimation of sires with poorer breeding values. Therefore whilst submission of all radiographs would be better, the BVA/KC scheme remains of high quality, scoring a large number of dogs with the majority of breeding stock. Such biases are present in many recording schemes, for example in preferential treatment of cows in dairy breeding.

This study clarified that the total hip score (of both left and right hips) was the appropriate statistic for genetic evaluation since investigation showed that left and right hips had near identical genetic parameters. The optimum weighting for individual hips, in principle, favours the hip that is richer in genetic information and this is related to heritabilities and phenotypic variances for each hip. However the demonstration of near perfect genetic concordance across hips indicates that analysis of total hip score averages out the environmental influences that differentiate the individual left and right hip score (note the environmental correlation was only 0.57). Furthermore, given the extent to which genetic influences are shared by both hips (the genetic correlation was 0.999) recording the worst hip only will add bias by recording the hip that has suffered from the most extreme deleterious environmental impact. This was supported by additional analysis which indicated that EBV for a measure of mean hip score was a better predictor of both mean and worst hip score than EBV for worst hip score (see supplementary Material S1 and Table S1).

The rate of genetic improvement estimated in this study is modest, equivalent to 0.43 genetic standard deviations p.a.; lower than that reported in Swedish Rottweilers from 1992–2002 (0.67) [16], but higher than that in US Labradors from 1970–2005 (0.37) [17]. Comparison between the US and UK studies are more straightforward since they consider the same breed/gene pool and, given the low selection intensity observed in the UK, the disparity of progress may be due to the recording schemes since the more refined scale of the BVA/KC was estimated to be 1.6 fold more heritable than the 7 point OFA scheme. Comparison with Swedish Rottweilers however is across gene-pools, and the reported heritability for the 5 point FCI scheme was marginally greater though with greater standard errors. Thus, whether the superior rate of improvement reported by the Swedish study is due to breed, to recording scale or to greater selection pressure is unclear.

To date any selection against hip dysplasia in the UK will have been accomplished using phenotypic hip score, and the BVA endorses such practice by recommending breeding from dogs with scores clearly below the breed mean, which is currently 15 (http://www.bva.co.uk/public/documents/chs_hip_scheme_breed_mean_scores.pdf). However, it is clear that the BVA recommendations are only just short of being met, since a score of 15 corresponds to the 81st–82nd percentile in our data, equivalent to avoiding only the worst 18–19% of animals for breeding – close to what is observed. At the current rate of progress (an improvement in mean EBV of 1.36×10^{-2} per annum), an ambitious but realistic target of a reduction in the median hip score from 10 to 5 would take over 44 years using phenotypic selection, or just over 37 years if selection was on EBV of dogs with a phenotypic hip score. Therefore, despite the improved accuracy of selection enabled by EBVs, there remains very slow selective progress against hip dysplasia. Even breeding below the median phenotype, i.e. best 50% of animals, would have resulted in progress over 2.5 fold greater than has been observed over the period 1996–2006. The selection intensity from breeding from the best 50% of scored animals using EBVs would be over 3 times higher than that achieved over 1996–2006 where breeding from dogs with scores less than the current breed mean was the guideline. These figures indicate that, even with the improved efficiencies afforded by EBV, adequate selection pressure is also vital in improving progress against hip dysplasia and that this could be achieved with more challenging guidelines.

Materials and Methods

BVA/KC hip score scheme

The BVA/KC hip-scoring scheme is voluntary and, to ensure skeletal maturity, restricted to dogs over a year old [23]. There is no upper age limit restricting participation, but dogs may only be scored once. Eight of the nine features considered in the scheme are scored 0–6 for each hip, and the ninth is scored 0–5 for each hip (a zero score indicating no signs of dysplasia in both cases) resulting in a score out of 53 for each hip, or 106 in total, which is considered to describe the general condition of the dog's hip joints. The nine features are scored on the detectable laxity of the joint, bone formation and the degree of any exostosis (abnormal bone growth) and wearing. A more detailed description of the scoring criteria is given by Gibbs [12].

Dog and pedigree data

Data on left, right and total hip score were obtained from the Kennel Club and restricted to Labrador Retrievers scored between 2000 and 2007 inclusive, since this restriction helped to minimise any diagnostic drift. Other data obtained for the same dogs were their sex, date of birth and date of radiograph. Data were also restricted to those records where sex was explicitly stated as male or female; coat colour was stated to be one of the 'permitted' colours (i.e. black, chocolate and yellow only); and the hip score was within the defined boundaries of 0 to 106. In the 'full' dataset the age at scoring was limited to within the boundaries of ≥ 1 and <4 years old (365 to 1459 days old inclusive) since over 90% of information available came from this relatively narrow age range and there would be an expectation of changing parameters over a wider period given the progressive nature of hip dysplasia. The resultant data set contained 25,243 single records of hip score from radiographs taken between 2000 and 2007 of dogs born between 1996 and 2006. The data were unevenly divided between the sexes with many more females than males scored, 75% to 25%. The fractions of each colour were close to those in the KC pedigree (black, 55 in study v 52% in KC; chocolate, 20 v 13%; yellow, 26 v 29%) indicating no obvious selective bias or stratification on the basis of coat colour. Records were distributed roughly equally over year of evaluation (max 2006 = 14.8%, min 2007 = 9.8%). The data records were linked to the KC Labrador pedigree database using their unique registration number. All ancestors of the dogs with hip score data were traced back to the founding generation, i.e. where the sire and dam are unrecorded, or to a maximum of four generations (great, great-grandsires/dams). As a result, the pedigree used in the initial analysis comprised 62,683 animals in total with 99.9% of grandparent identities of dogs with scores known. The coefficients of inbreeding were calculated using this restricted pedigree. Mean and standard deviation of inbreeding coefficients for dogs with data were 0.041 and 0.039 respectively.

Statistical Analysis

Mixed linear models were fitted to the data using ASREML [26] to estimate variance components for the hip score (H). Examination of the appropriate scale for analysis was undertaken given the skewed distribution of H (Figure 1). Preliminary analyses considered the family of power transformations [27] on 1+H, where the 1 was added to avoid the logarithm of zero – here without loss of generality, natural logarithms were used at all times. Transformations were assessed using the family of power transformations [28] (results not shown) with preference given to more readily interpretable scales of untransformed, square root, logarithmic, 1/square root and reciprocal. The optimum transformation was found to be $\log_e(1+H)$ and this form was used as the basis of all further analyses, however the final model was also fitted on the untransformed scale for purposes of comparison.

After resolving the scale for analysis, further preliminary models tested the hypothesis of genetic equivalence of left and right hip scores and the total hip scores of 1, 2 and 3 year olds. Subsequently, the significance of 'litter' and 'dam' random effects were determined using likelihood ratio tests. The full form of the linear model was as follows:

$$\mathbf{Y} = \mathbf{Xb} + \mathbf{Za} + \mathbf{Vd} + \mathbf{Wc} + \mathbf{e}$$

where **Y** is the vector of observations, **V, W, X** and **Z** are known incidence matrices, **b** is the vector of fixed effects, **a** is the vector of random additive genetic effects with the distribution assumed to be multivariate normal (MVN), with parameters $(0, \sigma^2_a\mathbf{A})$, **d** is the vector of random dam effects distributed MVN with parameters $(0, \sigma^2_d\mathbf{I_{dam}})$, **c** is the vector of random litter effects with the distribution assumed to be MVN, with parameters $(0, \sigma^2_c\mathbf{I_{litter}})$, **e** is the vector of residuals distributed MVN with parameters $(0, \sigma^2_e\mathbf{I})$. **I** represents an identity matrix of an appropriate size, **A** is the additive genetic relationship matrix, and σ^2 denotes the variance of each of the respective random effects. The fixed effects included in the model were: sex, inbreeding coefficient, age in days at evaluation, birth date measured as days since 1st Jan 1990, and year of evaluation. Age in days and absolute day of birth were fitted with random smoothing splines to model the temporal trends. Note that date of evaluation in days is the sum of birth date and age and cannot be fitted as an independent term.

Accuracies of EBV of parents and of individuals at birth and after scoring

Accuracies (r) of EBV were calculated as:

$$r = (1 - PEV/\sigma_a^2)^{0.5}$$

where PEV is the prediction error variance of each breeding value and σ^2_a is the estimated additive genetic variance obtained from the mixed model analysis. ASReml provides both the estimates of EBV and their associated PEV. Repeat analysis of the 'reduced' dataset using the final model described provided 'nascent' EBV with associated PEV for the 779 dogs born in 2006 for analysis of accuracies.

Assessment of potential progress using simulation of selection on EBVs and phenotypes

Simulation of selection for a single generation using both EBV and phenotypic hip score (H) was undertaken and the responses compared. The simulation produced 1000 matings between sires and dams sampled from the cohort born in 2005. Sires and dams were randomly selected with replacement from the lower x% of the distribution of either 1) phenotypic total hip score (H), or 2) EBV produced from the reduced dataset. The value of x varied from 90 to 10 in steps of 10. Each of these 18 combinations was replicated 1000 times. For each combination the difference in the overall mean of simulated nascent EBV of the offspring (½ EBV_{sire}+½ EBV_{dam}) and the mean EBV of all animals born in 2005 provided an estimate of response to selection after a single generation of selection.

Supporting Information

Material S1 Additional analysis indicating superiority of mean over worst hip score.

Table S1 The correlation of nascent EBVs with observed phenotypes for log-transformed AVRG and WORST, calculated for the 779 dogs born in 2006.

Acknowledgments

The authors are grateful to the BVA hip scoring panellists for data provided by their ongoing work.

Author Contributions

Conceived and designed the experiments: TWL SCB JAW. Performed the experiments: TWL. Analyzed the data: TWL JAW. Wrote the paper: TWL JAW.

References

1. Flint AP, Woolliams JA (2008) Precision animal breeding. Philos Trans R Soc Lond B Biol Sci 363: 573–590.
2. Higgins A, Nicholas FW (2008) The breeding of pedigree dogs: time for strong leadership. Vet J 178: 157–158.
3. Bateson P (2010) Independent inquiry into dog breeding. University of Cambridge. 65 p.
4. Lohi H, Nicholas FW (2009) Unlocking the genetic make-up of canine hip dysplasia: we can work it out. Vet J 181: 77–78.
5. Lust G (1997) An overview of the pathogenesis of canine hip dysplasia. J Am Vet Med Assoc 210: 1443–1445.
6. Ohlerth S, Busato A, Gaillard C, Fluckiger M, Lang J (1998) [Epidemiologic and genetic studies of canine hip dysplasia in a population of Labrador retrievers: a study over 25 years]. Dtsch Tierarztl Wochenschr 105: 378–383.
7. Wood JL, Lakhani KH, Rogers K (2002) Heritability and epidemiology of canine hip-dysplasia score and its components in Labrador retrievers in the United Kingdom. Prev Vet Med 55: 95–108.

8. Silvestre AM, Ginja MM, Ferreira AJ, Colaco J (2007) Comparison of estimates of hip dysplasia genetic parameters in Estrela Mountain Dog using linear and threshold models. J Anim Sci 85: 1880–1884.
9. Todhunter RJ, Mateescu R, Lust G, Burton-Wurster NI, Dykes NL, et al. (2005) Quantitative trait loci for hip dysplasia in a cross-breed canine pedigree. Mamm Genome 16: 720–730.
10. Brass W (1989) Hip dysplasia in dogs. Journal of small animal practice 30: 166–170.
11. Maki K (2004) Breeding against hip and elbow dysplasia in dogs [PhD Thesis]: University of Helsinki. 27 p.
12. Gibbs C (1997) The BVA/KC scoring scheme for control of hip dysplasia: interpretation of criteria. Vet Rec 141: 275–284.
13. Fluckiger M (2007) Scoring radiographs for canine hip dysplasia - The big three organisations in the world. European Journal of Companion Animal Practice 17: 135–140.
14. Willis MB (1997) A review of the progress in canine hip dysplasia control in Britain. J Am Vet Med Assoc 210: 1480–1482.
15. Leppanen M, Saloniemi H (1999) Controlling canine hip dysplasia in Finland. Prev Vet Med 42: 121–131.
16. Malm S, Fikse WF, Danell B, Strandberg E (2008) Genetic variation and genetic trends in hip and elbow dysplasia in Swedish Rottweiler and Bernese Mountain Dog. J Anim Breed Genet 125: 403–412.
17. Hou Y, Wang Y, Lust G, Zhu L, Zhang Z, et al. Retrospective analysis for genetic improvement of hip joints of cohort labrador retrievers in the United States: 1970–2007. PLoS One 5: e9410.
18. Falconer DS, Mackay TFC (1996) Introduction to Quantitative Genetics: Longman. 245 p.
19. Harris DL, Newman S (1994) Breeding for profit: synergism between genetic improvement and livestock production (a review). J Anim Sci 72: 2178–2200.
20. Leppanen M, Maki K, Juga J, Saloniemi H (2000) Estimation of heritability for hip dysplasia in German Shepherd Dogs in Finland. J Anim Breed Genet. pp 97–103.
21. Lewis T, Swift S, Woolliams JA, Blott S (2010) Heritability of premature mitral valve disease in Cavalier King Charles spaniels. Vet J: doi:10.1016/j.tvjl.2010.1002.1016.
22. Steinetz BG, Williams AJ, Lust G, Schwabe C, Bullesbach EE, et al. (2008) Transmission of relaxin and estrogens to suckling canine pups via milk and possible association with hip joint laxity. Am J Vet Res 69: 59–67.
23. Wood JL, Lakhani KH (2003) Effect of month of birth on hip dysplasia in Labrador Retrievers and Gordon setters. Vet Rec 152: 69–72.
24. Lindblad-Toh K, Wade CM, Mikkelsen TS, Karlsson EK, Jaffe DB, et al. (2005) Genome sequence, comparative analysis and haplotype structure of the domestic dog. Nature 438: 803–819.
25. Solberg TR, Sonesson AK, Woolliams JA, Meuwissen TH (2008) Genomic selection using different marker types and densities. J Anim Sci 86: 2447–2454.
26. Gilmour AR, Gogel BJ, Cullis BR, Thompson R, eds. (2006) ASReml user guide release 2.0: VSN International Ltd, Hemel Hempstead, HP1 1ES, UK. 372 p.
27. Box GEP, Cox DR (1964) An analysis of transformations. Journal of the Royal Statistical Society B 26: 211–252.
28. Darwash AO, Lamming GE, Woolliams JA (1997) Estimation of genetic variation in the interval from calving to postpartum ovulation of dairy cows. J Dairy Sci 80: 1227–1234.

5

Population-Based Rates of Revision of Primary Total Hip Arthroplasty

Kelly L. Corbett[1], Elena Losina[1,2,4], Akosua A. Nti[1], Julian J. Z. Prokopetz[1], Jeffrey N. Katz[1,2,3]*

1 Department of Orthopedic Surgery, Orthopedic and Arthritis Center for Outcomes Research, Brigham and Women's Hospital, Boston, Massachusetts, United States of America, 2 Division of Rheumatology, Immunology and Allergy, Brigham and Women's Hospital, Harvard Medical School, Boston, Massachusetts, United States of America, 3 Department of Epidemiology, Harvard School of Public Health, Boston, Massachusetts, United States of America, 4 Department of Biostatistics, Boston University School of Public Health, Boston, Massachusetts, United States of America

Abstract

Background: Most research on failure leading to revision total hip arthroplasty (THA) is reported from single centers. We searched PubMed between January 2000 and August 2010 to identify population- or community-based studies evaluating ten-year revision risks. We report ten-year revision risk using the Kaplan-Meier method, stratifying by age and fixation technique.

Results: Thirteen papers met the inclusion criteria. Cemented prostheses had Kaplan-Meier estimates of revision-free implant survival of ten years ranging from 88% to 95%; uncemented prostheses had Kaplan-Meier estimates from 80% to 85%. Estimates ranged from 72% to 86% in patients less than 60 years old and from 90 to 96% in older patients.

Conclusion: Data reported from national registries suggest revision risks of 5 to 20% ten years following primary THA. Revision risks are lower in older THA recipients. Uncemented implants may have higher ten-year rates of revision, regardless of age.

Editor: Francois Patrick Rannou, Hôpital Cochin, France

Funding: This study was funded by the National Institutes of Health (NIH). The funder had no role in study design, data collection and analysis, decision to publish, or preparation of the manuscript.

Competing Interests: The authors have declared that no competing interests exist.

* E-mail: jnkatz@partners.org

Introduction

Total hip arthroplasty (THA) is an efficacious and cost-effective intervention for reducing pain and improving function in patients with advanced hip arthritis [1,2,3,4]. Long-term studies of THA recipients have generally shown that the probability of surviving without undergoing a revision THA exceeds 90% at ten years and 80% at 25 years [1,5,6,7,8,9]. However, most of these reports have been from single referral centers or single surgeons, and most refer to only one type of implant [1,7,9,10,11]. Large national studies, especially population-based studies, provide a better framework for estimating implant survival rates that can more readily be generalized to the majority of patients receiving THA.

While randomized controlled trials are still considered the gold standard for evaluating medical outcomes, trials are both cost-prohibitive and impractical for evaluating the risk of long-term THA revision [2]. National or regional joint replacement registries have the potential to fill this gap in our understanding of long-term THA outcomes. Primary goals of registries include providing data on utilization patterns of total joint replacement and identifying risk factors for poor outcomes and poorly performing devices [2]. The national hip arthroplasty registries from Finland (origination date: 1980), Norway (1987), and Sweden (1979) have been crucial in defining the risks of subsequent revision surgery. By providing feedback to the healthcare community and identifying specific implants with poor results, the registries have also helped to improve the outcomes of THA [12]. Over the past few years, several additional countries have begun national joint registries: Denmark (1994), New Zealand (1997), Hungary (1998), Australia (1998), and Canada (2001).

The national THA registries have produced substantial research on the outcomes and failures of hip arthroplasty from individual countries. However, to our knowledge, the literature on the long-term revision rates following THA in national samples has not been reviewed systematically. Revision data, particularly from national samples, are needed to guide discussions of implant longevity and the risk of revision for elective THA. Health policymakers also need access to such data to anticipate revision volume and associated costs. The goal of this review is to summarize published data on primary THA revision rates over ten years in large national community-based or population-based studies. Additionally, we examine the influence of patient age and prosthesis fixation technique on THA revision rates.

Methods

Note: The protocol for this trial and supporting CONSORT checklist are available as supporting information; see PRISMA Checklist S1 and PRISMA Flow Diagram S1.

Search Strategy

We conducted a PubMed search to identify studies written in English that were published between January 2000 and August

2010. We did not include articles published prior to 2000 in order to reduce heterogeneity in biomaterials and process of care. We restricted the review to articles published in the peer-reviewed literature to ensure a high level of rigor and quality. We used PubMed hip arthroplasty MeSH Term keywords in combination with search terms relating to revision rates and prosthesis survival and failure. Our verbatim search query, performed August 10, 2010, was:

("Arthroplasty, Replacement, Hip/methods"[MAJR] OR "Arthroplasty, Replacement, Hip/statistics and numerical data"[MAJR]) AND ("revision rates" OR "revision rate" OR "rates of revision" OR "rate of revision" OR "prosthesis failure" OR "prosthesis survival")

We screened the title and abstract of each article identified for relevance to this literature review. To be included for further review, the studies had to discuss primary hip prosthesis failure leading to revision, provide long-term follow-up, and represent either population- or community-based samples. Single surgeon series, single hospital series, and collaborations between referral centers were excluded based on review of abstracts. Studies reporting only on specific failure mechanisms (e.g. dislocation or infection) were excluded, as were studies focused exclusively on either stem or cup failure (as opposed to failure of *any* component). For abstracts that passed this screening, the full length articles were retrieved and reviewed.

To ensure comparability of articles, minimize bias due to truncated follow-up, and incorporate the methods used in the majority of papers reporting prosthesis survival, we chose ten-year revision-free survival estimated by the Kaplan-Meier method as the primary outcome for our review. A key advantage of the Kaplan-Meier method is that it accounts for all persons who were lost to follow-up or died. We excluded studies that did not report the Kaplan-Meier ten-year survivorship of the prostheses (with survivorship defined as the patient surviving without undergoing revision of the THA).

Data Extraction and Analysis

We abstracted the following information from each eligible article: the number of patients who had had a primary THA, the calendar years during which the primary THAs were performed, the years during which the cohort was followed, the proportion of patients with osteoarthritis (OA), the definition of revision, the type of fixation method (cemented, uncemented, hybrid or not specified), the number of patients at risk at ten years, and the Kaplan-Meier based probability of revision-free survival at ten years. Additionally, we abstracted the age of the patients and whether the papers reported analyses for certain age brackets. The reports differed in their classification of "younger" patients. "Younger" denotes age less than 60 in one (Norwegian) registry and less than 55 in two (Finnish and Swedish) registries. Two authors abstracted each of the articles included in the review to ensure reliability. Any discrepancies were resolved through discussion with the senior author.

The principal outcome variable for this analysis was the Kaplan-Meier probability of revision-free implant survival at ten years. Some studies provided this parameter and others provided Kaplan-Meier plots from which we estimated the revision-free survival at ten years graphically. Two Swedish studies provided nine-year Kaplan-Meier estimates [12,13] and one Norwegian study provided eight-year estimates [14]. We transformed these to Kaplan-Meier ten-year estimates by assuming a constant annual risk of revision.

In general, studies reported on revision for any reason. Some of the Swedish [12,13] and Finnish [15] data report revision for aseptic loosening only. We note these instances in the text, tables and figures.

We used evidence tables and graphical techniques to describe the THA revision risks across national and regional registries and to examine revision risks in relevant subgroups defined by age and fixation technique (cemented vs. uncemented vs. hybrid). In circumstances where Kaplan-Meier ten-year revision-free survival values were given for subgroups defined by fixation status and age category, we derived summary estimates for fixation groups and for age groups by calculating weighted averages of Kaplan-Meier estimates across the relevant subgroups, with weights proportional to the number of patients in each subgroup.

The funding sources for this study had no role in design, analysis or reporting of results.

Results

Results of Search

The results of the search for papers on revision of primary THA in national samples are shown in Figure 1. Thirty-seven abstracts were identified. Of these, eighteen were excluded from further consideration because they failed to address hip prosthesis survival (1 abstract), did not rely on population- or community-based samples (8), focused on specific causes of revision (1) or because they provided incidence rates of the primary THA rather than revision rates (8). Nineteen abstracts were eligible for further analysis; these papers were retrieved and reviewed. Of these, six were excluded because the samples were not population- or community-based. Thirteen papers were used as a basis for the current review: six from the Finnish Arthroplasty Register [8,15,16,17,18,19], three from the Swedish Total Hip Replacement Register [12,13,20], three from the Norwegian Arthroplasty Register [14,21,22], and one from the Trent Regional Arthroplasty Study (TRAS) in England [23] (see Table 1). The Swedish, Norwegian, Finnish, and Trent Registers are described in Appendix S1 (see supporting information).

Revision Risk

Fixation. Our findings suggest that cemented implants have greater longevity when compared broadly to uncemented implants (Figure 2). Cemented prostheses had ten-year Kaplan-Meier estimates of revision-free survival ranging between 88% (95% CI not provided) in Finland to 95% (95% CI: 94.1, 96.3) in Norway. Uncemented prostheses had higher revision risks across the registers, with Kaplan-Meier ten-year revision-free survival estimates ranging from 80% in Finland (95% CI not provided) to 85% (95% CI: 84, 87) in Sweden. Hybrid prosthesis revision risks were only reported in the Swedish Register, precluding comparison of hybrid prosthesis survival data across countries. In Sweden, hybrid prosthesis survival with revision for aseptic loosening only as the endpoint had a 10-year survival of 92.7% (95% CI: 90.1, 95.4). Osteoarthritis was the only diagnosis included in these estimates of revision risk by fixation, with the exception of the English sample, which was 87% OA, and the uncemented Norwegian sample which ranged from 31 to 71% OA.

Age. The Kaplan-Meier ten-year revision-free survival estimates for younger patients ranged from 72% (95% CI: 67, 76) in Finland to 86% (95% CI: 84.5, 88.2) in Sweden (Figure 3). Revision risk was lower in older patients, with Kaplan-Meier ten-year revision-free survival estimates ranging from 90% (95% CI: 89, 91) in Finland to 97% (95% CI: 96.3, 97) in Sweden. The

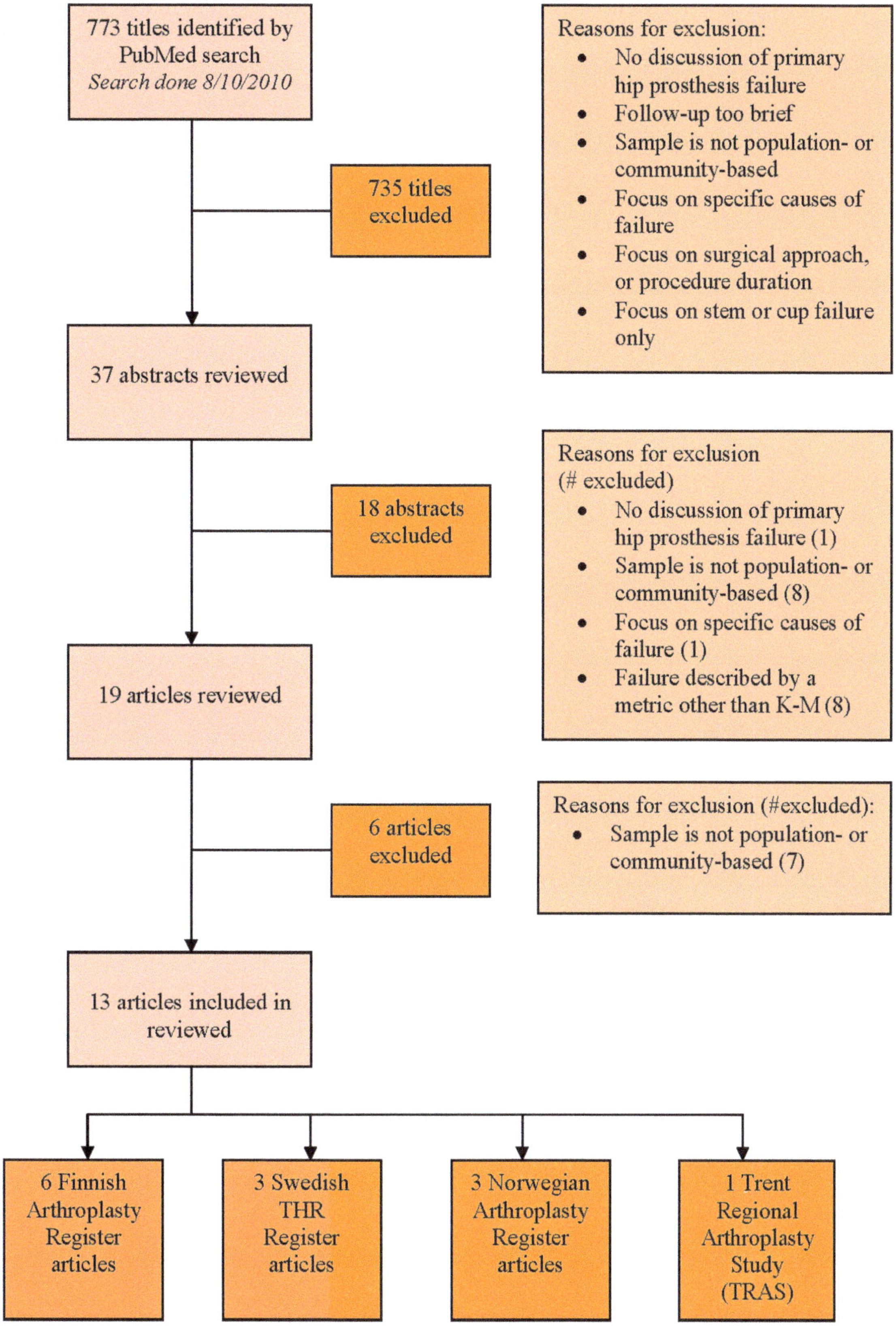

Figure 1. Manuscript search and selection process.

Table 1. Overview of papers included in the review.

Paper source (Citation #)	N	Years of operation	Years of follow-up	AR/N	Definition of survival endpoint	Definition of Revision	Country
Allami et al (2006) *Outcome of Charnley total hip replacement (23)*	1,198 (C)	1990	1990–2002	N/A	Revision for any reason	Removal of original components	England
Eskelinen et al (2006) *Uncemented Total Hip Arthroplasty (16)*	1410 (U)	1980–2003	1980–2005*	482/1410(.34)	Revision for any reason	Removal or exchange of any component	Finland
Maleka et al (2008) *Cemented total hip replacement for primary osteoarthritis (8)*	26347(C)	1980–2005	1980–2005*	10645/26347(.40)	Revision for any reason	Removal or exchange of the femoral head, liner or the whole implant	Finland
Makela et al (2008) *THA for primary osteoarthritis in patients fifty-five years or older (17)*	34296 (C) 12888 (U) 3784 (H)	1980–2004 1985–2004 1988–2004	1980–2005 1985–2004 1988–2004	10343/34296 (.30) 2750/12888 (.21) 344/3784 (.09)	Revision for any reason	Exchange or removal of the cup and/or stem or exchange of the liner	Finland
Makela (2010) *Cementless THA for primary osteoarthritis in patients aged 55 years and older (15)*	9,549 (C) 10,310 (U)	1980–2005	1980–2005	4447/9549 (.47) 2610/10310 (.25)	Revision due to aseptic loosening only	Surgical removal or exchange of the whole or part of the implant	Finland
Ogino et al (2008) *Total Hip Replacement in Patients eighty years of age and older (18)*	5047 (C) 399 (U) 729 (H)	1980–2004	1980–2004	N/A	Revision for any reason	Removal, exchange, or reimplantation of one, or both, of the prosthetic component	Finland
Puolakka et al (2001) *The Finnish Arthroplasty Register (19)*	4,609 (C) 5,519 (U)	1990–1994	1990–2000	N/A	Revision for any reason	Exchange or removal of part of a component, or the whole implant	Finland
Espehaug (2009) *18 years of results with cemented primary hip prostheses in the Norwegian ArthroplastyRegister (14)*	24728 (C) 37577 (C)	1987–1997 1998–2007	1987–2007 1998–2007	14622/24728 (.59) 4298/37577 (0.11)	Revision for any reason	Surgical removal or exchange of the whole or part of the implant	Norway
Furnes et al (2001), *Hip disease and the prognosis of total hip replacements (21)*	37215 (US) 11225 (C)	1987–1999	1987–1999	2384/37215 (.06) 703/11225 (.06)	Revision for any reason	Removal or exchange of a part of, or the whole implant	Norway
Hallan et al (2007) *Medium- and long-term performance of 11,516 uncemented primary femoral stems from the Norwegian arthroplasty register (22)*	8,444 (U)	1987–2005	1987–2006	N/A	Revision for any reason	Revision of any component (acetabular shell, liner or stem)	Norway
Hailer (2010) *Uncemented and cemented primary THA in the Swedish Hip Arthroplasty Register (20)*	161,413 (C) 8,953 (U)	1992–2007	1992–2007	N/A	Revision for any reason	Exchange or removal of any part of the cup or stem, or the entire implant	Sweden
Herberts and Malchau (2000), *Long-term registration has improved the quality of hip replacement (13)*	65,689 (C) 2645 (U)	1988–1997	1988–1997	N/A	Revision due to aseptic loosening only	Exchange or removal of one or both components of the prosthesis; Exchange of a liner or head component	Sweden
Malchau et al (2000), *The Swedish THR Register (12)*	2588 (CY) 56820(CO) 1004 (UY) 1083 (HY)	1992–2000 1992–2000 1992–2000 1992–2000	1992–2001* 1992–2001* 1992–2001* 1992–2001*	N/A	Revision due to aseptic loosening only	Exchange or removal of one or both components, or the implant	Sweden

C= cemented; CO= cemented old; CY=cemented young; U= uncemented; UY= uncemented young; H= hybrid; HY= hybrid young; US= unspecified;
AR/N= No. at risk at 10 yr/No. of primary operations;
*Estimate because years of follow-up were not given.

endpoint for these estimates was revision for any reason. These estimates were inclusive of all fixation methods (e.g. cemented, uncemented) and types of prostheses. The Norwegian reports excluded all diagnoses other than OA, while the Swedish sample was 75% OA and the Finnish sample was 78% OA.

Fixation and Age. To address the possibility that the main effects for fixation are confounded by age, we examined estimates of prosthesis revision risk in subgroups defined by fixation and age. These analyses are shown in Table 2. In younger and in older patients, cemented implants had lower revision risks than uncemented implants. Among both cemented and uncemented implants, revision risk was lower in older than in younger patients. The endpoint for these estimates was revision for any reason, except in the Swedish data, which report revision due to aseptic loosening only.

Discussion

Long-term clinical results of THA have been well-documented in the literature. However, the vast majority of studies report findings from individual referral centers. The comprehensive Scandinavian Registers have reported on prosthesis revision rates

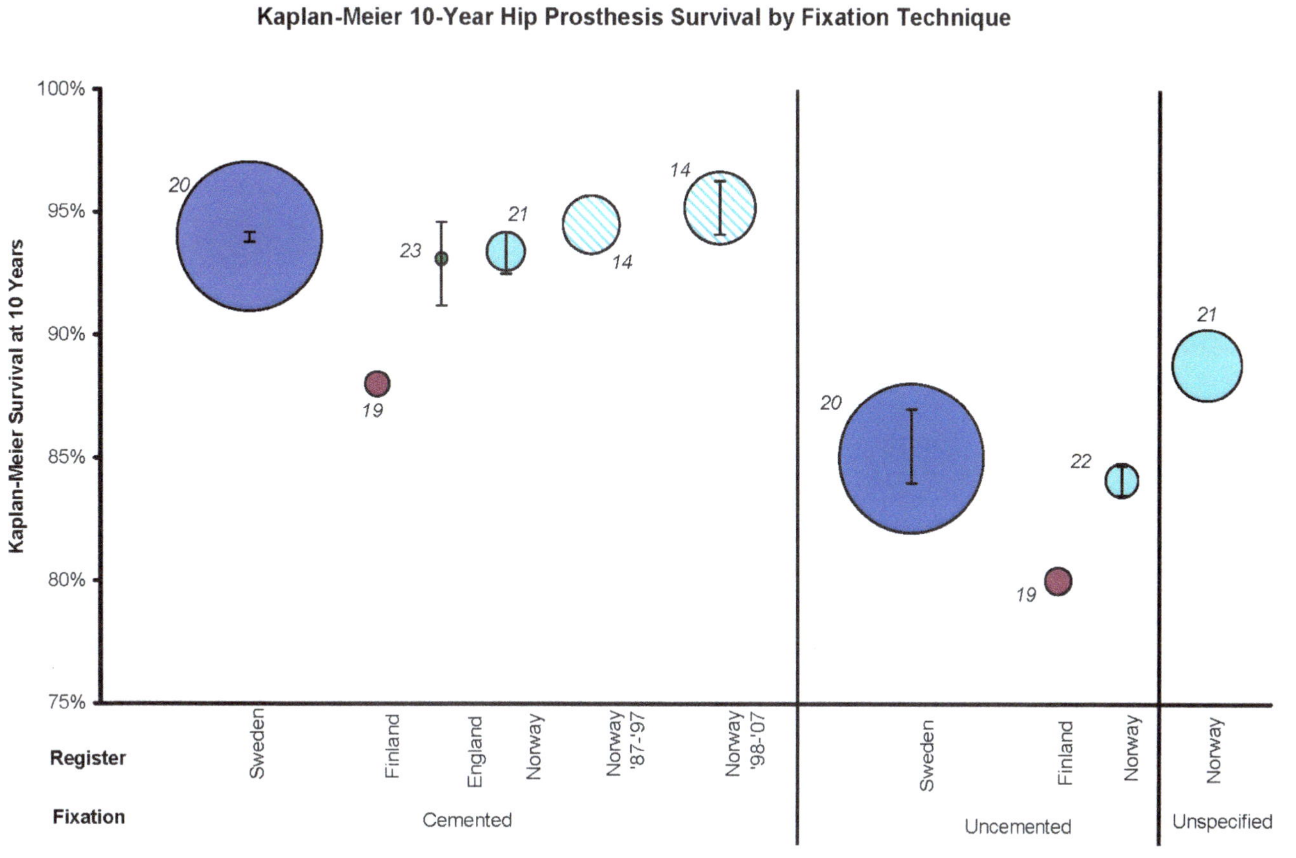

Figure 2. Kaplan-Meier ten-year hip prosthesis survival by fixation technique. Kaplan-Meier ten-year estimates are presented, stratified by national register and fixation technique. Circle area is proportional to the sample size. Error bars represent 95% CIs. All estimates use revision for any reason as the endpoint. Cemented Norway and cemented England are single prosthesis studies, including only Charnley implants. The K-M 10 for uncemented THA in Norway is the weighted average of nine [21,22] or ten [14] types of implant. All others are inclusive of all prosthesis brands. The Finnish K-M 10 data were estimated from K-M curves. Estimates are inclusive of all patient ages. 31% to 71% of the uncemented Norwegian sample, 87% of the English sample, and 100% of the remaining registers' samples were operated on for osteoarthritis. Each study reference is denoted next to the circle, representing the corresponding manuscript from which the Kaplan-Meier estimates were derived.

across entire countries, providing our best estimates of implant revision risk in large, national populations. However, to our knowledge, there has not been a systematic literature review of published articles describing THA survival rates from these large national or regional registries. We have summarized and compared findings from national and regional studies to describe the ten-year prosthesis survival following primary THA. We excluded papers with follow-up shorter than ten years, which prevented us from including data from the US Medicare population and the Danish Register. We did include three papers from Norway and Sweden with reported Kaplan-Meier rates of eight and nine years, respectively, from which we were able to extrapolate ten-year survival data, as described in the Methods section.

The findings suggest that both implant fixation and patient age influence prosthesis revision rates in large population- or community-based samples. Older patients with hip implants had revision-free implant survival rates that exceeded 90% at ten years, while the rates for younger patients ranged from 72 to 86%. Cemented implants had lower revision risk than uncemented implants in both younger and older patients. It is possible, however, that this finding is due to residual confounding by age and activity level, with uncemented implants used in younger, more active individuals.

Referral centers have documented greater than 90% revision-free implant survival at ten years, and greater than 80% revision-free implant survival at 25 years following primary THA [1,5,7,9]. Because of the heterogeneity in patient and hospital factors across large national and regional samples, it is not surprising to find somewhat higher revision rates in national registries than at referral centers. The data provided in the registry studies do not permit adjustment of revision rates for hospital or surgeon characteristics, such as procedure volume.

Methodological Challenges

Readers should be cautioned when interpreting implant revision data. By ten years postoperatively, the number of patients still at risk for revision THA may be quite small. Thus, revision-free survival estimates may be based on a minority of the entire sample. For example, Furnes et al reported that of 37,215 hips replaced in Norway for OA, inclusive of all ages and prostheses, the Kaplan-Meier ten-year revision-free implant survival estimate was 88.8% with revision for any reason as the endpoint. However, only 2,384 hips were still at risk at ten years, which means the K-M 10 estimate is based upon data from just 6% of the original sample. Patients become censored when they are revised, lost to follow-up or die, and they are seldom followed long enough to contribute ten-year survival data. In this example, the mean follow-up time

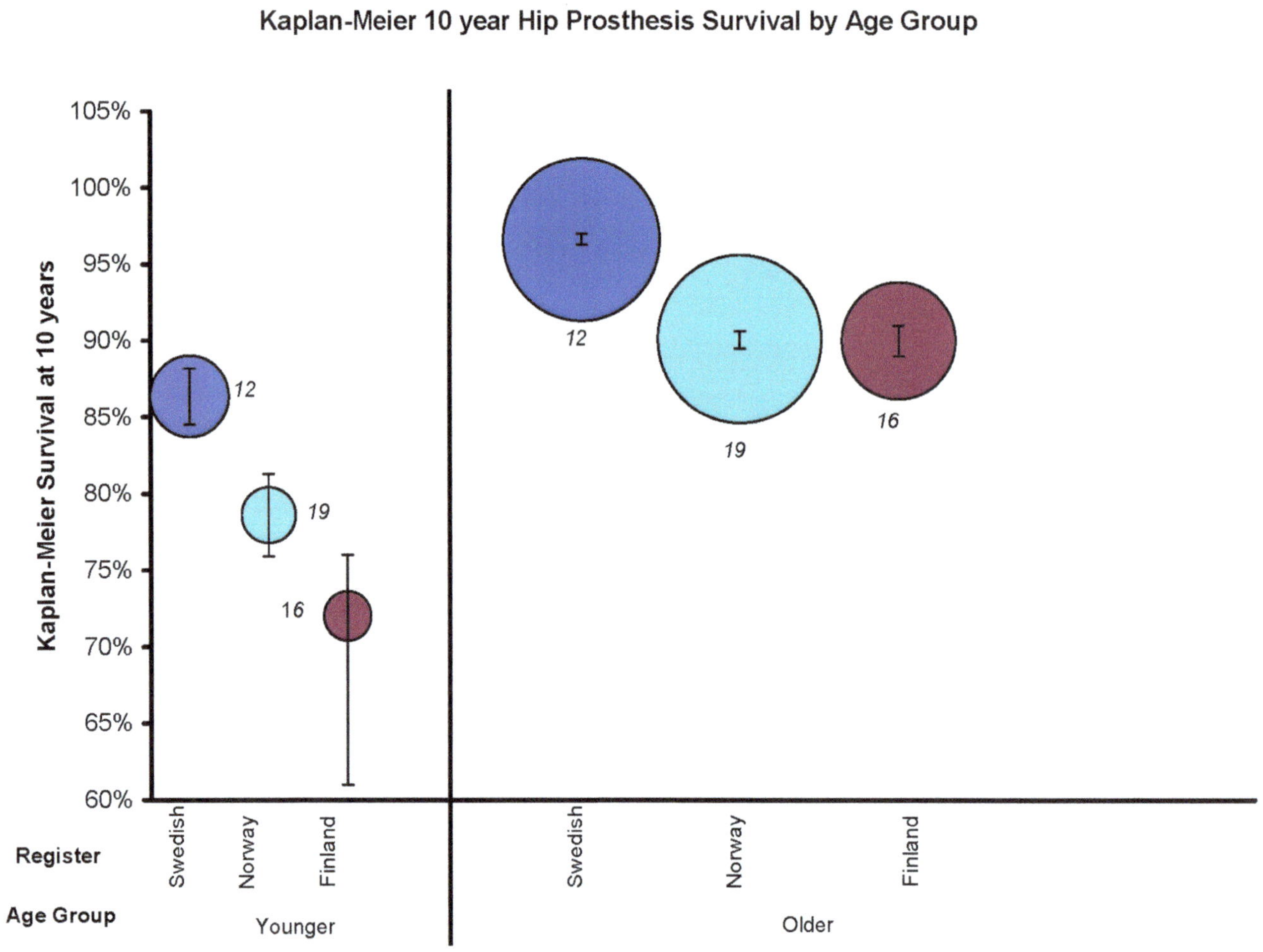

Figure 3. Kaplan-Meier ten-year hip prosthesis survival by age group. Kaplan-Meier ten-year estimates are stratified by register and age group. Circle area is proportional to the sample size. Error bars represent 95% CIs. Estimates are inclusive of all prosthesis types. The endpoint was revision for any reason, except for the Swedish studies, where it was revision due to aseptic loosening only. 75% of the Swedish sample, 78% of the Finnish sample, and 100% of the Norwegian sample were operated on for osteoarthritis. Each study reference is denoted next to the circle, representing the corresponding manuscript from which the Kaplan-Meier estimates were derived.

for the entire cohort was only 4.5 years. Thus, for the latter years of the K-M 10 estimates, only a fraction of the entire cohort was eligible to be analyzed [21]. Only six of the thirteen papers analyzed in this review provided information on the number of patients eligible for Kaplan-Meier analysis at ten years [8,14,15,16,17,21]. The proportion of original cohort members eligible for analysis at ten years in these four studies ranged from 6% to 59% (see Table 1).

Implicit in any discussion of revision rates is the definition of failure. The papers we analyzed all used revision as the endpoint. The majority of the papers provided data on revision for any reason, as well as on revision due specifically to aseptic loosening. We focused on revision for any reason, relying on this broader criterion because both patients and policy-makers consider any revision to be important, irrespective of the specific reason for prosthesis failure. However, two reports from the Swedish Register [12,13] and one report from the Finnish Register [15] only documented revision due to aseptic loosening (see Table 1), and we have indicated in any figure or table legends whether these more narrowly defined revision data have been used. Unless otherwise noted, all reported data compare survival rates in which the endpoint was revision for any reason.

Revision surgery is an unambiguous endpoint for a failed total hip replacement. However, revision rates do not capture implants that have failed clinically but have not been treated surgically. For example, this criterion would miss patients with painful, loose prostheses who do not seek medical attention, choose not to have revision, or are not offered revision because their general health is too unstable. Revision is a blunt measure that gives no information on clinical or radiographic outcome or patient satisfaction. Validation studies on the Swedish Register have indicated that clinical failure rates at ten years, as defined by radiographic loosening in combination with the Harris Hip Score and the Western Ontario and McMaster Osteoarthritis Index (WOMAC), are at least twice as high as the revision rates reported by the Register [4,13,24].

As implants and fixation techniques evolve over time, it is important to consider how changes might influence overall rates of revision. In Sweden, for example, modern cementing techniques were introduced in the late 1980s and fully established by the early 1990s. These changes improved the cementing process, and are acknowledged as among the reasons for a ten-year revision-free hip prosthesis survival rate of up to 94% [13]. Modern cementing techniques have only been documented in the Finnish Register

Table 2. Kaplan-Meier ten-year revision-free survival estimates by Fixation, Age and Register.

Fixation type	Age group	Register	N	% K-M 10	95% CI	Years of operation	Years of follow-up	Age of cohort	% OA
Cemented	Young	Sweden	2,588	88.8	(83.7, 92.7)	1992–2000	1992–2001*	<55	75
	Old	Sweden	56,820	96.2	(95.8, 96.7)	1992–2000	1992–2001*	≥55	75
		Finland	34,296	89.0	(89, 89)	1980–2004	1980–2005	≥55	100
		Weighted average	93,704	**93.5**					
Uncemented	Young	Sweden	1,004	94.7	(92.5, 96.9)	1992–2000	1992–2001*	<55	75
		Finland**	1,410	77		1980–2003	1980–2005*	<55	100
		Weighted average	2,414	**84.4**					
	Old	Finland^	7,145	86.0	(85, 88)	1986–2004	1986–2004	≥55	100
		Finland^	5,743	87.0	(86, 88)	1985–2004	1985–2004	≥55	100
		Weighted average	12,888	**86.4**					
Hybrid	Young	Sweden	1,083	92.2	(87.5, 97.1)	1992–2000	1992–2001*	<55	75
	Old	Finland	3,784	88.0	(86, 90)	1988–2004	1988–2004	≥55	100

*Estimate because years of follow-up were not given;
**Comprised from weighted averages of multiple implants;
^Note, these two studies from Finland involve different prostheses; the patient samples are independent;
Outcome here is revision due only to aseptic loosening for the Swedish Registry and revision for all indications for the other registries.

since 1996 [8]. We included papers published in 2000 or beyond to reduce the influence of such secular changes.

We limited the review to published studies in order to maintain a consistently high standard of methodological rigor. We acknowledge, however, that several registries in countries outside Scandinavia and England offer valuable unpublished data. For example, although the findings we report from Scandinavian countries document better prosthesis survival in cemented than in uncemented designs, data from the Australian Registry suggest that cemented and uncemented prostheses have similar survival [25]. The Australian Registry was established in 1998 and its website provides revision data on cases operated upon from 1999 to 2008. We did not include the Australian data in our formal analyses because they have not been published in a peer-reviewed journal. The discrepancy between Scandinavian and Australian registries in the performance of cemented vs. uncemented prostheses could reflect differences in control for potential confounders but may also reflect differences across countries in technique, materials, or indications.

The Australian data also show higher survival rates overall than many of the studies we included. Extrapolating from the Australian Registry's eight-year prosthesis survival rate of 95.1% by assuming a constant revision rate yields a ten-year survival rate of 94.1%, which is considerably higher than many of the survival rates reported in the Scandinavian Registries (Table 2). The Australian data reflect a more recent THA prosthesis survival experience, incorporating primary and revision hip replacements performed between 1998 and 2008. Similarly, the New Zealand National Joint Register reports a ten-year survival rate of 93.5% based on procedures performed between 1999 and 2008 [26]. Thus, the improved survival in the Australian and New Zealand data as compared with the Scandinavian experience may point to important secular changes. These observations from the antipodean registries suggest that published registry data may themselves have important limitations that should be appreciated before making broad inferences. The discrepancies between these data sources also urge caution in generalizing the Scandinavian experience.

Limitations

We acknowledge that these national estimates cannot adjust for differences between implant groups in factors such as activity level and weight, which may affect revision risk. It should also be noted that arthroplasty registers may report OA as the underlying diagnosis in some patients who in fact have mild developmental dysplasia [6,27]. Patients with dysplasia may have worse outcomes following THA than patients with OA, and this difference might skew the reported survival estimates [6,21]. Additionally, we recognize the inherent imprecision in estimating K-M 10 revision-free survival from curves when the actual data were not presented in tables [18,19]. The potential subjectivity of this approach is mitigated in part by having two independent abstractors, with any discrepancies resolved by the senior author.

Conclusion

These methodological challenges and limitations notwithstanding, we summarized ten-year prosthesis revision rates from international registry-based studies, a task that, to our knowledge, has not been done before. Our findings suggest that older patients who live for ten years following total hip arthroplasty experience a ten-year revision risk of about 10%, while younger patients have a somewhat greater risk of revision. As failure leading to revision is a critically important endpoint of THA from the standpoint of patients, surgeons and policy makers, these data will help anchor discussions of revision risks among these parties. Uncemented implants may be associated with greater revision risks in both age groups, although we cannot exclude confounding by age and activity level. Studies of implant failure are methodologically complex and should be accompanied by discussion of the definition of failure and detailed account of the actual number of subjects at risk at time points of interest.

Author Contributions

Conceived and designed the experiments: EL JNK. Analyzed the data: KLC EL AAN JJZP JNK. Wrote the paper: KLC JNK. Edited the paper: AAN JJZP.

References

1. Berry DJ, Harmsen WS, Cabanela ME, Morrey BF (2002) Twenty-five-year survivorship of two thousand consecutive primary Charnley total hip replacements: factors affecting survivorship of acetabular and femoral components. J Bone Joint Surg Am 84-A: 171–177.
2. Maloney WJ (2001) National Joint Replacement Registries: has the time come? J Bone Joint Surg Am 83-A: 1582–1585.
3. Soderman P, Malchau H, Herberts P (2000) Outcome after total hip arthroplasty: Part I. General health evaluation in relation to definition of failure in the Swedish National Total Hip Arthoplasty register. Acta Orthop Scand 71: 354–359.
4. Soderman P, Malchau H, Herberts P, Zugner R, Regner H, et al. (2001) Outcome after total hip arthroplasty: Part II. Disease-specific follow-up and the Swedish National Total Hip Arthroplasty Register. Acta Orthop Scand 72: 113–119.
5. Callaghan JJ, Templeton JE, Liu SS, Pedersen DR, Goetz DD, et al. (2004) Results of Charnley total hip arthroplasty at a minimum of thirty years. A concise follow-up of a previous report. J Bone Joint Surg Am 86-A: 690–695.
6. Eskelinen A, Remes V, Helenius I, Pulkkinen P, Nevalainen J, et al. (2005) Total hip arthroplasty for primary osteoarthrosis in younger patients in the Finnish arthroplasty register. 4,661 primary replacements followed for 0–22 years. Acta Orthop 76: 28–41.
7. Kavanagh BF, Wallrichs S, Dewitz M, Berry D, Currier B, et al. (1994) Charnley low-friction arthroplasty of the hip. Twenty-year results with cement. J Arthroplasty 9: 229–234.
8. Makela K, Eskelinen A, Pulkkinen P, Paavolainen P, Remes V (2008) Cemented total hip replacement for primary osteoarthritis in patients aged 55 years or older: results of the 12 most common cemented implants followed for 25 years in the Finnish Arthroplasty Register. J Bone Joint Surg Br 90: 1562–1569.
9. Wroblewski BM, Siney PD, Fleming PA (2002) Charnley low-frictional torque arthroplasty in patients under the age of 51 years. Follow-up to 33 years. J Bone Joint Surg Br 84: 540–543.
10. Aldinger PR, Thomsen M, Mau H, Ewerbeck V, Breusch SJ (2003) Cementless Spotorno tapered titanium stems: excellent 10–15-year survival in 141 young patients. Acta Orthop Scand 74: 253–258.
11. McLaughlin JR, Lee KR (2000) Total hip arthroplasty in young patients. 8- to 13-year results using an uncemented stem. Clin Orthop Relat Res. pp 153–163.
12. Malchau H, Herberts P, Eisler T, Garellick G, Soderman P (2002) The Swedish Total Hip Replacement Register. J Bone Joint Surg Am 84-A Suppl 2: 2–20.
13. Herberts P, Malchau H (2000) Long-term registration has improved the quality of hip replacement: a review of the Swedish THR Register comparing 160,000 cases. Acta Orthop Scand 71: 111–121.
14. Espehaug B, Furnes O, Engesæter LB, Havelin LI (2009) 18 years of results with cemented primary hip prostheses in the Norwegian Arthroplasty Register. Acta Orthopaedica 80: 402–412.
15. Makela KT, Eskelinen A, Paavolainen P, Pulkkinen P, Remes V (2010) Cementless total hip arthroplasty for primary osteoarthritis in patients aged 55 years and older. Acta Orthopaedica 81: 42–52.
16. Eskelinen A, Remes V, Helenius I, Pulkkinen P, Nevalainen J, et al. (2006) Uncemented total hip arthroplasty for primary osteoarthritis in young patients: a mid-to long-term follow-up study from the Finnish Arthroplasty Register. Acta Orthop 77: 57–70.
17. Makela KT, Eskelinen A, Pulkkinen P, Paavolainen P, Remes V (2008) Total hip arthroplasty for primary osteoarthritis in patients fifty-five years of age or older. An analysis of the Finnish arthroplasty registry. J Bone Joint Surg Am 90: 2160–2170.
18. Ogino D, Kawaji H, Konttinen L, Lehto M, Rantanen P, et al. (2008) Total hip replacement in patients eighty years of age and older. J Bone Joint Surg Am 90: 1884–1890.
19. Puolakka TJ, Pajamaki KJ, Halonen PJ, Pulkkinen PO, Paavolainen P, et al. (2001) The Finnish Arthroplasty Register: report of the hip register. Acta Orthop Scand 72: 433–441.
20. Hailer NP, Garellick G, Karrholm J (2010) Uncemented and cemented primary total hip arthroplasty in the Swedish Hip Arthroplasty Register. Acta Orthopaedica 81: 34–41.
21. Furnes O, Lie SA, Espehaug B, Vollset SE, Engesaeter LB, et al. (2001) Hip disease and the prognosis of total hip replacements. A review of 53,698 primary total hip replacements reported to the Norwegian Arthroplasty Register 1987–99. J Bone Joint Surg Br 83: 579–586.
22. Hallan G, Lie SA, Furnes O, Engesaeter LB, Vollset SE, et al. (2007) Medium- and long-term performance of 11,516 uncemented primary femoral stems from the Norwegian arthroplasty register. J Bone Joint Surg Br 89: 1574–1580.
23. Allami MK, Fender D, Khaw FM, Sandher DR, Esler C, et al. (2006) Outcome of Charnley total hip replacement across a single health region in England. The results at ten years from a regional arthroplasty register. J Bone Joint Surg Br 88: 1293–1298.
24. Soderman P (2000) On the validity of the results from the Swedish National Total Hip Arthroplasty register. Acta Orthop Scand Suppl 71: 1–33.
25. Australian Orthopaedic Association National Joint Replacement Registry (2010) Annual Report 2009. Available at http://www.dmac.adelaide.edu.au/aoanjrr/publications.jsp?section = reports2009.
26. The New Zealand Joint Registry (2010) Ten Year Report. Available at www.cdhb.govt.nz/njr/.
27. Harris WH (1986) Etiology of osteoarthritis of the hip. Clin Orthop Relat Res. pp 20–33.

6

Organizational Factors and Long-Term Mortality after Hip Fracture Surgery. A Cohort Study of 6143 Consecutive Patients Undergoing Hip Fracture Surgery

Caterina A. Lund[1], Ann M. Møller[1]*, Jørn Wetterslev[2], Lars H. Lundstrøm[2,3]

1 Department of Anaesthesia and Intensive Care, Herlev University Hospital, Herlev, Denmark, 2 Copenhagen Trial Unit, Centre for Clinical Intervention Research, Rigshospitalet, Copenhagen University Hospital, København, Denmark, 3 Department of Anaesthesia, Nordsjællands Hospital, Hillerød University Hospital, Hillerød, Denmark

Abstract

Objective: In hospital and health care organizational factors may be changed to reduce postoperative mortality. The aim of this study is to evaluate a possible association between mortality and 'length of hospital stay', 'priority of surgery', 'time of surgery', or 'surgical delay' in hip fracture surgery.

Design: Observational cohort study.

Setting: Prospectively and consecutively reported data from the Danish Anaesthesia Database were linked to The Danish National Registry of Patients and The Civil Registration System. Records on vital status, admittance, discharges, codes of diagnosis, anaesthetic and surgical procedures were retrieved.

Participants: 6143 patients aged more than 65 years undergoing hip fracture surgery.

Main Outcome Measures: All-cause mortality.

Results: The one year mortality was 30% (28–31%, 95% Confidence interval (CI)). In a multivariate model 'length of hospital stay' less than 10 days and more than 20 days are associated with mortality with hazard ratios of 1.34 (1.20–1.53 CI, $p<0.001$) and 1.27 (1.06–1.51 CI, $p<0.001$), respectively. 'Priority of surgery' categorized as 'non-scheduled' is associated with mortality with a hazard ratio of 1.31 (1.13–1.50 CI, $p<0.001$). Surgical delay and time of surgery are not significantly associated with mortality.

Conclusion: Non-scheduled surgery and length of hospital stay were associated with increased mortality. Confounding by indication may bias observational studies evaluating early and late discharge as well as priority; therefore cluster randomized clinical trials comparing different clinical set ups may be warranted evaluating health care organizational factors.

Editor: Jorge IF Salluh, D'or Institute of Research and Education, Brazil

Funding: These authors have no support or funding to report.

Competing Interests: The authors have declared that no competing interests exist.

* E-mail: ann.moeller@regionh.dk

Introduction

Mortality after hip fracture surgery is high and has been reported to range from 14 to 36% after one year [1]. To predict and reduce mortality after surgery for hip fracture, several patient related risk factors have been identified [1–4]. Most of these risk factors cannot be altered, whereas in hospital organizational risk factors may be changed in the individual hospital daily routine to reduce morbidity and mortality. However, the knowledge of the importance of different organizational factors remains inconclusive. The administrative management consist of interventions strongly depending on numerous conditions related to the patient, the physician etc. As an example both 'surgical delay' and 'length of hospital stay' is probably affected not only by organizational (i.e., the time required for the diagnostic procedures) but also clinical (i.e., the development of intercurrent adverse clinical events) factors. The impact of surgical delay on mortality is uncertain [5–16]. Furthermore, length of hospital stay has primarily been evaluated as an outcome measure [2;14;17;18] rather than a determinant for mortality. In this large cohort study with prospectively and consecutively recorded data, we evaluated the impact of factors partly categorized as organizational such as 'surgical delay', 'length of hospital stay', 'time of surgery' and 'surgical priority' on long-term mortality after hip fracture surgery.

Material and Method

The Danish National Board of Health, The Danish Data Protection Agency and The Danish Ethics Committees for Biomedical Research approved the registration of data in the Danish Anaesthesia Database. The Danish Data Protection Agency (Capital Region journal number 2007-58-0015) and the steering committee of the Danish Anaesthesia Database approved this study and provided access to the data for the analysis presented here. Since this is a database study, informed consent from the individual patient is not needed according to Danish legislation. Danish Database studies should not be sent for ethical approval, only be approved by the institutions mentioned above.

The data sources

The Danish Anaesthesia Database. Fourteen Danish departments of anaesthesia in 2005, and 25 departments in 2006–07, prospectively and consecutively reported data to the Danish Anaesthesia Database version 2 concerning all patients undergoing anaesthesia for surgery. The Danish Anaesthesia Database contains specific quantitative anaesthetic and surgical indicators describing the perioperative period. The departments (see Appendix I) are connected via the Internet to a central server hosted by The Unit for Clinical Quality, the Capital Region, Denmark. The information is recorded immediately after each anaesthesia and surgical procedure. The interface of the database is interactive and changes depending on the type of anaesthesia and surgery that is registered. All registered parameters are predefined and the interface to register was the same for all the registration sites as well as the rules of validation and the on-line user manual. Each patient entered into the database is registered with a unique identifying number from the centralized civil register. To construct the inpatient history, data from the different data sources were matched by this unique 10-digit national identification number that is assigned to every Danish citizen at birth. Furthermore, this unique identifier contains information regarding the patient's sex and date of birth and enables registration of each patient during the statistical analysis and prevents duplicates of anaesthesia records.

The National Registry of Patients. Contains information on admittance's, discharges, codes of diagnosis and surgical procedures from public hospitals in Denmark.

The Civil Registration System. Contains information on the vital status of all Danish citizens.

Data processing and study population

The cohort included patients recorded in the Danish Anaesthesia Database from January 2005 to November 2007 who were aged 65 or older and undergoing surgery following hip fracture. In the Danish Anaesthesia Database 10 634 patients were identified according to the "Nordic Classification of Surgical Procedures" records with codes for internal fixation (KNFJ50/1/2, KNFJ60/1/2, KNFJ70/1/2, KNFJ80/1/2) or arthroplasty (KNFB12, KNFB02, KNFB20, KNFB30, KNFB40). By using the patients unique identification number the codes of surgical procedure retrieved from the Danish Anaesthesia Database were linked with their corresponding diagnostic action codes in Nordic Classification of Surgical Procedures. We used codes from a Danish version of World Help Organization's "International Statistical Classification of Diseases and Related Health Problems version 10": DS720, DS721, DS722 to identify patients that had surgery for intracapsular, peritrochanteric or subtrochanteric fractures, respectively. Hereby we excluded 3907 patients who were treated with an arthroplasty for other reasons than acute fracture. A total of 424 patients were undergoing surgery because of hip fracture on more than one occasion, for these patients only the last record was included. The vital status of all patients was obtained by The Civil Registration System on January 14, 2008. For 28 foreign patients who were recorded in Danish Anaesthesia Database but had left Denmark before the vital status check in The Civil Registration System, the vital status was not available. These patients were excluded from the cohort. The final study population consisted of 6143 patients (figure 1).

Covariates

Covariates were obtained by the Danish Anaesthesia Database, the National Registry of Patients and the Civil Registration System. The covariates concerning organizational factors undergoing primary assessment were 'length of hospital stay', 'priority of surgery', 'time of surgery', and 'surgical delay'. Further, the following other covariates were retrieved for our assessments: age; sex; body mass index [19]; American Society of Anesthesiology classification of physical status [20]; day of admission; type of surgery; previous hip fracture surgery; type of fracture; duration of surgery; time of the year; type of hospital, type of anaesthesia and duration of surgery.

'Length of hospital stay' (LOS) was defined as the time between admission and discharge from the hospital. From a clinical point of view we anticipated, *a priori*, that a 'Length of hospital stay' of 10 days to two weeks would be recognized as usual and that 'Length of hospital stay' lesser than that would be anticipated as either fast recovery or if the patient dies as unsuccessful recovery and that 'Length of hospital stay' beyond 15 days would be recognized as a lengthy stay. Thus it was stratified as: 'length of hospital stay' <10 days, 10 to15 days, 16 to 20 days and 20 days < 'length of hospital stay'). Priority of surgery was defined as non-scheduled if a patient was anaesthetized without being planned for surgery the previous day. Otherwise surgery was categorized as scheduled. Time of surgery was categorized as 'dayshift' if start of surgery was between 08:00 and 16:00 or as 'nightshift' if start of surgery was between 16:00 and 08:00. The surgical delay was defined as the length of time between the admission to the department of surgery and the starting time of hip fracture surgery. We stratified surgical delay as: <12 hours; 12 to 23 hours; 24 to 47 hours; 48 to 71 hours; 72 to 95 hours; ≥96 hours. Age was categorized as (65 to 69 years; 70 to 79 years; 80 to 84 years; 85 to 89 years; ≥90 years). Body Mass Index was calculated as weight · height^{-2} (kilogram · meter^{-2}) and categorized as: underweight, Body Mass Index <18.5; normal, 18.5≤ Body Mass Index <25; overweight, 25≤ Body Mass Index <30; obesity, 30≤ Body Mass Index. Day of admission was categorized as 'week-end' if the patient was hospitalized Friday, Saturday or Sunday, while admission during rest of the week was categorized as 'not week-end'. Time of year was defined by the date of surgery according to the season. Type of surgery was categorized as either KNFB (arthroplasty) or KNFJ (internal fixation). 'Previous hip fracture surgery' was defined as the patients who were undergoing surgery because of hip fracture more than once during the time of observation and was categorized as 'Yes' or 'No'. Based upon international code of disease 10 codes: DS720, DS721, DS722 the type of fracture was categorized as intracapsular, peritrochanteric or subtrochanteric, respectively. Duration of surgery was measured in minutes, and categorized as: <60 minutes; 60 to 90 minutes; >90 minutes. Type of anaesthesia was defined as general, regional or combined general and regional. Hospitals were divided into 3 groups based on the number of operations performed during one year (2007) of observation and stratified as: (<100, 100 to 199, >199).

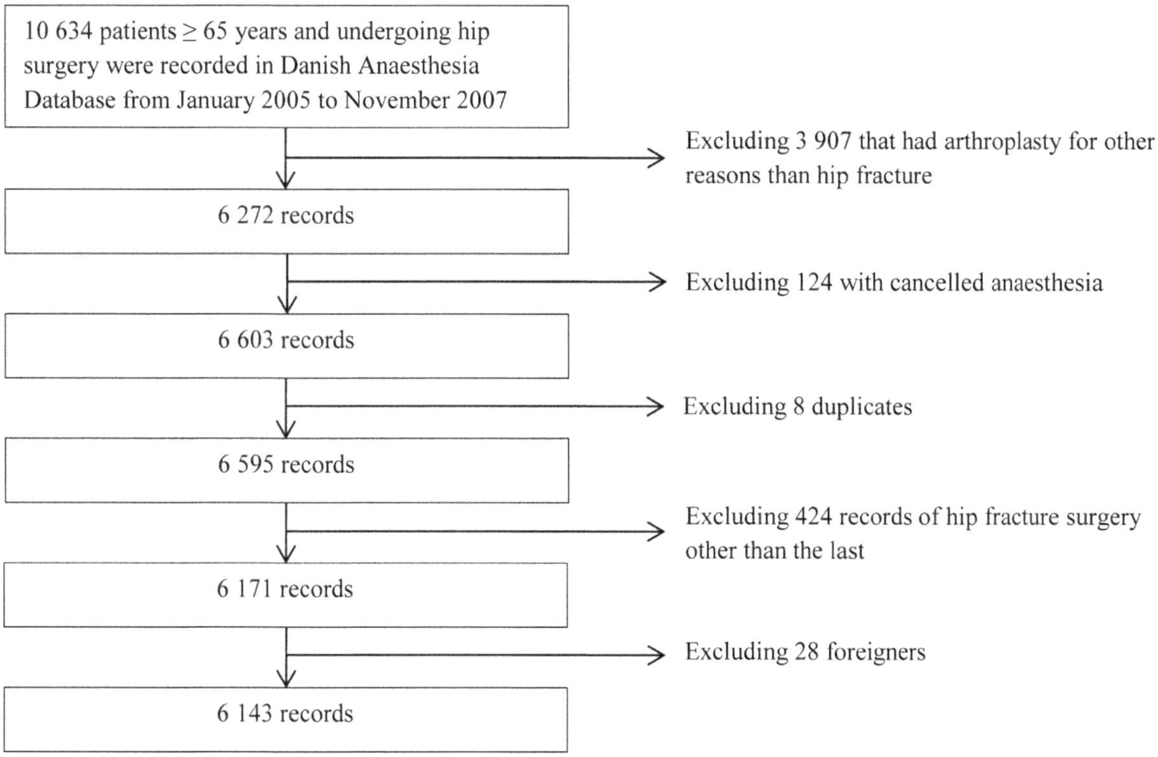

Figure 1. Selection of the study cohort.

Statistical Analysis

The overall mortality rates for two; six and 12 months were reported. The associations between death and the predefined covariates were assessed by Cox proportional hazards regression analysis. The primary analysis used start of the follow up at admission and a sensitivity analysis using start of follow-up after discharge from hospital. Initially, univariate regression analyses were performed. Subsequently, all significant covariates from the univariate analyses were included in a multivariate regression analysis. Backward stepwise regression was performed to identify a final Cox model. Survival functions were displayed for the organizational covariates contained in the final model. The assumption of proportional hazards was checked plotting cumulative hazard functions for different categories of 'length of hospital stay', 'priority of surgery' and sex. The cumulative hazard functions as well as the log minus log plots were very close to parallel and did not suggest violation of the assumption of proportional hazards. Because the association of 'length of hospital stay' with mortality may depend on the in-hospitality mortality, we performed a sensitivity analysis. Here we used the same co-variates as in our primary analyses, but excluded all patients who died during hospital admission. All estimates were reported with 95% confidence intervals.

The prevalence and pattern of missing data among all covariates were examined. If more than 10% of the patients had missing records for one or more covariates, the statistical method of multiple imputations for handling missing data [21–23] was used. Otherwise the results of the original dataset of complete cases were presented. For both the univariate and multivariate regression analyses we used a level for statistical significance of $p<0.05$. The data were analysed using the SPSS version 16.0 (SPSS Inc., Wacker Drive, Chicago, IL 60606-6307).

This study has been presented according to the STROBE-statement of reporting of an observational cohort study [24].

Ethical approval

The Danish Ethics Committees for Biomedical Research approved the registration of data in the Danish Anaesthesia Database.

Data sharing

No additional data available.

Results

From January 2005 to November 2007, 6 143 patients recorded in Danish Anaesthesia Database met the criteria for inclusion in this study. A total of 469 (7.6%) of the 6 143 patients had missing records for one or more covariates, whereas 5 674 patients had complete records without any missing data. The characteristics of the patients are shown in Table 1. The mortality rates after two, six and twelve months were 15.2% (14.3–16.1, 95% CI), 23.4% (22.2–24.6, 95% CI) and 29.8% (28.3–31.3, 95% CI), respectively. Performing Cox proportional hazards regression analysis, the median follow-up time was 9.8 months with a 90% inter percentile range from 0.3 to 30.8 months.

In our univariate Cox regression analyses 'length of hospital stay' and 'priority of surgery' were significant associated with mortality, while 'Time of surgery' ($P = 0.20$) and 'Surgical delay' ($P = 0.08$) were not significantly associated with mortality. Other

Table 1. Characteristics of the 6 143 patients.

Covariates		Number of patients (%)	Covariates		Number of patients (%)
Sex			**Priority of Surgery**		
	Male	1597 (26)		Scheduled	1097 (17.9)
	Female	4546 (74)		Non-scheduled	5046 (82.1)
	Missing	0		Missing	0
Age - years			**Time of Admission**		
	Age <70	786 (12.8)		Week-end	2367 (38.5)
	70≤ age <80	1538 (25.0)		Not week-end	3710 (60.4)
	80≤ age <85	1381 (22.5)		Missing	66 (1.1)
	85≤ age <90	1349 (22.0)	**Time of Year**		
	90≤ age	1089 (17.7)		Spring	1462 (23.8)
	Missing	0		Summer	1597 (26.0)
ASA				Autumn	1705 (27.8)
	ASA 1	428 (7.0)		Winter	1313 (21.4)
	ASA 2	3133 (51.0)		Missing	66 (1.1)
	ASA 3	2282 (37.1)	**Surgical delay - hours**		
	ASA 4–6	190 (3.1)		0–12	1151 (18.7)
	Missing	110 (1.8)		12–24	2115 (34.4)
Body Mass Index (BMI) - kg/m^2				24–48	2026 (33.0)
	BMI <18.5	742 (12.1)		48–72	425 (6.9)
	18.5≤ BMI <25	3643 (59.3)		72–96	163 (2.7)
	25≤ BMI <30	1253 (20.4)		>96	197 (3.2)
	30≤ BMI	312 (5.1)		Missing	66 (1.1)
	Missing	193 (3.1)	**Time of Surgery**		
Previous hip fracture surgery				Dayshift	4044 (65.8)
	Yes	406 (6.6)		Nightshift	2099 (34.2)
	No	5737 (93.4)		Missing	0
	Missing	0	**Duration of Surgery - minutes.**		
Type of fracture				<60	2517 (42.6)
	Intracapsular	3300 (53.7)		60–90	2060 (35.5)
	Peritrochanteric	2409 (39.2)		>90	1335 (21.7)
	Subtrochanteric	341 (5.6)		Missing	131 (2.1)
	Missing	93 (1.5)	**Type of Hospital - operations/years**		
Type of Operation				<100	556 (9.1)
	Internal fixation	3993 (65)		100–199	3133 (51.0)
	Arthroplasty	2148 (35)		>199	2286 (37.2)
	Missing	0		Missing	168 (2.7)
Type of Anaesthesia			**Length of hospital stay (LOS) - days**		
	Regional	3317 (54.0)		LOS <10	3810 (62.0)
	General	2389 (38.9)		10≤ LOS <15	1067 (17.4)
	Combined	424 (6.9)		15≤ LOS <20	443 (7.2)
	Missing	13 (0.2)		20≤ LOS	636 (10.4)
				Missing	187 (3.0)

ASA = American Society of Anesthesiology classification of physical status.

significant covariates were Gender; Type of operation; Previous hip fracture surgery; Type of anaesthesia; Type of hospital; Age; American Society of Anesthesiology classification of physical status; Body Mass Index and Type of fracture (Table 2).

In our subsequent multivariate Cox regression analysis 'length of hospital stay' and 'priority of surgery' remained statistically significant associated with increased mortality. In the multivariate model 'length of hospital stay' <10 days and a 20 days ≤ 'length of hospital stay' were associated with mortality with a hazard ratio of 1.34 (1.20–1.53, 95% CI, $p<0.001$) and 1.27 (1.06–1.51, 95% CI, $p = 0.008$), respectively. The hazard ratio of 'priority of surgery' categorized as 'Non-scheduled' was 1.31 (1.13–1.50, 95%

Table 2. Cox regression analyses.

Covariates	Univariate			Multivariate		
	Hazard ratio	95% C.I.	P value	Hazard ratio	95% C.I.	P value
Sex						
Female	Reference			Reference		
Male	1.47	1.34–1.62	<0.001	1.79	1.62–1.99	<0.001
Age - years						
Age <70	Reference			Reference		
70≤ age <80	1.58	1.29–1.95	<0.001	1.47	1.19–1.82	<0.001
80≤ age <85	2.12	1.73–2.60	<0.001	1.95	1.58–2.41	<0.001
85≤ age <90	2.95	2.42–3.60	<0.001	2.78	2.26–3.42	<0.001
90≤ age	4.26	3.49–5.19	<0.001	3.86	3.13–4.75	<0.001
ASA						
ASA 1	Reference			Reference		
ASA 2	2.46	1.84–3.28	<0.001	2.18	1.63–2.92	<0.001
ASA 3	4.84	3.63–6.45	<0.001	3.85	2.87–5.15	<0.001
ASA 4–6	9.43	6.76–13.16	<0.001	7.76	5.52–10.91	<0.001
Body Mass Index (BMI)						
BMI <18.5	1.43	1.26–1.61	<0.001	1.42	1.25–1.61	<0.001
18.5≤ BMI <25	Reference			Reference		
25≤ BMI <30	0.68	0.60–0.77	<0.001	0.73	0.64–0.84	<0.001
30≤ BMI	0.54	0.42–0.70	<0.001	0.61	0.47–0.79	<0.001
Previous hip fracture surgery						
No	Reference			Reference		
Yes	1.42	1.15–1.75	<0.001	1.26	1.01–1.57	0.040
Type of fracture						
Intracapsular	Reference			Reference		
Peritrochanteric	1.21	1.11–1.33	<0.001	NS		
Subtrochanteric	1.14	0.93–1.39	0.12	NS		
Type of operation						
Internal fixation	Reference			Reference		
Arthroplasty	0.80	0.72–0.88	<0.001	NS		
Type of anaesthesia						
Regional	Reference			Reference		
Combined	1.03	0.86–1.24	0.72	NS		
General	1.15	1.05–1.26	0.002	NS		
Priority of surgery						
Scheduled	Reference			Reference		
Non-scheduled	1.50	1.31–1.71	<0.001	1.31	1.13–1.50	0.003
Duration of surgery - minutes						
<60	Reference			Reference		
60–90	0.87	0.78–0.96	0.006	NS		
>90	0.77	0.68–0.86	<0.001	NS		
Length of hospital stay (LOS) - days						
LOS <10	1.40	1.23–1.60	<0.001	1.34	1.20–1.53	<0.001
10≤ LOS <15	Reference			Reference		
15≤ LOS <20	1.08	0.88–1.33	0.45	0.99	0.80–1.22	0.913
20≤ LOS	1.47	1.24–1.74	<0.001	1.27	1.06–1.51	0.008
Surgical delay - hours						
0–12	Reference					
12–24	0.89	0.78–1.01	0.08			

Table 2. Cont.

Covariates	Univariate			Multivariate		
	Hazard ratio	95% C.I.	P value	Hazard ratio	95% C.I.	P value
24–48	1.03	0.91–1.17	0.64			
48–72	1.02	0.84–1.24	0.82			
72–96	1.10	0.83–1.44	0.52			
>96	1.05	0.81–1.36	0.72			
Time of Surgery						
Dayshift	Reference					
Nightshift	1.07	0.98–1.18	0.20			

ASA = American Society of Anesthesiology classification of physical status; NS = non significant. Both Surgical delay, p = 0.08 and Time of Surgery, p = 0.20 were non significant in the univariate analysis. Other Non significant covariates in the univariate analyses were: Time of year, p = 0.67; Time of Admission, p = 0.25; Type of hospital, p = 0.19.

CI, p = 0.003). The final Cox model includes the following additional covariates: Sex; Previous hip fracture surgery; Type of hospital; Age; American Society of Anesthesiology classification of physical status and Body Mass Index (Table 2). The survival functions of 'length of hospital stay' and 'priority of surgery' are displayed in figure 2 and 3, respectively.

The impact of 'length of hospital stay' on mortality may depend on the in-hospitality mortality (2.0%, (1.6–2.4, 95% CI)). This possible influence was evaluated in an additional sensitivity analysis. With a similar statistical approach as in our primary analyses, we performed Cox regression analyses excluding all patients who died during hospital admission. This additional multivariate analysis did not show any noticeable differences compared with the original analyses, as 'length of hospital stay' < 10 and a 20≤ 'length of hospital stay' were associated with mortality with a hazard ratio of 1.32 (1.25–1.51, 95% CI, p< 0.001) and 1.25 (1.05–1.50, 95% CI, p = 0.014), respectively.

Discussion

We found that neither the surgical delay nor the time of surgery were associated with an increased risk of death. Non-scheduled surgery, early discharge ('length of hospital stay' <10 days), and

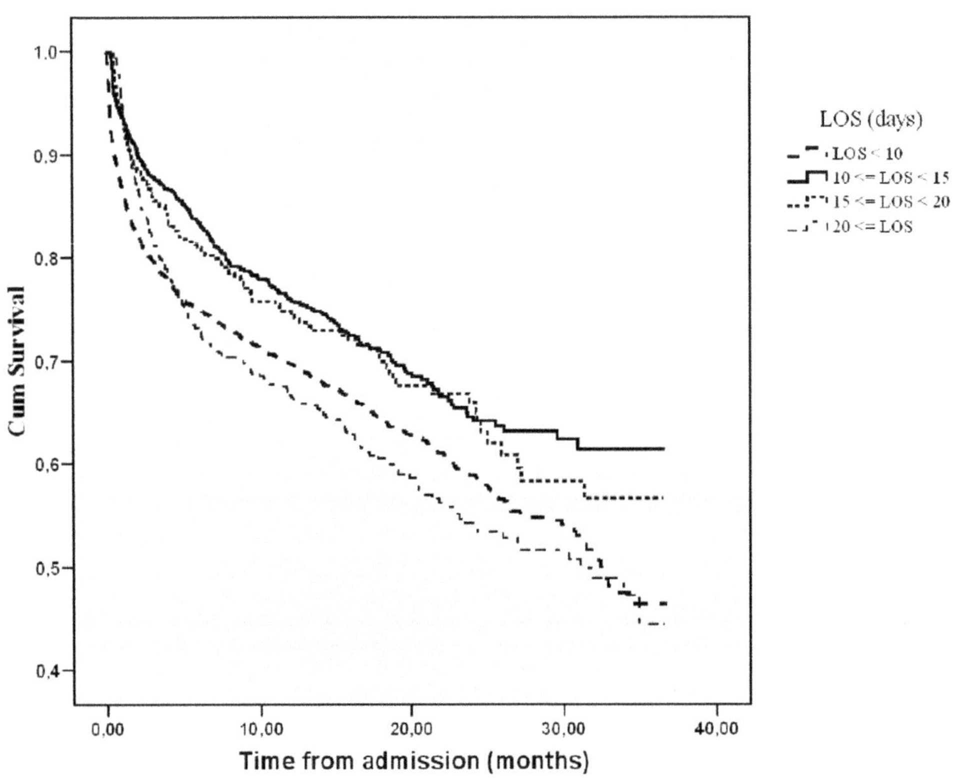

Figure 2. Survival function for 'Length of Hospital Stay' (LOS).

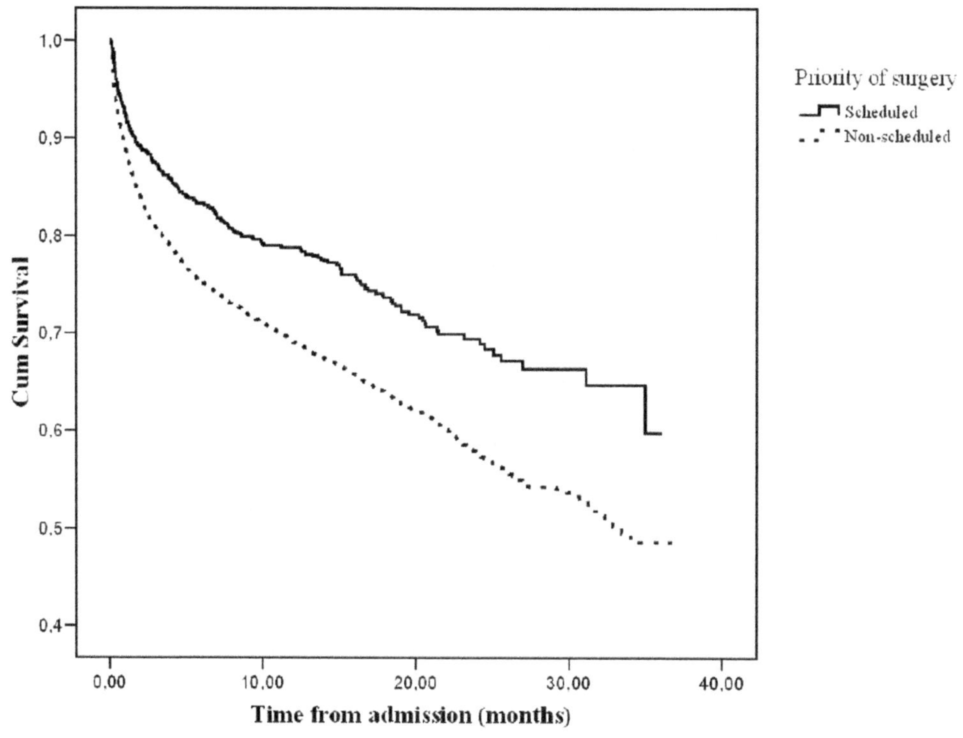

Figure 3. Survival Function for 'Priority of Surgery'.

late discharge, ('length of hospital stay' >20 days), were statistically significant risk factors for mortality after hip fracture surgery.

The present study is based upon a large cohort of patients with prospectively and consecutively collected data representing every-day experience from clinical practice. The Danish Anaesthesia Database requires all recorded indicators to be subjected to relevant rules of validation. This minimizes subsequent problems of missing and invalid data. The data from *The National Registry of Patients* and *The Civil Registration System* is of a high quality and the unique personal identification number almost ensuring complete follow up of data from Danish Anaesthesia Database concerning date of death after discharge from hospital. The data is recently collected and over a short period of time but with a long follow up time (up to 36.5 months).

There are several limitations in our assessment. Confounding by indication is well known to introduce bias in the results in any non-randomized study involving interventions [25]. In our assessment the 'organizational covariates' more and less reflect multiple factors. Especially 'length of hospital stay' may depend on various parameters other than organizational factors. Thus, the administrative management consist of interventions strongly depending on numerous conditions related to the patient, the comorbidity, the physician etc. It was not possible to acquire information of any administrative guidelines used by the participating departments these may strongly differ between patients within the same surgical department. As an example, the administrative and clinical choice of discharging a patient could depend on numerous variables not recorded in the Danish Anaesthesia Database, which may hereby bias our results. Even though, the American Society of Anesthesiology classification of physical status [26] was retrieved for our assessment, the mental status, residence and socio-economic status of the patients prior to the injury and after discharge are unknown. Furthermore, the mechanism of injury (pathological fracture, multiples and high energy trauma) and the time between the injury and admission (including inter-hospital transfer) are unknown [27]. All these various factors strongly affect 'length of hospital stay' and therefore it is important not to consider this covariate as a "pure" organizational factor. It was a further limitation that it was not possible to retrieve data about the patients' cognitive and functional status before fracture and there was no available information about patient's comorbidity in the database. Finally, we reported all-cause mortality. It would have been of interest to provide the cause of death in the patients during the time of observation, but these information were not contained in the database.

The mortality rates in our study exceed other estimates previously reported [1;7;8;14;28]. This might be due to the non-selected patient population including some patients with multiple co-existing diseases. In Denmark, all patients are treated in public hospitals. The present sample is therefore likely to be representative of the Danish population as a whole.

Despite of a trend, we did not find an association between surgical delay and mortality. The knowledge of the importance of surgical delay on mortality remains inconclusive. While some studies have found a decreased mortality with early surgery [6;16;28–31] others have not been able to find an association between surgical delay and mortality after hip fracture surgery [5;7;9;12;14;18;32–34]. Comparing the outcomes of these studies is difficult as the cut-offs and definitions of early and late surgery varies between studies. In most studies the number of patients included is small, but even in larger studies the results are ambiguous [7;9;16;28]. Despite of this it is considered good clinical practice in most countries to operate patients with hip fracture within 24 hours after admission. The largest study [6] on this subject included more than 100 000 patients and found an increased risk of death associated with delay. However, this study was limited to in-hospital mortality and therefore it is not comparable with our assessment focusing on long-term mortality. The majority of the patients (87%) in our assessment underwent surgery within 48 hours after admission. Hereby, our patient population differs from most other studies, where the interval of surgical delay was wider [1;8;12;13;16;28], making them difficult to compare. As an example, patients who in other studies would have been delayed for medical reasons, might have been included in the <48 hours group of our study. It will be difficult to estimate the effect of a possible gain of short delay in interaction with a possible disadvantage of not having optimized the medical status of selected patients.

Short surgical delay may increase the priority of patients with hip fracture on the surgery schedule and influence the time of surgery towards late shift with less experienced surgeons and staff. In our assessment 'The time of surgery' was not associated with an increased risk of death. This is in accordance with previous studies on this subject [35]. However, the number of patients undergoing surgery during night shift was limited, and therefore there may not be statistical power to detect a statistical significant association.

We found that patients who underwent non-scheduled surgery had a significant increased risk of mortality. It could indicate that the frailest patients had the highest priority or that the patients were not medically optimized enough for the operation. Thus our results may indicate that surgical precaution including meticulous planning is of importance.

We found that both 'length of hospital stay' <10 days and 'length of hospital stay' >20 days were independent risk factors for mortality. The increased risk of death with 'length of hospital stay' >20 days may be a marker for patients that had deterioration of pre-existing medical diseases or medical or surgical complications during admission. The increased risk of death with 'length of hospital stay' <10 days makes us hypothesize that some patients may be discharged too early without the implementation of relevant adjuvant interventions. Fast track systems [36;37] focuses on strategies to minimize the length of hospital stay. Short length of stay as an outcome measure might not be at guarantee of quality and cost effectiveness if the patients are not discharged following standardized and optimized discharge criteria. In a multidisciplinary rehabilitation strategy, it may be a goal to reduce the length of hospital stay. However, it is important to understand that discharge criteria with fast-track surgery should be the same as those of traditional care, but that the fast-track system may achieve the criteria sooner [36;37]. These interventions including good feeding, physical training, and regular medication may restore physical and mental abilities after general surgery. The increased risk of death with 'length of hospital stay' <10 days could suggest that the frailest patients were discharged quickly to nursing homes [38], however the American Society of Anesthesiology classification of physical status was included in the multivariate analysis to correct statistically for their functional status and level of disease. We were not able to retrieve information on clinical criteria for discharge as well as information on out of hospital clinical interventions after discharge. However, a recent national multicenter audit of hospital charts from hospitals in Denmark demonstrated significant variability in treatment and care of patients with hip fractures among the regions of Denmark [39].

In the effort of minimizing the risk of bias caused by confounding parameters, randomized trials are needed. In a randomized trial, it may be methodologically preferable randomizing patients individually [40]. However, in an attempt to assess the impact of the implementation of recommendations made at a departmental level, it may be difficult to conduct organizational interventions at an individual level. Consequently, a cluster-randomized design may be preferable [40;41], and hereby different clinical set ups may be compared.

In our large cohort, non-scheduled surgery, early and late discharge was demonstrated to be risk factors for mortality. The present study adds to previous studies dealing with the risk of hip fracture surgery. Confounding by indication is a major problem in observational studies to describe the effect of interventions. A cluster randomized clinical trial comparing different clinical set ups is warranted.

Author Contributions

Conceived and designed the experiments: CAL LHL JW AMØ. Analyzed the data: CAL LHL JW. Wrote the paper: LHL CAL JW AMØ.

References

1. Zuckerman JD (1996) Hip fracture. N Engl J Med; 334(23):1519–1525.
2. Clague JE, Craddock E, Andrew G, Horan MA, Pendleton N (2002) Predictors of outcome following hip fracture. Admission time predicts length of stay and in-hospital mortality. Injury; 33(1):1–6.
3. Holt G, Smith R, Duncan K, Finlayson DF, Gregori A (2008) Early mortality after surgical fixation of hip fractures in the elderly: an analysis of data from the scottish hip fracture audit. J Bone Joint Surg Br; 90(10):1357–1363.
4. Radcliff TA, Henderson WG, Stoner TJ, Khuri SF, Dohm M, et al. (2008) Patient risk factors, operative care, and outcomes among older community-dwelling male veterans with hip fracture. J Bone Joint Surg Am; 90(1):34–42.
5. Bergeron E, Lavoie A, Moore L, Bamvita JM, Ratte S, et al. (2006) Is the delay to surgery for isolated hip fracture predictive of outcome in efficient systems? J Trauma; 60(4):753–757.
6. Bottle A, Aylin P (2006) Mortality associated with delay in operation after hip fracture: observational study. BMJ; 332(7547):947–951.
7. Franzo A, Francescutti C, Simon G (2005) Risk factors correlated with post-operative mortality for hip fracture surgery in the elderly: a population-based approach. Eur J Epidemiol; 20(12):985–991.
8. Gdalevich M, Cohen D, Yosef D, Tauber C (2004) Morbidity and mortality after hip fracture: the mpact of operative delay. Arch Orthop Trauma Surg; 124(5):334–340.
9. Grimes JP, Gregory PM, Noveck H, Butler MS, Carson JL (2002) The effects of time-to-surgery on mortality and morbidity in patients following hip fracture. Am J Med; 112(9):702–709.
10. Kenzora JE, McCarthy RE, Lowell JD, Sledge CB (1984) Hip fracture mortality. Relation to age, treatment, preoperative illness, time of surgery, and complications. Clin Orthop Relat Res;(186):45–56.
11. Leung F, Lau TW, Kwan K, Chow SP, Kung AW (2010) Does timing of surgery matter in fragility hip fractures? Osteoporos Int; (Suppl 4):S529–S534.
12. Majumdar SR, Beaupre LA, Johnston DW, Dick DA, Cinats JG, et al. (2006) Lack of association between mortality and timing of surgical fixation in elderly patients with hip fracture: results of a retrospective population-based cohort study. Med Care; 44(6):552–559.
13. Moran CG, Wenn RT, Sikand M, Taylor AM (2005) Early mortality after hip fracture: is delay before surgery important? J Bone Joint Surg Am; 87(3):483–489.
14. Orosz GM, Magaziner J, Hannan EL, Morrison RS, Koval K, et al. (2004) Association of timing of surgery for hip fracture and patient outcomes. JAMA; 291(14):1738–1743.
15. Rogers FB, Shackford SR, Keller MS (1995) Early fixation reduces morbidity and mortality in elderly patients with hip fractures from low-impact falls. J Trauma; 39(2):261–265.
16. Sund R, Liski A (2005) Quality effects of operative delay on mortality in hip fracture treatment. Qual Saf Health Care; 14(5):371–377.
17. Lefaivre KA, Macadam SA, Davidson DJ, Gandhi R, Chan H, et al. (2009) Length of stay, mortality, morbidity and delay to surgery in hip fractures. J Bone Joint Surg Br; 91(7):922–927.
18. Siegmeth AW, Gurusamy K, Parker MJ (2005) Delay to surgery prolongs hospital stay in patients with fractures of the proximal femur. J Bone Joint Surg Br; 87(8):1123–1126.
19. Keys A, Fidanza F, Karvonen MJ, Kimura N, Taylor HL (1972) Indices of relative weight and obesity. J Chronic Dis; 25(6):329–343.
20. Owens WD, Felts JA, Spitznagel EL Jr (1978) ASA physical status classifications: a study of consistency of ratings. Anesthesiology; 49(4):239–243.
21. Rubin DB (1987) Multiple Imputations for Nonresponse in Surveys. J. Wiley & Sons, New York.
22. Schafer JL, Graham JW (2002) Missing data: our view of the state of the art. Psychol Methods; 7(2):147–177.

23. Schafer JL (1999) Multiple imputation: a primer. Stat Methods Med Res; 8(1):3–15.
24. von EE, Altman DG, Egger M, Pocock SJ, Gotzsche PC, et al. (2008) The Strengthening the Reporting of Observational Studies in Epidemiology (STROBE) statement: guidelines for reporting observational studies. J Clin Epidemiol; 61(4):344–349.
25. Deeks JJ, Dinnes J, D'Amico R, Sowden AJ, Sakarovitch C, et al. (2003) Evaluating non-randomised intervention studies. Health Technol Assess; 7(27):iii–173.
26. Bjorgul K, Novicoff WM, Saleh KJ (2010) American Society of Anesthesiologist Physical Status score may be used as a comorbidity index in hip fracture surgery. J Arthroplasty 2010; 25(6 Suppl):134–137.
27. Vidal EI, Moreira-Filho DC, Coeli CM, Camargo KR Jr, Fukushima FB, et al. (2009) Hip fracture in the elderly: does counting time from fracture to surgery or from hospital admission to surgery matter when studying in-hospital mortality? Osteoporos Int; 20(5):723–729.
28. Weller I, Wai EK, Jaglal S, Kreder HJ (2005) The effect of hospital type and surgical delay on mortality after surgery for hip fracture. J Bone Joint Surg Br; 87(3):361–366.
29. Bredahl C, Nyholm B, Hindsholm KB, Mortensen JS, Olesen AS (1992) Mortality after hip fracture: results of operation within 12 h of admission. Injury; 23(2):83–86.
30. Dorotka R, Schoechtner H, Buchinger W (2003) The influence of immediate surgical treatment of proximal femoral fractures on mortality and quality of life. Operation within six hours of the fracture versus later than six hours. J Bone Joint Surg Br; 85(8):1107–1113.
31. Simunovic N, Devereaux PJ, Sprague S, Guyatt GH, Schemitsch E, et al. (2010) Effect of early surgery after hip fracture on mortality and complications: systematic review and meta-analysis. CMAJ; 182(15):1609–1616.
32. Eiskjaer S, Ostgard SE (1991) Risk factors influencing mortality after bipolar hemiarthroplasty in the treatment of fracture of the femoral neck. Clin Orthop Relat Res; (270):295–300.
33. Parker MJ, Pryor GA (1992) The timing of surgery for proximal femoral fractures. J Bone Joint Surg Br; 74(2):203–205.
34. Rae HC, Harris IA, McEvoy L, Todorova T (2007) Delay to surgery and mortality after hip fracture. ANZ J Surg; 77(10):889–891.
35. Bosma E, de Jongh MA, Verhofstad MH (2010) Operative treatment of patients with pertrochanteric femoral fractures outside working hours is not associated with a higher incidence of complications or higher mortality. J Bone Joint Surg Br; 92(1):110–115.
36. Kehlet H, Wilmore DW (2002) Multimodal strategies to improve surgical outcome. Am J Surg; 183(6):630–641.
37. Kehlet H, Dahl JB (2003) Anaesthesia, surgery, and challenges in postoperative recovery. Lancet; 362(9399):1921–1928.
38. Holvik K, Ranhoff AH, Martinsen MI, Solheim LF (2010) Predictors of mortality in older hip fracture inpatients admitted to an orthogeriatric unit in oslo, norway. J Aging Health; 22(8):1114–1131.
39. Egerod I, Rud K, Specht K, Jensen PS, Trangbaek A, et al. (2010) Room for improvement in the treatment of hip fractures in Denmark. Dan Med Bull; 57(12):A4199.
40. Hahn S, Puffer S, Torgerson DJ, Watson J (2005) Methodological bias in cluster randomised trials. BMC Med Res Methodol; 5: 10.
41. Campbell MK, Elbourne DR, Altman DG (2004) CONSORT statement: extension to cluster randomised trials. BMJ; 328(7441):702–708.

7

Risk of Severe Knee and Hip Osteoarthritis in Relation to Level of Physical Exercise: A Prospective Cohort Study of Long-Distance Skiers in Sweden

Karl Michaëlsson[1,2*], Liisa Byberg[1,2], Anders Ahlbom[3], Håkan Melhus[2,4], Bahman Y. Farahmand[3]

1 Department of Surgical Sciences, Section of Orthopaedics, Uppsala University, Uppsala, Sweden, 2 Uppsala Clinical Research Center, Uppsala University, Uppsala, Sweden, 3 The Institute of Environmental Medicine, Karolinska Institutet, Stockholm, Sweden, 4 Department of Medical Sciences, Section of Clinical Pharmacology, Uppsala University, Uppsala, Sweden

Abstract

Background: To complete long-distance ski races, regular physical exercise is required. This includes not only cross-country skiing but also endurance exercise during the snow-free seasons. The aim of this study was to determine whether the level of physical exercise is associated with future risk of severe osteoarthritis independent of previous diseases and injuries.

Methodology/Principal Findings: We used a cohort that consisted of 48 574 men and 5 409 women who participated in the 90 km ski race Vasaloppet at least once between 1989 and 1998. Number of performed races and finishing time were used as estimates of exercise level. By matching to the National Patient Register we identified participants with severe osteoarthritis, defined as arthroplasty of knee or hip due to osteoarthritis. With an average follow-up of 10 years, we identified 528 men and 42 women with incident osteoarthritis. The crude rate was 1.1/1000 person-years for men and 0.8/1000 person-years for women. Compared with racing once, participation in ≥5 races was associated with a 70% higher rate of osteoarthritis (multivariable-adjusted hazard ratio (HR) 1.72, 95% confidence interval (CI) 1.33 to 2.22). The association was dose-dependent with an adjusted HR of 1.09, 95% CI 1.05 to 1.13 for each completed race. A faster finishing time, in comparison with a slow finishing time, was also associated with an increased rate (adjusted HR 1.51, 95% CI 1.14 to 2.01). Contrasting those with 5 or more ski races and a fast finish time to those who only participated once with a slow finish time, the adjusted HR of osteoarthritis was 2.73, 95% CI 1.78 to 4.18.

Conclusions/Significance: Participants with multiple and fast races have an increased risk of subsequent arthroplasty of knee and hip due to osteoarthritis, suggesting that intensive exercise may increase the risk.

Editor: Beverley Shea, Central Institute of Educational Technology, Canada

Funding: This work was supported by grants from the Swedish Research Council (K2006-73P-20267-01-4 and K2009-52x-13511-10-3). The funders had no role in study design, data collection and analysis, decision to publish, or preparation of the manuscript.

Competing Interests: The authors have declared that no competing interests exist.

* E-mail: karl.michaelsson@surgsci.uu.se

Introduction

Undoubtedly, participation in sports and exercise has a positive effect on health in most people [1–4]. Evidence shows that moderate habitual exercise at middle and old age does not increase the risk of developing osteoarthritis [5]. Nevertheless, it is well known that trauma or injury to the knee is associated with future osteoarthritis [6,7] and that vigorous sports activities increase the risk of acute joint injuries [7]. An important question is whether prolonged intensive exercise may lead to osteoarthritis [5]. Animal models indicate that moderate weight and non-weight bearing physical activity do lead to either reversible pathologic changes in cartilage composition or to osteoarthritis in some [8–10] but not all studies [11]. Research in humans has also been inconsistent: some studies indicate a higher risk of knee or hip osteoarthritis after previous sport participation, whereas others could not show this association [5,12–17]. We sought to delineate how the level of physical exercise independent of previous injuries affects the future risk of severe osteoarthritis in a large cohort of long-distance skiers.

Methods

Ethics statement

The study protocol was approved by the Regional Ethical Review Board, Karolinska Institutet, Stockholm, Sweden.

Study participants

The present cohort study is based on finishing Swedish participants in the 90 km long-distance cross-country ski marathon race Vasaloppet in Sweden (www.vasaloppet.se) which is held annually the first Sunday in March. We restricted the study base to participants of the main classical race. Vasaloppet is the oldest, longest, and largest cross-country ski race in the world. The first Vasaloppet was run in 1922 with 119 participants. Nowadays, more than 15 000 men and women annually take part in the main long race (www.vasaloppet.se). In the period 1924 to 1980, women were not allowed to participate in the race. Even if the participating number of women after the restriction period gradually increased during the 1980s, they are still in 2010 underrepresented (1:10 of the participants).

The vast majority of the participants are not competing on the elite levels but the best competitors have an extremely high physical capacity. There is also a close relationship between average speed or ranking in ski races and maximum aerobic power (VO_{2max}), r^2 values being in the range of 0.9 [18]. Winners of the Vasaloppet who finish the race in about 4 h have a VO_{2max} of 80 ml min^{-1} kg^{-1} or higher [19], whereas skiers who finish in 10–13 h, i.e., the slowest speed in the race, have VO_{2max} of at least 45 ml min^{-1} kg^{-1} or higher [20] compared with an average VO_{2max} of 36 and 33 ml min^{-1} kg^{-1} amongst men and women in the general population [21]. We have previously shown that participants in Vasaloppet report a higher leisure physical activity, lower frequency of smoking, obesity, high fat consumption, and physical and mental illness [4]. Accordingly, they have a reduced standardized mortality ratio, and the reduction is most pronounced for subjects who participated in several races and for deaths due to cardiovascular disease [4].

The Vasaloppet office provided information on all Swedish citizens (49 117 men and 5 443 women) that completed any of the 90 km Vasaloppet races from 1989–1998, including information on year of race and finishing time, as well as each participant's 10-digit Swedish identification number. The race in 1990 was cancelled because of thawing.

The records of all participants were matched to the National Patient Registry for identification of diagnoses through December 31, 2005. Information on date of death was attained from the Swedish Causes of Death Register. The cohort was also linked to the Swedish National Population Registry to collect information on emigration.

We excluded 463 individuals (439 men and 24 women) from the study base because prior to study entry (i.e., the last race) they had had a diagnosis of osteoarthritis (n = 225, with or without surgical procedure done), or a diagnosis of inflammatory joint disease, including rheumatoid arthritis (n = 235), or both (n = 3). Another 114 skiers with a diagnosis of secondary osteoarthritis were excluded from further analysis (104 men, 10 women). The remaining 53 983 participants formed our study base.

Exposures

Since those who participated in several races tended to ski faster races (Spearman rank correlation 0.45, $p<0.001$) and improvements in VO_{2max} are directly related to intensity, duration, and frequency of training [22], the number of successful participations in Vasaloppet and the finishing times in the period from 1989 through 1998, as continuous variables and in categories, were used as estimates of level of physical exercise [4]. Number of races and finishing time before 1989 or after 1998 were not considered in the exposure assessment. Nonetheless, it is important to emphasize that this exposure to exercise is not restricted to skiing, e.g. long-distance running and roller skiing are common activities during the preparation for the race when it is not possible to ski. The skiing season normally lasts 3 months. In our previous study we showed that regular strenuous leisure exercise was typically performed by 21% and strenuous exercise by 58% of the participants in Vasaloppet as compared with 4 and 25%, respectively, in the general population [4] Sixty-four percent of the participants had at least 4 h/week of regular training while only 17% of the population exercised 1.5 h or more per week.

Finishing time was, on average, about 8 h (range 4–13 h). As skiing conditions vary from year to year, we expressed finishing time relative to the winner time as previously defined [4] in four categories as 100–160, 161–200, 201–240 and 241% or more than the winner's time (year- and sex-specific). For those who had participated in several races, the lowest relative finishing time was used as exposure.

Outcomes

Information on knee and hip arthroplasty for osteoarthritis after the last race of the participant through 2005 were based on record linkage with the National Patient Registry. Severe knee and hip osteoarthritis were defined as previously described [23], i.e., as a first knee arthroplasty or high tibial osteotomy (procedures coded 8424, 8423, 8428, 8010, 8199 or NGB09, NGB19, NGB29, NGB39, NGB49, NGB99 and NGK59) in combination with a contemporaneous diagnosis of osteoarthritis (715 or M17 according to the International Classification of Disease (ICD) 9 and ICD-10, respectively). Only the first event was counted for patients with more than one knee arthroplasty. Severe hip osteoarthritis was defined as a first hip arthroplasty (procedures coded 8414, 8010, NFB09, NFB19, NFB29, NFB39, NFB49, NFB99) in combination with a contemporaneous diagnosis of hip osteoarthritis (715 or M16 according to ICD-9 and ICD-10, respectively). Patients with more than one hip arthroplasty were only counted once. The annually updated National Patient Registry covers all inpatient care in Sweden since 1987. and complete individual matching to the register is enabled by the personal registration number provided to all Swedish citizens [24]. It has been validated against the national Swedish arthroplasty registers and was estimated to include at least 95% of primary knee and hip arthroplasties [25].

Additional information

In order to assess and control for diseases and injuries before the last race and during follow-up, infectious arthritis; diabetes mellitus; other endocrine disorders; fractures; contusions, distortions, dislocations and other injury diagnoses were determined from the National Patient Registry to the end of follow-up by ICD-7 through ICD-10 codes, depending on the period of diagnosis ascertainment. The frequency of injuries associated with cross-country skiing is, however, low compared to most other athletic activities [26].

The cohort was linked to the censuses of 1960, 1970, 1980, and 1990 to retrieve information on occupation, educational level, and household income. Occupation was grouped into four categories (blue-collar, lower-middle white-collar, high white-collar, and entrepreneur). Education was grouped into three categories: low (elementary school), medium (secondary school), and high (university).

Statistical analyses

The number of person-years was ascertained individually for all participants in the cohort. The date of entry to the study was the date of the last race during the years 1989–1998. Date of the completion of follow-up was the first date of osteoarthritis diagnosis, date of death, date of emigration, or the end of follow-up on 31 December 2005, whichever came first.

Cox's proportional hazards regression models were used to assess hazard ratios with 95% confidence intervals for primary in-hospital treated osteoarthritis. Only the first event of each osteoarthritis category (hip or knee osteoarthritis) was considered for patients with more than one hospital stay.

We modelled osteoarthritis risk by number of successful races or by finishing time. The number of competitions was analyzed as a continuous variable or in four predefined [4] groups (one, two, three to four, and five or more races). Finishing time relative to the winning time was analyzed also in four predefined [4] categories. Similar results were obtained if we used average finishing time of the successful races instead of the relative fastest finishing time for those who participated in several races. We additionally considered the combined influence of successful races and finishing time on the association with future risk of osteoarthritis by contrasting those with several performed races (five or more races) and a fast finishing time (fastest category) to participants with only one finished, slow pace race.

Two models were fitted. The first one included age (continuous), sex, socioeconomic status by occupation and education as covariates. We extended this model to adjust our estimates for separate marker variables (all dichotomous) for concomitant disorders that can influence the risk of osteoarthritis and exercise level: infectious arthritis, diabetes mellitus, other endocrine disorders, fractures, dislocations, distortions, contusions, any other acute injury, and any other chronic injury.

Results

The characteristics of participants are shown in Table 1. During a total of 526 472 person-years of follow-up with an average follow-up of 10 years (range 0–16 years) per individual, 528 men and 42 women were treated with arthroplasty of the knee or hip due to osteoarthritis after their last ski race. As expected, the incidence of severe osteoarthritis increased with increasing age and

Table 1. Characteristics with incidence of osteoarthritis (OA) at the hip or the knee among participants in the cross-country ski race Vasaloppet.

	N participants	N cases with OA	Incidence OA per 1000 person-years
Total	53983	570	1.08
Age (years)			
15–29	15248	18	0.12
30–39	14589	56	0.39
40–49	12139	130	1.08
50–59	8997	221	2.66
≥60	3010	145	5.39
Mean age (SD)	*38.8 (12.3)*		
Successful races			
1	28012	214	0.73
2	10052	106	1.10
3–4	8648	105	1.35
≥5	7271	145	2.46
Finish time (% of winner time)			
100–160	9631	105	1.17
161–200	17504	206	1.22
201–240	16078	170	1.07
≥241	10770	89	0.81
Education			
Low	11511	189	1.69
Medium	23011	184	0.81
High	16344	173	1.08
Occupation			
Blue-collar	18449	210	1.15
Low-middle white-collar	18802	207	1.12
High white-collar	7529	98	1.34
Entrepreneur	2830	47	1.68
Medical conditions			
Dislocation	529	15	2.94
Distortion	1723	30	1.81
Contusion	861	17	2.04
Neurological disorder	118	2	1.96
Diabetes mellitus	169	2	1.22
Endocrine diseases	468	7	1.59
Fractures	3445	41	1.24
Chronic injuries	4049	93	2.49
Acute injuries	5940	93	1.66

with the crude occurrence of previous injuries. The distribution of participants and number of cases with incident severe osteoarthritis of the hip and knee during follow-up by year of the last race is provided in the Table S1. Most participants had their last race in the later part of the inclusion period.

Those who repeatedly had participated in the competition had a higher risk of osteoarthritis. Participants who had taken part in several races displayed an increased rate of hip or knee osteoarthritis with a 9% (hazard ratio 1.09, 95% CI 1.05 to 1.13) increase per successful race (Table 2). This estimate was only marginally influenced if co-morbidities, including previous injuries, were accounted for in the multivariable model (hazard ratio 1.08 per race, 95% CI 1.04 to 1.13). Using the same model and restraining the analysis to those with a last participation in the race in either of the last two years of the inclusion period (1997–1998), provided a similar estimate (hazard ratio 1.10 per race, 95% CI 1.04–1.16). In addition, restriction of the cohort to only those without an injury diagnosis still revealed a higher risk of osteoarthritis (hazard ratio 1.11 per race, 95% CI 1.06 to 1.16). Those who had participated in 5 or more races had a 72% (hazard ratio 1.72, 95% CI 1.33 to 2.22) higher rate of having a diagnosis of osteoarthritis of the knee or hip compared with participants who had taken part in only one race event.

The individual's race pace was also of importance (Table 3). For every category of a faster finishing time, we found a 13% (hazard ratio 1.13, 95% CI 1.03 to 1.23) increased rate of osteoarthritis of the knee or hip. Those who had a finishing time close to the winner (within 60% of his time) had a 50% (hazard ratio 1.51, 95% CI 1.14 to 2.01) increased rate of osteoarthritis of the knee or hip compared with the slowest competitors.

We finally contrasted those with 5 or more ski races and a fast finishing time to those who only participated once and did so with a slow finishing time (Table 4). The former intensive exercise category (5 or more ski races combined with a fast time), had a nearly three-fold increased rate of osteoarthritis of the knee or hip compared with those in the second category (those who participated only once with a slow finishing time), also after controlling for previous injuries. Notably, the hazard ratio for hip osteoarthritis alone was 3.15, 95% CI 1.79 to 5.52. Moreover, we found no evidence that those in the intensive exercise category had had more previous injuries (odds ratio by multivariable logistic regression 1.01, 95% CI 0.88 to 1.16).

Survival curves of knee or hip osteoarthritis by number of successful races and categories of finishing time are displayed in Figure 1. The survival curves have been adjusted for sex distribution (male to female ratio 10:1) and median age at study entry of cases (53 years). The 10-year probability to receive surgery for osteoarthritis was approximately 3% in participants with 5 or more successful ski races and in those with fastest average ski speed. The corresponding number for those in the contrasting categories with only one race performed or a low skiing speed was about 2%.

Discussion

Our data show a relation between the number of races completed and the time to completion and the risk of subsequent arthroplasty of the knee or hip due to osteoarthritis, suggesting that the intensive exercise required to most successfully complete the long-distance race Vasaloppet may be associated with an increased risk of osteoarthritis. The associations were independent of previous injuries identified from registry data.

There are no previous prospective investigations of this size that have examined intensive exercise and future risk of osteoarthritis. In a 9-year follow-up in 28 regular runners compared with matched controls, no radiological evidence of differences in osteophyte progression or narrowing of joint space by regular radiographs of the hips and knees was found [27]. In another small study with nine male triathletes and nine controls quantitative magnetic resonance imaging (MRI) was used for analysis of knee joint cartilage thickness [28]. A tendency of diminished cartilage volume was found at weight bearing sites in the athletes.

Prospective studies of individuals with less intensive physical activity level have presented conflicting results [12]. The most recent and thoroughly performed study from the Framingham Offspring cohort concluded that there was no association between regular physical activity level and development of knee osteoarthritis over a 9-year follow-up in 1 279 men and women with an average age of 53 years at baseline [29]. Few of these men and women reported performing intensive exercise. Earlier investigations based on the original Framingham study found that those who reported high physical activity had a higher future risk of radiographic signs of osteoarthritis [30,31]. Men investigated at the Cooper Clinic (Dallas, TX, US) who were younger than 50 years of age and who participated in high physical activity had an increased risk of self-reported but not physician-diagnosed osteoarthritis of the hip and knee [32]. When controlling for previous injuries in a later follow-up in the same cohort, no evident risk increase was noted [33]. No association between physical activity level and joint space narrowing or osteophyte occurrence

Table 2. Hazard ratios (HRs) and 95% confidence intervals (CIs) of osteoarthritis associated with number of successful races.

	Hip N = 356 cases		Knee N = 227 cases		Hip or knee N = 570 cases	
	HR[a] (95% CI)	HR[b] (95% CI)	HR[a] (95% CI)	HR[b] (95% CI)	HR[a] (95% CI)	HR[b] (95% CI)
Successful races						
1	1.00	1.00	1.00	1.00	1.00	1.00
2	1.25 (0.91–1.69)	1.24 (0.91–1.69)	1.41 (0.97–2.05)	1.38 (0.95–2.00)	1.33 (1.05–1.69)	1.32 (1.04–1.68)
3–4	1.34 (0.98–1.83)	1.31 (0.96–1.80)	1.35 (0.90–2.02)	1.31 (0.87–1.96)	1.33 (1.04–1.72)	1.31 (1.01–1.68)
≥5	1.59 (1.15–2.20)	1.59 (1.15–2.20)	1.83 (1.21–2.76)	1.73 (1.14–2.63)	1.72 (1.33–2.22)	1.68 (1.30–2.17)
Per race	1.08 (1.03–1.14)	1.08 (1.03–1.14)	1.09 (1.02–1.16)	1.08 (1.01–1.15)	1.09 (1.05–1.13)	1.08 (1.04–1.13)

[a]Adjusted for age (continuous), gender, education (low, medium, high) and occupation (blue-collar, lower-middle white-collar, high white-collar and entrepreneur).
[b]Adjusted for all variables in the model [a] and, in addition, the following diagnoses: any fracture, any acute injury, any chronic injury, any distortion, any dislocation, any contusion, any neurologic disease, infectious arthritis, diabetes mellitus, and any other endocrine disorder.

Table 3. Hazard ratios (HRs) and 95% confidence intervals (CIs) of osteoarthritis associated with finishing time.

	Hip N=356 cases		Knee N=227 cases		Hip or knee N=570 cases	
	HR[a] (95% CI)	HR[b] (95% CI)	HR[a] (95% CI)	HR[b] (95% CI)	HR[a] (95% CI)	HR[b] (95% CI)
Finishing time (% of winner time)						
≥241	1.00	1.00	1.00	1.00	1.00	1.00
201–240	1.20 (0.87–1.67)	1.21 (0.87–1.68)	0.99 (0.67–1.48)	1.00 (0.67–1.48)	1.13 (0.87–1.46)	1.13 (0.88–1.47)
161–200	1.26 (0.92–1.74)	1.25 (0.91–1.73)	0.99 (0.67–1.46)	0.97 (0.66–1.43)	1.17 (0.91–1.50)	1.15 (0.90–1.48)
100–160	1.54 (1.06–2.24)	1.53 (1.05–2.23)	1.41 (0.91–2.16)	1.34(0.87–2.07)	1.51 (1.14–2.01)	1.48 (1.11–1.97)
Per category	1.14 (1.01–1.27)	1.13 (1.01–1.26)	1.10 (0.96–1.26)	1.08 (0.94–1.24)	1.13 (1.03–1.23)	1.12 (1.02–1.22)

[a]Adjusted for age (continuous), gender, education (low, medium, high) and occupation (blue-collar, lower-middle white-collar, high white-collar and entrepreneur).
[b]Adjusted for all variables in the model [a] and, in addition, the following diagnoses: any fracture, any acute injury, any chronic injury, any distortion, any dislocation, any contusion, any neurologic disease, infectious arthritis, diabetes mellitus, and any other endocrine disorder.

was observed in the Chingford study [34]. In an Australian longitudinal study low physical activity conferred a reduced risk for radiological signs of knee osteoarthritis but only for the physical activity level during 20–29 years of age and not in the four other age categories [35]. Radiographic signs of knee osteoarthritis were associated with regular sports activities in a British cohort study of 354 participants but previous injuries were not adjusted for and progression of osteoarthritis was not influenced by regular sports participation [36].

Hence, self-reported physical activity has been used in most cohort studies. Some self-report measures have been validated and are thus feasible for use in large studies but the method is prone to misclassification and might not capture the type and true intensity of the physical exercise it is aimed to measure, leading to attenuated risk estimates. In addition, failure to account for previous injuries in the analysis or design of the study might overestimate the influence of high physical activity because these factors can act together. We have used the number of completed races and finishing time in a long-distance skiing competition as more objective estimates of physical exercise. Winners of the Vasaloppet belong to the group of world-class cross-country skiers. However, the vast majority of the participants do not compete on the elite levels. But even the slowest competitors in the Vasaloppet have a higher physical capacity and training load compared with the general population. We therefore also compared our incidences of osteoarthritis to the rates in the general population by data (generous support from Professor Gunnar Engström) from a large Swedish population-based cohort study well representing the distribution of body mass index, the prevalence of smoking and sociodemographic status and the average incidence of hip and knee joint replacement in Sweden [23]. With an identical definition of knee- and hip osteoarthritis in the studies, a similar age distribution, calendar period of observation and length of follow-up, the Mantel-Haenszel age- and sex-adjusted incidence rate ratio (IRR) of knee osteoarthritis among participants in Vasaloppet was 1.00, 95% CI 0.80 to 1.25 compared to the general population. The rate of hip osteoarthritis was, however, higher in our cohort (IRR 1.65, 95% CI 1.37 to 1.97), which indicates a conservative estimation of the risk for hip osteoarthritis by physical activity in the present study. Nevertheless, compelling evidence exists that a moderate and high VO_2max and physical activity reduce the risk of numerous chronic diseases and provide higher longevity [1,3]. There seems, however, only to be small additional benefits on longevity by vigorous exercise compared with moderate intensity training [1,3,37]. Our study suggests that intensive exercise might even harm joint cartilage. At the same time, restrained exercise may be a protective factor and is generally recommended for the patient with osteoarthritis [15]. In fact, moderate levels of exercise can even exert small short-time benefits of pain relief among those with osteoarthritis [38].

Major advantages with our design were the large study size, the individual personal registration number provided to all Swedish citizens that enabled linkage between registers with virtually no

Table 4. Hazard ratios (HRs) and 95% confidence intervals (CIs) of osteoarthritis associated with combination of finishing time and number of races.

		Hip N=72 cases		Knee N=49 cases		Hip or knee N=119 cases	
		HR[a] (95% CI)	HR[b] (95% CI)	HR[a] (95% CI)	HR[b] (95% CI)	HR[a] (95% CI)	HR[b] (95% CI)
Finish time (% of winner time)	**N races**						
≥241	**1**	1.00	1.00	1.00	1.00	1.00	1.00
100–160	**≥5**	3.11 (1.79 to 5.40)	3.18 (1.81 to 5.60)	1.95 (1.02 to 3.74)	1.96 (1.02 to 3.77)	2.73 (1.78 to 4.18)	2.74 (1.78 to 4.23)

[a]Adjusted for age (continuous), gender, education (low, medium, high) and occupation (blue-collar, lower-middle white-collar, high white-collar and entrepreneur).
[b]Adjusted for all variables in the model [a] and, in addition, the following diagnoses: any fracture, any acute injury, any chronic injury, any distortion, any dislocation, any contusion, any neurologic disease, infectious arthritis, diabetes mellitus, and any other endocrine disorder.

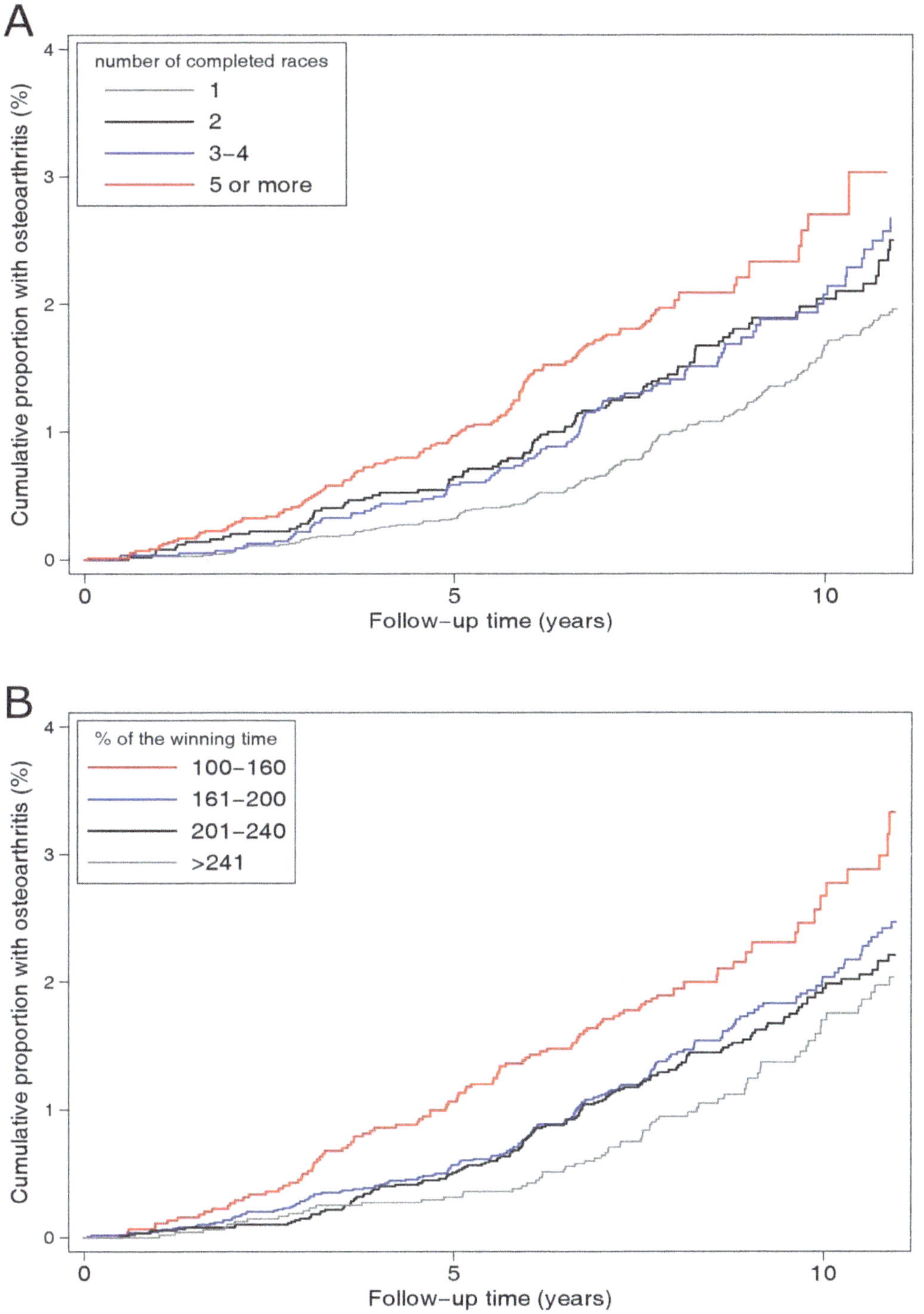

Figure 1. Age- and sex-adjusted survival curves of osteoarthritis by successful races (panel A) and finishing time (panel B).

loss at follow-up and no missing data, and the use of the combination of a diagnostic code for primary osteoarthritis with a surgical procedure code as a measure of a major clinical outcome. We were able to adjust our associations for injuries and exclude those with prevalent osteoarthritis. Our exposures are objective and they are closely related to, albeit proxy measures of, training intensity and duration [39]. Elite skiers do not only perform cross-country skiing exercises but also frequently long-distance running and roller skiing [39], a fact that only conservatively biases our estimates since previous injuries from any sports were identified by the register data.

Our study also has possible limitations. We did not have information on anthropometric measures, and excess body weight increases the risk of both hip and knee osteoarthritis [23]. Nevertheless, participants with many successful races combined with a fast race performance were those who were most likely to have a future diagnosis of severe osteoarthritis: these participants are not likely to have a higher body mass index than participants with low skiing speed. Our inclusion period and exposure assessment was limited to the period 1989 through 1998. Information regarding ski races before 1989 is lacking. The consequence of this conceivable misclassification of our exposures would tend to bias the results toward the null hypothesis. Most participants, however, had their last race during the later part of the inclusion period and this is also illustrated by our supplemental analysis when restricting the cohort to skiers with latest race participation in either of the two last years of the inclusion period. The effect was marginal on our estimates. By our register data, we might have overlooked mild cartilage injuries that might eventually have led to osteoarthritis. Such mild injuries are more likely to have occurred in the knee joint than in the more constrained hip joint [40], and in fact, the higher risk of hip osteoarthritis after intensive exercise in our study was not lower than that for knee osteoarthritis. Moreover, we found no significant evidence of higher frequency of registry reported injuries among participants with many races and a fast skiing speed compared to those with only one slow pace race. Indication bias is a further conceivable limitation if elite athletes had more easy access to health care. Surgery for severe osteoarthritis, however, is not unequally provided in the Swedish tax funded public health care system. The few privately funded operations done in Sweden are not reported to the National Patient register. Theoretically, genetic predisposition to both high physical performance capacity and an increased risk of osteoarthritis might be an underlying mechanism explaining our results. Indeed, both osteoarthritis [41] and exercise level [42] cluster in families and have a modest heritability [41,42]. Nevertheless, linkage and whole-genome analyses have not revealed chromosome sites or individual gene variants in common for osteoarthritis and athletic behaviour [41,43].

We conclude that intensive exercise, at a level required to complete multiple and fast long-distance skiing races, is associated with a higher risk of severe knee and hip osteoarthritis.

Supporting Information

Table S1 Distribution of participants and number of cases with incident severe osteoarthritis of the hip and knee during follow-up by year of the last race.

Author Contributions

Conceived and designed the experiments: KM BF. Performed the experiments: KM BF. Analyzed the data: KM BF. Contributed reagents/materials/analysis tools: KM BF AA. Wrote the paper: KM LB AA HM BF.

References

1. Manson JE, Greenland P, LaCroix AZ, Stefanick ML, Mouton CP, et al. (2002) Walking compared with vigorous exercise for the prevention of cardiovascular events in women. N Engl J Med 347: 716–725.
2. Sui X, LaMonte MJ, Laditka JN, Hardin JW, Chase N, et al. (2007) Cardiorespiratory fitness and adiposity as mortality predictors in older adults. JAMA 298: 2507–2516.
3. Byberg L, Melhus H, Gedeborg R, Sundstrom J, Ahlbom A, et al. (2009) Total mortality after changes in leisure time physical activity in 50 year old men: 35 year follow-up of population based cohort. BMJ 338: b688.
4. Farahmand BY, Ahlbom A, Ekblom O, Ekblom B, Hallmarker U, et al. (2003) Mortality amongst participants in Vasaloppet: a classical long-distance ski race in Sweden. J Intern Med 253: 276–283.
5. Hunter DJ, Eckstein F (2009) Exercise and osteoarthritis. J Anat 214: 197–207.
6. Lohmander LS, Englund PM, Dahl LL, Roos EM (2007) The long-term consequence of anterior cruciate ligament and meniscus injuries: osteoarthritis. Am J Sports Med 35: 1756–1769.
7. Gelber AC, Hochberg MC, Mead LA, Wang NY, Wigley FM, et al. (2000) Joint injury in young adults and risk for subsequent knee and hip osteoarthritis. Ann Intern Med 133: 321–328.
8. Venn G, Billingham ME, Hardingham TE (1995) Increased proteoglycan synthesis in cartilage in experimental canine osteoarthritis does not reflect a permanent change in chondrocyte phenotype. Arthritis Rheum 38: 525–532.
9. Arokoski J, Jurvelin J, Kiviranta I, Tammi M, Helminen HJ (1994) Softening of the lateral condyle articular cartilage in the canine knee joint after long distance (up to 40 km/day) running training lasting one year. Int J Sports Med 15: 254–260.
10. Kiviranta I, Tammi M, Jurvelin J, Arokoski J, Saamanen AM, et al. (1992) Articular cartilage thickness and glycosaminoglycan distribution in the canine knee joint after strenuous running exercise. Clin Orthop Relat Res. pp 302–308.
11. Newton PM, Mow VC, Gardner TR, Buckwalter JA, Albright JP (1997) Winner of the 1996 Cabaud Award. The effect of lifelong exercise on canine articular cartilage. Am J Sports Med 25: 282–287.
12. Hart LE, Haaland DA, Baribeau DA, Mukovozov IM, Sabljic TF (2008) The relationship between exercise and osteoarthritis in the elderly. Clin J Sport Med 18: 508–521.
13. Creamer P, Hochberg MC (1997) Osteoarthritis. Lancet 350: 503–508.
14. Felson DT, Lawrence RC, Dieppe PA, Hirsch R, Helmick CG, et al. (2000) Osteoarthritis: new insights. Part 1: the disease and its risk factors. Ann Intern Med 133: 635–646.
15. Vignon E, Valat JP, Rossignol M, Avouac B, Rozenberg S, et al. (2006) Osteoarthritis of the knee and hip and activity: a systematic international review and synthesis (OASIS). Joint Bone Spine 73: 442–455.
16. Lievense AM, Bierma-Zeinstra SM, Verhagen AP, Bernsen RM, Verhaar JA, et al. (2003) Influence of sporting activities on the development of osteoarthritis of the hip: a systematic review. Arthritis Rheum 49: 228–236.
17. Buckwalter JA, Martin JA (2004) Sports and osteoarthritis. Curr Opin Rheumatol 16: 634–639.
18. Åstrand P-O, Rodahl K (1986) Textbook of Work Physiology. New York: McGraw-Hill Book Company.
19. Lee IM, Paffenbarger Jr. RS (2000) Associations of light, moderate, and vigorous intensity physical activity with longevity. The Harvard Alumni Health Study. Am J Epidemiol 151: 293–299.
20. Forsberg A, Holmberg H, Woxnerud K (2002) Improve your fitness. Farsta.
21. Engström L, Ekblom B, Forsberg A, Koch M, Seger J (1993) Lifestyle - function -health. Ödeshög: Danagårds.
22. Pollock ML (1977) Submaximal and maximal working capacity of elite distance runners. Part I: Cardiorespiratory aspects. Ann N Y Acad Sci 301: 310–322.
23. Lohmander LS, Gerhardsson de Verdier M, Rollof J, Nilsson PM, Engstrom G (2009) Incidence of severe knee and hip osteoarthritis in relation to different measures of body mass: a population-based prospective cohort study. Ann Rheum Dis 68: 490–496.
24. Ludvigsson JF, Otterblad-Olausson P, Pettersson BU, Ekbom A (2009) The Swedish personal identity number: possibilities and pitfalls in healthcare and medical research. Eur J Epidemiol 24: 659–667.
25. Soderman P, Malchau H, Herberts P, Johnell O (2000) Are the findings in the Swedish National Total Hip Arthroplasty Register valid? A comparison between the Swedish National Total Hip Arthroplasty Register, the National Discharge Register, and the National Death Register. J Arthroplasty 15: 884–889.
26. Renstrom P, Johnson RJ (1989) Cross-country skiing injuries and biomechanics. Sports Med 8: 346–370.
27. Lane NE, Oehlert JW, Bloch DA, Fries JF (1998) The relationship of running to osteoarthritis of the knee and hip and bone mineral density of the lumbar spine: a 9 year longitudinal study. J Rheumatol 25: 334–341.
28. Muhlbauer R, Lukasz TS, Faber TS, Stammberger T, Eckstein F (2000) Comparison of knee joint cartilage thickness in triathletes and physically inactive volunteers based on magnetic resonance imaging and three-dimensional analysis. Am J Sports Med 28: 541–546.
29. Felson DT, Niu J, Clancy M, Sack B, Aliabadi P, et al. (2007) Effect of recreational physical activities on the development of knee osteoarthritis in older adults of different weights: the Framingham Study. Arthritis Rheum 57: 6–12.
30. Felson DT, Zhang Y, Hannan MT, Naimark A, Weissman B, et al. (1997) Risk factors for incident radiographic knee osteoarthritis in the elderly: the Framingham Study. Arthritis Rheum 40: 728–733.
31. McAlindon TE, Wilson PW, Aliabadi P, Weissman B, Felson DT (1999) Level of physical activity and the risk of radiographic and symptomatic knee osteoarthritis in the elderly: the Framingham study. Am J Med 106: 151–157.
32. Cheng Y, Macera CA, Davis DR, Ainsworth BE, Troped PJ, et al. (2000) Physical activity and self-reported, physician-diagnosed osteoarthritis: is physical activity a risk factor? J Clin Epidemiol 53: 315–322.
33. Hootman JM, Macera CA, Helmick CG, Blair SN (2003) Influence of physical activity-related joint stress on the risk of self-reported hip/knee osteoarthritis: a new method to quantify physical activity. Prev Med 36: 636–644.
34. Hart DJ, Doyle DV, Spector TD (1999) Incidence and risk factors for radiographic knee osteoarthritis in middle-aged women: the Chingford Study. Arthritis Rheum 42: 17–24.

35. Szoeke CE, Cicuttini FM, Guthrie JR, Clark MS, Dennerstein L (2006) Factors affecting the prevalence of osteoarthritis in healthy middle-aged women: data from the longitudinal Melbourne Women's Midlife Health Project. Bone 39: 1149–1155.
36. Cooper C, Snow S, McAlindon TE, Kellingray S, Stuart B, et al. (2000) Risk factors for the incidence and progression of radiographic knee osteoarthritis. Arthritis Rheum 43: 995–1000.
37. Leitzmann MF, Park Y, Blair A, Ballard-Barbash R, Mouw T, et al. (2007) Physical activity recommendations and decreased risk of mortality. Arch Intern Med 167: 2453–2460.
38. Fransen M, McConnell S (2008) Exercise for osteoarthritis of the knee. Cochrane Database Syst Rev. CD004376.
39. Rusko HK (1992) Development of aerobic power in relation to age and training in cross-country skiers. Med Sci Sports Exerc 24: 1040–1047.
40. Garstang SV, Stitik TP (2006) Osteoarthritis: epidemiology, risk factors, and pathophysiology. Am J Phys Med Rehabil 85: S2–11; quiz S12-14.
41. Spector TD, MacGregor AJ (2004) Risk factors for osteoarthritis: genetics. Osteoarthritis Cartilage 12(Suppl A): S39–44.
42. Carlsson S, Andersson T, Lichtenstein P, Michaelsson K, Ahlbom A (2006) Genetic effects on physical activity: results from the Swedish Twin Registry. Med Sci Sports Exerc 38: 1396–1401.
43. De Moor MH, Spector TD, Cherkas LF, Falchi M, Hottenga JJ, et al. (2007) Genome-wide linkage scan for athlete status in 700 British female DZ twin pairs. Twin Res Hum Genet 10: 812–820.

8

Differential Genetic Regulation of Canine Hip Dysplasia and Osteoarthritis

Zhengkui Zhou[1,2,3], Xihui Sheng[2,3,4], Zhiwu Zhang[5]*, Keyan Zhao[6], Lan Zhu[7], Gang Guo[8], Steve G. Friedenberg[3], Linda S. Hunter[3], Wendy S. Vandenberg-Foels[3], William E. Hornbuckle[3], Ursula Krotscheck[3], Elizabeth Corey[3], Nancy S. Moise[3], Nathan L. Dykes[3], Junya Li[2], Shangzhong Xu[2], Lixin Du[2], Yachun Wang[8], Jody Sandler[9], Gregory M. Acland[10], George Lust[10], Rory J. Todhunter[3]

1 College of Animal Science and Technology, Northwest A&F University, Yangling, China, **2** Institute of Animal Science, Chinese Academy of Agricultural Sciences, Beijing, China, **3** Department of Clinical Sciences, College of Veterinary Medicine, Cornell University, Ithaca, New York, United States of America, **4** Department of Animal Science and Technology, Beijing University of Agriculture, Beijing, China, **5** Institute for Genomic Diversity, Cornell University, Ithaca, New York, United States of America, **6** Department of Computational Biology and Statistics, Cornell University, Ithaca, New York, United States of America, **7** Department of Statistics, Oklahoma State University, Stillwater, Oklahoma, United States of America, **8** Department of Animal Science, China Agricultural University, Beijing, China, **9** Guiding Eyes for the Blind, Yorktown Heights, New York, United States of America, **10** Baker Institute for Animal Health, Cornell University, Ithaca, New York, United States of America

Abstract

Background: Canine hip dysplasia (HD) is a common polygenic trait characterized by hip malformation that results in osteoarthritis (OA). The condition in dogs is very similar to developmental dysplasia of the human hip which also leads to OA.

Methodology/Principal Findings: A total of 721 dogs, including both an association and linkage population, were genotyped. The association population included 8 pure breeds (Labrador retriever, Greyhounds, German Shepherd, Newfoundland, Golden retriever, Rottweiler, Border Collie and Bernese Mountain Dog). The linkage population included Labrador retrievers, Greyhounds, and their crosses. Of these, 366 dogs were genotyped at ~22,000 single nucleotide polymorphism (SNP) loci and a targeted screen across 8 chromosomes with ~3,300 SNPs was performed on 551 dogs (196 dogs were common to both sets). A mixed linear model approach was used to perform an association study on this combined association and linkage population. The study identified 4 susceptibility SNPs associated with HD and 2 SNPs associated with hip OA.

Conclusion/Significance: The identified SNPs included those near known genes (*PTPRD, PARD3B*, and *COL15A1*) reported to be associated with, or expressed in, OA in humans. This suggested that the canine model could provide a unique opportunity to identify genes underlying natural HD and hip OA, which are common and debilitating conditions in both dogs and humans.

Editor: Amanda Ewart Toland, Ohio State University Medical Center, United States of America

Funding: The study was supported by National Institutes of Health (1R21AR055228-01A1), National Science Foundation (#0606461), Chinese National Key Technologies R&D Program (No.2006BAD04A01, No.2006BAD01A10, No.2008BADB2B03, No.2008AA101010), National Department Public Benefit Research Foundation of China (No. nyhyzx07-035), National Natural Science Foundation of China (No. 30871774), Waltham Center for Pet Nutrition, Cornell Advanced Technology in Biotechnology, and the Collaborative Research Grant Program, Department of Clinical Sciences, and the Baker Institute for Animal Health in the College of Veterinary Medicine, Cornell University. The funders had no role in study design, data collection and analysis, decision to publish, or preparation of the manuscript.

Competing Interests: The authors have declared that no competing interests exist.

* E-mail: zz19@cornell.edu

These authors contributed equally to this work.

Introduction

The high relevance of canine diseases to those in humans, and the intrinsic importance of dogs to humans as special companions with a shared environment, makes the dog an attractive species to discover genes underlying the homologous, relevant diseases in humans. An important shared condition is hip dysplasia (HD) and osteoarthritis (OA), both of which are remarkably similar in their clinical expression and pathogenesis in both man and dog [1,2,3]. Shared phenotypic characteristics of human and canine HD are hip joint laxity accompanied by hip subluxation. The secondary effect of HD is OA which results in lameness and physical disability due to hip pain [4,5,6].

Canine HD, a complex trait, is a major veterinary problem occurring with a frequency up to 75% in mixed and pure breed dogs [7] of the approximately 70 million dogs in American households. Human HD, referred to as developmental dysplasia of the hip (DDH), occurs with a frequency ranging from 5~13% [8]. Hip OA prevalence was ~5% for individuals over 60 years old [9,10]. Genetic predisposition and transmission models for DDH have been described [11,12]. A locus linked to DDH spanning a 4 Mb region on HSA17q21 was recently identified [13].

Complex traits and diseases of dogs, many of which are models of homologous human conditions, are now exploitable for molecular genetic dissection [14,15,16,17]. Surveys of single nucleotide polymorphisms (SNPs) within and across dog breeds reveal haplotype structures that are ideal for mapping complex traits and diseases [18]. Targeted genotyping or genome wide association studies have identified the *IGF1* gene responsible for canine body size[19], and genes associated with hair coat variation [20], degenerative myelopathy[21], and the retrogene *RFGF4* associated with the chondrodystrophoid phenotype [22].

Quantitative trait loci (QTL) influencing canine HD have shown some convergence of QTL location across studies and breeds. The challenge remains to identify the mutations that collectively underlie HD and OA in order to understand the molecular pathogenesis of these diseases and develop marker and gene based tests and novel treatments. To improve the resolution of QTL mapping for HD and OA in dogs, we extended our linkage population (Greyhound, Labrador retriever and their crosses) to include six additional breeds to reduce the extent of linkage disequilibrium (LD) between the mutation and SNPs in a genome-wide association study (GWAS). Among the 6 SNPs identified, three of them are adjacent to *COL15A1, PARD3B,* and *PTPRD* that have also been linked, or associated, with human OA. Candidate genes were suggested for the other three SNPs.

Results

The GWAS on a linkage and association joint population identified 2 loci underlying hip OA and 4 loci underlying HD with plausible positional candidate genes (**Table 1 and Figure 1**). The joint population contained 721 dogs from eight breeds and the crosses between two of the breeds (**Figure S1**). Canine HD was measured as the Norberg angle (NA) on all the breeds and crosses (**Figure S2**) and OA was measured only in Labrador retrievers, Greyhounds, and their cross breed offspring. The genotypes included 3,324 SNPs from targeted areas on 8 chromosomes (**Figure S3**) and 21,455 SNPs covering the whole genome (**Figure S4**).

We tested the power of GWAS and the veracity of the genotype calls by mapping two known genes controlling Mendelian coat color. Among the genotyped dogs were 185 Labrador retrievers of which 101 were black, 78 were yellow, and 6 were chocolate. Black Labrador retrievers are fixed at the K locus enabling the genotype at the *MC1R* locus to be expressed [23,24]. The *MC1R* gene causes yellow coat color in Labrador retrievers homozygous for the *MC1R* mutation. *MC1R* is located at 66.692398–66.693344 Mb on canine chromosome CFA05. When GWAS was performed on a binary trait defined as yellow versus the others (black or chocolate), SNP BICF23260560, 2 Kb away from *MC1R*, had the strongest association ($P = 1\times10^{-18}$). The *TYRP1* gene, located at 36.344658–36.363203 Mb on CFA11, causes chocolate coat color in black dogs [25]. When GWAS was performed on a binary trait defined as black versus chocolate, SNP BICF2P1415909, 509 Kb away from the *TYRP1* gene, showed significant association ($P = 3\times10^{-7}$).

For the traits of primary interest, we identified two SNPs associated with hip OA and four SNPs associated with HD in dogs. The associations were determined at the probability threshold at which the declared SNPs could be identified with a distinguishably different distribution compared to the rest of the SNPs [26] on quantile-quantile (QQ) plots. The probability thresholds were 3×10^{-6}, and 5×10^{-5} for HD and hip OA, respectively.

One of the associated SNPs, at base pair 17.299306 Mb on CFA37, is near *PARD3B* which is associated with knee OA in humans [27]. However, *NRP2* lies at 17.293709–17.405724 Mb and is nearer the associated SNP locus than *PARD3B*. There may be as yet unknown genes in this interval. We identified a locus strongly associated ($P = 4.9\times10^{-8}$) with hip OA at 48.092910 Mb on CFA17 (**Figure 1**). The nearest known gene in the region is *REG3A* (47.930245–47.932143 Mb), 160 Kb from this locus, and which encodes a pancreatic secretory protein involved in cell proliferation or differentiation [28].

For canine HD, we discovered 4 SNPs; two of these SNPs were on CFA03 and CFA30 in which QTL for HD had been previously identified [29,30]. and the other two SNPs were on CFA11 where QTL had also been previously identified [30,31]. The locus at 57.517597 Mb on CFA11 is located near *COL15A1* contributing to OA in human patients [32]. The other three SNPs had no known genes associated with human HD or OA. The corresponding positional candidate genes are *EVC, EVC2* [33], *PTPRD* [34], and *MAGP1*[35].

Discussion

Many human and canine diseases are thought to have related causes, and localizing disease genes in dogs is likely to be substantially easier than in humans [36,37]. This is the first SNP-based, GWAS reported for canine HD and hip OA in dogs. Our goals were to resolve QTL mapping to near gene level while

Table 1. The associated SNPs and nearby candidate genes for hip dysplasia and osteoarthritis[a].

SNP	Chr	Position (bp)	Allele (Risk/nonrisk)	*P* value	MAF	Distance to gene (Mb)	Notable Nearby Gene
Hip dysplasia							
BICF2S2459425	3	74720873	G/A	6.74×10^{-8}	0.354	0.900	*EVC, EVC2*
BICF2P550340	11	32935770	T/A	3.27×10^{-6}	0.220	0.64	*PTPRD*
BICF2S23432143	11	57517597	G/A	9.35×10^{-7}	0.394	1.577	*COL15A1*
BICF2P799261	30	13883057	C/T	1.06×10^{-6}	0.135	0.109	*MAGP1*
Osteoarthritis							
BICF2G630205523	17	48092910	T/G	4.90×10^{-8}	0.277	0.060	*REG3A*
BICF2P1242205	37	17299306	C/A	4.20×10^{-5}	0.3148	0.070	*PARD3B*

[a]The SNPs are categorized by traits (hip dysplasia or osteoarthritis). The chromosome (Chr), position in base pair (bp), minor allele frequency (MAF), and distance to the candidate genes are listed for each SNP.

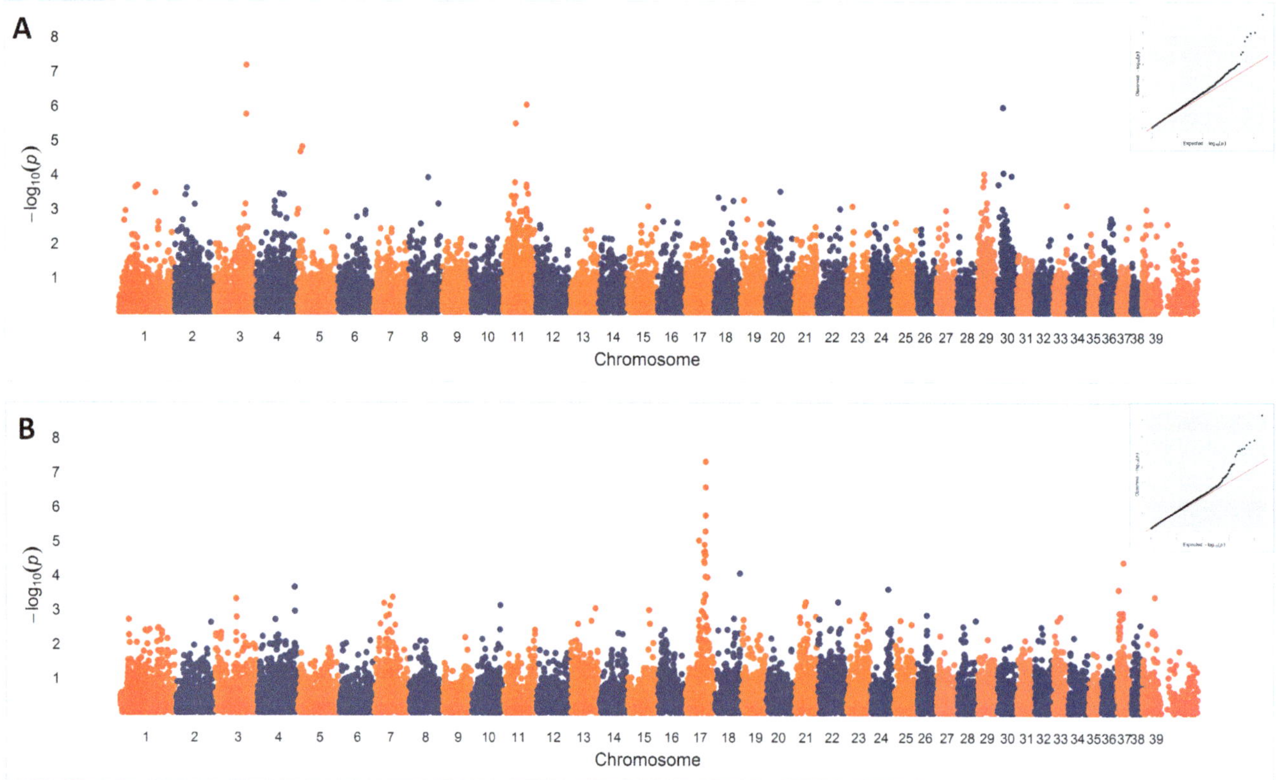

Figure 1. Manhattan and Quantile-Quantile (QQ) plots. The plots summarize the genome-wide association results for hip dysplasia (A) and hip osteoarthritis (B). The genome-wide *P* values ($-\log_{10}$ *P*) of the F test for the SNP effect are plotted against position on each chromosome. The inset shows QQ plots of the observed *P* values versus the expected *P* values under the null hypothesis that there was no association.

maintaining low risk of false positive findings (FPF) [38,39]. In so doing, we may have overlooked some contributory loci. One of our strategies to balance the resolution and FPF was to use both ancient LD and genetic linkage retained in the crossing process. A proportion of association in our study relied on genetic linkage (recent LD) retained in the 4-generation crosses between Labrador retrievers and Greyhounds. These crosses composed 30% and 20% of the total dogs in the genome-wide screen and customized fine mapping study, respectively. The down side of the linkage population is that the extent of recent LD is much broader than ancient LD [40]. The associated SNPs we declared might be a few genes away from the causal mutations. The advantage of the linkage population is that it was used to break down the spurious associations due to population structure and cryptic relationships.

To further eliminate the potential associations due to population structure, we fitted the first 10 principal components (PCs) derived from all the SNP genotypes as covariates to capture false association due to the population structure. This sacrificed statistical power for any mutations with effects confounded with the population structure in this study. The population structure was clearly revealed by the first two PCs derived from each set of SNPs. All the dogs from within a pure breed were clustered together in the scatter plots of the first and second PCs. All the F_1 dogs of Greyhound/Labrador retriever breedings were positioned genetically between their respective parental breeds. The back-cross of the F_1 to Labrador retriever was closer to Labrador retrievers and the backcross of F_1 to Greyhound was genetically closer to Greyhound as expected (**Fig. S5**). Both sets of SNP genotypes showed substructure within the Labrador retriever breed. The substructure reflected the multiple sources of Labrador retriever for these studies; cohorts from the Guiding Eyes for Blind in Yorktown Heights NY, the Baker Institute for Animal Health at the College of Veterinary Medicine, and the dogs admitted to the Cornell University Hospital for Animals for diagnosis and treatment of lameness related to HD and hip OA.

To eliminate the spurious associations due to cryptic relationships among individual dogs, we fitted a random effect for dog groups clustered by kinship among individual dogs [41]. The kinship was derived from all the SNPs to capture unequal relatedness among dogs. This statistical model had higher statistical power than the approach that considered population structure only and the approach that considered both population structure and individual relationship without grouping [41]. The statistical power of the linkage population was 65% for a causal mutation which explained 2% of the phenotypic variation when using the linkage population only under assumption that the minor allele frequency (MAF) of the mutation is at a middle level (30%) [41].

The MAF of the SNPs from each set followed a uniform distribution (**Fig. S4**). Both sets of SNPs were informative with respective to heterozygosity. The heterozygosities showed a bimodal distribution with two peaks toward 0 and 0.5, respectively. This trend is similar to practical [42,43,44] and theoretical observations [45] under assumptions of the neutral theory. The mean and median heterozygosity of the 21,455 Illumina SNPs were 0.30 and 0.32, respectively. There were 4.3% SNPs with heterozygosity greater than 0.5 and 6.4% SNPs with heterozygosity less than 0.02. The mean and median heterozygosity of the customized 3,324 SNPs were 0.26 and 0.28, respectively including 2% SNPs with heterozygosity greater than 0.5 and 7.5% SNPs with heterozygosity less than 0.02.

Although the associated SNPs declared in this study had support from previous QTL linkage mapping, the current study had limited statistical power, and consequently revealed only a subset of the QTLs (10–20) reported previously [29,30,46], which indicated that both HD and OA were underpinned by a complex genetic model with multiple QTLs, instead of a simple genetic model for traits such as body size [47]. We previously reported HD loci through linkage analysis in a Labrador retriever/Greyhound cross breed pedigree at 63 and 64 cM on CFA11 and 18 cM on CFA30 [30]. The associated loci on CFA11 and 30 for HD in **Table 1** refine the location of the loci from linkage analysis. In our previous linkage studies for HD, we used 3 HD phenotypes including the NA and their PCs. We also used chromosome-wide, not genome-wide, permutation to establish the significance of the LOD scores. In this report, we had the most power for the NA as all the dogs had this measurement. Other loci showed possible association but we declared only those loci that had strong association signals and that had support from previous studies. Several loci linked to HD in German Shepherd Dogs were reported on CFA03 including one at ~79 Mb [29] but these may not be identical to the CFA03 locus in our report.

Hip OA is heritable in the Labrador retriever/Greyhound cross breeds [48] and Portuguese Water Dog [46]. Linkage was found to hip OA in the Labrador retriever cross breed pedigree [49] but a significant association in the current GWAS was not discovered in the linked regions. The hip OA (acetabular osteophytes) locus reported on CFA03 in Portuguese Water Dogs was between ~42 and 46 Mb [50] which was far from the SNP locus we reported at ~74 Mb for HD. Similarly, although GWAS for human height only found QTLs explaining 5% of total variation, the heritability of human height was ~ =80%) [51].

Sample size (dogs with both genotype and phenotype), sample selection from the available population, inclusion of different dogs in the linkage studies, GWAS and fine mapping (each of which only included a subset of common dogs), marker density and distribution, and marker informativeness each both enhanced and limited the statistical power of the current study. The majority of the customized SNPs were focused on the targeted regions. A few of them were spread to cover the remainder of the LOD score profile in our previous linkage studies. The power to detect association for hip OA in our report was a limiting factor as only 99 dogs were available for this analysis and only the Labrador retrievers and the crosses to Greyhounds were included for this phenotype. Within dog breeds on average, LD is extensive (0.5–1.0 Mb), whereas across breeds, the extent of LD is less than 10 Kb [18,19,52]. Labrador retrievers are diversified even within breed as illustrated in **Figure S5**. The LD, on average, was less than 0.3 (R^2) for a pair of SNPs 30 Kb and 10 Kb apart in Labrador retriever and across all breeds respectively (**Fig. S4**). The mean and median marker interval for the genome-wide SNPs was 107 Kb and 70 Kb, respectively. The mean and median marker interval for the 3,324 customized SNPs was 150 Kb and 46 Kb, respectively (**Fig. S4**). This density, in hindsight, especially for the Illumina Beadarray, was not sufficient to take full advantage of the genetic architecture in the whole genome. We expect that the current population would have more statistical power to reveal more SNPs associated with HD and hip OA if more dense markers were applied through new genotyping technology such as application of the version 2 canine Illumina Beadarray or genotyping by sequencing [53] and if more dogs were included in the GWAS.

The statistical model in which we fitted SNP genotypes across all breeds had the advantage of identifying mutations segregating in all the breeds and in the same linkage phase to the associated SNPs. However, the statistical model had low statistical power for a QTN that was in a different linkage phase from Labrador retrievers which comprised ~50% of the individuals. An alternative mapping approach would be to treat the SNPs as confounded within breed. This statistical approach may be necessary to discover private SNPs associated with causal genes for a particular breed.

Despite the loss of statistical power in an effort to avoid false positive findings, six SNPs were identified with association. Among the positional candidate genes, *EVC* and *EVC2*, near SNPs associated with HD on CFA03, cause Ellis–van Creveld syndrome (EVC, MIM 225500) [33], a rare autosomal recessive chondrodysplasia also called chondroectodermal or mesoectodermal dysplasia. The two genes, 2.6 Kb apart, encode novel proteins with no significant homology to each other or to any other proteins. *PTPRD* (protein tyrosine phosphatase receptor type D gene), associated with HD on CFA11, encodes a member of the protein tyrosine phosphate (PTP) family. Protein tyrosine phosphatases (*PTPs*) are signaling molecules that regulate cell growth, differentiation, mitotic cycle, and oncogenic transformation. *PTPRD* belongs to the family of type IIa receptor-like protein tyrosine phosphatases[54]. It is highly expressed in human knee OA cartilage and is associated with restless legs syndrome [34,55].

On CFA11, SNP BICF2S23432143 at 57.517597 Mb is near nicotinamide adenine dinucleotide (*NAD*) and a gene at ~57.6 Mb identified as bA113O24.1 which is similar to IGF receptor binding proteins, based on sequence similarity. This is a positional candidate gene because *IGF1* is an anabolic growth factor for chondrocytes and *IGF*1 polymorphisms are responsible for size variation in Portuguese Water dogs and other breeds [19]. Reduced growth rate of Labrador retrievers through caloric restriction reduced phenotypic expression of HD and the accompanying hip OA [56,57,58]. *COL15A1*, 1.58 Mb away from SNP BICF2S23432143 on CFA11,was reported as a new positional candidate gene in genome-wide expression profiling in human OA articular cartilage[32]. *COL15A1* encodes a protein which is prominently expressed in newly-formed blood vessels indicating a possible role in angiogenesis and neovascularization. Femoral caput vascularization must occur before mineralization can proceed in the secondary center of ossification [59,60].

An interesting positional candidate gene for HD near SNP BIC2P799261 on CFA30 is microfibril-associated protein 1 (*MFAP1*) which encodes the MFAP1 protein[61]. The microfibril associated proteins and the smaller microfibrillar associated glycoproteins appear to play roles in microfibril structure and function. Microfibrils are found in the extracellular matrices of most tissues where they serve several functional roles, including the binding and sequestration of growth factors, supplying informational signals through receptor signaling, and providing the basic structural elements for elastic fiber assembly which is important to joint capsule and ligament function. The nonglycosylated *MFAP1*, a 57 kDa protein processed to 32 kDa, was immunolocalized to microfibrils in aorta, nuchal ligament, and zonule [61]. *MFAP1* is located near *FBN1* and mutations in both genes are causal for Marfan syndrome. We are especially interested in the microfibrillary composition of the fibrous hip joint capsule as hip laxity is an important contributor, or predisposing factor, to HD. A mutation in intron 30 of *FBN2* on CFA11contributed to HD in dogs homozygous for the deletion[62]. In the cited report [62], as the degree of HD worsened in Labrador retrievers, the *FBN2* mRNA isolated from their hip capsule increased significantly consistent with developing OA. Those dogs with incipient hip OA had significantly increased *FBN2* mRNA in their hip joint capsules compared to those dogs without OA. However, dogs homozygous for the *FBN2* deletion haplotype had significantly less *FBN2* mRNA in their femoral head articular cartilage. This gene expression analysis was confounded by the incipient hip OA in HD dogs but the current data warrant further exploration for its role in HD.

SNP BICF2G630205523 on CFA17 was strongly associated with hip OA suggesting that the nearest gene *REG3A* may also play a role in canine hip OA. *REG3A* (regenerating islet derived gamma 3) was originally identified as a pancreatitis associated protein (*PAP*) released by the acini during acute pancreatitis. It is a secreted C-type lectin, reported to be upregulated in primary hepatocellular carcinomas [28]. Several functional studies demonstrated that *REG3A* may be involved in cell recognition and adhesion and in the protection of cells from oxidative stress-induced apoptosis[63]. *REG3A* possesses anti-inflammatory properties and is a signaling molecule in the *MAPK* pathway. This association offers a potential mechanism by which chondrocytes might regulate their response to injury and thereby influence the progression of hip OA.

In a GWAS for knee OA in women, SNP rs1207421, significantly associated with OA, mapped to HSA2q33(chr2:205976100) located in the *PARD3B* (par-3 partitioning defective 3 homolog B) gene [27]. In our study, its homologous gene in dog was associated with hip OA. In humans, rs1207421 is also adjacent to a previously reported linkage peak for hip OA at HSA2q31.1 in humans [64]. Moreover, this SNP was positioned in the middle of a genome-wide linkage peak mapped in extended early-onset OA families [65] making it likely that the genomic region near this marker harbors OA-susceptibility genes.

The identification of functional mutations in these candidate genes associated with canine HD or hip OA further suggest that the dog is suited for comparative mapping of homologous complex traits and diseases in humans [19,21,22]. No genes have yet been associated with DDH, yet positional candidate genes for HD in the dogs in our study included loci reported to be associated with human OA either through GWAS or expression studies. This raises the question of whether some of the loci associated with human hip OA contributed to a primary malformation of the hip that led to secondary hip OA. As many as 20–50% of people with hip OA in middle age had undetected DDH as neonates [9]. The earlier a developmental disease is expressed, the more likely it is to be genetic in origin assuming that primary trauma has been ruled out as a contributing factor. The secondary OA superimposed on a primary heritable defect itself affects gene expression which should be considered in microarray, transcriptome sequencing, or individual quantitative reverse transcriptase expression studies as we found in our effort to measure *FBN2* expression in hip tissues with incipient OA as a result of prior HD. Our data suggested that the rapidity of the articular response to injury seems to also be governed genetically and independently of the primary trait.

Materials and Methods

Dog Populations and Radiographic Methods

A total of 721 dogs from the 2,716 dogs in the HD archive [66] for this study contained a linkage population and an association population (**Figure S1** and **Table S1**). The linkage population consisted of two breeds (dysplastic Labrador retriever and non dysplastic Greyhound) and their crosses. The association population was comprised of eight breeds (Labrador retriever, Greyhound, German Shepherd, Newfoundland, Golden retriever, Rottweiler, Border Collie and Bernese Mountain Dog).

The pelves of these dogs were radiographed following physical maturity (i.e. older than 8 months of age) (**Figure 2**). Hip dysplasia was measured by the Norberg angle (NA) which is a continuous trait ranging from ~50° (a subluxated hip) to ~120° (a phenotypically unaffected hip), see **Figure S2** and **Table S2–S3**. The NA was treated as a continuous trait in the statistical modeling. The worst hip (the minimum) between measurements on left and right from each dog was used in the statistical analyses.

The presence or absence of hip OA was determined on dysplastic Labrador retrievers and their crosses to unaffected Greyhounds. Hip OA was defined radiographically, as osteophytes on the acetabular rim and periphery of the femoral head and neck or at autopsy, as fibrillation and erosion of the articular cartilage of the femoral head and acetabulum, increased synovial fluid volume, and hypertrophy of the teres ligament and fibrous joint capsule [67]. We used a synovial fluid volume >0.3 ml, a displacement volume of the round ligament of the femoral head >0.8 ml, and a perifoveal articular cartilage lesion of fibrillation or ulceration as incontrovertible evidence of the presence of hip OA. Hip OA was defined in two ways. The majority of dogs used in the analyses for hip OA had postmortem evidence of OA which was defined above and by Lust et al. [67,68]. A small portion of dogs were scored from the radiographic evidence of hip OA based on the OFA hip score assigned by a board certified radiologist. Dogs with any acetabular osteophytes, osteophytes around the femoral head or enthesiophytes on the femoral neck were determined to have hip OA [69]. Based on these gross observations, we then assigned dogs affected with hip OA as cases and unaffected as controls. Of the 99 dogs evaluated for hip OA, 50 were unaffected (controls) and 49 had OA (cases) (**Table S4**). The coat color was recorded for the 185 Labrador retriever dogs. Cornell Institutional Animal Care and Use Committee approved all of the studies (Protocol approval numbers were 2005-0151 (Cornell Medical Genetic Archive) and 2006-0187 (Hip Dysplasia and OA Genetics).

Selection of Dogs and SNP Genotyping

The 721 dogs were genotyped on two different SNP platforms. One was the Illumina CanineSNP20 Bead array containing ~ 22,000 loci distributed across the entire canine genome. The other array was customized with ~3,500 SNPs chosen from the regions in eight chromosomes (2, 3, 5, 11, 18, 19, 29, and 30) harboring QTLs for HD and some for hip OA identified in previous studies [30,49,70]. The SNPs for custom genotyping were chosen from the CanFam 2.0 database provided by the Broad Institute at Harvard/MIT (http://www.broadinstitute.org/science/projects/mammals-models/dog/dog-snps-canfam-20). The custom SNPs were chosen to maximize the number of Labrador retriever origin SNPs and intragenic SNPs. The physical order of the custom SNPs selected were alternated by breed to span the QTL linkage interval defined by the LOD score profile (personal communication, Kerstin Lindblad-Toh, 2007). The QTL intervals for chromosome 05, 18, and 19, were linked to hip OA [49] while those on chromosomes 02, 03, 11, 29 and 30 were linked to HD based on microsatellite screening [70]. The SNPs for genotyping were chosen to be denser under the LOD score linkage peak and less dense on either side of the estimated peak LOD score position (**Figure. S3**).

We selected one SNP every ~45 Kb in the following locations on the canine genome: CFA03, between 55–75 Mb; CFA11, between 4–31 and 38–65 Mb; CFA 29, between 9–31 Mb; CFA30, between 13–39 Mb. Each of these chromosomes including CFA11 and 29 harbored at least 1 QTL contributing to canine HD. In aggregate, these regions comprise 122 Mb. From the Broad canine SNP data base, the most valid SNPs (those identified by capitalization) were chosen. Where ever possible, we included SNPs derived from Labrador retrievers as Labrador

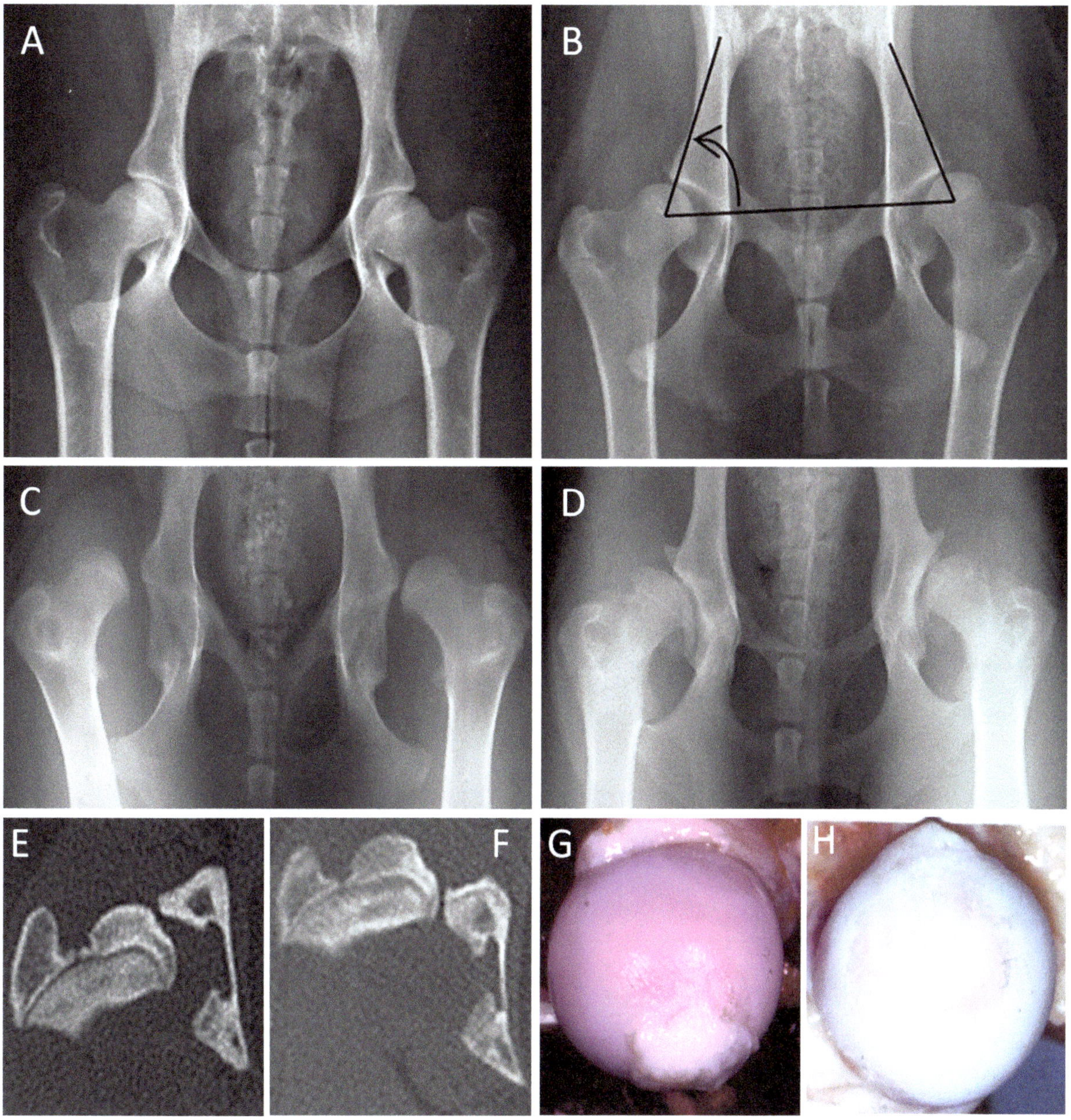

Figure 2. Radiographs and computed tomography (CT) images of the canine hip joint. A: Unaffected hips. B: Moderate hip dysplasia. The arrow indicates the included angle which is the Norberg angle. C: Severely affected hip dysplasia with luxation. D: Severe secondary osteoarthritis as a result of previous hip dysplasia. E: A CT image of a hip with moderate hip dysplasia illustrating the subluxation and impingement of the femoral head on the lateral acetabular rim when the dog is imaged with its hips in a weight bearing position. F: A CT image of a dog with severe hip dysplasia characterized by complete luxation. G: The gross appearance of a femoral head from a hip joint moderately affected with HD and early secondary OA with articular cartilage fibrillation in the perifoveal area and hypertrophy of the teres ligament. H: A femoral head from a severely affected hip with full thickness articular cartilage erosion and loss of the teres ligament due to mechanical abrasion and enzymatic degradation. These affected hips are painful.

retrievers or their crosses comprised the most common breeds among our genotypes dogs. We attempted to select at least one SNP within the boundaries of each gene in our target regions. Additionally, among the 902 genes in our target regions, we selected SNPs within 534 of the 902 genes in our target regions ; the remainder had no intragenic SNPs in the Broad database.

In total, we selected 2,799 SNPs across the four chromosomes described above. By breed, these SNPs represent: 31% boxer, 26% poodle, 5% Labrador retriever (enriched from 1% in the Broad database), 4% German shepherd, and the remainder miscellaneous breeds (e.g., Bedlington terrier, Portuguese water dog, Akita).

To fine map the hip OA locus, we selected 592 SNPs on 4 chromosomes at 4 loci: CFA02 between 10–60 Mb, CFA05 between 40–70 Mb, CFA18 between 3–30 Mb, and CFA19 between 3–15 Mb. These correspond to regions where our microsatellite screen showed association with hip OA. On average, we selected 1 SNP every 181 Kb. These SNPs arose from 13% Labradors, 11% Boxers, 8% Malamutes, 8% Portuguese water dogs, and 60% other breeds. Of the 861 genes in these regions, we had SNPs within 377 genes or 44% of them. The SNPs were selected from the Broad Harvard/MIT web site. The customized genotyping used Molecular Inversion Probe Technology [71].

There were 366 and 551 dogs genotyped with the Illumina array and the customized array, respectively. Genotypes were obtained on 196 dogs across both arrays. All the genotyped dogs had at least one phenotype for HD. However, only 99 dogs were phenotyped for OA. The 48 dogs with OA phenotype that were genotyped on the customized array were included in the dogs that were genotyped on the Illumina array (**Table S1, S2, S3**). DNA was extracted from whole blood collected in Na-EDTA using either phenol-chloroform or the Puregene (Gentra) protocol [30]. Physical locations of candidate genes were based on the UCSC web browser (http://genome.ucsc.edu/cgi-bin/hgGateway).

The majority (92.3%) of the Illumina SNPs had call rate of 100%. There was 99.46% of SNPs with call rate above 95%. For the customized SNP array, 84.9% of SNPs had a call rate above 95%. SNPs with missing calls above 45% were removed. We also removed SNPs with minor allele frequency (MAF) below 1% [72]. The final analysis contained 21,455 SNPs for the Illumina array and 3,324 SNPs for the customized array. For the Illumina SNP array, the mean and median MAF were 0.2394 and 0.2399, respectively. For the customized SNP array, the mean and median MAF were 0.2205 and 0.2110, respectively (**Fig. S4**). There were 111 SNPs in common between the two sets of SNP arrarys. The concordance rate was 99.999% of the 111 common SNPs genotyped on 196 dogs.

Statistical analysis

A compressed mixed linear model was used for the association analysis. This approach is superior to other approaches with respect to minimizing false positive finding due to population structure and cryptic relationships accompanied by increased statistical power [41]. The fixed effects in the model included sex, age and the first ten principal components (PCs) derived from all the SNPs. The PCs were calculated from the numerical genotypes coded as 0 or 2 for the two homozygote classes, or 1 for the heterozygote class. Because the first two PCs captured the breed structure (**Figure S5**), we did not include breed as a co-factor in the model. The random effect was the groups clustered based on the kinship among individual dogs. The kinship among individuals was derived from all the SNPs. Individuals were clustered into groups which contained 3 individual dogs on average based on the optimization from our previous study [41].

The genotype of each SNP was treated as a fixed effect, one SNP at a time. The *P* values resulting from the *F* test were used to indicate the association strength. The majority of the SNPs from the two sets were analyzed independently. The 111 common SNPs underwent a joint analysis by combining all 721 dogs together. For the 196 dogs genotyped with both SNP sets, there were two sets of PCs and kinships. We used the SNPs from the Illumina array in the joint analysis. As the PCs derived from the two DNA arrays do not exactly reflect the same genetic components, we fitted PC nested within the two SNP sets. For the gap in kinship between the dogs genotyped on only one of the arrays, we used their pedigree based kinship. We used the visual approach [26] to determine whether there was an excess of significant associations by comparing the *P* values for the association tests to those expected under the null distribution using Quantile-Quantile (QQ) plots.

Supporting Information

Figure S1 The linkage and association joint population.

Figure S2 Distribution of phenotyped dogs on Norberg Angle measurements.

Figure S3 The chromosome coverage of the customized SNP array.

Figure S4 The properties of single nucleotide polymorphisms (SNPs)

Figure S5 Population structure of linkage and association joint population.

Table S1 Number of dogs categorized by breed, phenotype and SNP platforms.

Table S2 Distribution of Norberg Angle measurements (number of dogs).

Table S3 Number of dogs with Norberg Angle measurements categorized by study population and SNP array.

Table S4 Total number of dogs with hip osteoarthritis _OA_ records categorized by study population and SNP array.

Author Contributions

Conceived and designed the experiments: Z. Zhang GL RJT. Performed the experiments: GG SGF LSH WSVF EC NSM. Analyzed the data: Z. Zhou XS. Contributed reagents/materials/analysis tools: KZ LZ GG SGF LSH WSVF WEH UK EC NSM NLD JL SX LD YW JS GMA GL RJT. Wrote the paper: Z. Zhang Z. Zhou RJT.

References

1. Nakamura S, Ninomiya S, Nakamura T (1989) Primary osteoarthritis of the hip joint in Japan. Clin Orthop Relat Res. pp 190–196.
2. Yoshimura N, Campbell L, Hashimoto T, Kinoshita H, Okayasu T, et al. (1998) Acetabular dysplasia and hip osteoarthritis in Britain and Japan. Br J Rheumatol 37: 1193–1197.
3. Parentin F, Sangalli A, Mottes M, Perissutti P (2001) Stickler syndrome and vitreoretinal degeneration: correlation between locus mutation and vitreous phenotype. Apropos of a case. Graefes Arch Clin Exp Ophthalmol 239: 316–319.
4. Clements DN, Carter SD, Innes JF, Ollier WE (2006) Genetic basis of secondary osteoarthritis in dogs with joint dysplasia. Am J Vet Res 67: 909–918.
5. Smith GK, Mayhew PD, Kapatkin AS, McKelvie PJ, Shofer FS, et al. (2001) Evaluation of risk factors for degenerative joint disease associated with hip dysplasia in German Shepherd Dogs, Golden Retrievers, Labrador Retrievers, and Rottweilers. J Am Vet Med Assoc 219: 1719–1724.
6. Todhunter RJ, Grohn YT, Bliss SP, Wilfand A, Williams AJ, et al. (2003) Evaluation of multiple radiographic predictors of cartilage lesions in the hip joints of eight-month-old dogs. Am J Vet Res 64: 1472–1478.
7. Breur G, Lust G, Todhunter R (2001) Genetics of hip dysplasia and other orthopedic diseases. In: The genetics of the dog (eds A Ruvinsky and J Sampson). Wallingford, Oxon, UK: CAB International. pp 267–298.

8. Jacobsen S (2006) Adult hip dysplasia and osteoarthritis. Studies in radiology and clinical epidemiology. Acta Orthop Suppl 77: 1–37.
9. Weinstein SL (1987) Natural history of congenital hip dislocation (CDH) and hip dysplasia. Clin Orthop Relat Res. pp 62–76.
10. Jacobsen S, Sonne-Holm S (2005) Hip dysplasia: a significant risk factor for the development of hip osteoarthritis. A cross-sectional survey. Rheumatology (Oxford) 44: 211–218.
11. Cilliers HJ, Beighton P (1990) Beukes familial hip dysplasia: An autosomal dominant entity. American Journal of Medical Genetics 36: 386–390.
12. Stevenson DA, Mineau G, Kerber RA, Viskochil DH, Schaefer C, et al. (2009) Familial predisposition to developmental dysplasia of the hip. J Pediatr Orthop 29: 463–466.
13. Feldman G, Dalsey C, Fertala K, Azimi D, Fortina P, et al. (2009) The Otto Aufranc Award: Identification of a 4 Mb region on chromosome 17q21 linked to developmental dysplasia of the hip in one 18-member, multigeneration family. Clin Orthop Relat Res 468: 337–344.
14. Lark KG, Chase K, Sutter NB (2006) Genetic architecture of the dog: sexual size dimorphism and functional morphology. Trends in Genetics 22: 537–544.
15. Ostrander EA, Wayne RK (2005) The canine genome Genome Res 15: 1706–1716.
16. Mosher DS, Quignon P, Bustamante CD, Sutter NB, Mellersh CS, et al. (2007) A Mutation in the Myostatin Gene Increases Muscle Mass and Enhances Racing Performance in Heterozygote Dogs. PLoS Genet 3: e79.
17. Parker HG, Ostrander EA (2005) Canine Genomics and Genetics: Running with the Pack. PLoS Genet 1: e58.
18. Lindblad-Toh K, Wade CM, Mikkelsen TS, Karlsson EK, Jaffe DB, et al. (2005) Genome sequence, comparative analysis and haplotype structure of the domestic dog. Nature 438: 803–819.
19. Sutter NB, Bustamante CD, Chase K, Gray MM, Zhao K, et al. (2007) A Single IGF1 Allele Is a Major Determinant of Small Size in Dogs. Science 316: 112–115.
20. Cadieu E, Neff MW, Quignon P, Walsh K, Chase K, et al. (2009) Coat Variation in the Domestic Dog Is Governed by Variants in Three Genes. Science 326: 150–153.
21. Awano T, Johnson GS, Wade CM, Katz ML, Johnson GC, et al. (2009) Genome-wide association analysis reveals a SOD1 mutation in canine degenerative myelopathy that resembles amyotrophic lateral sclerosis. Proc Natl Acad Sci U S A 106: 2794–2799.
22. Parker HG, VonHoldt BM, Quignon P, Margulies EH, Shao S, et al. (2009) An Expressed Fgf4 Retrogene Is Associated with Breed-Defining Chondrodysplasia in Domestic Dogs. Science 325: 995–998.
23. Kerns JA, Cargill EJ, Clark LA, Candille SI, Berryere TG, et al. (2007) Linkage and segregation analysis of black and brindle coat color in domestic dogs. Genetics 176: 1679–1689.
24. Candille SI, Kaelin CB, Cattanach BM, Yu B, Thompson DA, et al. (2007) A -defensin mutation causes black coat color in domestic dogs. Science 318: 1418–1423.
25. Schmutz SM, Berryere TG, Goldfinch AD (2002) TYRP1 and MC1R genotypes and their effects on coat color in dogs. Mamm Genome 13: 380–387.
26. Rivadeneira F, Styrkarsdottir U, Estrada K, Halldorsson BV, Hsu YH, et al. (2009) Twenty bone-mineral-density loci identified by large-scale meta-analysis of genome-wide association studies. Nat Genet 41: 1199–1206.
27. Valdes AM, Loughlin J, Timms KM, van Meurs JJ, Southam L, et al. (2008) Genome-wide association scan identifies a prostaglandin-endoperoxide synthase 2 variant involved in risk of knee osteoarthritis. Am J Hum Genet 82: 1231–1240.
28. Choi B, Suh Y, Kim WH, Christa L, Park J, et al. (2007) Downregulation of regenerating islet-derived 3 alpha (REG3A) in primary human gastric adenocarcinomas. Exp Mol Med 39: 796–804.
29. Marschall Y, Distl O (2007) Mapping quantitative trait loci for canine hip dysplasia in German Shepherd dogs. Mammalian Genome 18: 861–870.
30. Todhunter RJ, Mateescu R, Lust G, Burton-Wurster NI, Dykes NL, et al. (2005) Quantitative trait loci for hip dysplasia in a cross-breed canine pedigree. Mammalian Genome 16: 720–730.
31. Zhu L, Zhang Z, Feng F, Schweitzer P, Phavaphutanon J, et al. (2008) Single nucleotide polymorphisms refine QTL intervals for hip joint laxity in dogs. Anim Genet 39: 141–146.
32. Karlsson C, Dehne T, Lindahl A, Brittberg M, Pruss A, et al. (2010) Genome-wide expression profiling reveals new candidate genes associated with osteoarthritis. Osteoarthritis Cartilage 18: 581–592.
33. Tompson SW, Ruiz-Perez VL, Blair HJ, Barton S, Navarro V, et al. (2007) Sequencing EVC and EVC2 identifies mutations in two-thirds of Ellis-van Creveld syndrome patients. Hum Genet 120: 663–670.
34. Schormair B, Kemlink D, Roeske D, Eckstein G, Xiong L, et al. (2008) PTPRD (protein tyrosine phosphatase receptor type delta) is associated with restless legs syndrome. Nat Genet 40: 946–948.
35. Liu W, Faraco J, Qian C, Francke U (1997) The gene for microfibril-associated protein-1 (MFAP1) is located several megabases centromeric to FBN1 and is not mutated in Marfan syndrome. Hum Genet 99: 578–584.
36. Karlsson EK, Baranowska I, Wade CM, Salmon Hillbertz NH, Zody MC, et al. (2007) Efficient mapping of mendelian traits in dogs through genome-wide association. Nat Genet 39: 1321–1328.
37. Karlsson EK, Lindblad-Toh K (2008) Leader of the pack: gene mapping in dogs and other model organisms. Nat Rev Genet 9: 713–725.
38. Moonesinghe R, Khoury MJ, Janssens AC (2007) Most published research findings are false-but a little replication goes a long way. PLoS Med 4: e28.
39. Ioannidis JPA (2005) Why most published research findings are false. Plos Medicine 2: 696–701.
40. Lou XY, Todhunter RJ, Lin M, Lu Q, Liu T, et al. (2003) The extent and distribution of linkage disequilibrium in a multi-hierarchic outbred canine pedigree. Mamm Genome 14: 555–564.
41. Zhang Z, Ersoz E, Lai CQ, Todhunter RJ, Tiwari HK, et al. (2010) Mixed linear model approach adapted for genome-wide association studies. Nat Genet 42: 355–360.
42. Makarieva AM (2001) Variance of protein heterozygosity in different species of mammals with respect to the number of loci studied. Heredity 87: 41–51.
43. Higashino A, Osada N, Suto Y, Hirata M, Kameoka Y, et al. (2009) Development of an integrative database with 499 novel microsatellite markers for Macaca fascicularis. BMC Genet 10: 24.
44. Rogers J, Garcia R, Shelledy W, Kaplan J, Arya A, et al. (2006) An initial genetic linkage map of the rhesus macaque (Macaca mulatta) genome using human microsatellite loci. Genomics 87: 30–38.
45. Fuerst PA, Chakraborty R, Nei M (1977) Statistical studies on protein polymorphism in natural populations. I. Distribution of single locus heterozygosity. Genetics 86: 455–483.
46. Chase K, Lawler DF, Adler FR, Ostrander EA, Lark KG (2004) Bilaterally asymmetric effects of quantitative trait loci (QTLs): QTLs that affect laxity in the right versus left coxofemoral (hip) joints of the dog (Canis familiaris). Am J Med Genet A 124: 239–247.
47. Boyko AR, Quignon P, Li L, Schoenebeck JJ, Degenhardt JD, et al. A simple genetic architecture underlies morphological variation in dogs. PLoS Biol 8: e1000451.
48. Bliss S, Todhunter RJ, Quaas R, Casella G, Wu R, et al. (2002) Quantitative genetics of traits associated with hip dysplasia in a canine pedigree constructed by mating dysplastic Labrador Retrievers with unaffected Greyhounds. Am J Vet Res 63: 1029–1035.
49. Mateescu RG, Burton-Wurster NI, Tsai K, Phavaphutanon J, Zhang Z, et al. (2008) Identification of quantitative trait loci for osteoarthritis of hip joints in dogs. Am J Vet Res 69: 1294–1300.
50. Chase K, Lawler DF, Carrier DR, Lark KG (2005) Genetic regulation of osteoarthritis: A QTL regulating cranial and caudal acetabular osteophyte formation in the hip joint of the dog (Canis familiaris). Am J Med Genet A 135: 334–335.
51. Yang J, Benyamin B, McEvoy BP, Gordon S, Henders AK, et al. (2010) Common SNPs explain a large proportion of the heritability for human height. Nat Genet 42: 565–569.
52. Lee JW, Waldron DF, Van Vleck LD (2000) Parameter estimates for greasy fleece weight of Rambouillet sheep at different ages. J Anim Sci 78: 2108–2112.
53. Mardis ER (2008) The impact of next-generation sequencing technology on genetics. Trends Genet 24: 133–141.
54. Uetani N, Chagnon MJ, Kennedy TE, Iwakura Y, Tremblay ML (2006) Mammalian motoneuron axon targeting requires receptor protein tyrosine phosphatases sigma and delta. J Neurosci 26: 5872–5880.
55. Tsuritani K, Takeda J, Sakagami J, Ishii A, Eriksson T, et al. (2009) Cytokine receptor-like factor 1 is highly expressed in damaged human knee osteoarthritic cartilage and involved in osteoarthritis downstream of TGF-beta. Calcif Tissue Int 86: 47–57.
56. Kealy RD, Lawler DF, Ballam JM, Lust G, Biery DN, et al. (2000) Evaluation of the effect of limited food consumption on radiographic evidence of osteoarthritis in dogs. J Am Vet Med Assoc 217: 1678–1680.
57. Kealy RD, Lawler DF, Ballam JM, Lust G, Smith GK, et al. (1997) Five-year longitudinal study on limited food consumption and development of osteoarthritis in coxofemoral joints of dogs. J Am Vet Med Assoc 210: 222–225.
58. Kealy RD, Lawler DF, Monti KL, Biery D, Helms RW, et al. (1993) Effects of dietary electrolyte balance on subluxation of the femoral head in growing dogs. Am J Vet Res 54: 555–562.
59. Madsen JS, Svalastoga E (1994) Inclination and anteversion of collum femoris in hip dysplasia and coxarthritis. Acta Vet Scand 35: 115–119.
60. Todhunter RJ, Zachos TA, Gilbert RO, Erb HN, Williams AJ, et al. (1997) Onset of epiphyseal mineralization and growth plate closure in radiographically normal and dysplastic Labrador retrievers. J Am Vet Med Assoc 210: 1417–1418.
61. Yeh H, Chow M, Abrams WR, Fan J, Foster J, et al. (1994) Structure of the human gene encoding the associated microfibrillar protein (MFAP1) and localization to chromosome 15q15-q21. Genomics 23: 443–449.
62. Friedenberg SG, Zhu L, Zhang Z, Van den Berg Foels W, Schweitzer PA, et al. (2010 (accepted)) A fibrillin 2 haplotype associated with canine hip dysplasia and incipient osteoarthritis. Am J Vet Res.
63. Ortiz EM, Dusetti NJ, Vasseur S, Malka D, Bodeker H, et al. (1998) The pancreatitis-associated protein is induced by free radicals in AR4-2J cells and confers cell resistance to apoptosis. Gastroenterology 114: 808–816.
64. Ikegawa S (2007) New gene associations in osteoarthritis: what do they provide, and where are we going? Curr Opin Rheumatol 19: 429–434.
65. Meulenbelt I, Min JL, van Duijn CM, Kloppenburg M, Breedveld FC, et al. (2006) Strong linkage on 2q33.3 to familial early-onset generalized osteoarthritis and a consideration of two positional candidate genes. Eur J Hum Genet 14: 1280–1287.

66. Zhang Z, Zhu L, Sandler J, Friedenberg SS, Egelhoff J, et al. (2009) Estimation of heritabilities, genetic correlations, and breeding values of four traits that collectively define hip dysplasia in dogs. American Journal of Veterinary Research 70: 483–492.
67. Lust G, Todhunter RJ, Erb HN, Dykes NL, Williams AJ, et al. (2001) Repeatability of dorsolateral subluxation scores in dogs and correlation with macroscopic appearance of hip osteoarthritis. American Journal of Veterinary Research 62: 1711–1715.
68. Lust G, Todhunter RJ, Erb HN, Dykes NL, Williams AJ, et al. (2001) Comparison of three radiographic methods for diagnosis of hip dysplasia in eight-month-old dogs. Journal of the American Veterinary Medical Association 219: 1242–1246.
69. Lust G (1997) An overview of the pathogenesis of canine hip dysplasia. J Am Vet Med Assoc 210: 1443–1445.
70. Phavaphutanon J, Mateescu RG, Tsai KL, Schweitzer PA, Corey EE, et al. (2009) Evaluation of quantitative trait loci for hip dysplasia in Labrador Retrievers. American Journal of Veterinary Research 70: 1094–1101.
71. Hardenbol P, Baner J, Jain M, Nilsson M, Namsaraev EA, et al. (2003) Multiplexed genotyping with sequence-tagged molecular inversion probes. Nat Biotechnol 21: 673–678.
72. Maffia M, Acierno R, Cillo E, Storelli C (1996) Na(+)-D-glucose cotransport by intestinal BBMVs of the Antarctic fish Trematomus bernacchii. Am J Physiol 271: R1576–1583.

9

Pathway-Based Association Analyses Identified TRAIL Pathway for Osteoporotic Fractures

Yin-Ping Zhang[1]*, Yao-Zhong Liu[2], Yan Guo[3], Xiao-Gang Liu[3], Xiang-Hong Xu[3], Yan-Fang Guo[3], Yuan Chen[3], Feng Zhang[1], Feng Pan[3], Xue-Zhen Zhu[4], Hong-Wen Deng[2,3,4]*

1 The Key Laboratory of Environment and Genes Related to Diseases, Xi'an Jiaotong University College of Medicine, Ministry of Education, Xi'an, Shaanxi, People's Republic of China, **2** Department of Biostatistics, Tulane University School of Public Health and Tropical Medicine, New Orleans, Louisiana, United States of America, **3** The Key Laboratory of Biomedical Information Engineering, Xi'an Jiaotong University School of Life Science and Technology, Ministry of Education and Institute of Molecular Genetics, Xi'an, Shaanxi, People's Republic of China, **4** University of Shanghai for Science and Technology, Shanghai, People's Republic of China

Abstract

Introduction: Hip OF carries the highest morbidity and mortality. Previous studies revealed that individual genes/loci in the Tumor Necrosis Factor (TNF) -Related Apoptosis-Inducing Ligand (*TRAIL*) pathway were associated with bone metabolism. This study aims to verify the potential association between hip OF and TRAIL pathway.

Methods: Using genome-wide genotype data from Affymetrix 500 K SNP arrays, we performed novel pathway-based association analyses for hip OF in 700 elderly Chinese Han subjects (350 with hip OF and 350 healthy matched controls).

Results: The TRAIL pathway achieved a significant p value ($p = 0.01$) for association with hip OF. Among the 38 genes in the TRAIL pathway, seven genes achieved nominally significant association with hip OF ($p<0.05$); the *TNFSF10* (*TRAIL*) gene obtained the most significant p value ($p = 1.70 \times 10^{-4}$). SNPs (*rs719126*, *rs6533015*, *rs9594738*, *rs1805034*, *rs11160706*) from five genes (*CFLAR*, *NFKB1*, *TNFSF11*, *TNFRSF11A*, *TRAF3*) of the pathway had minor alleles that appear to be protective to hip OF. SNPs (*rs6445063* and *rs4259415*) from two genes (*TNFSF10* and *TNFRSF10B*) of the pathway had minor alleles (A) that are associated with an increased risk of hip OF, with the ORs (odds ratios) of 16.51 (95%CI:3.83–71.24) and 1.37 (95%CI:1.08–1.74), respectively.

Conclusions: Our study supports the potential role of the TRAIL pathway in the pathogenesis of hip OF in Chinese Han population. Further functional study of this pathway will be pursued to determine the mechanism by which it confers risk to hip OF.

Editor: Ioannis P. Androulakis, Rutgers University, United States of America

Funding: Investigators of this work were partially supported by grants from National Institutes of Health (R01 AR050496, R21 AG027110, R01 AG026564, P50 AR055081, 5R03TW008221, 5R01AR057049, and R21 AA015973). The study was also benefited from grants from Guanghua Foundation (GH0203416), Xi'an Jiaotong University, Shaanxi Province (2010K16-01), National Natural Science Foundation of China (81000363, 31000554), Huo Ying Dong Education Foundation, and China Scholarship Council, Programs Foundation of Ministry of Education of China (20100201120058), Shanghai Leading Academic Discipline Project (S30501), a grant from Ministry of Education to ShangHai University of Science and Technology, and startup fund from University of Shanghai for Science and Technology. No additional external funding received for this study. The funders had no role in study design, data collection and analysis, decision to publish, or preparation of the manuscript.

Competing Interests: The authors have declared that no competing interests exist.

* E-mail: cathyzh@mail.xjtu.edu.cn (Y-PZ); hdeng2@tulane.edu (H-WD)

Introduction

The prevalence of osteoporotic fractures (OF), especially hip OF, has now become a significant public health burden due to the associated high morbidity, mortality and tremendous health care cost [1,2] The incidence of hip OF will reach 6.27 million worldwide with a resultant cost of >$34 billion by the year 2050 [1]. The major demographic change of hip OF will occur in Asia. In 1990, 26% of hip OF worldwide occurred in Asia, and this rate could rise to 37% by the year 2025 and to 45% by the year 2050 [2]. Genetic factors play an important role in susceptibility to hip OF [3,4]. However, to date, the genetic determination of hip OF is still largely unknown.

A pathway-based association analysis approach is based on gene set enrichment analysis. The method ranks genes/SNPs genome-wide by the significance of association with a disease phenotype to generate a gene list, then uses a statistic enrichment score (*ES*) to examine whether a particular group of genes/SNPs within a certain functional pathway is enriched at the top (or bottom) of the list more than would be expected by chance [5]. This approach considers critical information about the interaction of a set of functionally related genes and their joint effects, and could potentially improve the power to detect genetic variants working in functional pathways. The method may play a major role in genetic analyses of complex diseases; for a pathway that contributes to a disease's risk, a single genetic variant within that pathway may have only limited contribution to the risk that might not be detectable (in regular genetic association analyses) if not otherwise be detected at the whole pathway level. Recently, through this new powerful approach, we have identified two novel pathways for wrist BMD and femur geometry in US whites [6,7].

Previous studies revealed importance in the pathogenesis of bone metabolism for several individual genes/loci, or their transcripts and proteins in Tumor Necrosis Factor (TNF)-Related Apoptosis-Inducing Ligand (TRAIL) pathway, for example, *TRAIL*, *TRAILR1*, *TRAILR2*, *CFLAR*, *RANK*, and *OPG* [8,9,10]. However, it is unknown if the TRAIL pathway may contribute to osteoporotic fracture risk at the whole pathway level. We therefore undertook a novel, pathway-based association study to assess contribution of the pathway to hip OF risk.

Materials and Methods

Subjects

The study was approved by the institutional review board of Xi'an Jiaotong University. After signing an informed consent agreement, all subjects were assisted to complete a structured questionnaire including anthropometric variables, lifestyles, and medical history.

The sample consisted of 700 elderly Chinese Han subjects, including 350 with osteoporotic (low trauma) hip fractures (including 124 males and 226 females) and 350 controls (including 173 males and 177 females) (see Table 1 for the basic characteristics of these subjects). All the subjects were unrelated Chinese Han adults living in the city of Xi'an and its neighboring areas. Inclusion criteria for cases were (i) onset age >55 years, all female subjects were postmenopausal women; (ii) age <80 years to minimize the effect due to age, since previous studies showed that approximately half of females aged 80 years or older have fractures [11]; (iii) minimal or no trauma fractures, usually due to falls from standing height or less; (iv) fracture site at femoral neck or inter-trochanter regions; (v) hip fracture was identified/confirmed through diagnosis of orthopedic surgeons/radiologists according to radiological reports and X-rays. Patients with pathological fractures and high-impact fractures (such as due to motor vehicle accidents) were excluded.

Healthy control subjects were selected from our established large database. They were geographically matched to the cases. Inclusion criteria for controls were: (i) age at exam >55 years, without any fracture histories (all female controls were postmenopausal); and (ii) not suffering from chronic diseases and conditions that might potentially affect bone mass, structure, or metabolism. The criteria may ensure that controls are less likely to suffer OF during their remaining life span compared with the general populations. The diseases/conditions mentioned above included chronic disorders involving vital organs (heart, lung, liver, kidney, brain), serious metabolic diseases (diabetes, hypo- and hyper-parathyroidism, hyperthyroidism, etc.), other skeletal diseases (Paget disease, osteogenesis imperfecta, rheumatoid arthritis, etc.); chronic use of drugs affecting bone metabolism (e.g., hormone replacement therapy, corticosteroid therapy, anti-convulsant drugs), and malnutrition conditions (such as chronic diarrhea, chronic ulcerative colitis). In addition, subjects taking anti-resorptive or bone anabolic agents/drugs, such as bisphosphonates were also excluded.

Table 1. Characteristics of the study subjects.

	Case (n = 350)	Control (n = 350)
Age (years)	69.35 (7.41)	69.54 (6.09)
Weight (kg)	59.15 (12.05)	59.61 (10.84)
Height (cm)	162.84 (8.31)	159.41 (9.20)

Note: Data are shown as mean (standard deviation).

Genotyping and quality control

Genomic DNA was extracted from peripheral blood leukocytes using a commercial isolation kit (Gentra systems, Minneapolis, MN, USA) following the standard protocols. SNP genotyping was performed using Affymetrix Human Mapping 500 K array set (Affymetrix, Santa Clara, CA, USA). Genotyping calls were determined from the fluorescent intensities using the dynamic model (DM) algorithm [12] as well as the B-RLMM (Bayesian Robust Linear Model with Mahalanobis Distance Classifier) algorithm [13]. DM calls were used for quality control of the genotyping experiment. BRLMM calls were used for the following pathway-based analyses. SNPs with a sample call rate <90%, with allele frequencies extremely deviating from Hardy-Weinberg equilibrium ($p<10^{-7}$) and having a minor allele frequency (MAF) <0.01 in the total sample were discarded. The final SNP number for the analyses is 371,258. This SNP set covers 14,642 genes and yielded an average marker spacing of ~7.9 kb throughout the human genome. Among these SNPs, 350 belong to the genes of the TRAIL pathway.

Statistical Analysis

Statistical analyses on individual SNPs were first conducted by the Wald test implemented in Plink (version 1.03) [14] with age and sex as covariates. The main procedures of pathway-based analysis [15] are briefly summarized as follows:

(1) Generation of gene-phenotype association rank and calculation of *ES*: Among all the SNPs of a given gene G_i, the SNP achieving the smallest p value in the single-marker association tests was used to represent the magnitude of association evidence of the gene. We ranked all genes by sorting their statistic values from the largest to smallest, denoted as a vector of the gene list L ($r_1, r_2, \ldots, r_N$). "N" equals to the total gene number contained in the GeneChip® Human Mapping 500 K set arrays. "r" represents the gene-phenotype association statistic value. Then, a weighted Kolmogorov-Smirnov-like running-sum enrichment score (ES^S) was calculated in Equation 1. For the given pathway S composed of N_S genes, by walking down the gene list L, we increased the running-sum statistic for the pathway when we encountered a gene in the S and decreased it when we encountered a gene not in the *S*.

$$ES^S = \max_{1 \leq i \leq N} \left\{ \sum_{G_{j^*} \in S, j^* \leq i} \frac{|r_{(j^*)}|^p}{N_R} - \sum_{G_{j^*} \notin S, j^* \leq i} \frac{1}{N - N_S} \right\}, \quad (1)$$

Where $N_R = \sum_{G_{j^*} \in S} |r_{j^*}|$ and parameter p (designated as 1 here) is designed to give higher weight to genes with extreme statistic values. The magnitude of the increment depends on the correlation of the gene with the phenotype. In short, ES^S is the maximum deviation from zero encountered in the random walk. It will be high if the association signal is enriched at the top of list L, reflected by the significance level of observed ES^S (i.e. nominal p value).

(2) Permutation and nominal significance assessment: The phenotype data was shuffled and permutation (*per*) was done

to compute a ES^S_{per} through repeating steps (1)~(2) to estimate the nominal p value. A total of 1,000 permutations were done to create a histogram of the corresponding enrichment scores $ES^S_{per,null}$ for the given pathway/gene set S. The nominal p value was estimated as the percentage of permutations whose ES^S_{per} were greater than the observed ES^S.

To detect possible population stratification that may lead to spurious association results, we used Structure 2.2 software (http://pritch.bsd.uchicago.edu/software.html) to investigate the potential population substructure/stratification of the sample. The program uses a Markov chain Monte Carlo (MCMC) algorithm to cluster individuals into different cryptic sub-populations on the basis of multi-locus genotype data [16]. We performed the analysis assuming the number of population strata k = 2 and using 1,000 un-linked SNPs randomly selected genome-wide. To confirm the results achieved through Structure 2.2, we further tested population stratification in our sample using EIGENSOFT 2.0 software that uses both principal component analysis and a genomic control approach to correct possible statistical bias caused by ancestral differences [17,18]. Reported p value was adjusted by the λ value estimated by genomic control method.

Results

Characteristics of study subjects

Basic characteristics of the 700 subjects are presented in Table 1. The STRUCTURE program revealed that all subjects in this Chinese sample were clustered together and could not be assigned into any subgroups, indicating that there was no significant population stratification within the sample. We also performed analysis using EIGENSOFT [17] and confirmed the homogeneity of the sample revealed by Structure; there is only one principal component that is significant in the principal component analysis ($p<0.001$), suggesting only one population ancestry existing for our sample. Finally, we used the genomic control method [18] to estimate the λ value, which equals to 1.02, suggesting again there is no population stratification in the sample.

Pathway-based association analysis

The TRAIL pathway, annotated by the Ambion GeneAssist Pathway Atlas (Table 2), achieved a high NES of 1.76 with a p value of 0.01. Among the 38 genes in the TRAIL pathway, the gene with the most significant p value is *TNFSF10* (*TRAIL*, $p = 1.70\times10^{-4}$) (Table 3). Another six genes in the TRAIL pathway, which also contribute positively to the *ES* (i.e., the genes that ranked before or at the point of *ES*, also denoted as "leading edge genes"), are: *CFLAR* (*c-FLIP*, *FLIP*, $p = 3.17\times10^{-3}$), *TNFSF11* (*RANKL*, $p = 6.06\times10^{-3}$), *TNFRSF11A* (*RANK*, $p = 7.63\times10^{-3}$), *TNFRSF10B* (*TRAILR2*, $p = 1.07\times10^{-2}$), *TRAF3* ($p = 1.67\times10^{-2}$), and *NFKB1* (*NF-κB1*, $p = 2.04\times10^{-2}$). Among the 38 genes in the TRAIL pathway, 4 genes, *NFKBIE*, *IKBKG*, *RELB*, *DIABLO*, were not covered by Affymetrix 500 k Array Set, and the SNPs of the *XIAP* and *APAF1* genes were discarded for failure of passing the quality control criteria (Table 3).

For the top SNP of each gene, the effect size of the minor allele is expressed by odds ratio (OR) derived from logistic regression analyses. The OR value is interpreted in the standard manner. A value of 1.0 indicates no effect. A value greater than 1.0 indicates that the minor allele is associated with an increased hip OF risk, and a value less than 1.0 implies that the minor allele is associated with a decreased risk, hence may be protective. Among the 7 SNPs representing the 7 leading edge genes, 5 SNPs had the protective minor allele. They are: *rs719126* of the *CFLAR* gene (minor allele A, OR = 0.05, 95%CI: 0.01–0.36), *rs6533015* of the *NFKB1* gene (minor allele C,OR = 0.76, 95%CI: 0.60–0.96), *rs9594738* of the *TNFSF11* gene (minor allele C, OR = 0.55, 95%CI: 0.36–0.84), *rs1805034* of the *TNFRSF11A* gene (minor allele C, OR = 0.72, 95%CI: 0.57–0.92), and *rs11160706* of the *TRAF3* gene (minor allele A, OR = 0.75, 95%CI: 0.60–0.95). The other two SNPs, *rs6445063* in the *TNFSF10* (*TRAIL*) gene and *rs4259415* in the *TNFRSF10B* (*TRAILR2*) gene, had a minor allele "A" with OR values of 16.51 (95%CI: 3.83–71.24) and 1.37 (95%CI: 1.08–1.74), respectively. The minor alleles of these two SNPs are significantly associated with an increased risk of hip OF ($P<0.05$) (Table 3).

Discussion

In this study, the TRAIL pathway was shown to be significantly associated with hip OF ($p = 0.01$) according to the pathway-based association analysis. This is the first time that the TRAIL pathway is implicated as an underlying factor for hip OF in Chinese. The pathway may contribute to bone mass variation via regulating osteoclast metabolism; previous findings have shown that the TRAIL pathway play roles in modulating the differentiation, function, survival and/or apoptosis of osteoclasts [19,20], which may in turn accelerate bone resorption and consequently the susceptibility to hip OF. The core process of TRAIL and the functional interactions among the genes in the TRAIL pathway are depicted in Figure 1.

TRAIL, also known as *Apo2L*, is a widely recognized member of the tumor necrosis factor (TNF) ligand family [21,22]. *TRAIL* is a typical type II membrane protein, binds to aggregates type I transmembrane receptors with cytoplasmic death domains (DD), which ultimately activate a protease cascade leading to apoptosis [23]. Interacting with five different receptors of the TNF receptor superfamily, *TRAILR1*, *TRAILR2*, *TRAILR3*, *TRAILR4* and *OPG*, the ligand is expressed constitutively in a wide range of tissues [22,24,25], including bone-related cells, such as osteoclast or osteoclast precursors. The binding of *TRAIL* to *TRAILR2* (DR5), which contains a conserved death domain (DD), may induce the apoptosis of osteoclast [19]. This may play an important role in the etiology of hip OF. *TRAIL* induces apoptosis in human differentiated osteoclasts by means of *TRAILR2*, and activates an intracellular pathway involving caspase-8 and Bid cleavage in the active forms [19]. However, in this study, SNP *rs6445063* from *TNFSF10 (TRAIL) gene* and SNP *rs4259415* from *TNFRSF10B* (*TRAILR2*) gene of the pathway had minor alleles (A) that are associated with an increased risk of hip OF, with the ORs (odds ratios) of 16.51 (95%CI:3.83–71.24) and 1.37 (95%CI:1.08–1.74), respectively. SNP *rs6445063* is located on chromosome 3q26.31 and has never been studied previously. SNP *rs4259415* is located on chromosome 8p21.3 and functions as intronic enhancer. According to the FASTSNP program (http://fastsnp.ibms.sinica.edu.tw), a change of "G→A" at *rs4259415* may lead to alter the binding sites for transcription factor from GATA-1 to CdxA and TATA, which may change the function of apoptosis related *TRAILR2* gene and accordingly alter the apoptosis of osteoclast. Furthermore, the apoptosis induced by death receptors can be modulated at several levels. Intracellular anti-apoptotic molecules can block the apoptotic signaling pathway. Soluble receptors inhibit TRAIL-mediated apoptosis in part by increasing baseline levels of CFLAR (c-FLIP), which competes with caspase-8 for binding to FADD, and inhibits active caspases [26]. Increased c-FLIP levels following exposure to soluble factors may decrease the apoptosis of osteoclast. Intracellular

Table 2. Component genes in the TRAIL pathway.

Gene Symbol	Gene ID	Genome Location	Full name	Protein Name
APAF1	317	12q23	apoptotic peptidase activating factor 1	APAF1
BID	637	22q11.1	BH3 interacting domain death agonist	BID
CBL	867	11q23.3	Cas-Br-M (murine) ecotropic retroviral transforming sequence	c-Cbl
REL	5966	2p13-p12	v-rel reticuloendotheliosis viral oncogene homolog (avian)	c-Rel
CASP3	836	4q34	caspase 3, apoptosis-related cysteine peptidase	Caspase3
CASP8	841	2q33-q34	caspase 8, apoptosis-related cysteine peptidase	Caspase8
CASP9	842	1p36.21	caspase 9, apoptosis-related cysteine peptidase	Caspase9
CYCS	54205	7p15.3	cytochrome c, somatic	CytoC
DAP3	7818	1q22	death associated protein 3	DAP3
TNFRSF10C	8794	8p22-p21	tumor necrosis factor receptor superfamily, member 10c, decoy without an intracellular domain	DCRI
TNFRSF10D	8793	8p21	tumor necrosis factor receptor superfamily, member 10d, decoy with truncated death domain	DCR2
FADD	8772	11q13.3	Fas (TNFRSF6)-associated via death domain	FADD
CFLAR	8837	2q33-q34	CASP8 and FADD-like apoptosis regulator	c-FLIP, FLIP
NFKBIA	4792	14q13	nuclear factor of kappa light polypeptide gene enhancer in B-cells inhibitor, alpha	I-KappaB-Alpha
NFKBIB	4793	19q13.1	nuclear factor of kappa light polypeptide gene enhancer in B-cells inhibitor, beta	I-KappaB-Beta
NFKBIE	4794	6p21.1	nuclear factor of kappa light polypeptide gene enhancer in B-cells inhibitor, epsilon	I-KappaB-Epsilon
CHUK	1147	10q24-q25	conserved helix-loop-helix ubiquitous kinase	IKK-Alpha
IKBKB	3551	8p11.2	inhibitor of kappa light polypeptide gene enhancer in B-cells, kinase beta	IKK-Beta
Gene Symbol	**Gene ID**	**Genome Location**	**Full name**	**Protein Name**
IKBKE	9641	1q32.1	inhibitor of kappa light polypeptide gene enhancer in B-cells, kinase epsilon	I-KK-Epsilon
IKBKG	8517	Xq28	inhibitor of kappa light polypeptide gene enhancer in B-cells, kinase gamma	I-KK-Gamma
NFKB1	4790	4q24	nuclear factor of kappa light polypeptide gene enhancer in B-cells 1	NF-KappaB1
NFKB2	4791	10q24	nuclear factor of kappa light polypeptide gene enhancer in B-cells 2 (p49/p100)	NF-KappaB2
TNFRSF11B	4982	8q24	tumor necrosis factor receptor superfamily, member 11b	OPG
TNFSF11	8600	13q14	tumor necrosis factor (ligand) superfamily, member 11	RANKL
PARP1	142	1q41-q42	poly (ADP-ribose) polymerase 1	PARP
TNFRSF11A	8792	18q22.1	tumor necrosis factor receptor superfamily, member 11a, NFKB activator	RANK
RELA	5970	11q13	v-rel reticuloendotheliosis viral oncogene homolog A (avian)	RelA
RELB	5971	19q13.32	v-rel reticuloendotheliosis viral oncogene homolog B	RelB
DIABLO	56616	12q24.31	diablo homolog (Drosophila)	SMAC
TRAF1	7185	9q33-q34	TNF receptor-associated factor 1	TRAF1
TRAF2	7186	9q34	TNF receptor-associated factor 2	TRAF2
TRAF3	7187	14q32.32	TNF receptor-associated factor 3	TRAF3
TRAF4	9618	17q11-q12	TNF receptor-associated factor 4	TRAF4
TRAF6	7189	11p12	TNF receptor-associated factor 6	TRAF6
TNFSF10	8743	3q26	tumor necrosis factor (ligand) superfamily, member 10	TRAIL
TNFRSF10A	8797	8p21	tumor necrosis factor receptor superfamily, member 10a	TRAILR1
TNFRSF10B	8795	8p22-p21	tumor necrosis factor receptor superfamily, member 10b	TRAILR2
XIAP	331	Xq25	X-linked inhibitor of apoptosis	XIAP

Note: (1) TRAIL, TNF-Related Apoptosis-Inducing Ligand.
(2) The Gene ID was retrieved from NCBI GenBank (http://www.ncbi.nlm.nih.gov/Genbank/).

anti-apoptotic molecules can also divert the apoptosis signaling into alternative responses, i.e., the proliferation/survival of osteoclast via activating NF-κB [20]. Although lack of bone phenotype in mice with gene deletion of *TRAIL* was observed by Sedger et al [27], Yen et al [28] showed that *TRAIL* can induce osteoclast formation via direct engagement with the *TRAIL* death receptor. Yen et al [28,29] suggested that TRAIL-induced osteoclastogenesisis was dependent on activation of NF-κB, ERK, and p38 MAP kinase and TRAF6 dependent. However *TRAF6* was not found to contribute positively to the ES as *TRAF3* in this study, suggests that there may be other factors that also can function in this capacity.

Table 3. Association Results for the SNPs of Top Significance for Each Gene in the TRAIL Pathway.

Gene	SNP	Chr.	Physical location	Role	P value	Allele[a]	MAF[b]	OR (95%CI)[c]
APAF1	-	12	-	-	-	-	-	-
BID	rs424708	22	16588746	Downstream	0.07899	C	0.012	0.35 (0.11–1.13)
CBL	rs4938638	11	118580639	Downstream	0.3039	C	0.127	0.84 (0.60–1.17)
REL	rs842627	2	60994311	Downstream	0.08129	A	0.127	1.38 (0.96–1.99)
CASP3	rs4862379	4	185849707	Downstream	0.1001	C	0.081	1.40 (0.94–2.09)
CASP8	rs6723097	2	201954124	Intron	0.4147	C	0.468	0.91 (0.73–1.14)
CASP9	rs2042369	1	15715831	Intron	0.1818	A	0.039	0.66 (0.36–1.22)
CYCS	rs10239907	7	24905619	Upstream	0.1457	C	0.290	1.20 (0.94–1.53)
DAP3	rs821551	1	152501653	Intron	0.3871	A	0.180	0.88 (0.67–1.17)
TNFRSF10C	rs10111172	8	23025036	Intron	0.24	C	0.173	0.84 (0.64–1.12)
TNFRSF10D	rs4278155	8	23052724	Intron	0.4	C	0.441	0.91 (0.73–1.13)
FADD	rs11604809	11	69722984	Downstream	0.9726	C	0.466	1.00 (0.81–1.23)
CFLAR	**rs719126**	**2**	**201726075**	**Intron**	**0.00317**	**A**	**0.015**	**0.05 (0.01–0.36)**
NFKBIA	rs10132268	14	35017365	Upstream	0.1129	A	0.431	1.19 (0.96–1.46)
NFKBIB	rs2241704	19	44088175	Intron	0.9237	A	0.120	0.98 (0.71–1.37)
NFKBIE	-	6	-	-	-	-		-
CHUK	rs7909855	10	101957202	Intron	0.2635	C	0.460	0.88 (0.70–1.10)
IKBKB	rs10094577	8	42206733	Upstream	0.4423	C	0.013	0.68 (0.25–1.83)
IKBKE	rs2871360	1	203065616	Downstream	0.2916	C	0.428	0.89 (0.71–1.11)
IKBKG	-	X	-	-	-	-		-
NFKB1	**rs6533015**	**4**	**103712711**	**Upstream**	**0.02041**	**C**	**0.336**	**0.76 (0.60–0.96)**
NFKB2	rs11574851	10	104150949	Coding exon	0.4637	C	0.058	1.20 (0.74–1.96)
TNFRSF11B	rs7816831	8	119792244	Upstream	0.07085	C	0.201	1.29 (0.98–1.69)
TNFSF11	**rs9594738**	**13**	**41850145**	**Upstream**	**0.00606**	**C**	**0.080**	**0.55 (0.36–0.84)**
PARP1	rs3219058	1	222879529	Intron	0.1564	C	0.318	0.85 (0.67–1.07)
TNFRSF11A	**rs1805034**	**18**	**58178221**	**Coding exon**	**0.00763**	**C**	**0.314**	**0.72 (0.57–0.92)**
RELA	rs1466462	11	65175940	Intron	0.7124	A	0.193	0.95 (0.72–1.25)
RELB	-	19	-	-	-	-		-
DIABLO	-	12	-	-	-	-		-
TRAF1	rs2416804	9	120755950	Intron	0.7757	C	0.472	1.03 (0.83–1.28)
Gene	SNP	Chr.	Physical location	Role	P value	Allele[a]	MAF[b]	OR (95%CI)[c]
TRAF2	rs2811757	9	137071341	Intron	0.4854	A	0.131	0.88 (0.61–1.26)
TRAF3	**rs11160706**	**14**	**102431489**	**Intron**	**0.01667**	**A**	**0.341**	**0.75 (0.60–0.95)**
TRAF4	rs4794836	17	24106837	Downstream	0.4349	A	0.253	1.10 (0.87–1.40)
TRAF6	rs2201845	11	36512834	Downstream	0.3038	C	0.040	0.74 (0.42–1.31)
TNFSF10	**rs6445063**	**3**	**173676334**	**Downstream**	**0.00017**	**A**	**0.024**	**16.51 (3.83–71.24)**
TNFRSF10A	rs6557634	8	23116201	Intron	0.1974	C	0.022	1.65 (0.77–3.51)
TNFRSF10B	**rs4259415**	**8**	**22957513**	**Intron**	**0.0107**	**A**	**0.298**	**1.37 (1.08–1.74)**
XIAP	-	X	-	-	-	-		-

Note: (1) The SNPs significantly associated with hip OF are shown in bold.
(2) [a]Minor allele of each SNP.
(3) [b]Minor allele frequency calculated in our sample.
(4) [c]Per-allele effect size of the minor allele is expressed by odds ratio (OR) and the 95% confidence interval of OR.

As the soluble decoy receptor of *TRAIL*, *OPG* was originally identified as a decoy receptor for *RANKL* [30] later found to be able to bind *TRAIL* [31]. *OPG* acts as antagonist for osteoclast apoptosis induced by *TRAIL*. But when *OPG* binds to the *RANKL* on the surface of osteoblast/bone matrix, it prevents *RANKL* from binding to its receptor, RANK, which inhibits the formation, activation and survival of multinucleated osteoclasts. In this process, the *RANKL/OPG* ratio is an important determinant of bone mass and skeletal integrity [32]. Up-regulation of the *RANKL* gene increases the RANKL/OPG ratio and enhances bone loss

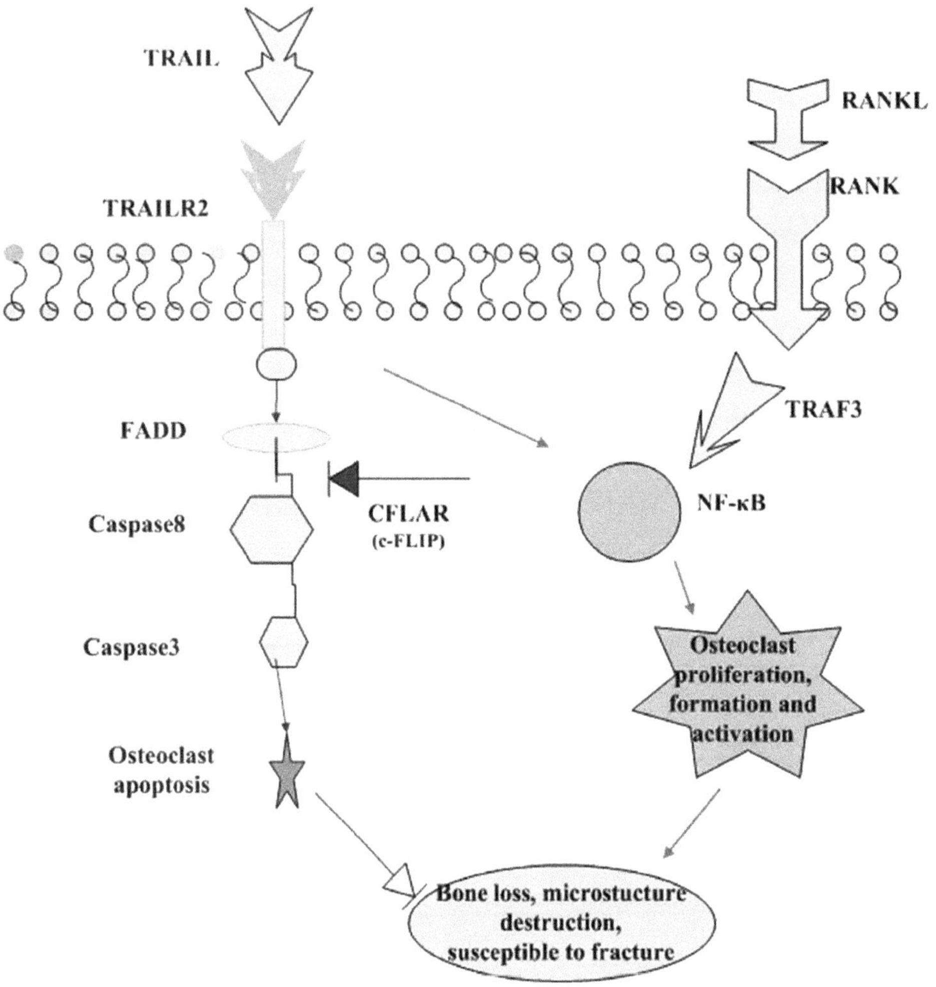

Figure 1. TRAIL pathway and the gene-gene interaction. The binding of TRAIL to TRAILR2 may induce the apoptosis of osteoclast. Increased c-FLIP levels may decrease the apoptosis of Osteoclast. The osteoclast apoptosis signal transduced by TRAIL/TRAILR2 was transformed to activate NF-κB. A key step in downstream signaling of RANKL/RANK is binding of TRAFs to RANK. Stimulation of RANK also results in strong NF-κB activation. NF-κB1(p50) is an important signal for osteoclast development and osteoclast function.

[32]. Our study found a significant association of SNPs (*rs9594738* and *rs1805034*) of *RANKL* and *RANK* with hip OF.

NF-κB1 (p50) is a subunit of NF-κB transcriptional factor complex. The balance of survival (anti-apoptotic) and death (apoptotic) signals through NF-κB activation cascades results in normal bone homeostasis and healthy remodeling [33]. NF-κB activation through RANK/RANKL signal pathway is closely related with osteoporosis and the bone resorbing activity of osteoclasts [34]. After *RANKL* binds to *RANK*, a key step in downstream signaling is binding of TRAFs to specific sites of the cytoplasmic domain of *RANK* [20,35,36]. Stimulation of *RANK* results in strong *NF-κB* activation. *NF-κB1(p50)* is an important signal for osteoclast development and osteoclast function. Moreover, NF-κB can be activated in many signal cascades related to bone metabolism, e.g., NF-κB activation through the Fas/FasL system leads to enhanced osteoclastogenesis and reduced apoptosis, and it may also cause apoptotic cell death in osteoblasts [37].

Population stratification is an important source of spurious association in genetic association studies [38,39]. However, these factors are unlikely to exist in our sample to interfere with our pathway-based association results. Our cohort came from an apparently homogenous Chinese north-west Han ethnicity population, living in Xi'an city and its neighboring areas. More importantly, in the analyses using Structure 2.2 [40], all subjects used in our study consistently clustered together as a single group, suggesting no significant population substructure. In the analysis using EIGENSTRAT [17], the measure for population stratification, λ, was very close to 1, which also suggests no stratification in our cohort. For the above reasons, our association results are unlikely to be plagued by spurious associations due to population admixture/stratification.

In summary, we applied a pathway-based analysis method to identify functional gene sets associated with hip OF. The significant enrichment of the TRAIL pathway genes among the top ranking genes associated with hip OF, together with the pathway's functional relevance to bone metabolism, strongly supports the important role of TRAIL in human hip OF risk. Further detailed and specific functional studies of the TRAIL pathway will be pursued to provide new insights into the etiology of hip OF.

Acknowledgments

We thank all the study subjects for volunteering to participate in the study.

Author Contributions

Conceived and designed the experiments: Y-PZ H-WD. Performed the experiments: Y-PZ YG X-HX YC FP X-ZZ. Analyzed the data: X-GL Y-FG FZ. Wrote the paper: Y-PZ Y-ZL.

References

1. Cooper C, Campion G, Melton LJ, 3rd (1992) Hip fractures in the elderly: a world-wide projection. Osteoporosis international : a journal established as result of cooperation between the European Foundation for Osteoporosis and the National Osteoporosis Foundation of the USA 2: 285–289.
2. Gullberg B, Johnell O, Kanis JA (1997) World-wide projections for hip fracture. Osteoporosis international : a journal established as result of cooperation between the European Foundation for Osteoporosis and the National Osteoporosis Foundation of the USA 7: 407–413.
3. Tranah GJ, Taylor BC, Lui LY, Zmuda JM, Cauley JA, et al. (2008) Genetic variation in candidate osteoporosis genes, bone mineral density, and fracture risk: the study of osteoporotic fractures. Calcified tissue international 83: 155–166.
4. Styrkarsdottir U, Halldorsson BV, Gretarsdottir S, Gudbjartsson DF, Walters GB, et al. (2008) Multiple genetic loci for bone mineral density and fractures. The New England journal of medicine 358: 2355–2365.
5. Curtis RK, Oresic M, Vidal-Puig A (2005) Pathways to the analysis of microarray data. Trends in biotechnology 23: 429–435.
6. Zhang L, Guo YF, Liu YZ, Liu YJ, Xiong DH, et al. (2010) Pathway-based genome-wide association analysis identified the importance of regulation-of-autophagy pathway for ultradistal radius BMD. J Bone Miner Res 25(7): 1572–80.
7. Chen Y, Xiong DH, Guo YF, Pan F, Zhou Q, et al. (2010) Pathway-based genome-wide association analysis identified the importance of EphrinA-EphR pathway for femoral neck bone geometry. Bone 46: 129–136.
8. Vaira S, Alhawagri M, Anwisye I, Kitaura H, Faccio R, et al. (2008) RelA/p65 promotes osteoclast differentiation by blocking a RANKL-induced apoptotic JNK pathway in mice. The Journal of clinical investigation 118: 2088–2097.
9. Sanjay A, Houghton A, Neff L, DiDomenico E, Bardelay C, et al. (2001) Cbl associates with Pyk2 and Src to regulate Src kinase activity, alpha(v)beta(3) integrin-mediated signaling, cell adhesion, and osteoclast motility. The Journal of cell biology 152: 181–195.
10. Yao GQ, Sun BH, Insogna KL, Weir EC (2000) Nuclear factor-kappaB p50 is required for tumor necrosis factor-alpha-induced colony-stimulating factor-1 gene expression in osteoblasts. Endocrinology 141: 2914–2922.
11. Ross PD (1998) Risk factors for osteoporotic fracture. Endocrinol Metab Clin North Am 27: 289–301.
12. Di X, Matsuzaki H, Webster TA, Hubbell E, Liu G, et al. (2005) Dynamic model based algorithms for screening and genotyping over 100 K SNPs on oligonucleotide microarrays. Bioinformatics (Oxford, England) 21: 1958–1963.
13. Rabbee N, Speed TP (2006) A genotype calling algorithm for affymetrix SNP arrays. Bioinformatics (Oxford, England) 22: 7–12.
14. Purcell S, Neale B, Todd-Brown K, Thomas L, Ferreira MA, et al. (2007) PLINK: a tool set for whole-genome association and population-based linkage analyses. Am J Hum Genet 81: 559–575.
15. Subramanian A, Tamayo P, Mootha VK, Mukherjee S, Ebert BL, et al. (2005) Gene set enrichment analysis: a knowledge-based approach for interpreting genome-wide expression profiles. Proceedings of the National Academy of Sciences of the United States of America 102: 15545–15550.
16. Pritchard JK, Stephens M, Donnelly P (2000) Inference of population structure using multilocus genotype data. Genetics 155: 945–959.
17. Price AL, Patterson NJ, Plenge RM, Weinblatt ME, Shadick NA, et al. (2006) Principal components analysis corrects for stratification in genome-wide association studies. Nat Genet 38: 904–909.
18. Devlin B, Roeder K (1999) Genomic control for association studies. Biometrics 55: 997–1004.
19. Colucci S, Brunetti G, Cantatore FP, Oranger A, Mori G, et al. (2007) The death receptor DR5 is involved in TRAIL-mediated human osteoclast apoptosis. Apoptosis 12: 1623–1632.
20. Feng X (2005) Regulatory roles and molecular signaling of TNF family members in osteoclasts. Gene 350: 1–13.
21. Pitti RM, Marsters SA, Ruppert S, Donahue CJ, Moore A, et al. (1996) Induction of apoptosis by Apo-2 ligand, a new member of the tumor necrosis factor cytokine family. The Journal of biological chemistry 271: 12687–12690.
22. Wiley SR, Schooley K, Smolak PJ, Din WS, Huang CP, et al. (1995) Identification and characterization of a new member of the TNF family that induces apoptosis. Immunity 3: 673–682.
23. Pan G, O'Rourke K, Chinnaiyan AM, Gentz R, Ebner R, et al. (1997) The receptor for the cytotoxic ligand TRAIL. Science (New York, NY) 276: 111–113.
24. Chamoux E, Houde N, L'Eriger K, Roux S (2008) Osteoprotegerin decreases human osteoclast apoptosis by inhibiting the TRAIL pathway. J Cell Physiol 216: 536–542.
25. Zauli G, Rimondi E, Nicolin V, Melloni E, Celeghini C, et al. (2004) TNF-related apoptosis-inducing ligand (TRAIL) blocks osteoclastic differentiation induced by RANKL plus M-CSF. Blood 104: 2044–2050.
26. Tschopp J, Irmler M, Thome M (1998) Inhibition of Fas death signals by FLIPs. Current Opinion in Immunology 10: 552–558.
27. Sedger LM, Glaccum MB, Schuh JCL, Kanaly ST, Williamson E, et al. (2002) Characterization of the in vivo function of TNF-alpha-related apoptosis-inducing ligand, TRAIL/Apo2L, using TRAIL/Apo2L gene-deficient mice. European Journal of Immunology 32: 2246–2254.
28. Yen ML, Tsai HF, Wu YY, Hwa HL, Lee BH, et al. (2008) TNF-related apoptosis-inducing ligand (TRAIL) induces osteoclast differentiation from monocyte/macrophage lineage precursor cells. Molecular Immunology 45: 2205–2213.
29. Hsu PN, Huang SC (2009) TNF-related apoptosis-inducing ligand (TRAIL) induces osteoclast differentiation from monocyte/macrophage lineage precursor cells via TRAF-6 dependent pathway. The Journal of Immunology 182: 14.
30. Lacey DL, Timms E, Tan HL, Kelley MJ, Dunstan CR, et al. (1998) Osteoprotegerin ligand is a cytokine that regulates osteoclast differentiation and activation. Cell 93: 165–176.
31. Emery JG, McDonnell P, Burke MB, Deen KC, Lyn S, et al. (1998) Osteoprotegerin is a receptor for the cytotoxic ligand TRAIL. The Journal of biological chemistry 273: 14363–14367.
32. Grimaud E, Soubigou L, Couillaud S, Coipeau P, Moreau A, et al. (2003) Receptor activator of nuclear factor kappaB ligand (RANKL)/osteoprotegerin (OPG) ratio is increased in severe osteolysis. Am J Pathol 163: 2021–2031.
33. Xu JK, Wu HF, Ang ESM, Yip K, Woloszyn M, et al. (2009) NF-kappa B modulators in osteolytic bone diseases. Cytokine & Growth Factor Reviews 20: 7–17.
34. Wakeyama H, Akiyama T, Takahashi K, Amano H, Kadono Y, et al. (2007) Negative feedback loop in the Bim-caspase-3 axis regulating apoptosis and activity of osteoclasts. Journal of bone and mineral research : the official journal of the American Society for Bone and Mineral Research 22: 1631–1639.
35. Hauer J, Pèuschner S, Ramakrishnan P, Simon U, Bongers M, et al. (2005) TNF receptor (TNFR)-associated factor (TRAF) 3 serves as an inhibitor of TRAF2/5-mediated activation of the noncanonical NF-kappaB pathway by TRAF-binding TNFRs. Proceedings of the National Academy of Sciences of the United States of America 102: 2874–2879.
36. Darnay BG, Ni J, Moore PA, Aggarwal BB (1999) Activation of NF-kappa B by RANK requires tumor necrosis factor receptor-associated factor (TRAF) 6 and NF-kappa B-inducing kinase - Identification of a novel TRAF6 interaction motif. Journal of Biological Chemistry 274: 7724–7731.
37. Mogi M, Ozeki N, Nakamura H, Togari A (2004) Dual roles for NF-kappa B activation in osteoblastic cells by serum deprivation: osteoblastic apoptosis and cell-cycle arrest. Bone 35: 507–516.
38. Thomas DC, Witte JS (2002) Point: population stratification: a problem for case-control studies of candidate-gene associations? Cancer epidemiology, biomarkers & prevention : a publication of the American Association for Cancer Research, cosponsored by the American Society of Preventive Oncology 11: 505–512.
39. Chanock SJ, Manolio T, Boehnke M, Boerwinkle E, Hunter DJ, et al. (2007) Replicating genotype-phenotype associations. Nature 447: 655–660.
40. Pritchard JK, Stephens M, Donnelly P (2000) Inference of population structure using multilocus genotype data. Genetics 155: 945–959.

10

Retrospective Analysis for Genetic Improvement of Hip Joints of Cohort Labrador Retrievers in the United States: 1970–2007

Yali Hou[1]☯, Yachun Wang[1]☯, George Lust[2], Lan Zhu[3], Zhiwu Zhang[4]*, Rory J. Todhunter[5]

1 College of Animal Science & Technology, China Agricultural University, Beijing, China, **2** Baker Institute for Animal Health, College of Veterinary Medicine, Cornell University, Ithaca, New York, United States of America, **3** Department of Statistics, Oklahoma State University, Stillwater, Oklahoma, United States of America, **4** Institute for Genomic Diversity, Cornell University, Ithaca, New York, United States of America, **5** Department of Clinical Sciences, College of Veterinary Medicine, Cornell University, Ithaca, New York, United States of America

Abstract

Background: Canine Hip Dysplasia (CHD) is a common inherited disease that affects dog wellbeing and causes a heavy financial and emotional burden to dog owners and breeders due to secondary hip osteoarthritis. The Orthopedic Foundation for Animals (OFA) initiated a program in the 1960's to radiograph hip and elbow joints and release the OFA scores to the public for breeding dogs against CHD. Over last four decades, more than one million radiographic scores have been released.

Methodology/Principal Findings: The pedigrees in the OFA database consisted of 258,851 Labrador retrievers, the major breed scored by the OFA (25% of total records). Of these, 154,352 dogs had an OFA hip score reported between 1970 and 2007. The rest of the dogs (104,499) were the ancestors of the 154,352 dogs to link the pedigree relationships. The OFA hip score is based on a 7-point scale with the best ranked as 1 (excellent) and the worst hip dysplasia as 7. A mixed linear model was used to estimate the effects of age, sex, and test year period and to predict the breeding value for each dog. Additive genetic and residual variances were estimated using the average information restricted maximum likelihood procedure. The analysis also provided an inbreeding coefficient for each dog. The hip scores averaged 1.93 ($\pm$SD = 0.59) and the heritability was 0.21. A steady genetic improvement has accrued over the four decades. The breeding values decreased (improved) linearly. By the end of 2005, the total genetic improvement was 0.1 units, which is equivalent to 17% of the total phenotypic standard deviation.

Conclusion/Significance: A steady genetic improvement has been achieved through the selection based on the raw phenotype released by the OFA. As the heritability of the hip score was on the low end (0.21) of reported ranges, we propose that selection based on breeding values will result in more rapid genetic improvement than breeding based on phenotypic selection alone.

Editor: Amanda Ewart Toland, Ohio State University Medical Center, United States of America

Funding: The study was supported by National Institutes of Health (1R21AR055228-01A1), Chinese National Key Technologies R&D Program (No.2006BAD04A01, No.2006BAD14B07) and Chinese National Department Public Benefit Research Foundation (No. NYHYZX07-035). The funders had no role in study design, data collection and analysis, decision to publish, or preparation of the manuscript.

Competing Interests: The authors have declared that no competing interests exist.

* E-mail: zz19@cornell.edu

☯ These authors contributed equally to this work.

Introduction

There are an estimated 60–70 million pet dogs in USA households. The selective crossing, and then line breeding, that generated pure dog breeds inadvertently caused fixation of recessive alleles that predispose to inherited disorders. Canine Hip Dysplasia (CHD) is a developmental disease that is expressed between 2 and 6 months of age for most medium and large dog breeds. It is a major veterinary medical problem with estimates of over 40% dysplastic dogs in some large breeds [1] and up to 75% as reported by the Orthopedic Foundation for Animals (OFA) (www.offa.org). Inherited developmental traits like hip and elbow dysplasia cause much of the osteoarthritis that plagues dogs as they age and could be prevented by better breeding practices. Treatment of a chronic disease like hip osteoarthritis, which results from hip dysplasia, has both a financial and emotional impact when it requires lifelong therapy or surgery. Pelvic radiographic examination of anesthetized or deeply sedated dogs in a ventro-dorsal position has been used in attempts to improve hip joint conformation and thus reduce the occurrence of hip dysplasia in dogs [2,3,4,5,6].

Canine hip dysplasia is a complex trait which can be characterized by at least four measurements. The OFA hip score [2] is the most popular measurement used in North America. The other three measurements are the Norberg angle (NA) [7], the distraction index (DI; PennHip^{TM}) [4] and the dorsolateral subluxation (DLS) score [6,8]. Here we focus on a single method established by the Orthopedic Foundation for Animals (OFA) [2]. The OFA established a registry to certify dogs based on their hip conformation. Their scoring system includes the grades of excellent, good and fair for so-called unaffected dogs, a borderline grade, and grades of mild, moderate and severe for dogs with hip dysplasia (www.offa.org/hipgrade).

Selective breeding using normal dogs can reduce the frequency of hip dysplasia especially when selection of breeders is based on breeding values for hip dysplasia [9,10]. In a previous report [11], analysis of OFA data suggested that for the period of 1970–1990 hip joint phenotypes improved in particular breeds. The percentage of dogs that were classified as excellent increased over this time. This phenotypic improvement has continued in their most recent analysis of OFA hip scores between 1989 and 2003 in the Labrador retriever, the Golden retriever, the German shepherd dog, the Bernese mountain dog, the rottweiler and other breeds combined [12]. The question that remains is whether the improvement underlying the phenotypic change has a genetic basis. Such a conclusion would offer support for the voluntary resource that the OFA provided because improvement in genetic hip quality should be sustainable.

Recently the genetic trends of the four measurements of CHD (OFA score, NA, DLS and DI) were reported for the Labrador retriever dogs in the breeding program of the Guiding Eyes for Blind in Yorktown Heights NY which formed part of a larger study [13]. Hip radiographic measurements (phenotypes) and pedigree information were jointly used to predict the genetic basis underlying each hip radiographic phenotype. Application of breeding values has previously been used for successful genetic improvement in livestock [14] and to reduce the incidence and severity of hip dysplasia in closed colonies of dogs [10]. In a recent report [13], the application of hip breeding values to the selection process of the Guiding Eyes for the Blind has resulted in genetic improvement in hip conformation. To extend this idea to the general population of pure breed registered dogs, we used hip phenotypes based on ventrodorsal pelvic radiographs of Labrador retriever dogs in the public OFA database (OFA scores) to evaluate whether the genetic improvement accrued over a period of almost four decades. Our hypothesis was that there was no improvement in the predicted breeding value for OFA scores over the four decades.

We analyzed the pedigree and hip joint phenotypes of Labrador retrievers in the OFA database for the period of 1970–2007 and predicted the hip score breeding value for each dog to verify if there was genetic improvement over this period. These breeding values and inbreeding coefficients are available to the public through a searchable webpage (www.vet.cornell.edu/research/bvhip) to enhance selection criteria for dog owners, breeders, and buyers of Labrador retrievers.

Results

Effect of Time Period

The number of dogs scored by OFA increased linearly each year since 1974. The increase reached a plateau in 1996 (Fig. 1). As most dogs were screened at 24 or more months of age, there was a two or more year of lag between the year of birth and the year in which the hips were scored. The OFA started reporting phenotype data in 1974. The founders of these dogs can be traced back to dogs born in 1970. The youngest dogs scored in 2007 were born in 2005. The dogs born in 2006 and 2007 have not been scored yet by the time this study made the final cut on scoring date. Because the number of dogs screened increased each year and the lag between year of birth and year of scoring was over two years, the number of dogs scored before 1997 was larger than the number of dogs that were born in the same year. The average number of dogs scored per year was 8,368 at the plateau with a standard deviation of 421.

During the last four decades, the OFA experienced four time periods when records were released under different policies. In period I (1970–1984), only the unaffected dogs were released as "Normal". In the first half year of period II (1985), the release policy was as for in period I. In the second half year, the OFA started to release unaffected dogs with detailed categories. The policy was continued in the period III (1986–2000). In period IV (1986–2007), both affected and unaffected dogs were released with detailed categories (Table 1). No significant difference was found for the least square means across the four time periods (Table 2). This indicated that the scoring standard has been consistently followed over the past four decades. The OFA hip scores averaged 1.93 with a standard deviation of 0.59 among all the dogs investigated.

The Contribution of Sires versus Dams

There were many less sires than dams for breeding dogs. Consequently, the average number of progeny per sire was 1.63 times of the number of progeny per dam. The variation of number of progeny per sire was much larger (6 fold) than the variation of number of progeny per dam (Table 3). The maximum number of progeny per sire was about 24 fold of the maximum number of progeny per dam (807 vs. 34). As the selection intensity among sires was higher than the intensity among dams, the selection of sires played a larger role in changing the genetic basis of CHD.

Age and Sex Effect

The OFA score increased with age. The score measured on 37–60 month old dogs was significantly higher ($P<0.05$) than the score measured on 24 month old dogs (Table 4). No significant difference ($P>0.05$) in OFA hip scores was found between male and female dogs (Table 5).

Variance Components and Heritability

The estimates of genetic and residual variance were 0.0729 and 0.2760, respectively. Consequently, OFA score in these Labrador retrievers had phenotypic variance of 0.3489 and a estimated heritability of 0.21 (Table 6).

Phenotypic and Genetic Trends

Both the phenotypic scores and the predicted breeding values improved steadily over the last four decades (Fig. 2). The phenotypic mean of OFA hip scores exhibited greater fluctuations than the breeding values. The breeding values improved linearly after integration of pedigree information and absorbing the influence of factors such as age when the radiographs were recorded. The improvement of breeding values was still found for dogs born between 1970 and 1983 even though the OFA scores in the public OFA database remained constant over that period. The selection based on the indicator of "normal" dogs still fostered genetic improvement. The total change in hip breeding values over the four decades was 0.1 units for the dogs born in 2005 compared to dogs born in 1970.

A joint distribution of breeding values and their accuracies is displayed for the 258,851 Labrador retrievers in Fig. 3. A lower breeding value indicates better hip joint conformation as lower OFA scores indicate better hip conformation. The higher accuracy, the more precision for the corresponding breeding value because more dogs are used for its prediction. The dogs in

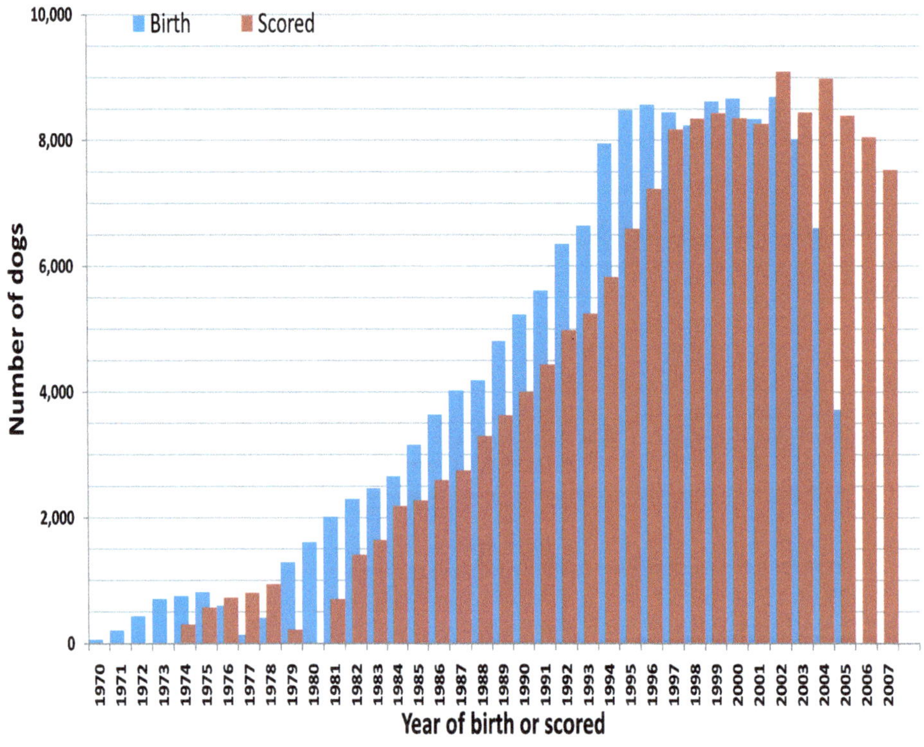

Figure 1. Distribution of dogs born and scored between 1970 and 2007. There were 154,352 Labrador retrievers scored by the Orthopedic Foundation for Animals (OFA) during this period. The number of dogs are indicated by the blue bars for the year that the dogs were born and by the red bars for the year that the dogs were scored. Both the minimum and the median age of scoring were two years old. The lag between the birth year and scoring year was over two years.

the upper right corner of the plot in Fig. 3 have the most accurate and desirable hip joint conformation. The correlation between the breeding value and its accuracy was −0.32. This correlation ($P<0.01$) indicated that selection for hip quality had been employed upon the dogs in this database as suggested [12]. The dogs with lower breeding values (better hip conformation) in the upper right corner have been more intensively used to generate progeny. Consequently, these dogs achieved higher accuracy as more progeny were available upon which to make accurate estimates.

Table 1. Numerical coding and distribution of Orthopedic Foundation for Animals (OFA) scores*.

Category	Score	Time period				Total
		1970–1984	1985	1986–2000	2001–2007	
NORMAL	2	9,482	1,260			10,742
EXCELLENT	1		140	16,386	12,811	29,337
GOOD	2		740	57,019	39,501	97,260
FAIR	3		128	10,452	5,664	16,244
BOARDLINE	4				93	93
MILD	5				321	321
MODERATE	6				272	272
SEVERE	7				83	83
TOTAL		9,482	2,268	83,857	58,745	154,352

*The OFA scores were reported between 1970 and 2007. Four time periods were categorized according to the year the pelvic radiographs were taken and reported in the public OFA database based on record release policy.

Inbreeding

The average inbreeding coefficient was 0.85% for the dogs born in 2005. The founder dogs born in 1970–1973 were considered as unrelated and had inbreeding coefficients of zero. The average increment of inbreeding was 0.0283% per year over the past forty years (Fig. 4).

Discussion

Our goal was to determine if improvement in hip phenotypes, as has been reported in the OFA database over the last four decades [11,12], has been accompanied by improvement in a breed's genetic potential for nondysplastic hip conformation. We used as the prototype breed the Labrador retriever as one of the most popular breeds in North America. To do this, the pedigree and hip score information in the public OFA database were combined to derive hip breeding values. Our analysis clearly showed that irregular improvement in hip quality has been accompanied by steady improvement in the hip breeding values. The trend was negative as a better hip was classified with a lower OFA score in this analysis. According to Fig. 2, the total change in hip breeding value was 0.1 units which was 17% of the total phenotypic standard deviation (0.59). In the period of 2001–2007, when all seven categories of OFA scores were reported, the proportion of excellent hips was 22%. The cutoff for having an excellent hip score would be 0.77 standard deviations above the mean for the underlying breeding value. Under the assumption that the underlying breeding value had a normal distribution, the

Table 2. Statistics of Orthopedic Foundation for Animals (OFA) scores over the four time periods.

Period	N	Percent	Phenotypic mean	Phenotypic SD	LS Mean	LS Error
1970–1984	9,482	6.14	2.0000	0.0000	0.1178 ns	0.1251
1985	2,268	1.47	1.9947	0.3438	0.0931 ns	0.1144
1986–2000	83,857	54.33	1.9292	0.5613	0.1012 ns	0.0774
2001–2007	58,745	38.06	1.9219	0.6845	0.0000 ns	0.0000

ns - no significant difference at the level of 5%.
LS - least squares.
SD - standard deviation.

improvement of 17% of the standard deviation implied that the proportion of excellent hips in the public OFA data base would be increased to 27%. This meant that the proportion of excellent hips increased 24% during the last four decades. Thus, even for a database biased toward better hip conformation, measureable improvement could be achieved. The challenge is how to use this publicly available data most efficiently to maximize genetic improvement [15,16,17].

When dogs are bred as part of closed breeding colonies for a specific purpose, the decision of which dogs to breed is often made by staff geneticists. Breeding decisions then take many traits into account including those particular to the musculoskeletal system. When breeding decisions are made based on the breeding values for a particular trait like CHD, further reduction in unwanted traits can be achieved [10,13,18] compared to when decisions are made based on phenotype alone. Several investigators have advocated the application of hip breeding values to breeding decisions including Ginja et al. [19] most recently. However, individual dog breeders do not have access, for the most part, to a large diverse group of potential male and female dogs from which to breed. Most have a few female and male dogs and may search for a suitable mate. Individuals who plan to purchase a pure breed dog often do not have the time or the expertise to search public databases in order to find litters of puppies for which full pedigrees and hip radiographs are available. Based on our analysis, we are encouraged to deliver these hip breeding values and related inbreeding coefficients derived from the public OFA database to the breeders and dog owners to educate their choice of a mate or purchase of a dog, respectively. We reason that integration of this information into a user-friendly web based format will encourage more rapid improvement in Labrador retriever hip quality than the current *ad hoc* system (see Figure S1).

Bias in the Data Base

The phenotypic data reported in the public OFA database was highly biased against CHD reporting. Only the dogs with excellent, good or fair hip scores were publicly reported in the period from 1970 to 2000. All the dogs were reported as "normal" until the second half year in 1985. Starting from 2001, the dysplastic dogs and dogs with borderline scores were reported (Table 1). In the OFA database (www.offa.org) accessed on August 31, 2009, 18% of Labrador retrievers were reported as dysplastic in the breed statistic summary. Yet when complete information of publicly identified dogs was accessed for the analysis reported here, less than 1% of dogs were dysplastic (OFA scores of mile, moderate and severe hip dysplasia). This indicated that a minor proportion of dysplastic dogs were reported in the publicly accessible part of the OFA database. Although this was not the best way of breeding against CHD, it implied that selection was applied as the reported dogs had more chances to breed. This is equivalent to the situation in livestock breeding. Individuals from undesirable families are usually omitted for phenotyping to reduce cost. Nevertheless, with the collected information, including the dog's pedigree, age, and sex, useful information for analysis was still extracted. Even though the OFA database is biased toward unaffected hips due to the optional nature of public submissions, taken together our results are encouraging. The statistical properties of breeding values resulting from the mixed model approach still hold for a population under selection. These properties are called best linear unbiased prediction (BLUP) [20]. Clearly, the more complete the pedigree and phenotype information included in the calculation of the breeding value, the more accurate the estimate.

Table 3. The statistics of number of progeny per sire and per dam.

	N	mean	SD	SE	Min	Max
Sire	54,454	3.0252	10.7064	0.0459	1	807
Dam	88,698	1.8569	1.7400	0.0058	1	34

Popular Sire Effects

There was a strong sire effect in that as many as 807 puppies were bred by a single sire while the largest number of puppies produced by a single dam was 34. The variation of number of progeny per sire was six fold of the variation of the number of progeny per dam (Table 3). Using breeding values, several prospective sires or dams would be ranked by hip breeding values [13] and then selected according to many other traits deemed important to a particular breeder. Such a selection would inevitably lead to the "popular sire effect" because it is likely that the dogs with best hip quality would be used as sires more often. Actually, this trend already exists, even with the current selection on phenotypes. There are 104 dogs with accuracy>75% and breeding values <-0.25. Among these dogs, there were only two females, the rest (102) were males. The value of these dogs would increase accordingly. It is clear from the OFA data analyzed herein over the last four decades that many more offspring (24-fold more in this study) are produced per sire than per dam. Hence it is also important to provide inbreeding coefficients for each dog. Inbreeding coefficients did increase steadily over the analyzed years which is not unexpected if breeders continue to select the better hipped dogs for breeding. It is possible that even though breeders may carefully select a dog with which to breed that is a popular sire that inadvertent propagation of undesirable clandes-

Table 4. Statistics of Orthopedic Foundation for Animals (OFA) scores grouped by age.

Age (month)	N	Percent	Phenotypic mean	Phenotypic SD	LS Mean*	LS Error
24	38,766	25.12	1.9137	0.5951	-0.0221^{b}	0.0091
25–29	55,100	35.70	1.9244	0.5856	-0.0137^{ab}	0.0080
30–36	29,703	19.24	1.9549	0.5927	0.0096^{ab}	0.0066
37–60	30,783	19.94	1.9453	0.6026	0.0000^{a}	0.0000

*with different subscript indicating significantly different at 5% level.
LS – least squares.
SD – standard deviation.

tine traits may ensue. As dog breeders make breeding decisions based on many factors, it is unlikely that deleterious inbreeding would occur in a large diverse breed like the Labrador retriever. In breeds with small effective population size however, attention to maintenance of genetic diversity would be important. Education in the best practice of the use of breeding values will be essential to maximize genetic diversity. Eventually, breeding values could be weighted for many qualities thought to be important to the breed. Some like orthopedic traits will be more easily quantified than others like behavior or hunting characteristics.

Heritability

The heritability of OFA hip score in this study estimated at 0.21 is consistent with other reports that have used this, or a similar hip scoring system, but lower compared to other radiographic methods used to estimate heritability of CHD [21]. Selection on phenotypes is as accurate as the selection on breeding values only when heritability is close to one. Therefore, we reason that selection of dogs based on breeding values would improve hip quality more rapidly compared to selection based on raw OFA hip scores [9,14,22]. When radiographic methods that emphasize hip laxity in which the hips are imaged in a neutral position are used to estimate heritability in pedigrees, the estimates can be higher [13,23]. Heritability estimates are also affected by the pedigree on which the calculations are made and missing information on the phenotype (as in this study) and the pedigree relatives. Fig. 1 shows that more dogs were born (i.e. had relatives in their pedigrees) than were reported as scored in the public OFA data until the late 1990's and this is consistent with comparisons to records of litters registered by the American Kennel Club [11] in which most dogs registered are not recorded with hip scores in the OFA database. Additionally, the expression of complex traits like CHD is also influenced by non genetic (environmental) factors like plane of nutrition, exercise and score variation among radiologists. Although the average concordance rate among the radiologists was reasonably good as reported by the OFA (74%), including the radiologist in the model would improve the accuracy. The estimate of heritability made on dogs in closed breeding colonies in which the environment is controlled is likely to be higher than the estimates made on the entire breed in a country.

Selection Pressure

Selection pressure placed upon breeders based on traits with higher heritability will likely result in more rapid gain than selection pressure based on traits with lower heritability. Selection pressure based on the distraction index has been reported to markedly reduce the incidence of CHD in a closed population of Labrador retrievers and German shepherd dogs [10]. Our studies have shown the OFA score and the NA are highly genetically correlated while the DI and the DLS score are also highly genetically correlated but that the genetic correlations between these two groups of hip phenotypes are only moderate [13]. Therefore, selection pressure based on the OFA score will likely not result in as rapid gain as if selection pressure was also exerted based on either the DI or the DLS score which have higher heritability [23]. At present, there is no publicly accessible database for the DI or the DLS score. So for now, breeders and prospective purchasers must avail themselves of individual dog phenotype and related pedigree information to which they have access from breeders or be given access to publicly available hip scores and integrated pedigree information (breeding values) based on the public OFA database.

Modest improvement in hip score breeding values occurred through voluntary self-reporting and any voluntary improvements breeders have made in their breeding decisions. It is also possible that competition from PennHIP™, who also uses the extended hip radiograph to assess hip conformation, and reports a dog's DI relative to the breed as a whole, has improved hip conformation in American Labrador retrievers. Once breeders and prospective

Table 5. Statistics of Orthopedic Foundation for Animals (OFA) scores grouped by sex.

Sex	N	Percent	Phenotypic mean	Phenotypic SD	LS Mean	LS Error
Male	51,010	33.05	1.9317	0.5936	1.9944^{ns}	0.0296
Female	103,342	66.95	1.9318	0.5926	1.9865^{ns}	0.0295

ns – no significant difference at level of 5%.
LS – least squares.
SD – standard deviation.

Table 6. Estimates of variance components and heritability*.

	σ_a^2	σ_e^2	σ_p^2	h^2
Estimate	0.0729	0.2760	0.3489	0.2086
Standard error	0.0020	0.0019	0.0014	0.0055

*The phenotypic variance (σ_p^2) was decomposed into the additive genetic variance (σ_a^2) and the residual variance (σ_e^2). The heritability (h^2) was calculated as the ratio of the additive genetic variance over the phenotypic variance.

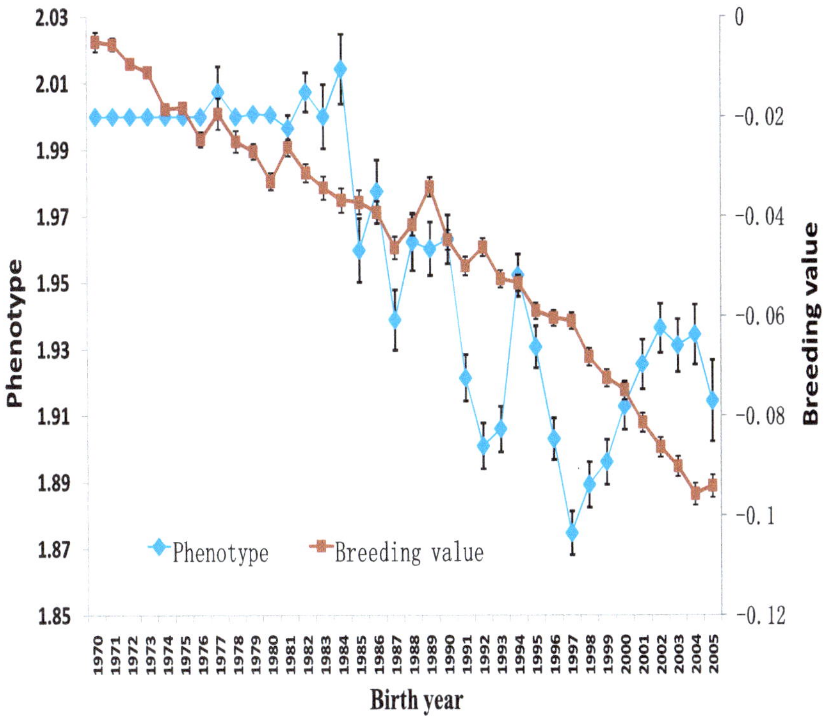

Figure 2. The phenotypic and genetic trends in last four decades. The trends are presented by the mean (± standard error) within each year for Orthopedic Foundation for Animals (OFA) score (the vertical axis on the left) and breeding value (the vertical axis on the right) for the 258,851 Labrador retrievers born between 1970 and 2005.

Labrador retriever owners are provided breeding values based on the OFA scores, we anticipate that more rapid gain in hip conformation will ensue as suggested by Kaneene et al. [12] who suggested more use of progeny testing. However, progeny testing for a complex trait requires the evaluation of many offspring (maybe as many as 15–20) to best estimate a dog's genetic potential. The provision of breeding values would obviate this step in selection of the best breeding dogs with reasonable accuracy for good hip conformation (see Figure S2). As some of these dogs have a DNA sample available for genotyping (www.caninehealthinfo.org), the application of these breeding values will also be used in studies leading to identification of contributing genes and to establish genomic prediction for susceptibility or resistance to CHD.

Materials and Methods

Dogs

The OFA database provides selection criteria for pet dog breeders and owners to lower the incidence of inherited disease. By the end of 2007, there were 1,411,127 entries reported in the public OFA database, 266,805 of which belonged to Labrador retriever dogs. There were 168,617 records on hip scores. The rest (98,188) were the records on other traits such as elbow dysplasia. Additionally, 14,265 hip records were removed for data quality control. The final data set used for the analysis contained 154,352 dogs each with one hip score record. The pedigrees recorded in the OFA data base provided an additional 104,499 ancestors (without hip scores) which were used to establish kinship among dogs with hip scores. The total number of dogs included in this analysis was 258,851. The trait records and pedigrees used in this retrospective study were available in the public domain and no live animals were used in the study.

Replicate dogs, dogs recorded with incorrect sex (such as female sire or male dam), or recorded as born earlier than a parent were also removed. These reasons lead to the deletion of 5,514 records. The most common age for scoring was 24 months (24%) and 71% of dogs were scored between 24 and 60 month. The rest (5%) of the dogs (8,751) scored before 24 months or after 60 months of age were removed from the analysis as part of data quality control.

As most of the dogs were scored at 2 years old, a lag of two year existed from the last date on which a dog was born (end of 2005) to when it was scored at the end of 2007. Therefore, the latest records used in the analysis dated from the end of 2007.

Hip Phenotypes

Hip radiographs were taken by a veterinarian with the dog in the hip-extended, supine position (www.offa.org/hipproc) and were mailed to the OFA by the owner. The radiographs were independently evaluated by 3 randomly selected board-certified radiologists from a pool of 20–25, with concordance rates averaging 74% over 1.8 million radiographs, according to the OFA. Dogs were scored into seven categories: excellent, good, and fair hip conformation, borderline, then mild, moderate and severe hip dysplasia and each score was given a numerical value from 1 (excellent hip conformation) to 7 (severe hip dysplasia). The first three categories (excellent, good and fair) are considered by many as "normal" dogs. The last three categories (mild, moderate and severe) are considered "dysplastic" dogs.

From 1970 to mid 1985, only records of the normal dogs were released as "normal". From mid 1985 to 2000, the "normal" dogs were released with their hip score categories (excellent, good and fair). From 2001, all seven score categories were released. Based on the record release policy, four time periods were grouped correspondingly, with year of 1985 as a separate group (Table 1).

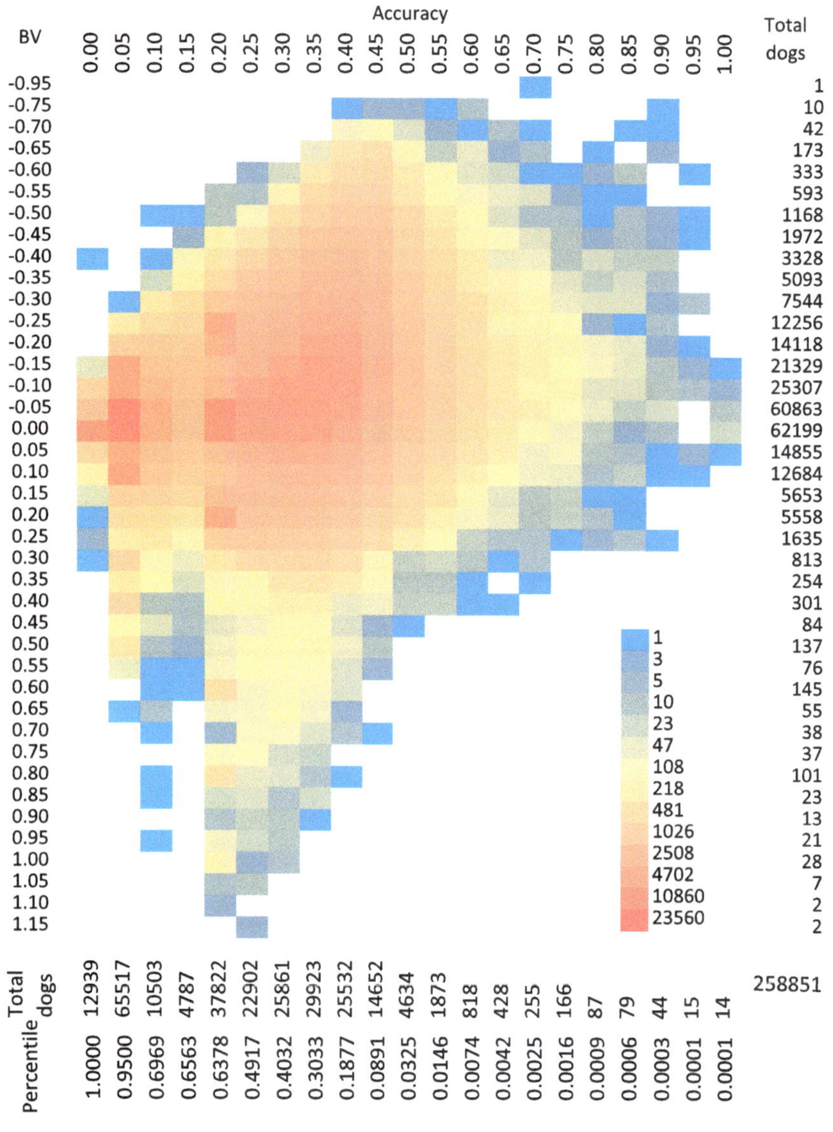

Figure 3. The joint and marginal distribution of breeding value and accuracy. Breeding value (BV) is displayed on the vertical axis and its accuracy is plotted on the horizontal axis for the 258,851 Labrador retrievers born between 1970 and 2005. The marginal distributions of BV and accuracy are indicated by both the total number of dogs and percentile at each category. The dogs on the upper right with lower BV (better hip) and higher accuracy are the most ideal for breeding against hip dysplasia.

A numerical value of 2 was assigned to the combined category of "normal" for the only category reported in the first time period. Four test year periods were formed based on the record releasing policy of OFA: 1770–1984, 1985, 1986–2000 and 2000–2007.

The earliest ancestors were born in 1970. There were no further pedigrees that could be traced back further for the ancestors born between 1970 and 1973. These ancestors were therefore considered as founders with inbreeding coefficient of zero.

Statistical Model

A single trait mixed linear model was employed to estimate the variance components (additive genetic variance and residual variance) and to predict breeding values for each dog in the pedigree. The model can be illustrated in matrix notation:

$$\mathbf{y}=\mathbf{X}\boldsymbol{\beta}+\mathbf{Z}\mathbf{u}+\mathbf{e}$$

where $\mathbf{y}$ is the vector of observed phenotypes (OFA hip scores); $\boldsymbol{\beta}$ is the vector of fixed effects including the effects of sex, age, test year period, and test year nested within test year period; dogs were grouped into four levels based on age: 24, 25–29, 30–36 and 37–60 months, and $\mathbf{u}$ is the vector of the animal genetic effects. The prediction of $\mathbf{u}$ is called BLUP. It is also called the breeding value in animal and plant breeding; $\mathbf{e}$ is the vector of random residuals; and $\mathbf{X}$ and $\mathbf{Z}$ are incidence matrices associating $\boldsymbol{\beta}$ and $\mathbf{u}$ with $\mathbf{y}$. It was assumed that $\mathbf{u}\sim N(0,\mathbf{A}\sigma_a^2)$ and $\mathbf{e}\sim N(0,\mathbf{I}\sigma_e^2)$, where $\mathbf{A}$ is the matrix of additive genetic relationships derived from identity by descent [24,25], σ_a^2 is the additive genetic variance, $\mathbf{I}$ is an identity matrix, and σ_e^2 is the residual variance. Average information restricted maximum likelihood (AI-REML) method was used to estimate the variance components. The analysis was executed using the DMU Package [26,27].

The accuracy of the breeding value was derived from Prediction Error Variance (PEV) and the additive (σ_a^2) genetic variance by

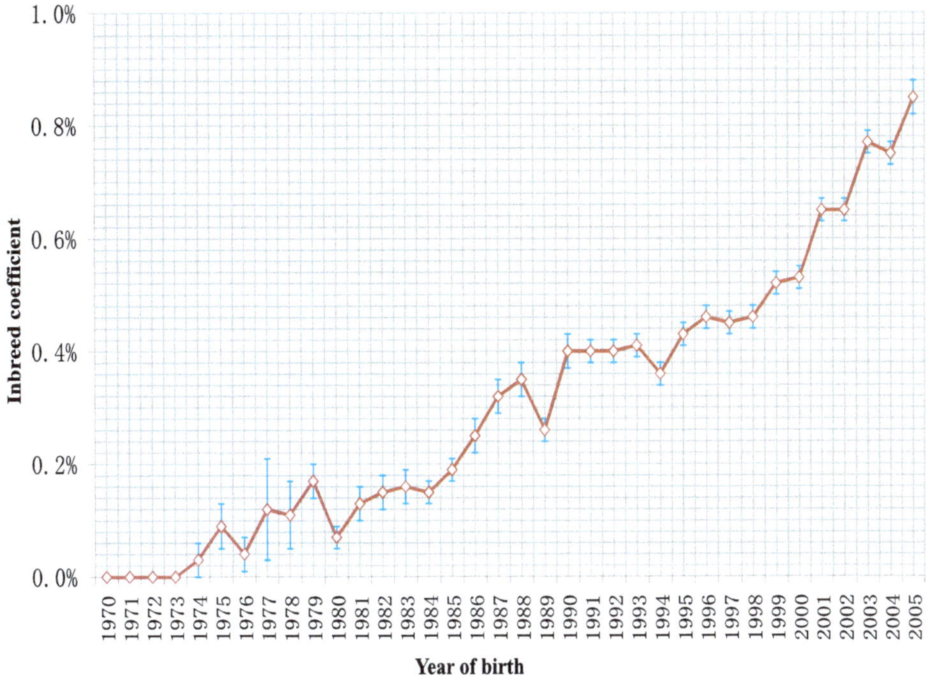

Figure 4. Trend of inbreeding coefficients. The trend is presented by the mean (± standard error) within each year for the 258,851 Labrador retrievers born between 1970 and 2005.

using the formula as follows:

$$\text{Accuracy} = \text{square root } \left(1\text{-PEV}/\sigma_a^2\right)$$

The maximum accuracy equals 1 and the minimum equals 0 [26,27]. The inbreeding coefficient for each dog equals the diagonal element of the A matrix by subtracting one.

URLs. The breeding values, accuracy and inbreeding coefficient of the 258,851 Labrador retrievers can be accessed at the World Wide Web as follows: www.vet.cornell.edu/research/bvhip

Supporting Information

Figure S1 User interface

Figure S2 Search results

Acknowledgments

The authors thank Cathy French and Marie Stewart for the website development to host breeding values on hip dysplasia.

Author Contributions

Conceived and designed the experiments: GL LZ ZZ RJT. Performed the experiments: YH YW. Analyzed the data: YH. Contributed reagents/materials/analysis tools: YW ZZ. Wrote the paper: GL LZ ZZ RJT.

References

1. Corley EA (1992) Role of the Orthopedic Foundation for Animals in the control of canine hip dysplasia. Vet Clin North Am Small Anim Pract 22: 579–593.
2. Fluckiger MA, Friedrich GA, Binder H (1999) A radiographic stress technique for evaluation of coxofemoral joint laxity in dogs. Vet Surg 28: 1–9.
3. Henricson B, Norberg I, Olsson SE (1966) On the etiology and pathogenesis of hip dysplasia: a comparative review. J Small Anim Pract 7: 673–688.
4. Smith GK (1997) Advances in diagnosing canine hip dysplasia. Journal of the American Veterinary Medical Association 210: 1451–&.
5. Farese JP, Lust G, Williams AJ, Dykes NL, Todhunter RJ (1999) Comparison of measurements of dorsolateral subluxation of the femoral head and maximal passive laxity for evaluation of the coxofemoral joint in dogs. American Journal of Veterinary Research 60: 1571–1576.
6. Farese JP, Todhunter RJ, Lust G, Williams AJ, Dykes NL (1998) Dorsolateral subluxation of hip joints in dogs measured in a weight-bearing position with radiography and computed tomography. Veterinary Surgery 27: 393–405.
7. Henry GA (1992) Radiographic development of canine hip dysplasia. Veterinary Clinics of North America: Small Animal Practice 22: 559–578.
8. Lust G, Todhunter RJ, Erb HN, Dykes NL, Williams AJ, et al. (2001) Repeatability of dorsolateral subluxation scores in dogs and correlation with macroscopic appearance of hip osteoarthritis. American Journal of Veterinary Research 62: 1711–1715.
9. Swenson L, Audell L, Hedhammar A (1997) Prevalence and inheritance of and selection for hip dysplasia in seven breeds of dogs in Sweden and benefit: Cost analysis of a screening and control program. Journal of the American Veterinary Medical Association 210: 207–&.
10. Leighton EA (1997) Genetics of canine hip dysplasia. Journal of the American Veterinary Medical Association 210: 1474–1479.
11. Kaneene JB, Mostosky UV, Padgett GA (1997) Retrospective cohort study of changes in hip joint phenotype of dogs in the United States. J Am Vet Med Assoc 211: 1542–1544.
12. Kaneene JB, Mostosky UV, Miller R (2009) Update of a retrospective cohort study of changes in hip joint phenotype of dogs evaluated by the OFA in the United States, 1989–2003. Veterinary Surgery 38: 398–405.
13. Zhang Z, Zhu L, Sandler J, Friedenberg SS, Egelhoff J, et al. (2009) Estimation of heritabilities, genetic correlations, and breeding values of four traits that collectively define hip dysplasia in dogs. American Journal of Veterinary Research 70: 483–492.
14. Van Vleck LD (1991) C. R. Henderson: farm boy, athlete, and scientist. J Dairy Sci 74: 4082–4096.
15. Wood JL, Lakhani KH (2003) Effect of month of birth on hip dysplasia in labrador retrievers and Gordon setters. Vet Rec 152: 69–72.

16. Wood JL, Lakhani KH, Dennis R (2000) Heritability of canine hip-dysplasia score and its components in Gordon setters. Prev Vet Med 46: 87–97.
17. Wood JL, Lakhani KH, Dennis R (2000) Heritability and epidemiology of canine hip-dysplasia score in flat-coated retrievers and Newfoundlands in the United Kingdom. Prev Vet Med 46: 75–86.
18. Janutta V, Hamann H, Distl O (2008) Genetic and phenotypic trends in canine hip dysplasia in the German population of German shepherd dogs. Berl Munch Tierarztl Wochenschr 121: 102–109.
19. Ginja MM, Gonzalo-Orden JM, Melo-Pinto P, Bulas-Cruz J, Orden MA, et al. (2008) Early hip laxity examination in predicting moderate and severe hip dysplasia in Estrela mountain dog. J Small Anim Pract 49: 641–646.
20. Henderson CR (1984) Applications of Linear Models in Animal Breeding. GuelphOntario, Canada: University of Guelph.
21. Zhu L, Zhang Z, Friedenberg S, Jung SW, Phavaphutanon J, et al. (2009) The long (and winding) road to gene discovery for canine hip dysplasia. The Veterinary Journal 181: 97–110.
22. Gianola D, Heringstad B, Odegaard J (2006) On the quantitative genetics of mixture characters. Genetics 173: 2247–2255.
23. Todhunter RJ, Bliss SP, Casella G, Wu R, Lust G, et al. (2003) Genetic structure of susceptibility traits for hip dysplasia and microsatellite informativeness of an outcrossed canine pedigree. J Hered 94: 39–48.
24. Emik LO, Terrill CE (1949) Systematic procedures for calculating inbreeding coefficients. J Hered 40: 51–55.
25. Cruden D (1949) The computation of inbreeding coefficients for closed populations. J Hered 40: 248–251.
26. Madsen P, Jensen J (2007) A user's Guide to DMU. Denmark: University of Aarhus version 6, release 4.7: Faculty of Agricultural Sciences, Denmark.
27. Madsen P, Sørensen P, Su G, Damgaard LH, Thomsen H, et al. (2006) DMU - a package for analyzing multivariate mixed models. 8th World Congress on Genetics Applied to Livestock Production, Belo Horizonte, Brazil, 13–18 August Communication No 07-06.

11

Outcome of Hemiarthroplasty and Total Hip Replacement for Active Elderly Patients with Displaced Femoral Neck Fractures: A Meta-Analysis of 8 Randomized Clinical Trials

Yiqiong Zhao¶, Dong Fu¶, Kai Chen, Guodong Li, Zhengdong Cai, Yan Shi, Xiaobing Yin*

The Tenth People's Hospital Affiliated with Tong Ji University Shanghai, China

Abstract

Background: Displaced fracture of the femoral neck has been a common clinical problem, especially in aged patients. However, the optimal treatment choice remains controversial. The purpose of this study is to conduct a systematic review of randomized clinical trials assessing the results of hemiarthroplasty and total hip replacement in patients undergoing either alternative using meta-analysis.

Methods: A literature search for randomized clinical trials was conducted through Medline, Embase and Cochrane library between 1969 and 2013 with no restrictions. Additional relevant articles were referred as source of information by way of manual searches on major orthopedic journals. Upon the search, two authors independently evaluated study quality and relevant data was extracted.

Results: A total of 8 studies with 983 patients were included in this meta-analysis. After pooling the available data, a significant dominance of Harris hip score was found for total hip replacement compared with hemiarthroplasty (SMD: −7.11, 95%:−10.70,−3.53) one year postoperatively and the advantage kept over (SMD: −6.91, 95%:−12.98, −0.85) two years after surgery. A trend toward a higher dislocation rate was found in total hip replacement group (RR: 0.46, 95%: 0.21, 1.02), of which the difference was considered insignificant. The risk of revision in group hemiarthroplasty appeared to be more than two folds higher than that after total hip replacement (RR: 4.14, 95%CI: 2.09, 8.19).

Conclusion: Even though there is a higher rate of dislocation after total hip replacement, this disadvantage could be accounted for, on the basis of a better functional score and the lower revision rate. However, from the results, it stands to reason that total hip replacement should be strongly suggested in elderly active patients with femoral neck fracture.

Editor: Gregory Tranah, San Francisco Coordinating Center, United States of America

Funding: The authors have no support or funding to report.

Competing Interests: The authors have declared that no competing interests exist.

* E-mail: fudongshenanfang@126.com

¶ YZ and DF are co-first authors on this work.

Introduction

Displacement of femoral neck (fracture) in the elderly has become a worldwide health concern. The trend of rise in incidence with increasing age is alarming, and it is predicted that the total number of patients suffering femoral fracture would rise to 6.26 million per year by 2050 worldwide [1]. Treatment choices for femoral neck fractures in elderly patients include internal fixation, hemiarthroplasty (HA) and total hip replacement (THR). The option should be determined by the fracture typing, the patients' condition, functional demands and their medical and mental ability to cope with surgery [2,3]. Currently, the optimal initial treatment of choice osteosynthesis which resulted in nonunion or avascular necrosis is fast given way to arthroplasty. It is recommended that Osteosynthesis should be favoured in young patients with displaced intracapsular fractures [4], relative to elderly patients who are medically fit for arthroplasty [5]. Arthroplasty is commonly used either as hemiarthroplasty or total hip arthroplasty. Although both two prosthetic replacement methods are widely accepted, the preferred treatment for displaced intracapsular fracture in elderly patients is currently of subject of debate among orthopedic surgeons. Theoretically, the results from previous prospective studies and meta-analysis [6,7] which comparing the outcome of hemiarthroplasty and total hip replacement in patients with fracture of the femoral neck have equally been inconsistent. The purpose of this study is to evaluate the evidence from previous randomized clinical studies by summarizing it quantitatively with a meta-analysis approach.

Methods

Search Strategy

Computer literature search was conducted in Medline, Embase and Cochrane databases without special limitations, and articles ahead of publication were also included. The following Medical Subject Headings (MeSH) and terms were used in searching: "femoral neck fracture", "hip fracture", "arthroplasty", "total hip replacement", "prosthesis replacement" and "elderly". Moreover, keywords in headers and abstracts in related journals were also used in the searches (e.g. Journal of Bone and Joint Surg). The reference list of each comparative study and previous reviews were hand searched to find additional studies. If the necessary data for analysis was absent or insufficient, we tried to contact the authors by e-mail. All processes in this review were in accordance with the standards of quality for meta-analysis [8].

Eligibility Criteria

Citations selected from the primary search were screened for eligibility by two independent authors. We included the studies if they met all following criteria: 1 age >55 years; 2 displaced hip fracture (Garden III, IV); 3 mental health and independent walking prior to the fracture; 4 the intervention included hemiarthroplasty or total hip replacement regardless of whether internal fixation was compared in the trial; 5 pathologic and old fractures, patients with advanced rheumatoid arthritis or metastatic diseases were excluded. A controversy was cross-checked and resolved by a third author to reach a final consensus. This was done primarily to exclude experimental bias as much as possible thereby improving consistency.

Data Extraction

Data were extracted independently by two authors subsequently after all the eligible studies were recruited. The following variables were recorded: last name of the first author, country where the study was performed, year of publication, participant sex and age, sample size, surgical approach. Outcome measurements including hip function (Harris hip score), revision (reasons) and dislocation rate and some parameters about the surgery (e.g. duration of surgery, blood loss, transfusion) were also recorded in detail.

Statistical Analysis

Study-specific RR (relative risks) and associated 95% (CI) confidence intervals accounting for discontinuous variables within the study were pooled using a random-effects model, which considered both within-study and between-study variation. Standardized mean difference (SMD) or weighted mean difference (WMD) were used for continuous variables for which a fixed effect model was used initially, and if the P value of heterogeneity test was < 0.1 or $I^2 > 50\%$, the random effect model replaced the previous modality.

Statistical heterogeneity among studies was evaluated by both Q^2 test [9] and I^2 test [10]. Sensitivity was performed to evaluate the stability of the results. Subgroup analysis was conducted if the data was present.

An estimation of potential publication bias was assessed by the funnel plot, in which the SE (standardized effect) of log (RR) of each study was plotted against its log (RR). The result was assessed by the method of Egger's linear regression test, a linear regression approach to assess asymmetry on the natural logarithm scale of the RR. All statistical analysis were performed with STATA software (version 11.1; Stata Corporation, College Station, Texas) and Review Manager (version 5.0.0 for Windows, The Cochrane Collaboration, The Nordic Cochrane Centre, Copenhagen, 2008).

Literature Search

A flow chart of the studies recruited in our review was shown in Figure 1. We identified 163 potential citations (112 from Pubmed; 26 from Embase; 11 from the Cochrane Randomized Trials Databases; and 14 from relevant journals) aiming at comparing hemiarthroplasty and total replacement for the treatment of femoral neck fracture in elderly patients. After reading the articles, as well as communicating with the first author to get additional studies or data, 12 of the 163 citations were selected for application. Four studies belonging to the same institution were conducted with different follow-up and only the recent studies were selected. As a result, eight articles including a total of 983 patients (526 in the hemiarthroplasty group and 457 in the total hip replacement group) were used in the final analysis (details shown in Table 1).

Study Characteristics

The eight studies on arthroplasty (hemiarthroplasty and total hip replacement) were published between 2000 and 2013 (Table 1). Out of the eight studies, three were conducted in the United Kingdom, the other five trials were completed in USA, Holland, Germany, Italy and Sweden respectively. At baseline, there were no significant differences between the groups of hemiarthroplasty and total hip replacement.

All eight trials have adequate sequence generation for randomization. Allocation concealment by either a sealed-envelope technique [11,12] or computer automation based distribution [13,14] was performed in four studies while the remained four were unclear [15–18]. In terms of blinding, it was "unclear" for four trials, "no" for two [11,15] and "yes" for two [14,16]. All the randomized trials were free of selective reporting. Whether these eight trials were free of other elements of bias could not be found.

Results

Harris hip score

HSS at 3 m, 6 m, 1 y, 2 y, 3 y and 5 y postoperatively were recorded and comparison between group HA and THR based on the available score 1 y and 2 y after surgery was performed. A greater likelihood of higher Harris hip score was observed in the total hip replacement group compared to the hemiarthroplasty group (SMD: −7.11, 95%:−10.70,−3.53). This dominance kept over time (SMD: −6.91, 95%:−12.98, −0.85) two years after surgery. Both results demonstrated significant differences.

Dislocation rate

Six studies provided information about dislocation. The Review Manage Software will exclude the categorical variables automatically if the value of incidence is 0% in both groups. Except one study in which no dislocation occurred in either group, a total of 5 studies with 691 patients were included for analysis. A trend toward a higher dislocation rate was found in total hip replacement group (RR: 0.46, 95%: 0.21, 1.02) with a low heterogeneity ($I^2 = 14\%$, $p = 0.32$) Figure 2.

Revision rate

Based on the five studies providing available data, the risk of revision in group hemiarthroplasty appeared to be more than two folds higher than that after total hip replacement (RR: 4.14, 95%CI: 2.09, 8.19)with a low heterogeneity ($I^2 = 19\%$, $p = 0.30$) Figure 3. Reasons for revision surgery in HA group were erosion 78.1% (25/32), peri-prosthetic fracture 9.4% (3/32), acetabulum osteoarthritis 3.1% (1/32) and deep infection 9.4% (3/32). While in THA group, infection, femoral stem subsidence, acetabulum

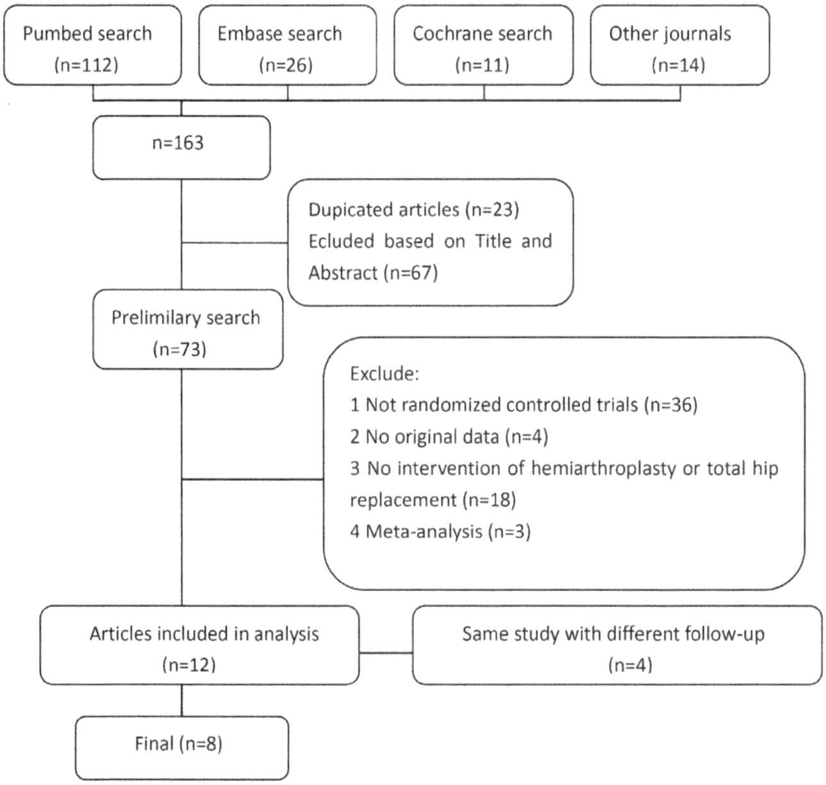

Figure 1. Flow chart of the studies recruited in this meta-analysis.

osteoarthritis and dislocation occupied 36.4% (4/11), 9.1% (1/11), 9.1% (1/11) and 45.5% (5/11) respectively.

Discussion

The goal of any surgical treatment for elderly and independent patients with displaced fractures of the femoral neck is to return them as quickly as possible to pre-injure functional status as well as minimize the risk of dislocation or reoperation. Total hip replacement and hemiarthroplasty are two primary treatment choices for those patients and each of these methods has its associated advantages and disadvantages.

Two meta-analysis [6,7] evaluated the optimal type of arthroplasty before this study was initiated. Both studies concluded that total hip replacement was associated with a better overall result compared to hemiarthroplasty in the management of elderly patients, but it remained to be further confirmed, due to insufficient evidence backing the claim. An obvious limitation of their studies was that the conclusion was based on relatively small studies. This current meta-analysis summarized the results of randomized controlled trials, including eight randomized clinical studies on hemiarthroplasty and total hip replacement with a total of 983 patients. This meta-analysis up to now is associated with the largest number of patients. The results indicated that total hip replacement had a potential advantage on the whole, compared to hemiarthroplasty.

Harris hip score

As one of the most important measurement tools, Harris hip score was used to investigate the living status of patients. From three independent studies [14,18,19], we extracted that hip function reached its peak one year after surgery. Our result favored the total hip replacement because hip function improved significantly compared to the hemiarthoplasty group within 1year and 2year after surgery. Cadossi et al noted from 3 m to 3 y postoperatively, the higher HHS transferred from HA to THR and the dominance of THR seemed to be increasingly evident. Similar result was reported by Hedbeck with the same duration of follow-up (Table 2). Avery et al [17] showed the functional score had declined in both groups between three and nine years and the dominance in the THR group had also decreased nine years after surgery as a result of the older age, prosthetic degeneration and other complications. Hemiarthroplasty was often accompanied with acetabular erosion and protrusion particularly in young patients under 60 years [17,20]. According to our analysis, erosion accounted for 78.1% revision surgery of patients in HA group while no erosion case was found in THP group. Theoretically, acetabular erosion was associated with hip pain and poor function. This phenomenon would be increasingly apparent with the longer follow-up.

Dislocation rate

Dislocation of the prosthesis has been the major concern after a primary total hip replacement [19,21]. We tried to find a relationship between surgical approach and dislocation. However, it was impossible as mixed surgical approaches were used in each group. A higher rate of dislocation was reported previously in total hip replacement [16,18]. In patients using a posterolateral approach during the surgery, reported incidence of dislocation ranged between 13% to 22% [18,22–24]. Potential risk factors leading to dislocation include component design, operative approach, and around soft-tissue tensioning [25]. In our series,

Table 1. Summary of studies that compared groups of patients treated with HA and THA.

author	year	location	Male/Female	Surgical approach	Type	Age(year)	No(P)	Follow up (month)	Surgical Time(min)	Blood loss	Dislocation	revision
Cadossi, et al	2013	German	13/28	straight lateral	HA Bipolar	84.2	37	28.6	81	<500 ml 7/26#	NG	NG
			8/34		THA PCU	82.3	41	30.1	75.4	<500 ml 15/27	NG	NG
Giannini, et al	2011	Italy	NG	NG	HA Bipolar	84.2	26	12	71.6	380	NG	NG
					THA PCU	82.3	26	12	76.7	460	NG	NG
Hedbeck, et al	2011	Sweden	6/54	anterolateral	HA Bipolar	80.7±5.1	60	48	NG	NG	0	0 (HA)
			13/47		THR	80.5±5.1	60	48	NG	NG	0	1 (THA) for infection
Avery, et al	2011	UK	9/32	transgluteal lateral	HA Unipolar	75.83	41	103	NG	NG	0	1 for erosion 3 for peri-prosthetic fracture(HA)
			8/32		THA PCA	74.2	40	106	NG	NG	3	1 for femoral stem subsidence (THA)
Vanden, et al	2010	Holland	22/115	anterolateral posterolateral	HA Bipolar	80.3	137	60	<90 min 110	<500 ml 111	0	5 for erosion 1 for acetabulum osteoarthritis (HA)
			25/90		THA	82.1	115	60	<90 min 75	<500 ml 70	8	1 for acetabulum osteoarthritis 1 for infection(THA)
Macaulay, et al	2008	USA	9/14	Posterolateral direct lateral	Uni(Bi)polar	77±9	23	12	82.0±35.1	5.4±2.8(Unit)	0	0 (HA)
			10/7		THA	82±7	17	12	89.1±35.8	7.7±5.5(Unit)	1	1 for dislocation(THA)
Keating, et al	2006	UK	57/54	lateral posterior	Uni(Bi)polar	75.4±7	111	24	58.5	NG	2/69#	NG
			17/52		THA	75.2±6	69	24	79.7	NG	3/69	NG
Kasetti, et al	2000	UK	NG	posterolateral	HA Bipolar	82.06	91	156	NG	NG	12	19 for acetabular erosion, loosening, heterotopic ossification 3 for deep infection)(HA)
					THA	81.03	89	156	NG	NG	18	2 for infection; 4 for dislocation)(THA)

Abbreviations: NG = not given; HA = hemoarthroplasty; THA = total hip arthroplasty; PCU = acetabular polycarbonate-urethane cup; PCA = polyethylene cemented acetabular;
No(p) = number of patients;
means patients available for the clinical data.

Study or Subgroup	Hemiarthroplasty Events	Hemiarthroplasty Total	Total hip replacement Events	Total hip replacement Total	Weight	Risk Ratio M-H, Random, 95% CI
Avery 2011	0	41	3	40	7.0%	0.14 [0.01, 2.62]
Hedbeck 2011	0	60	0	60		Not estimable
Kasetti 2000	12	91	18	89	62.0%	0.65 [0.33, 1.27]
Keating 2006	2	69	3	69	17.5%	0.67 [0.11, 3.87]
Macaulay 2008	0	23	1	17	6.1%	0.25 [0.01, 5.79]
Vanden 2010	0	137	8	115	7.4%	0.05 [0.00, 0.85]
Total (95% CI)		**421**		**390**	**100.0%**	**0.46 [0.21, 1.02]**
Total events	14		33			

Heterogeneity: Tau² = 0.15; Chi² = 4.66, df = 4 (P = 0.32); I² = 14%
Test for overall effect: Z = 1.91 (P = 0.06)

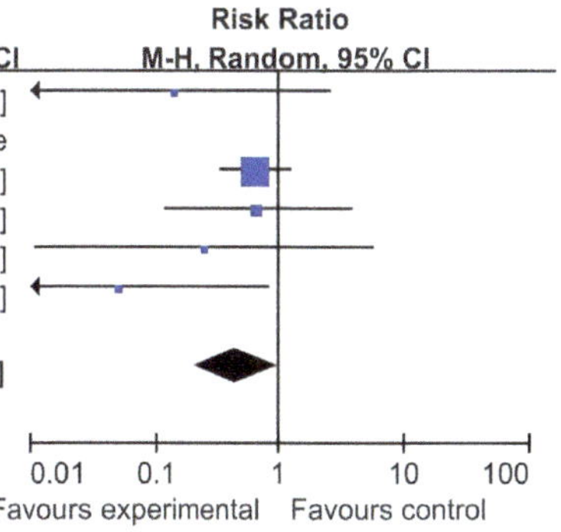

Figure 2. Statistical analysis of dislocation between HA (hemiarthroplasty) and THA (total hip arthroplasty) with Review Manager.

the modular femoral component with a 28 mm head was used in three studies, a 32 mm head in two studies and the remained were unknown. Dislocation rates for all approaches decrease as femoral head size increases from 22 mm to 32 mm [19]. However, of these five studies, no significant difference was observed between two different sizes of the femoral head and dislocation incidence. The reason which might explain this fact is that size 28 mm and 32 mm are two most commonly used head and any more increase in head size will produce a higher wear rate and subsequent aseptic loosening rate [26]. Surgical approach has been an important factor that influences the stability of hip joint. Woo and Morrey et al [25] reported a much higher dislocation rate for the posterior approach (5.8%) than that for anterolateral approach (2.3%) ($p<0.01$). In this review, six studies provided the data about dislocation. Hedback noticed no occurrence of dislocation in patients with anterolateral approach in either group, thus confirming that dislocation is not a major problem when an anterolateral approach is used [14,21,27,28]. When the posterolateral approach was used, the highest dislocation rate in both groups among the six trials was observed (Table 1). However, the dislocation rate of THR with a posterior soft tissue repair was significantly lower than that without a posterior soft tissue repair in the posterolateral approach [29]. Consequently, if posterior structures could not be preserved and repaired as much as possible, anterolateral approach might be chosen for major patients just as recommended by Enocson [27].

Erosion and Revision

Acetabular erosion is a very severe complication of both unipolar and bipolar HA (reaching to 36% and 26% of hips, respectively) after five years of follow-up postoperatively which often leading to revision surgery [30–32]. In younger patients, this change would be more frequent because of more activity. Acetabular erosion has been considered to be one important factor influencing the functional outcome. The majority of the patients receiving hemiarthroplasty experienced revision surgery which might result from the degeneration of acetabular cartilage or erosion of the prosthesis [16,30]. In the hemiarthroplasty group, the bipolar prosthesis usually had a better result than the unipolar prosthesis [15]. In this study, a bipolar component was used in 90% of the patients undergoing hemiarthroplasty and a monopolar component for the other 10% of the patients. Even though, the revision rate of HA group appeared to be more than two folds higher than that after THR, 78% resulted from erosion in HA group. When we linked the data from 12 month to 156 month of five inclusive studies, another interesting and obvious finding was that compared to HA, THR revealed notable dominance of relatively lower increasing rate of revision with the passage of time. Patients who had a 'secondary' total hip replacement for a failed hemiarthroplasty would feel much better than those who retained their hemiarthroplasty (e.g less pain and better functional outcome). But they were less likely to restore their independency than those who undertook the same procedure initially [17]. Possible reasons might be the experience of suffering two surgeries at different periods and more complications after the secondary surgery. To reduce the rate of erosion, revision and subsequent bad functional results, THR should replace HA from the beginning in some patients.

Other measurements

Blood loss and Transfusion. Patients who underwent THR had a slightly higher blood loss than those in HA group (460 vs

Study or Subgroup	hemiarthroplasy Events	hemiarthroplasy Total	Total hip replaement Events	Total hip replaement Total	Weight	Odds Ratio M-H, Random, 95% CI
Avery 2011	4	41	1	40	14.2%	4.22 [0.45, 39.49]
Hedbeck 2011	0	60	1	60	7.4%	0.33 [0.01, 8.21]
Kasetti 2000	22	91	6	89	47.3%	4.41 [1.69, 11.49]
Macaulay 2008	0	23	1	17	7.2%	0.23 [0.01, 6.11]
Vanden 2010	6	137	2	115	23.9%	2.59 [0.51, 13.08]
Total (95% CI)		**352**		**321**	**100.0%**	**2.58 [1.04, 6.40]**
Total events	32		11			

Heterogeneity: Tau² = 0.22; Chi² = 4.92, df = 4 (P = 0.30); I² = 19%
Test for overall effect: Z = 2.04 (P = 0.04)

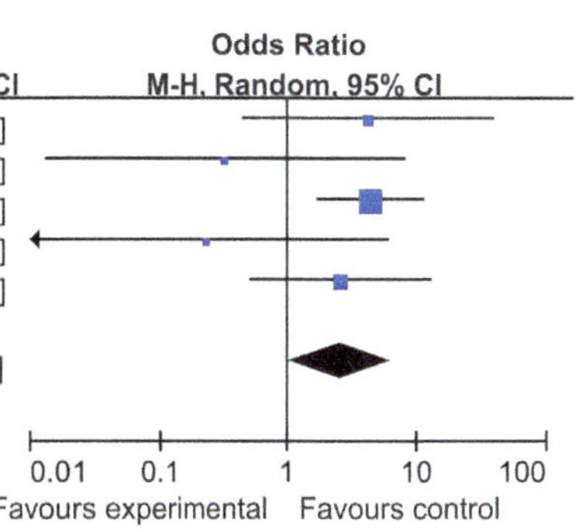

Figure 3. Statistical analysis of dislocation between HA (hemiarthroplasty) and THA (total hip arthroplasty) with Review Manager.

Table 2. Summary of HSS of included five studies that compared groups of patients treated with HA and THA.

author	Type	No (P)	HSS					
			3month	6month	1year	2year	3year	5year
Cadossi, et al	HA	37	74.0 (43.7 to 93)	NG	73.1 (40 to 97.4)	71.9 (30 to 93)	71.3 (45 to 93)	NG
	THR	41	72.3 (50.3 to 98)	NG	74.7 (56 to 98)	75.0 (55 to 98)	78.7 (55 to 98)	NG
Giannini, et al	HA	26	71.6	NG	75.5	NG	NG	NG
	THR	26	74.	NG	80.7	NG	NG	NG
Hedbeck, et al	HA	60	NG	NG	79.4±12.3	77.9±12.5	75.2±15.4	NG
	THR	60	NG	NG	87.2±9.4	87.2±10.1	89.0±8.1	NG
Vanden, et al	HA	137	NG	NG	73.9 (23 to 100)	NG	NG	71.9 (33 to 99)
	THR	115	NG	NG	76.0 (44 to 100)	NG	NG	75.2 (45 to 96)
Macaulay, et al	HA	23	NG	77.1±12	80.6±14.3	81.1 ±11.7	NG	NG
	THR	17	NG	76.1±26.5	84.2±12.0	84.0±12.2	NG	NG

Abbreviations: No(P) = number of knees(patients); HSS = Harris hip score; NG = not given; HA=Hemiarthroplasty; THA: Total Hip Arthroplasty.

320 ml) in the study of Giannini et al. Hedbeck et al reported a smaller proportion of patients who had blood loss over 500 ml in the hemiarthroplasty group (64.3% vs. 93.3%). Macaulay et al noted that more blood transfusion was needed in THR compared to HA (7.7 vs 5.5 unit). However, Cadossi et al recently got an opposite result that more patients undertaking THR had blood loss of less than 500 ml. Total to say, no advantage in either group was observed in this review and more studies providing unified, concrete values are needed.

Surgical time. The mean duration of surgery was a litter longer in THR. Vander et al divided surgical time into three periods and the results were less than one hour (35.2% vs. 9.5%), one to one and a half hour (52.8% vs.61.9%), more than one and a half hour (12% vs. 28.6%) in the HA and THR group respectively. Keating, Macaulay, Giannini observed longer mean surgical time in THR group, while Cadossi found a decrease of 5.6 minutes in THR group. An important possible factor explaining this difference was that with the development of technique and prosthesis, the surgery of THR tended to be more convenient and time saving. Of course, individual differences could not be ignored too.

However, we failed to calculate whether there was a significant difference between these two groups regarding blood loss and surgical time as a result of various value forms. (Table 1)

Strengths and Limitations of This Analysis

Meta-analysis is an effective tool for revealing trends that might not be apparent in a single study. Pooling the data from different high quality studies increases the confidence of the findings regarding the parameters which were addressed in the included studies. The current analysis met the methodological standard with no or low heterogeneity. The number of total patients were large enough and all participants met the including criteria. All of our evaluations were based on randomized controlled trials, which minimize the possibility of recall or selection bias.

To our knowledge, this review is the most current report on this topic. Here, we only included RCTs, the patients were balanced distribution between the two groups. This enhanced the credibility of our statistical result. Despite these advantages, the limitations should be acknowledged separately. Firstly, necessary data were not provided in each trial which may lead to less accuracy of the final conclusion. Secondly, because the number of studies involved in this analysis was relatively small, some of the subgroup analyses were not performed (e.g. age, sex and country). Another important limitation for generalizing our results was that we could not assessed the health-related quality according to some index scores like EQ-5D because of limited data. So the results should be verified by more centers with a longer follow-up in further trials.

Conclusion

An obvious advantage was found in Harris hip score, revision ratewith significant difference for the total hip replacement. Even though dislocation rate was a little higher in THR, it could be treated with manipulative reduction in most cases. Regarding all these results, it could be concluded that total hip replacement should be the first choice of treatment in elderly and independent patients with fracture of the femoral neck.

Author Contributions

Conceived and designed the experiments: YZ DF. Performed the experiments: KC GL ZC. Analyzed the data: YS XY. Contributed reagents/materials/analysis tools: YZ XY. Wrote the paper: YZ DF GL ZC YS XY.

References

1. Riggs BL, Melton LJ III (1995) The worldwide problem of osteoporosis: insights afforded by epidemiology. Bone 17: 505s–511s.
2. Parker MJ, Gurusamy K (2006) Internal fixation versus arthroplasty for intracapsular proximal femoral fractures in adults. Cochrane Database Syst Rev: Cd001708.
3. Parker MJ, Gurusamy KS, Azegami S (2010) Arthroplasties (with and without bone cement) for proximal femoral fractures in adults. Cochrane Database Syst Rev: Cd001706.
4. Bhandari M, Devereaux PJ, Swiontkowski MF, Tornetta P III, Obremskey W, et al. (2003) Internal fixation compared with arthroplasty for displaced fractures of the femoral neck. A meta-analysis. J Bone Joint Surg Am 85-a: 1673–1681.
5. Parker MJ, Khan RJ, Crawford J, Pryor GA (2002) Hemiarthroplasty versus internal fixation for displaced intracapsular hip fractures in the elderly. A randomised trial of 455 patients. J Bone Joint Surg Br 84: 1150–1155.
6. Goh SK, Samuel M, Su DH, Chan ES, Yeo SJ (2009) Meta-analysis comparing total hip arthroplasty with hemiarthroplasty in the treatment of displaced neck of femur fracture. J Arthroplasty 24: 400–406.
7. Liao L, Zhao J, Su W, Ding X, Chen L, et al. (2012) A meta-analysis of total hip arthroplasty and hemiarthroplasty outcomes for displaced femoral neck fractures. Arch Orthop Trauma Surg 132: 1021–1029.
8. Stroup DF, Berlin JA, Morton SC, Olkin I, Williamson GD, et al. (2000) Meta-analysis of observational studies in epidemiology: a proposal for reporting. Meta-analysis Of Observational Studies in Epidemiology (MOOSE) group. Jama 283: 2008–2012.
9. Wu R, Li B (1999) A multiplicative-epistatic model for analyzing interspecific differences in outcrossing species. Biometrics 55: 355–365.
10. Higgins JP, Thompson SG, Deeks JJ, Altman DG (2003) Measuring inconsistency in meta-analyses. Bmj 327: 557–560.
11. Cadossi M, Chiarello E, Savarino L, Tedesco G, Baldini N, et al. (2013) A comparison of hemiarthroplasty with a novel polycarbonate-urethane acetabular component for displaced intracapsular fractures of the femoral neck: a randomised controlled trial in elderly patients. Bone Joint J 95-b: 609–615.
12. Macaulay W, Nellans KW, Iorio R, Garvin KL, Healy WL, et al. (2008) Total hip arthroplasty is less painful at 12 months compared with hemiarthroplasty in treatment of displaced femoral neck fracture. Hss j 4: 48–54.
13. van den Bekerom MP, Hilverdink EF, Sierevelt IN, Reuling EM, Schnater JM, et al. (2010) A comparison of hemiarthroplasty with total hip replacement for displaced intracapsular fracture of the femoral neck: a randomised controlled multicentre trial in patients aged 70 years and over. J Bone Joint Surg Br 92: 1422–1428.
14. Keating JF, Grant A, Masson M, Scott NW, Forbes JF (2006) Randomized comparison of reduction and fixation, bipolar hemiarthroplasty, and total hip arthroplasty. Treatment of displaced intracapsular hip fractures in healthy older patients. J Bone Joint Surg Am 88: 249–260.
15. Giannini S, Chiarello E, Cadossi M, Luciani D, Tedesco G (2011) Prosthetic surgery in fragility osteopathy. Aging Clin Exp Res 23: 40–42.
16. Hedbeck CJ, Enocson A, Lapidus G, Blomfeldt R, Tornkvist H, et al. (2011) Comparison of bipolar hemiarthroplasty with total hip arthroplasty for displaced femoral neck fractures: a concise four-year follow-up of a randomized trial. J Bone Joint Surg Am 93: 445–450.
17. Avery PP, Baker RP, Walton MJ, Rooker JC, Squires B, et al. (2011) Total hip replacement and hemiarthroplasty in mobile, independent patients with a displaced intracapsular fracture of the femoral neck: a seven- to ten-year follow-up report of a prospective randomised controlled trial. J Bone Joint Surg Br 93: 1045–1048.
18. Ravikumar KJ, Marsh G (2000) Internal fixation versus hemiarthroplasty versus total hip arthroplasty for displaced subcapital fractures of femur—13 year results of a prospective randomised study. Injury 31: 793–797.
19. Berry DJ, von Knoch M, Schleck CD, Harmsen WS (2005) Effect of femoral head diameter and operative approach on risk of dislocation after primary total hip arthroplasty. J Bone Joint Surg Am 87: 2456–2463.
20. Soreide O, Skjaerven R, Alho A (1982) The risk of acetabular protrusion following prosthetic replacement of the femoral head. Acta Orthop Scand 53: 791–794.
21. Tidermark J, Ponzer S, Svensson O, Soderqvist A, Tornkvist H (2003) Internal fixation compared with total hip replacement for displaced femoral neck fractures in the elderly. A randomised, controlled trial. J Bone Joint Surg Br 85: 380–388.
22. Waaler Bjornelv GM, Frihagen F, Madsen JE, Nordsletten L, Aas E (2012) Hemiarthroplasty compared to internal fixation with percutaneous cannulated screws as treatment of displaced femoral neck fractures in the elderly: cost-utility analysis performed alongside a randomized, controlled trial. Osteoporos Int 23: 1711–1719.
23. Johansson T, Jacobsson SA, Ivarsson I, Knutsson A, Wahlstrom O (2000) Internal fixation versus total hip arthroplasty in the treatment of displaced femoral neck fractures: a prospective randomized study of 100 hips. Acta Orthop Scand 71: 597–602.
24. Jonsson B, Sernbo I, Carlsson A, Fredin H, Johnell O (1996) Social function after cervical hip fracture. A comparison of hook-pins and total hip replacement in 47 patients. Acta Orthop Scand 67: 431–434.
25. Woo RY, Morrey BF (1982) Dislocations after total hip arthroplasty. J Bone Joint Surg Am 64: 1295–1306.
26. Halley D, Glassman A, Crowninshield RD (2004) Recurrent dislocation after revision total hip replacement with a large prosthetic femoral head. A case report. J Bone Joint Surg Am 86-a: 827–830.
27. Enocson A, Hedbeck CJ, Tidermark J, Pettersson H, Ponzer S, et al. (2009) Dislocation of total hip replacement in patients with fractures of the femoral neck. Acta Orthop 80: 184–189.
28. Enocson A, Tidermark J, Tornkvist H, Lapidus LJ (2008) Dislocation of hemiarthroplasty after femoral neck fracture: better outcome after the anterolateral approach in a prospective cohort study on 739 consecutive hips. Acta Orthop 79: 211–217.
29. Suh KT, Park BG, Choi YJ (2004) A posterior approach to primary total hip arthroplasty with soft tissue repair. Clin Orthop Relat Res: 162–167.
30. Rodriguez-Merchan EC (2002) Displaced intracapsular hip fractures: hemi-arthroplasty or total arthroplasty? Clin Orthop Relat Res: 72–77.
31. Baker RP, Squires B, Gargan MF, Bannister GC (2006) Total hip arthroplasty and hemiarthroplasty in mobile, independent patients with a displaced intracapsular fracture of the femoral neck. A randomized, controlled trial. J Bone Joint Surg Am 88: 2583–2589.
32. Poignard A, Bouhou M, Pidet O, Flouzat-Lachaniette CH, Hernigou P (2011) High dislocation cumulative risk in THA versus hemiarthroplasty for fractures. Clin Orthop Relat Res 469: 3148–3153.

12

The Epidemic of Hip Fractures: Are We on the Right Track?

Klaas A. Hartholt[1,2], Christian Oudshoorn[1], Stephanie M. Zielinski[2], Paul T. P. W. Burgers[2], Martien J. M. Panneman[3], Ed F. van Beeck[4], Peter Patka[2], Tischa J. M. van der Cammen[1]*

1 Department of Internal Medicine - Section of Geriatric Medicine, Erasmus MC, University Medical Center Rotterdam, Rotterdam, The Netherlands, **2** Department of Surgery-Traumatology, Erasmus MC, University Medical Center Rotterdam, Rotterdam, The Netherlands, **3** Consumer and Safety Institute, Amsterdam, The Netherlands, **4** Department of Public Health, Erasmus MC, University Medical Center Rotterdam, Rotterdam, The Netherlands

Abstract

Background: Hip fractures are a public health problem, leading to hospitalization, long-term rehabilitation, reduced quality of life, large healthcare expenses, and a high 1-year mortality. Especially older adults are at greater risk of fractures than the general population, due to the combination of an increased fall risk and osteoporosis. The aim of this study was to determine time trends in numbers and incidence rates of hip fracture-related hospitalizations and admission duration in the older Dutch population.

Methods and Findings: Secular trend analysis of all hospitalizations in the older Dutch population (≥65 years) from 1981 throughout 2008, using the National Hospital Discharge Registry. Numbers, age-specific and age-adjusted incidence rates (per 10,000 persons) of hospital admissions and hospital days due to a hip fracture were used as outcome measures in each year of the study. Between 1981 and 2008, the absolute number of hip fractures doubled in the older Dutch population. Incidence rates of hip fracture-related hospital admissions increased with age, and were higher in women than in men. The age-adjusted incidence rate increased from 52.0 to 67.6 per 10,000 older persons. However, since 1994 the incidence rate decreased (percentage annual change −0.5%, 95% CI: −0.7; −0.3), compared with the period 1981–1993 (percentage annual change 2.3%, 95% CI: 2.0; 2.7). The total number of hospital days was reduced by a fifth, due to a reduced admission duration in all age groups. A possible limitation was that data were obtained from a linked administrative database, which did not include information on medication use or co-morbidities.

Conclusions: A trend break in the incidence rates of hip fracture-related hospitalizations was observed in the Netherlands around 1994, possibly as a first result of efforts to prevent falls and fractures. However, the true cause of the observation is unknown.

Editor: William John Taylor, University of Otago, New Zealand

Funding: Grants from The Netherlands Organization for Health Research and Development (ZonMw, project number 170.885.607 and 170.882.503) and a grant from NutsOhra (project number T-0602-43) were received. The funders had no role in study design, data collection and analysis, decision to publish, or preparation of the manuscript.

Competing Interests: A grant from NutsOhra (project number T-0602-43) was received.

* E-mail: t.vandercammen@erasmusmc.nl

Introduction

Fall incidents and fall-related injuries among older people are a major public health problem in ageing societies worldwide [1,2,3]. Of people aged ≥65 years approximately one third fall each year [4,5,6,7]. Especially older individuals are at an increased risk of sustaining fractures after a low energetic trauma, *e.g.* a fall incident, due to underlying medical conditions, especially osteoporosis [8].

Osteoporosis, a highly prevalent condition in the older population, is characterized by low bone mass and micro-architectural deterioration of bone tissue. Osteoporosis results in an increased bone fragility and increased susceptibility to fractures [8]. Typical sites of osteoporotic fractures include those of the hip, wrist, vertebrae, and upper arm [9]. Approximately 85% of all hip fractures occur in individuals aged ≥65 years [10]. Hip fractures are, more than any other type of fracture, associated with a loss of independence [11], morbidity [12], and mortality [13].

Besides the health impact on the individual patient, the socioeconomic impact of osteoporosis and of hip fractures in particular is substantial [14]. Hip fractures are currently leading to nearly half (46%) of all injury related healthcare costs in older adults in the Netherlands [15,16]. In a global perspective, the annual estimated worldwide direct and indirect costs of hip fractures amounted to $34.8 billion in 1990, and are expected to rise to an estimated $131 billion by 2050 [17]. With the expected continuing ageing of populations worldwide [18], it might be expected that the number of hip fractures will increase accordingly, making it necessary to prepare our healthcare systems for this burden.

In order to optimize healthcare use and healthcare planning in an ageing society, accurate numbers in hip fracture incidence are mandatory. The aim of this study was to provide secular trends of age- and gender specific numbers, incidence rates and length of hospital stay (LOS) of hip fractures in the older Dutch population.

Materials and Methods

For this study all data of hospital admissions due to a hip fracture in persons aged ≥65 years were collected from 1981 throughout 2008 in the Netherlands. The data were retrieved from Statistics Netherlands (CBS, The Hague, The Netherlands), which combines information of the National Medical Registration (LMR) [19] and the National Hospital Discharge Registry. Data regarding hospital admissions, admission diagnosis, LOS in days, age, and gender are stored in this database. The LMR database has a high nationwide coverage and nearly all admissions are stored in this database (less than five percent missing). Hospital admissions data and population numbers were verified with the national Birth-Registry [19]. The Birth-Registry is used to identify individual patients in the National Medical Registry. Data were corrected for missing values by the Statistics Netherlands, and extrapolated to full national coverage [20]. A uniform classification and coding system is used by the LMR for all hospitals and did not change during the study period. Official coding clerks register the diagnosis and injury mechanism of all hospital admissions, based on data obtained from medical records. Throughout the study period, a hip fracture was defined by using the International Classification for Diseases, 9th revision of the World Health Organization, code 820. Older persons were defined as persons aged 65 years and older. Demographic numbers were retrieved from the Statistics Netherlands. In this study the mid-year population was used. The medical ethical review board of the Erasmus MC, University Medical Center, Rotterdam, approved the study (MEC-2010-402) and provided a waiver for 'informed consent', because the data were retrieved from a large public accessible database, containing anonymous data on admissions, which cannot be traced to individuals.

Numbers of hospitalizations due to hip fractures were specified for age and gender. The age-specific incidence rates were calculated in 5-year age groups using the number of hip fractures in that specific age group, divided by the population size within that specific age-group for male and female patients, and was expressed per 10,000 persons in that age-group. Age-adjusted incidence rates allowed us to compare the incidence rate for a standardized population during the study period, and were performed by 'Direct Standardization' to correct for demographic changes throughout the study period. Growth in the numbers of hospital admissions and LOS were calculated in percentages compared to the index year 1981.

Data were analyzed using a Poisson regression analysis for annual growth in overall hospital admissions for older persons, corrected for population size and age composition. In order to model the trend in hospital admissions, a linear regression model with Poisson error and log link was built with log (mid year population size of each year of the study) as offset factor. To assess if the annual growth changed during the study period for both genders, the Joinpoint Regression Program, Version 3.4.3. (Statistical Research and Applications Branch, National Cancer Institute, USA) was used. This program showed the necessity for assuming a spline instead of a simple linear model, for men and women separately, and determines where to place the knot. The spline function accommodated two piecewise linear fits, connected with one another at the knot. Comparison of these two periods enabled us to detect and quantify changes in the secular trend in admission rates such as stagnation or an increase in admission rates. The best knot was found to be January 1, 1994. The parameter for calendar year, corrected for gender and age-group was transformed into Percentage Annual Change (PAC). The analysis including splines yielded estimates of annual changes in admission rates within each period (1981–1993 and 1994–2008). All statistical analyses were performed using the Statistical Package for the Social Sciences (SPSS) software (version 16.1.1). A p-value <0.05 was considered statistically significant.

Results

During the study period from 1981 throughout 2008, 355,320 patients aged ≥65 years were admitted due to a hip fracture in the Netherlands. The annual number of hip fracture-related hospitalizations doubled in both men and women, from 7,614 cases in 1981 to 16,049 cases in 2008 (Table 1). The male:female ratio remained 1:3 throughout the study period. The crude incidence rate increased, from 46.4 per 10,000 older adults in 1981 to 66.5 per 10,000 in 2008 (an increase of 43.3% compared to 1981), and peaked in 1995 (70.4 per 10,000 older adults). For older men the crude incidence rate increased from 27.6 to 39.5 (an increase of 43.3%) and for older women from 59.5 to 86.8 (an increase of 46.0%) from 1981 to 2008 respectively.

Gender and age-specific incidence rates of hip fracture-related hospital admissions are shown in Table 2. For men and women aged 65–74 years the age-specific incidence rates of hip fractures did not change significantly when comparing 2008 to 1981. However, a strong increase (>50%) in the incidence rate of hospital admissions due to hip fracture was seen in men aged ≥80 years since 1981, up to an increase of 127% in men aged ≥95 years (from 156.3 per 10,000 in 1981 to 354.7 per 10,000 in 2008). Age-specific incidence rates for women aged ≥75 years showed growth of one sixth to a quart.

The overall age-adjusted incidence rate of hip fractures increased (Figure 1) from 52.0 per 10,000 older adults in 1981 to 62.7 in 2008 (an increase of 20.6%). Throughout the study period, the age-adjusted incidence rate for women (68.6 per 10,000 older women in 1981 and 79.9 in 2008) remained twice as high compared to men (27.9 per 10,000 older men in 1981 and 37.8 in 2008).

The PAC, change per year, of the age-adjusted incidence rate was 1.13% (CI 95%: 0.80; 1.45) for men versus 0.52% (CI 95%: 0.24; 0.81) for women over the whole study period. A joint-point regression analysis showed that the change in age-adjusted incidence rates was not constant over time and could be divided into two phases: first, the incidence of hospital admissions due to a hip fracture in older patients increased between 1981 and 1993,

Table 1. Population Characteristics of Persons Aged ≥65 Years, Number, Incidence and mean Admission Duration of Hip Fracture-Related Hospitalizations in Persons Aged ≥65 Years (The Netherlands, 1981–2008).

Characteristic	1981	1986	1991	1996	2001	2006	2008
Population ≥65 year (*1,000)	1,642	1,769	1,934	2,061	2,175	2,330	2,415
Female (%)	59.0%	61.2%	60.2%	59.8%	58.9%	57.6%	57.0%
Admissions overall (n)	7,614	9,958	12,565	14,508	14,810	15,249	16,049
- men (n)	1,857	2,281	2,879	3,326	3,385	3,845	4,105
- women (n)	5,757	7,677	9,686	11,182	11,425	11,404	11,944
Incidence rate†	46.4	56.3	65.0	70.4	68.1	65.4	66.5
Mean admission duration, day	37.0	32.1	30.0	23.8	23.1	15.4	14.0

†Crude incidence rate, expressed per 10,000 older adults.

Table 2. Incidence Rates of Hip Fracture-Related Hospital Admissions per 10,000 Persons in the Older Dutch Population (1981–2008).

	65–69 year		70–74 year		75–79 year		80–84 year		85–89 year		90–94 year		≥95 year	
Year	Men	Women	Men	Women	Men	Women	Men	Women	Men	Women	Men	Women	Men	Women
1981	10.2	16.6	16.6	29.5	31.9	58.8	57.7	113.1	89.7	209.8	156.2	272.4	156.3	319.4
1986	11.0	19.6	20.3	34.6	34.8	66.9	65.1	128.6	107.3	229.7	190.0	303.5	233.7	349.2
1991	12.2	21.7	20.7	40.0	41.9	78.9	77.9	134.0	141.1	235.5	220.4	369.9	296.4	379.3
1996	12.2	21.8	24.4	45.5	45.6	82.0	86.3	147.2	148.1	240.0	211.0	363.5	269.0	410.9
2001	9.1	18.0	18.4	38.3	45.1	81.5	80.9	144.6	148.3	241.4	237.3	338.1	345.1	369.3
2006	9.8	15.8	16.9	32.5	38.2	72.1	85.3	138.2	159.6	229.7	265.5	326.1	372.3	385.1
2008	9.1	16.8	18.1	32.2	38.9	70.1	81.1	139.3	161.6	237.5	275.7	325.5	354.7	388.2
Change*	−11%	1%	9%	9%	22%	19%	41%	23%	80%	13%	77%	19%	127%	22%
(95% CI)	(−24; 5)	(−10; 14)	(−5; 26)	(−1; 20)	(8; 37)	(11; 28)	(25; 58)	(16; 31)	(58; 106)	(6; 21)	(47; 112)	(8; 32)	(55; 233)	(0; 48)

*change is 2008 compared to 1981; 95% CI:, 95% Confidence Interval.

and second, decreased between 1994 and 2008 (Figure 1). The annual growth in men was 2.46% (CI 95%: 1.98; 2.94) and in women 2.16% (CI 95%: 1.89; 2.43) in the period 1981–1993. The PAC decreased in the period 1994–2008 to a negative annual growth of −0.34% (CI 95%: −0.86; 0.19) in men and −0.64% (CI 95%: −0.83; −0.46) in women.

Also the mean LOS decreased throughout the study period in both men and women, from 37.0 days in 1981 to 14.0 days in 2008 (Figure 2). The admission duration decreased over 60% in male and female patients of 65–79 years. Reduction in LOS was smaller in the older patient groups. In patients ≥80 years the LOS per admission was reduced by a third. In general, the LOS was age-related: the higher the age, the longer the admission duration (Figure 2). Although the total number of hip fracture-related hospital admissions increased, the total number of hospital-bed-days decreased due to a reduced LOS per admission. The total numbers of hospital-bed-days are shown in Figure 3 and decreased from 281,396 days in 1981 to 224,002 days in 2008 (a decrease of 20%). For all men aged ≥65 years, the total number of hospital days decreased with 8% (from 62,980 days in 1981 to 58,146 days in 2008). In women aged 65–79 years, a reduction of 54% in hospital days was seen (from 94,903 days in 1981 to 43,474 days in 2008). In women aged ≥80 years the number of hospital days increased until 1991 to 194,264 days and from there on started to decrease, with the total number of hospital days in 2008 (122,382 days) just below (−1%) the total number of hospital days in 1981 (123,513 days).

Discussion

In order to determine trends in hip fractures in the older Dutch population, all hip fracture-related hospitalizations were analyzed from 1981 throughout 2008. The age-adjusted incidence rates of hip fractures increased until the end of 1993 in the population ≥65 years. After that year, a trend break was observed and the incidence rates started to decrease. Although an encouraging

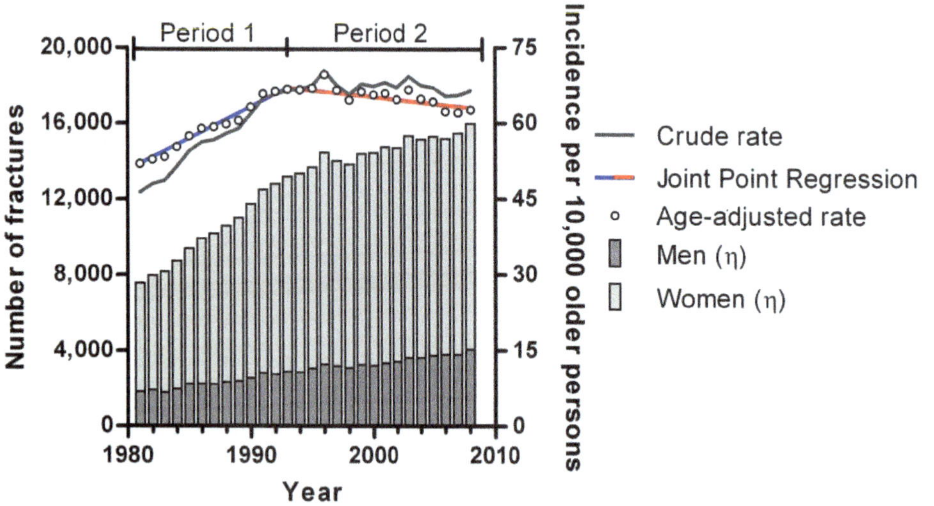

Figure 1. Absolute Numbers, Crude and Age-Specific Incidence Rates of Hip Fracture-Related Hospitalizations in the Dutch Population ≥65 years (1981–2008). Period 1 (blue line): 1981–1993, percentual annual change 2.30%, (95% CI: 2.00; 2.59). Period 2 (red line): 1994–2008, percentual annual change −0.50% (95% CI: −0.70; −0.30).

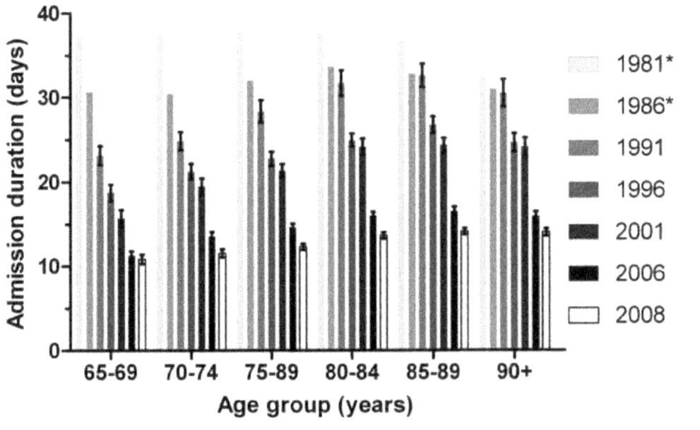

Figure 2. Mean Hospital Admission Duration in Persons Aged ≥65 Years due to a Hip Fracture in the Netherlands between 1981–2008. * No SD data were available before 1991.

decrease in the age-adjusted incidence rates was observed, the absolute number of hip fractures continued to increase due to a rising number of older persons in the population.

Comparable trends of decreasing incidence rates for hip fracture-related hospitalizations since the mid-nineties have been reported in several countries around the globe, such as the United States [21], Canada [22], and Finland [23]. However, not all findings across western countries are consistent. A recent study from Germany failed to demonstrate a decline in hip fracture incidence rates [24]. Since most studies on hip fracture incidence from multiple countries point in the same direction, there might be a causal explanation for this observation. However, there is no simple answer to this question, because risk factors for hip fractures are multifactorial, as mentioned by Leslie *et al.* [22] Important developments over the last two decades include: the increasing awareness of falls [25,26], the implementation of guidelines for the diagnosis and treatment of osteoporosis [27,28], increasing availability and use of bisphosphonates [29], and an improvement of calcium intake and vitamin D status, although the latter is argued by some [22]. Other nationwide changes, such as the prevention and improved treatment of cardiovascular diseases in the general population may also have contributed to the observed trend break. A large Finnish twin-study recently demonstrated that cardiovascular diseases are associated with the

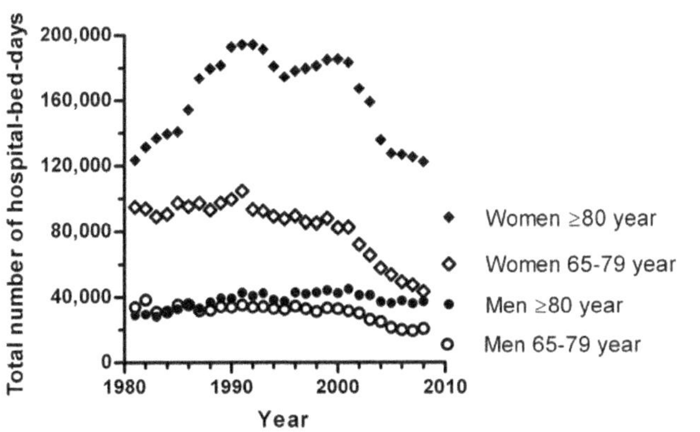

Figure 3. Total Number of Hip Fracture-Related Hospital-Bed-Days in Persons of ≥65 Years in the Netherlands between 1981–2008.

development of hip fractures [30]. However, the exact mechanism behind this association is not clear yet [30]. Another possibility might be that general health [31] and bone quality [32] have improved since smoking has been discouraged. The proportion of smokers is decreasing rapidly in the Netherlands [31,33] as well as in other countries [34,35]. Furthermore, the Statistics Netherlands (CBS) reported that the mean body weight has increased in the Dutch population [33]. An increased Body Mass Index is associated with a lower fracture risk [36].

A remarkable difference was observed between the younger and older age-groups. Whereas incidence rates decreased in persons <80 years, the incidence rate stabilized in females aged ≥80 years, and continued to increase in males ≥80 years. This finding is worrisome because the population of 80 years and over is the fastest growing segment in the ageing population [37] and because mortality and morbidity associated with hip fractures are greater for the oldest old, and are higher in men than in women in the first year after sustaining a hip fracture [38,39]. A possible explanation for this observation might be that life expectancy increased more rapidly in men compared to women over the past decades, resulting in a smaller gap in life expectancy between men and women [40]. Consequently, men have become more vulnerable for age-related (co)morbidities, such as osteoporosis and hip fractures, which were previously frequently seen in older women. This assumption is supported by a previous report on a more rapid increase in fall-related injures, hospitalizations, and mortality in older men than in older women in the Netherlands over the past decades [1,41]. Another possible explanation might be that osteoporosis in men is frequently underdiagnosed and undertreated [42].

The number of hospital-bed-days per admission is considered to be one of the most important determinants of total costs per hip fracture in an individual patient [43]. Therefore, a reduced LOS is necessary in order to reduce hospital care demands and to limit related healthcare costs. During the study period the LOS decreased by two-thirds. Several factors might have contributed to this impressive reduction: the rapid improvement of surgical and anesthetical care over the last decades, resulting in less invasive surgical procedures; the introduction of new hip prostheses, and implants; protocols for early timed surgery after a hip fracture; better pain management and better post-operative care with early mobilization; early discharge to designated rehabilitation places and skilled nursing homes; and the implementation of hip fracture treatment guidelines [44,45,46]. In addition, during the final years of the study period a change in the financing structure of Dutch hospitals, which was introduced in 2004, may have led to a further decline in LOS.

A strength of the present study is the availability of population-based in-hospital data, covering a period of 28 years. The Dutch healthcare system is characterized by full health insurance coverage and full accessibility for the whole population during the study period. Since 1981 absolute numbers of hip fracture related hospital admissions and hospital-bed-days in all hospitals in the Netherlands have been recorded with nearly complete national coverage in a highly accurate electronic database. Throughout the study period, the coding system of the National Medical Registry did not change and no major policy changes were introduced in the Netherlands which might have affected the increase in admission rates. However, this study has some limitations. A possible limitation is that these data describe the situation in one country, which may not directly translate to other western countries, because of differences in healthcare system characteristics and demographics. Nevertheless, since hip fracture trends [21,22,47] in other western populations are comparable with the trends in the Netherlands, there is no reason to assume that hip fractures trends will be substantially different in other countries. This study is based on a linked administrative database, which does not contain clinical data regarding underlying diagnosis, co-morbidity, injury severity, lifestyle, or medication use of the patients. This limits the interpretation of the causal mechanisms behind the observed trends. Furthermore, readmissions in one calendar year were not excluded and could potentially lead to some 'double registration'. However, it is unlikely that readmissions influenced our results, since readmissions for injuries constitute at the most 2.6% (at the maximum) in the Netherlands, as was found in a study by Polinder *et al.* [48]

In summary, the increase in hip fracture incidence rates slowed down between 1981 and 1993, and the incidence rates started to decrease over the last 14 years. However, incidence rates nowadays remain higher than in 1981, suggesting that there is still room for improvement. Furthermore, the continuing increasing incidence rates in the oldest men is a worrying trend that deserves specific attention, since the group of persons aged 80 years and older are the fastest growing segment of aging societies. With the expected ageing of societies worldwide, continued attention is needed in order to cope with the demand of hip fracture related care in the near future.

Author Contributions

Conceived and designed the experiments: KAH TJMvdC. Performed the experiments: KAH MJMP. Analyzed the data: KAH MJMP CO PP TJMvdC. Contributed reagents/materials/analysis tools: KAH CO SMZ PTPWB. Wrote the paper: KAH CO SMZ PTPWB MJMP EFvB PP TJMvdC. Approved final version: KAH CO SMZ PTPWB MJMP EFvB PP TJMvdC.

References

1. Hartholt KA, van der Velde N, Looman CW, van Lieshout EM, Panneman MJ, et al. (2010) Trends in fall-related hospital admissions in older persons in the Netherlands. Arch Intern Med 170: 905–911.
2. Kannus P, Parkkari J, Koskinen S, Niemi S, Palvanen M, et al. (1999) Fall-induced injuries and deaths among older adults. Jama 281: 1895–1899.
3. Hartholt KA, Stevens JA, Polinder S, van der Cammen TJM, Patka P (2011) Increase in fall-related hospitalizations in the United States, 2001–2008. J Trauma;E-pub ahead of print; DOI: 10.1097/TA.0b013e31821c36e7.
4. Stalenhoef PA, Crebolder HFJM, Knotnerus JA, van der Horst FGEM (1997) Incidence, risk factors and consequences of falls among elderly subjects living in the community. The European Journal of Public Health 7: 328–334.
5. Hoidrup S, Sorensen TI, Gronbaek M, Schroll M (2003) Incidence and characteristics of falls leading to hospital treatment: a one-year population surveillance study of the Danish population aged 45 years and over. Scand J Public Health 31: 24–30.
6. Dijcks BP, Neyens JC, Schols JM, van Haastregt JC, de Witte LP (2005) [Falls in nursing homes: on average almost two per bed per year, resulting in a fracture in 1.3%]. Ned Tijdschr Geneeskd 149: 1043–1047.
7. Gibson RE, Harden M, Byles J, Ward J (2008) Incidence of falls and fall-related outcomes among people in aged-care facilities in the Lower Hunter region, NSW. N S W Public Health Bull 19: 166–169.
8. [No authors listed] (1993) Consensus development conference: diagnosis, prophylaxis, and treatment of osteoporosis. Am J Med 94: 646–650.
9. Curran D, Maravic M, Kiefer P, Tochon V, Fardellone P (2010) Epidemiology of osteoporosis-related fractures in France: A literature review. Joint Bone Spine 77: 546–551.
10. Braithwaite RS, Col NF, Wong JB (2003) Estimating hip fracture morbidity, mortality and costs. J Am Geriatr Soc 51: 364–370.
11. Boonen S, Singer AJ (2008) Osteoporosis management: impact of fracture type on cost and quality of life in patients at risk for fracture I. Curr Med Res Opin 24: 1781–1788.
12. Chrischilles EA, Butler CD, Davis CS, Wallace RB (1991) A model of lifetime osteoporosis impact. Arch Intern Med 151: 2026–2032.
13. van Staa TP, Dennison EM, Leufkens HG, Cooper C (2001) Epidemiology of fractures in England and Wales. Bone 29: 517–522.
14. Kanis JA, Johnell O (2005) Requirements for DXA for the management of osteoporosis in Europe. Osteoporos Int 16: 229–238.
15. Hartholt KA, van Beeck EF, Polinder S, van der Velde N, van Lieshout EMM, et al. (2010) Societal consequences of falls in the older population: injuries, healthcare costs and long term reduced quality of life. J Trauma;E-pub ahead of print, DOI: 10.1097/TA.0b013e3181f6f5e5.
16. Meerding WJ, Mulder S, van Beeck EF (2006) Incidence and costs of injuries in The Netherlands. Eur J Public Health 16: 272–278.
17. Johnell O (1997) The socioeconomic burden of fractures: today and in the 21st century. Am J Med 103: 20S–25S; discussion 25S–26S.
18. United Nations (2007) World Population Prospects, The 2006 Revision. New York, .
19. van der Stegen R, Ploemacher J (2009) [Discription of methods for statistics by diagnoses in time by using the LMR (1981–2005)]. The Hague: Statistics Netherlands (CBS). 9 p.
20. Statistics Netherlands (CBS) (2009) [Health care use and hospital admission statistics in The Netherlands]. Den Haag: Centraal Bureau voor de Statistiek. Health care use and hospital admission statistics in The Netherlands.
21. Brauer CA, Coca-Perraillon M, Cutler DM, Rosen AB (2009) Incidence and mortality of hip fractures in the United States. Jama 302: 1573–1579.
22. Leslie WD, O'Donnell S, Jean S, Lagace C, Walsh P, et al. (2009) Trends in hip fracture rates in Canada. Jama 302: 883–889.
23. Kannus P, Niemi S, Parkkari J, Palvanen M, Vuori I, et al. (2006) Nationwide decline in incidence of hip fracture. J Bone Miner Res 21: 1836–1838.
24. Icks A, Haastert B, Wildner M, Becker C, Meyer G (2008) Trend of hip fracture incidence in Germany 1995–2004: a population-based study. Osteoporos Int 19: 1139–1145.
25. Dutch Institute for Healthcare Improvement (CBO) (2004) [Guideline "For the prevention of fall incidents in the elderly population"]. Alphen aan de Rijn: Van Zuiden Communications B.V. 83 p.
26. Gillespie LD, Robertson MC, Gillespie WJ, Lamb SE, Gates S, et al. (2009) Interventions for preventing falls in older people living in the community. Cochrane Database Syst Rev. CD007146.
27. Dutch Institute for Healthcare Improvement (CBO) (2002) [Osteoporosis: second reviewed guideline]. Utrecht: van Zuiden Communications B.V. 156 p.
28. Kern LM, Powe NR, Levine MA, Fitzpatrick AL, Harris TB, et al. (2005) Association between screening for osteoporosis and the incidence of hip fracture. Ann Intern Med 142: 173–181.
29. Hollingworth SA, Gunanti I, Nissen LM, Duncan EL (2010) Secondary prevention of osteoporosis in Australia: analysis of government-dispensed prescription data. Drugs Aging 27: 255–264.
30. Sennerby U, Melhus H, Gedeborg R, Byberg L, Garmo H, et al. (2009) Cardiovascular diseases and risk of hip fracture. Jama 302: 1666–1673.
31. Draper H, Frenken F (2008) [The number of smokers is still declining; the quantity of sold cigarettes has been stabilized]. Statistics Netherlands (CBS). The Hague, The Netherlands.
32. Law MR, Hackshaw AK (1997) A meta-analysis of cigarette smoking, bone mineral density and risk of hip fracture: recognition of a major effect. Bmj 315: 841–846.
33. Statistics Netherlands (CBS) (2010) [Health, life style and healthcare use]. The Hague: Statistics Netherlands.
34. National Center for Chronic Disease Prevention and Health Promotion (2010) Tobacco Use: Targeting the Nation's leading killer. Atlanta: Centers for Disease Control and Prevention. pp 1–4.
35. Patja K, Hakala S, Boström G, Nordgren P, Haglund M (2009) Trends of tobacco use in Sweden and Finland: Do differences in tobacco policy relate to tobacco use? Scand J Public Health. pp 153–160.
36. De Laet C, Kanis JA, Oden A, Johanson H, Johnell O, et al. (2005) Body mass index as a predictor of fracture risk: a meta-analysis. Osteoporos Int 16: 1330–1338.
37. Statistics Netherlands (CBS) (2009) [Population prognosis]. The Hague: Statistics Netherlands, Population and prognosis from 1969 until 2040.
38. Khosla S, Amin S, Orwoll E (2008) Osteoporosis in men. Endocr Rev 29: 441–464.
39. Haentjens P, Magaziner J, Colon-Emeric CS, Vanderschueren D, Milisen K, et al. (2010) Meta-analysis: excess mortality after hip fracture among older women and men. Ann Intern Med 152: 380–390.
40. Bruggink J, Knoops K, Nusselder W, van Gool C (2010) [Healthy life expectancy]. Bilthoven, the Netherlands: National Institute for Public Health and the Environment (RIVM). 3 p.
41. Hartholt KA, Polinder S, van Beeck EF, van der Velde N, van Lieshout EMM, et al. (2011) End of the spectacular decrease in fall-related mortality rate: men are catching up. Am J Public Health: In press.
42. Curtis JR, McClure LA, Delzell E, Howard VJ, Orwoll E, et al. (2009) Population-based fracture risk assessment and osteoporosis treatment disparities by race and gender. J Gen Intern Med 24: 956–962.
43. Haentjens P, Lamraski G, Boonen S (2005) Costs and consequences of hip fracture occurrence in old age: an economic perspective. Disabil Rehabil 27: 1129–1141.
44. van Vught AB, van Balen R, van der Cammen TJM, Go PMNYH, Heetveld MJ, et al. (2007) [Guideline: Treatment of proximal femural fractures in older adults]. Utrecht: The Netherlands Surgical Society.

45. Weller I, Wai EK, Jaglal S, Kreder HJ (2005) The effect of hospital type and surgical delay on mortality after surgery for hip fracture. J Bone Joint Surg Br 87: 361–366.
46. Saltzherr TP, Borghans HJ, Bakker RH, Go PM (2006) [Proximal femur fractures in the elderly in The Netherlands during the period 1991–2004: incidence, mortality, length of hospital stay and an estimate of the care capacity needed in the future]. Ned Tijdschr Geneeskd 150: 2599–2604.
47. Kannus P, Niemi S, Parkkari J, Sievanen H, Palvanen M (2009) Declining incidence of low-trauma knee fractures in elderly women: nationwide statistics in Finland between 1970 and 2006. Osteoporos Int 20: 43–46.
48. Polinder S, Meerding WJ, Lyons RA, Haagsma JA, Toet H, et al. (2008) International variation in clinical injury incidence: exploring the performance of indicators based on health care, anatomical and outcome criteria. Accid Anal Prev 40: 182–191.

13

The Effect of Disease Site (Knee, Hip, Hand, Foot, Lower Back or Neck) on Employment Reduction Due to Osteoarthritis

Eric C. Sayre[1,2,3]*, Linda C. Li[1,4], Jacek A. Kopec[1,2], John M. Esdaile[1,5], Sherry Bar[6], Jolanda Cibere[1,5]

1 Arthritis Research Centre of Canada, Vancouver, British Columbia, Canada, **2** School of Population and Public Health, University of British Columbia, Vancouver, British Columbia, Canada, **3** Department of Medicine, University of British Columbia, Vancouver, British Columbia, Canada, **4** Department of Physical Therapy, University of British Columbia, Vancouver, British Columbia, Canada, **5** Division of Rheumatology, Department of Medicine, University of British Columbia, Vancouver, British Columbia, Canada, **6** Primary Health Care, British Columbia Ministry of Health Services, Victoria, British Columbia, Canada

Abstract

Background: Osteoarthritis (OA) has a significant impact on individuals' ability to work. Our goal was to investigate the effects of the site of OA (knee, hip, hand, foot, lower back or neck) on employment reduction due to OA (EROA).

Methods and Findings: This study involved a random sample of 6,000 patients with OA selected from the Medical Service Plan database in British Columbia, Canada. A total of 5,491 were alive and had valid addresses, and of these, 2,259 responded (response rate = 41%), from which 2,134 provided usable data. Eligible participants were 19 or older with physician diagnosed OA based on administrative data between 1992 and 2006. Data of 688 residents were used (mean age 62.1 years (27 to 86); 60% women). EROA had three levels: no reduction; reduced hours; and total cessation due to OA. The (log) odds of EROA was regressed on OA sites, adjusting for age, sex, education and comorbidity. Odds ratios (ORs) represented the effect predicting total cessation and reduced hours/total cessation. The strongest effect was found in lower back OA, with OR = 2.08 (95% CI: 1.47, 2.94), followed by neck (OR = 1.59; 95% CI: 1.11, 2.27) and knee (OR = 1.43; 95% CI: 1.02, 2.01). We found an interaction between sex and foot OA (men: OR = 1.94; 95% CI: 1.05, 3.59; women: OR = 0.89; 95% CI = 0.57, 1.39). No significant effect was found for hip OA (OR = 1.33) or hand OA (OR = 1.11). Limitations of this study included a modest response rate, the lack of an OA negative group, the use of administrative databases to identify eligible participants, and the use of patient self-reported data.

Conclusions: After adjusting for socio-demographic variables, comorbidity, and other OA disease sites, we find that OA of the lower back, neck and knee are significant predictors for EROA. Foot OA is only significantly associated with EROA in males. For multi-site combinations, ORs are multiplicative. These findings may be used to guide resource allocation for future development/improvement of vocational rehabilitation programs for site-specific OA.

Editor: Isabelle Boutron, University Paris 7, France

Funding: Dr. Sayre is supported by a Canadian Arthritis Network (CAN) Postdoctoral Fellowship Award. Dr. Li is supported by a Canadian Institutes of Health Research (CIHR) New Investigator Award, and an American College of Rheumatology Research and Education Foundation Health Professional New Investigator Award. This study was supported by funding from the Arthritis Society British Columbia and Yukon Division (TAS; http://www.arthritis.ca/) and the Healthy Heart Society (http://www.healthyheart.bc.ca/). The funders had no role in study design, data collection and analysis, decision to publish, or preparation of the manuscript.

Competing Interests: The authors have declared that no competing interests exist.

* E-mail: esayre@arthritisresearch.ca

Introduction

Osteoarthritis (OA) is one of the top reasons for long-term disability and employment loss [1,2]. Identifying which groups are at high risk of work loss due to arthritis is an important first step in developing vocational rehabilitation, or work loss prevention programs [3–6]. Studies have looked at disability associated with OA of various sites, including knees [7,8], hips [9], knees and hips [10,11], and hands [12]. Many studies measured an overall effect of OA (or even just "arthritis") at any site [13–16]. The majority referred to employment loss due to OA when describing the effects of disability, but these studies focused their analyses on pain and function (e.g., Western Ontario and McMaster Universities (WOMAC) scales), rather than loss of gainful employment. They used impairment or disability measures like the pain and function scales on the WOMAC as a surrogate of employment reduction. This has made it challenging to interpret the actual impact of OA on gainful employment from many previous studies. Also, while there are studies that have treated foot OA [17,18], neck and/or spine OA [19–21], multiple site OA [22], or pain due to those conditions as outcomes, there do not appear to be *direct* studies of the impact on employment loss due to OA at those sites specifically.

Previous studies of vocational strategies in musculoskeletal diseases have highlighted the differences between strategies that address disability associated with different joints [3–6]. However, they also highlight the relative dearth of vocational rehabilitation programs designed for neck or back OA. For example, Hammond et al (2008) described vocational rehabilitation for musculoskeletal diseases of the hand, knee and hip, including both exercise and assistive devices designed to improve function [3]. Roos et al (2006) described foot supportive devices [23]. Vliet Vlieland et al (2009) reviewed the recent literature on vocational rehabilitation programs in patients with chronic arthritis and found that interventions employed in the early stages of threatened work ability point to a favorable effect. However, the review did not discuss the effectiveness of these programs for patients with OA at specific joints [4]. In a systematic review, Brosseau et al (2003) considered a number of exercise programs for hip and knee OA, but hand, foot, lower back and neck OA were not included [5]. In a review of thermotherapy for OA, Brosseau et al (2003) considered knee OA only [6]. The apparent dearth of vocational devices and strategies designed for site-specific OA, particularly neck or back OA, may in part be due to a lack of studies demonstrating the direct impact of OA at these sites on paid employment loss. Besides vocational rehabilitation programs per se, there are also a variety of assistive devices designed to help those with OA reduce pain or improve function, thereby indirectly improving their chances of maintaining employment [3]. Devices have been developed for musculoskeletal diseases at various sites, including hand (e.g., splint for trapeziometacarpal OA) [24], foot (e.g., orthotics for plantar fasciitis) [23], neck (e.g., resting and immobilizing the neck with a cervical collar) [25], knee or hip [26]. Therapeutic exercises have been developed for before or after surgical intervention [27,28]. While all these approaches have shown varying success at restoring function, none is a cure-all, and employment loss due to osteoarthritis continues to be an unfortunate reality for many with this disease [4].

Like the strategies designed to help those with OA, the effect of OA at each site on paid employment loss is an important question. The purpose of this study was to assess the effects of locations of OA, including the knee, hip, hand, foot, lower back and neck, on the time lost in gainful employment in a combined multivariable model. By including these six important sites in one model, controlling for each other, socio-demographic variables and comorbidity, and allowing for interaction terms, we aim to gain a better understanding of how OA impacts one's ability to work for pay, on a level of detail not yet achieved in other studies.

Methods

Ethics Statement

Informed consent to participate was not obtained by written or verbal agreement, but was obtained by undocumented "implied consent"; the cover letter included with the survey explained that returning the questionnaire implied consent. Implied consent is an acceptable practice for population surveys. The study protocol was approved by the University of British Columbia Behavioral Research Ethics Board (Application number: B04-0289). Their statement was:"The Annual Renewal for Study have been reviewed [*sic*] and the procedures were found to be acceptable on ethical grounds for research involving human subjects." Data were analyzed anonymously.

Data collection

This study is conducted within the British Columbia OA survey, where an initial random sample of 6,000 people with OA, or hip/knee replacement surgeries due to OA, was selected after stratifying by the five health authorities (Vancouver Coastal, Vancouver Island, Fraser, Interior and Northern) [29]. Five hundred and one surveys were returned unopened due to incorrect addresses and eight persons were reported deceased. This left a sample of 5,491 persons.

Random selection was conducted by the BC Ministry of Health Services (MoHS) using administrative billing data for outpatient physician visits (Medical Services Plan Fee-For-Service Database) and hospitalization (Discharge Abstract Database). Individuals were included if they: (1) met the case definitions for OA or hip/knee replacement surgeries between April 1, 1992 and March 31, 2006 (Table 1); (2) had at least two medical visits for OA or one hospitalization within a 365-day period; (3) were age 19 or older on March 31, 2006; (4) were living in BC; and (5) were alive (i.e., no date of death recorded on the MoHS OA administrative database at the time of sampling). The case date was defined as the first date by which the case definition was met.

Three mailings were conducted in 2007 by the MoHS. All participants received a survey package, including an information letter, a questionnaire booklet, and a stamped return envelope during the first mailing (June 20). Reminder cards were sent to everyone at two weeks (July 5) and four weeks (July 19). To protect confidentiality, the MoHS assigned an identification number to all participants. The researchers did not have access to the personal contact information.

The survey included questions about health status (e.g., OA, comorbidities), health services utilization (e.g., visits to a physician, physical therapist, or surgeries), use of medications and supplements (e.g., acetaminophen, non-steroidal anti-inflammatory drugs (NSAIDs), glucosamine), alternative therapies (e.g., water therapy, acupuncture), current and past employment status, and socio-demographic variables.

The locations of OA were determined with the following questions: 1) "What type of arthritis do you have? If you have had joint replacement surgery, please indicate the type of arthritis you had before the surgery"; and 2) "In which joint(s) do/did you have arthritis?" Employment reduction due to OA (EROA) was determined by the series of questions listed in Figure 1. From these we created a 3-level ordinal variable measuring EROA, with the levels "no reduction", "reduced hours" and "total cessation due to OA". This structure was pre-specified to reflect the best available information. Our assumptions were that those who had experienced either no reduction or total cessation due to OA would clearly know that, but those with a partial reduction of hours due to OA could have difficulty quantifying the reduction beyond saying that it was between none and total.

Confounding variables specified *a priori* include sex, age, education, and comorbidities. Age was divided into four groups: 24–54; 55–64; 65–74; and 75+. Education was split into four levels: less than high school; high school; some postsecondary (included "trades certificate, vocational school diploma, apprenticeship" or "non-university certificate below Bachelor's level"); and Bachelor's degree plus (included "Bachelor's degree" and "university degree, certificate or diploma above Bachelor's degree"). Age was divided into four groups: 24–54; 55–64; 65–74; and 75+. Comorbidity was collected as a count of comorbid conditions including: diabetes; kidney and/or bladder problems; fibromyalgia; high blood pressure; lung problems; osteoporosis; heart problems; intestinal or stomach ulcers; cancer; liver problems; bowel disorder; and depression.

Data analysis

The models were fit as proportional odds cumulative logit models [30]. In this model, the effects of the explanatory variables on the odds of being at or above each level of EROA are estimated. Explanatory variables included the six sites of OA, and were also adjusted for age group, sex, education and comorbidity.

Table 1. Osteoarthritis and hip/knee replacement surgeries case definitions.

Osteoarthritis (OA)		
Rule:	One hospitalization or two medical visits in 365 days with an OA diagnostic code	
Diagnostic codes:		
ICD-9	715	Osteo-arthrosis and allied disorders
ICD-10	M15	Polyarthrosis
	M16	Coxarthrosis [arthrosis of hip]
	M17	Gonarthrosis [arthrosis of knee]
	M18	Arthrosis of first carpometacarpal joint
	M19	Other arthrosis
Exclusions:	None	
Hip or knee replacements		
Rule:	At least one hospitalization coded with a hip or knee replacement procedure code	
Procedure codes:		
CCP	934.1	Total knee replacement
	935	Total hip replacement
CCI	1.VA.53-LA-PN	Implant dual comp prosthetic hip OA
	1.VA.53-PN-PN	Implant dual comp prosthetic hip robotic OA
	1.VA.53	Implant sing, dual or tri comp prosthetic knee OA
Exclusions:	Exclude the above procedures if any of the following diagnostic codes exist on the discharge abstract	
ICD-9	800–999	Fractures
	E800–869, E880–E928, E950–E999	Non-medical injury
	140–208	Malignant neoplasms
	235–239	Neoplasm uncertain behavior
ICD-10	S00–S99, V01–V99, W00–W99, X93–99	Non-medical injury
	C00–C97	Malignant neoplasms
	D37–D48	Neoplasm uncertain behavior

Non-proportional odds (i.e., when an effect is dependent on which level of EROA is being considered) were tested (at alpha = 0.05) in all models on a per-variable basis. We included interaction terms between response levels (reduced hours or total cessation due to OA) and each variable. We used the Type III score test for generalized estimating equations models. Statistically significant interactions would lead to rejection of the proportional odds assumption for that variable. Other two-way interactions were selected (at alpha = 0.05) from between the six sites of OA, age group, sex and education. Effects were estimated as odds ratios which (in a proportional odds cumulative logit model) simultaneously estimate the effect of the variable on the odds of reduced hours/total cessation compared to no reduction, as well as on the odds of total cessation compared to no reduction/reduced hours. Model fit was assessed with scaled deviance and c statistics. All statistical analyses were done using SAS version 9.1.3.

Results

Of the 5,491 questionnaires, 2,259 responded (response rate = 41%), from which 2,134 provided usable data, and 1,713 reported that they had been told by a health professional that they had OA. Of these, 1,004 subjects did not provide answers to the employment questions, and an additional 21 subjects had missing data on age, sex or education. This left a total of 688 participants with complete responses to the outcome and explanatory variables. The sample had a mean age of 62.1 years (ranged from 27 to 86). Table 2 lists sample distributions of sex, age group, education, each of the six sites of OA and OA site count from the six sites considered in this study, both overall and split according to employment reduction due to OA. Sixty percent of the sample was female, 36.8% were 65 years old or older and 32.8% had at least some postsecondary education. Nearly a quarter had less than a high school diploma. Overall percentages with OA at each site range from 30.8% (foot) to 65.8% (knee). OA site count (Table 2) ranges from 0 to 6, although all subjects met the eligibility criteria for OA. Subjects who indicated none of the six sites we are studying had the opportunity to indicate site of OA in an "other" field. 97.4% indicated OA in at least one of the six sites; 67% had OA in 2 or more sites, and nearly half of the sample had OA in 3 or more sites. Considering this, there are sufficient degrees of freedom for estimating interaction terms.

Of the 1,713 who reported that they had been told by a health professional that they had OA, 1,025 were excluded from the analysis due to missing variables primarily on employment. In order to investigate the potential impact of this on our study findings, we tabulated sample distributions (Table 3) of age, sex and education in the excluded subjects. The results indicate that those who were not included were generally older (42% of the excluded were 75+ vs. 13% of the included) and less educated (6% of the excluded had a Bachelor's degree plus vs. 13% of the included). Sex was similar in proportion (63% of the excluded

In the past year, have you worked for pay? (This includes working for others for wages, salary, or commission, or being self-employed such as in your own business, farm or profession):

❑ Yes ❑ No ⇒ If no, go to question 16.

If you have worked for pay in the past year, did you reduce the amount that you worked because of your arthritis? (Please check (✓) all that apply).

❑	No	❑	Yes, I have completely stopped work because of my arthritis	❑	Yes, I have missed_____ days of work because of my arthritis
❑	Yes, I have reduced the number of hours I work by ________hours a week	❑	Yes, I have reduced the number of weeks that I work by _____ weeks/year	❑	Yes, I have changed the kind of work I do because of my arthritis
❑	Yes, I have changed how I do my work	❑	Other (please specify): ________________________________		

If you have not worked for pay, are you: (Please check (✓) all that apply).

❑	Retired because of arthritis	❑	Volunteering	❑	Retired, but not because of arthritis
❑	Not working because of arthritis	❑	Staying at home to care for my family or house	❑	Not working because of other medical reasons
❑	Student	❑	Unemployed, but looking for work	❑	Other (please specify): ____________________

Figure 1. Questions for determining employment reduction due to osteoarthritis.

were female vs. 60% of the included), however all three differences were statistically significant at the alpha = 0.05 level, as measured with a chi-square test.

All variables passed the Type III score test for proportional odds. Scaled deviance divided by degrees of freedom was 1.15, which is not much greater than 1, indicating reasonable fit. The c statistic was 0.733, substantially better than 0.5. Table 4 lists the odds ratios with 95% confidence intervals (CIs) from the model. The odds ratios (95% CI) of OA at individual sites range from 1.11 (0.78, 1.57) for hand OA to 2.08 (1.47, 2.94) for lower back OA. The only significant interaction remaining in the model is sex by foot OA, with women having 0.46 times the OR for foot OA compared to men. For women, the effect of foot OA is 0.89 (0.57, 1.39). Therefore the only significant effects of OA site are in the knee (OR = 1.43, 95% CI = 1.02, 2.01), lower back and neck (OR = 1.59, 1.11, 2.27) for both sexes, and in the foot for males only (OR = 1.94, 95% CI = 1.05, 3.59). Hand and hip (OR = 1.33, 95% CI = 0.95, 1.87) were not significant for either sex in the multivariable model.

Among the controlling variables, only comorbidity is significant, with 1.34 times the odds of higher EROA levels for every additional comorbid condition (of those we counted). Sex, age and education all fell in their expected directions according to the common literature for these variables [13,14,16], though none were statistically significant. Specifically, EROA was directionally associated with lower education, older age and being female.

Finally, we performed *post-hoc* analyses to investigate the effect of keeping subjects with joint replacements in the data. Eighty-seven subjects (12.6%) in the analysis sample had a knee replacement, 80 (11.6%) had a hip replacement and 28 (4.1%) indicated "other joint" replacement. Chi-square tests were used to assess the association between joint replacement and EROA, and the results indicated a reverse effect, that joint replacement is associated with higher EROA. To confirm that this effect was free of confounders, we fit proportional odds models predicting higher EROA from joint replacement variables together in one model, adjusting for age, sex, education and comorbidity. The reverse effect remained, and was highly significant for knee (OR = 2.02, 95% CI = 1.27, 3.22) and other joint replacement (OR = 3.47, 95% CI = 1.52, 7.88), although just non-significant for hip (OR = 1.57, 95% CI = 0.97, 2.53).

Discussion

This exploratory analysis provides evidence on the unique contribution of OA sites on employment reduction, with the largest effect found in OA of the lower back. Two-way interactions between sites were not significant, indicating that the effects of each site on EROA were independent of other affected sites. This means that the effects of multiple OA sites on EROA are multiplicative (in odds ratios), and confidence intervals of ORs for multi-site OA can be obtained using the covariance matrix of the parameter estimates. For example, the OR for the effect on EROA due to OA in the knee, hip and foot simultaneously is 3.71, 95% CI = 2.32, 5.93. This is an important finding because while the individual effects of OA at the hip and hand are not significant, they contribute to raising the odds of employment reduction in patients with OA in multiple sites.

We did not exclude subjects who had had joint replacement surgery, which may raise questions about the effects, when those who have a degenerated joint replaced are generally less disabled post-surgery. However, our finding that EROA and previous joint replacement surgery are positively correlated in our data suggests that keeping these subjects in our sample does not bias the results,

Table 2. Distribution of sample characteristics, overall and by level of Employment Reduction due to OA.

Variable	Overall	Employment reduction due to OA		
n (%)	(N=688)	No reduction (N=382)	Reduced hours (N=80)	Total cessation due to OA (N=226)
Sex				
Female	410 (59.6)	220 (57.6)	43 (53.8)	147 (65.0)
Male	278 (40.4)	162 (42.4)	37 (46.3)	79 (35.0)
Age group				
24–54	161 (23.4)	108 (28.3)	25 (31.3)	28 (12.4)
55–64	274 (39.8)	150 (39.3)	41 (51.3)	83 (36.7)
65–74	165 (24.0)	76 (19.9)	10 (12.5)	79 (35.0)
75+	88 (12.8)	48 (12.6)	4 (5.0)	36 (15.9)
Education				
Less than high school	154 (22.4)	72 (18.8)	3 (3.8)	79 (35.0)
High school	308 (44.8)	169 (44.2)	37 (46.3)	102 (45.1)
Some postsecondary	135 (19.6)	79 (20.7)	28 (35.0)	28 (12.4)
Bachelor's degree plus	91 (13.2)	62 (16.2)	12 (15.0)	17 (7.5)
*OA site				
Knee	453 (65.8)	235 (61.5)	57 (71.3)	161 (71.2)
Hand	343 (49.9)	165 (43.2)	38 (47.5)	140 (61.9)
Lower back	272 (39.5)	109 (28.5)	29 (36.3)	134 (59.3)
Hip	259 (37.6)	121 (31.7)	28 (35.0)	110 (48.7)
Neck	231 (33.6)	92 (24.1)	26 (32.5)	113 (50.0)
Foot	212 (30.8)	97 (25.4)	24 (30.0)	91 (40.3)
†OA site count				
0	18 (2.6)	11 (2.9)	3 (3.8)	4 (1.8)
1	210 (30.5)	157 (41.1)	20 (25.0)	33 (14.6)
2	145 (21.1)	89 (23.3)	20 (25.0)	36 (15.9)
3	136 (19.8)	62 (16.2)	18 (22.5)	56 (24.8)
4	78 (11.3)	33 (8.6)	10 (12.5)	35 (15.5)
5	56 (8.1)	14 (3.7)	6 (7.5)	36 (15.9)
6	45 (6.5)	16 (4.2)	3 (3.8)	26 (11.5)

*Percentages add up to more than 100% due to multiple OA sites.
†Only counting knee, hip, hand, foot, lower back and neck.

and rather, it ensures a more representative distribution of OA severity (since subjects with more severe disease are the ones who need joint replacement).

Our results are comparable with those reported by previous studies. In 2005, Dahaghin et al (2005) found that "... positive radiographic hand osteoarthritis was a poor explanation for hand pain ... or hand disability" [12]. This is consistent with our findings in which hand OA had the lowest odds ratio in our model, and not significantly different from unity. Bother-Scheepers et al (2004) found that patients with lumbar spine degeneration reported more limitation in activities than those without lumbar spine degeneration [21], which is consistent with our finding of an increased OR for lower back OA. Rytter et al (2007) found a positive but non-significant association between knee complaints lasting more than 30 days during the past 12 months and exclusion from employment among floor layers (OR = 1.4, 95% CI = 0.6, 3.5) [7]. Their estimate exactly matches the point estimate for knee OA in our multivariable model with an OR of 1.43, although our result was statistically significant. Heijbel et al (2005) found that the most common reasons for sick leave in the public sector were long-lasting musculoskeletal problems, especially neck/shoulder and low back pain [20]. Discounting foot OA (which is only important in males in our model), lower back and neck OA have the two highest effects in our results. In a less direct example relating our findings to the existing literature, when selecting interactions, the foot OA by hip OA interaction was approaching statistical significance (p-value = 0.054). To further investigate this, we fit an alternative model in which this interaction was allowed in instead of the sex by foot OA interaction. In that model with only the one interaction retained, the interaction was significant, and the estimate indicated that the presence of foot OA reduces the effect of hip OA (or vice versa), or put another way, that the effect of both hip and foot OA together was no worse than either one alone. That neither interaction was significant when the sex by foot OA interaction term was included is possibly related to differences in prevalence; females exhibit more OA at all sites except the knee in our data, at which the sexes show equal prevalence. Nevertheless, consistent with existing literature, the

Table 3. Distribution of sample characteristics in excluded subjects (N = 1,025).

Variable	n (%)
Sex	
Female	648 (63.2)
Male	350 (34.1)
Missing	27 (2.6)
Age group	
24–54	73 (7.1)
55–64	169 (16.5)
65–74	340 (33.2)
75+	426 (41.6)
Missing	17 (1.7)
Education	
Less than high school	253 (24.7)
High school	470 (45.9)
Some postsecondary	208 (20.3)
Bachelor's degree plus	66 (6.4)
Missing	28 (2.7)

idea that foot OA may not independently impact disability due to OA has been discussed previously (Menz et al, 2005) [31].

This study has implications to policy. Allocating limited health care resources (including vocational counselors, rehabilitation therapists and assistive devices), is a challenge. Understanding which disease sites significantly affect paid employment loss may better inform such decisions. For instance, hand OA is not significantly associated with EROA, but lower back and neck OA are important determinants in both sexes. This is consistent with a relative dearth of vocational rehabilitation programs designed for OA of the lower back and neck, and would seem to suggest an area in need of additional research. Secondly, that the effect of foot OA is significant in males but not in females (and that the difference is significant) may imply a sex inequality with respect to either the utilization or effectiveness of assistive devices or exercise programs for feet, as far as their capacity to reduce EROA (which in turn may be related to the more physical nature of some men's jobs). This also may indicate an area for further research: how can existing vocational therapies and assistive devices be improved or reallocated to better serve men with OA of the foot? Finally, that knee OA remains significantly associated with EROA suggests that despite the knee being the most common site of OA in weight-bearing joints, there remains room to improve or add to existing programs and assistive devices for knee OA.

Table 4. Odds ratios from the proportional odds cumulative logit model for employment reduction due to OA.

Variable	Odds ratio (95% CI)
Knee OA	1.43 (1.02, 2.01)
Hip OA	1.33 (0.95, 1.87)
Hand OA	1.11 (0.78, 1.57)
Foot OA	1.94 (1.05, 3.59)
Lower back OA	2.08 (1.47, 2.94)
Neck OA	1.59 (1.11, 2.27)
Female*Foot OA	0.46 (0.22, 0.96)
Sex	
Female	1.21 (0.82, 1.80)
Male	1
Age group	
24–54	0.87 (0.48, 1.56)
55–64	1.41 (0.83, 2.40)
65–74	1.66 (0.96, 2.85)
75+	1
Education	
Less than high school	1.45 (0.96, 2.18)
High school	1
Some postsecondary	0.72 (0.46, 1.10)
Bachelor's degree plus	0.66 (0.39, 1.11)
Comorbidity	1.34 (1.19, 1.51)

This study has a number of limitations. While OA was confirmed via our case definition and administrative records, site(s) of OA were collected by self-report. This cannot generally be considered as accurate as a doctor's diagnosis of OA at each site, and sites were not independently confirmed to have OA. In addition, we did not differentiate the sites of hand OA, which commonly affects the carpometacarpal (CMC) joint of the thumb, the proximal interphalangeal (PIP) and distal interphalangeal (DIP) joints of fingers. It may be argued that moderate to severe OA in the CMC joints is more problematic than that in the fifth DIP joint, since the former might affect gripping and writing [32]. Another limitation is that our response rate is low. Out of 1,713 subjects with OA who responded to the OA survey, only 688 (40%) were eventually analyzed in our models due to missing or inconsistent reporting of the employment-related variables. Chi-square tests between included and excluded groups revealed no significant differences in the prevalence of knee, hip, hand or lower back OA, but those who were included in the analysis showed somewhat higher (statistically significant) levels of foot OA (31% vs. 25%) and neck OA (34% vs. 27%). We did find statistically significant differences between included/excluded subjects on socio-demographic variables. Specifically, excluded subjects (primarily due to missing employment variables) were generally older and less educated. Finally, since our sample included only individuals who had an OA-related physician visit based on records on the provincial administrative database, we do not have a control group that does not have OA. Our data do however have a large number of subjects with OA in multiple sites, and as such our models can still effectively estimate the effects of multiple OA site(s) on EROA. Nevertheless, in order to estimate these effects for a general population (i.e., to compare the odds of EROA in those with OA at various sites against those without any OA), one would require a control group. Administrative data in the USA frequently present a limitation related to the mixture of insured and uninsured persons seeking treatment, potentially biasing which patients end up being recorded. However, in British Columbia, >99% are covered by Medical Services Plan (MSP) coverage, so this limitation is not present in our data. On the other hand, MSP data do reflect other limitations of administrative data, for example, the fact that visits for other musculoskeletal conditions or pain may be coded as being for OA, and vice versa. To address this issue, we only include those who had at least two OA-related visits or one major procedure due to OA in our case definition. The similar strategy was also used by Lacaille et al

[33] to identify people with rheumatoid arthritis using administrative data. In summary, we find that employment reduction due to OA is dependent on the site(s) affected by OA. This study may offer new insights into areas in the highest need of improvement in the workplace both in terms of ergonomics and other accommodations for those with disabling OA (e.g., better chairs or keyboards), as well as vocational rehabilitation programs and assistive devices. As the proportionality of our model indicates, such efforts could potentially reduce the impact of osteoarthritis on patients' ability to continue at a full or reduced capacity to participate in gainful employment, versus having to reduce or cease employment altogether.

Author Contributions

Conceived and designed the experiments: LCL JAK JE SB JC. Performed the experiments: LCL JAK SB. Analyzed the data: ECS. Wrote the paper: ECS LCL JAK JE SB JC.

References

1. Badley EM (1995) The effect of osteoarthritis on disability and health care use in Canada. J Rheumatol 43: S19–S22.
2. Gobelet C, Luthi F, Al-Khodairy AT, Chamberlain MA (2007) Work in inflammatory and degenerative joint diseases. Disabil Rehabil 29: 1331–1339.
3. Hammond A (2008) Rehabilitation in musculoskeletal diseases. Best Pract Res Clin Rheumatol 22: 435–449.
4. Vlieland TPMV, de Buck PDM, van den Hout WB (2009) Vocational rehabilitation programs for individuals with chronic arthritis. Curr Opin Rheumatol 21: 183–8.
5. Brosseau L, MacLeay L, Welch V, Tugwell P, Wells GA (2003) Intensity of exercise for the treatment of osteoarthritis. Cochrane Database Syst Rev 2003 Issue 2. Art. No.: CD004259. DOI: 10.1002/14651858.CD004259.
6. Brosseau L, Yonge KA, Robinson V, Marchand S, Judd M, et al. (2003) Thermotherapy for treatment of osteoarthritis. Cochrane Database Syst Rev 2003 Issue 4. Art. No.: CD004522. DOI: 10.1002/14651858.CD004522.
7. Rytter S, Jensen LK, Bonde JP (2007) Knee complaints and consequences on work status; a 10-year follow-up survey among floor layers and graphic designers. BMC Musculoskelet Disord 8: 93–93.
8. Chen JC, Linnan L, Callahan LF, Yelin EH, Renner JB, et al. (2007) Workplace policies and prevalence of knee osteoarthritis: the Johnston County Osteoarthritis Project. Occup Environ Med 64: 798–805.
9. Hirata S, Ono R, Yamada M, Takikawa S, Nishiyama T, et al. (2006) Ambulatory physical activity, disease severity, and employment status in adult women with osteoarthritis of the hip. J Rheumatol 33: 939–945.
10. Gupta S, Hawker GA, Laporte A, Croxford R, Coyte PC (2005) The economic burden of disabling hip and knee osteoarthritis (OA) from the perspective of individuals living with this condition. Rheumatology 44: 1531–1537.
11. Palmer KT, Milne P, Poole J, Cooper C, Coggon D (2005) Employment characteristics and job loss in patients awaiting surgery on the hip or knee. J Occup Environ Med 62: 54–57.
12. Dahaghin S, Bierma-Zeinstra SMA, Reijman M, Pols HAP, Hazes JMW, et al. (2005) Prevalence and determinants of one month hand pain and hand related disability in the elderly (Rotterdam study). Ann Rheum Dis 64: 99–104.
13. Abasolo L, Carmona L, Lajas C, Candelas G, Blanco M, et al. (2008) Prognostic factors in short-term disability due to musculoskeletal disorders. Arthritis Care Res 59: 489–496.
14. Kaptein SA, Gignac MAM, Badley EM (2009) Differences in the Workforce Experiences of Women and Men With Arthritis Disability: A Population Health Perspective. Arthritis Care Res 61: 605–613.
15. Gignac MAM, Cao XS, Lacaille D, Anis AH, Badley EM (2008) Arthritis-Related Work Transitions: A Prospective Analysis of Reported Productivity Losses, Work Changes, and Leaving the Labor Force. Arthritis Care Res 59: 1805–1813.
16. Thomas E, Peat G, Harris L, Wilkie R, Croft PR (2004) The prevalence of pain and pain interference in a general population of older adults: cross-sectional findings from the North Staffordshire Osteoarthritis Project (NorStOP). Pain 110: 361–368.
17. Besse JL, Leemrijse T, Themar-Noel C, Tourne Y, Pilliard D, et al. (2006) Congenital club foot: treatment in childhood, outcome and problems in adulthood. Rev Chir Orthop Reparatrice Appar Mot 92: 175–192.
18. Jennings MB (1994) Comparison of piroxicam and naproxen in osteoarthritis of the foot. J Am Podiatr Med Assoc 84: 348–354.
19. Muraki S, Yoshimura N, Oka H, Mabuchi A, En-Yo Y (2007) The association of radiographic osteoarthritis of knee and lumbar spine with pain: The research on osteoarthritis against disability (ROAD) study. Calcif Tissue Int 80: S67–S67.
20. Heijbel B, Josephson M, Jensen I, Vingard E (2005) Employer, insurance, and health system response to long-term sick leave in the public sector: Policy implications. J Occup Rehabil 15: 167–176.
21. Botha-Scheepers SA, Riyazi N, Kroon HM, Slagboom E, Meulebelt I, et al. (2004) Pain and disability in the lower extremities in patients with osteoarthritis (OA) at multiple sites are associated with lumbar spine OA, the number of oa joints, range of motion and psychological factors. Ann Rheum Dis 63: S72–S72.
22. Min JL, Meulenbelt I, Riyazi N, Kloppenburg M, Houwing-Duistermaat JJ, et al. (2005) Association of the Frizzled-related protein gene with symptomatic osteoarthritis at multiple sites. Arthritis Rheum 52: 1077–1080.
23. Roos E, Engstrom M, Soderberg B (2006) Foot orthoses for the treatment of plantar fasciitis. Foot Ankle Int 27: 606–611.
24. Carreira AG, Jones A, Natour J (2007) Effectiveness assessment of a functional splint for patients with trapeziometacarpal osteoarthritis in the dominant hand. Ann Rheum Dis 66: S659–S659.
25. Hostler D, Colburn D, Seitz SR (2009) A Comparison of Three Cervical Immobilization Devices. Prehosp Emerg Care 13: 256–60.
26. Gravlee JR, Van Durme DJ (2007) Braces and splints for musculoskeletal conditions. Am Fam Physician 75: 342–348.
27. Klobas L, Axelsson S, Tegelberg A (2006) Effect of therapeutic jaw exercise on temporomandibular disorders in individuals with chronic whiplash-associated disorders. Acta Odontol Scand 64: 341–347.
28. Levine B, Kaplanek B, Jaffe WL (2009) Pilates Training for Use in Rehabilitation after Total Hip and Knee Arthroplasty: A Preliminary Report. Clin Orthop Relat Res 467: 1468–1475.
29. Li L, Kopec JA, Cibere J, Sayre EC, Esdaile J (2008) British Columbia Osteoarthritis Survey. Final Report to the British Columbia Ministry of Health, April, 2008.
30. Hosmer DW, Lemeshow S (2000) Applied Logistic Regression (Second Ed.). Malden: John Wiley & Sons, Inc. 288 p.
31. Menz HB, Morris ME (2005) Determinants of disabling foot pain in retirement village residents. J Am Podiatr Med Assoc 95: 573–579.
32. Wilder FV, Barrett JP, Farina EJ (2006) Joint-specific prevalence of osteoarthritis of the hand. Osteoarthritis Cartilage 14: 953–957.
33. Lacaille D, Anis AH, Guh DP, Esdaile JM (2005) Gaps in care for rheumatoid arthritis: a population study. Arthritis Rheum 53: 241–248.

14

Difference in the Recruitment of Hip and Knee Muscles between Back Squat and Plyometric Squat Jump

Norihide Sugisaki[1,2]*, Sadao Kurokawa[3], Junichi Okada[4], Hiroaki Kanehisa[5]

1 Center for Environment, Health and Field Sciences, Chiba University, Kashiwa, Chiba, Japan, **2** Waseda Institute for Sport Sciences, Waseda University, Tokorozawa, Saitama, Japan, **3** Center for Liberal Arts, Meiji Gakuin University, Yokohama, Kanagawa, Japan, **4** Faculty of Sport Sciences, Waseda University, Tokorozawa, Saitama, Japan, **5** National Institute of Fitness and Sports in Kanoya, Kanoya, Kagoshima, Japan

Abstract

Athletes who aim to improve both muscular endurance and power often perform exercises that involve similar joint actions under different lifting conditions, such as changes in the load or speed, which are implemented at different times during a periodized exercise program or simultaneously. The prescribed exercises are considered to recruit the same muscles even if the lifting conditions differ to each other. The present study aimed to clarify this by examining whether the recruitment of individual hip and knee muscles during the squat exercise differs between lifting conditions adopted for muscular endurance and power training regimens. Moderately trained men performed back squats (BS), with a load of approximately 60% of one repetition maximum, as a muscular endurance training exercise, and they performed plyometric squat jumping (PSJ) for power training. During each exercise, the lower limb joint torques and the recruitment of five hip and knee muscles were determined with inverse-dynamics and T2-weighted magnetic resonance imaging, respectively. While the maximal and mean knee joint torques were greater during PSJ than during BS ($p<0.01$), the T2 values for the quadriceps femoris muscle did not differ between the exercises. In contrast, the T2 values of the gluteus maximus and hip adductor muscles were higher during PSJ ($p<0.05$) than during BS, although there was no significant difference in the mean hip extension torque between the two exercises. The current results indicate that the individual use of the agonist muscles differs between BS and PSJ, and it does not always correspond with the joint kinetics during the exercises. Therefore, in addition to the exercise type, the lifting condition should also be taken into consideration as a determinant of the major muscles trained during a resistance exercise.

Editor: Amir A. Zadpoor, Delft University of Technology (TUDelft), Netherlands

Funding: This study was supported by JSPS Grant-in-Aid for Scientific Research (24700667), (http://www.jsps.go.jp/j-grantsinaid/index.html). The funders had no role in study design, data collection and analysis, decision to publish, or preparation of the manuscript.

Competing Interests: The authors have declared that no competing interests exist.

* Email: sugisaki@chiba-u.jp

Introduction

The muscular endurance and power generation capabilities of the lower body are essential factors of fitness in not only athletes but also in the untrained populations. In general, exercises aimed to improve muscular endurance are performed at a relatively slow speed with a load corresponding to 15−20 repetitions maximum (RM) or 50−65% of one repetition maximum (1 RM) [1–5]. Exercises aimed at improving muscular power are generally performed at a high speed (explosive motion) with a relatively low load (e.g., 30–60% of 1 RM) [6–8] or without load (i.e., body weight plyometric exercise) [1,9]. Depending on the circumstances, athletes who aim to improve both muscular endurance and power often perform exercises that involve similar joint actions such as hip and knee extension and flexion, with different lifting conditions as mentioned above, in different training periods of a periodized program or simultaneously [1,2,10,11]. Both lifting conditions are considered to recruit (i.e. train) the same muscles because the major muscles involved are usually designated according to the event of exercise without regard to the lifting conditions, e.g., the gluteus maximus (GM), hamstrings (Ham), and quadriceps femoris muscles for squat exercises [12]. However, no study has examined whether the same muscles are recruited during an exercise performed under different lifting conditions. Clarifying this will be useful for designing an effective training program that aims to improve both muscular endurance and power.

Physical movements are usually achieved by forces produced by more than one muscle (i.e., synergist muscles). Synergist muscles differ in several ways, including the fiber type distribution [13], muscle architecture [14], and recruitment patterns [15]. Voigt et al. [15] reported that the soleus muscle dominated the plantar flexion movement in slow motion, while the activity of the gastrocnemius muscle increased in rapid motion. Considering these findings, it is natural to assume that the differences in lifting conditions between the muscular endurance and power training regimens produce a different synergist muscle use, even when exercises with almost similar joint involvement and motions are adopted.

The standard approach to evaluating muscular recruitment during exercise involves the use of surface electromyography (EMG). However, surface EMG has several disadvantages. For example, the detectable region is limited to a small part of the muscle, and it is difficult to detect deep muscle activity. In addition, the surface EMG signal of a small muscle could be affected by crosstalk from nearby muscles [16]. Furthermore, there are problems with surface EMG recordings during dynamic movements, such as a shift of the muscle relative to the electrode position and greater signal variability due to the rapid recruitment of motor units [17]. Several studies have provided evidence to support the use of transverse relaxation time (T2) measurements from magnetic resonance (MR) images of muscles as an alternative approach to assessing the recruitment of exercised muscles. It has been established that the increase in signal intensity and T2 of the muscles is associated with the exercise intensity [18] and osmotically driven shifts of fluid into an intracellular compartment (i.e., metabolic response) [19]. Furthermore, recent studies have revealed that regional increases in T2 after exercise training corresponded with the hypertrophic changes induced after chronic resistance training [20]. These findings indicate that the quantification of the exercise-induced increase in T2 is useful to evaluate the recruitment of individual muscles during an exercise with relation to the differences in the lifting conditions.

In the present study, we performed two experiments, which aimed to clarify the differences in the joint torque (Experiment 1) and recruitment of the thigh and hip muscles (Experiment 2) between the back squat (BS), with a load programmed for improving muscular endurance, and plyometric repeated squat jumping (PSJ) as a power training exercise. BS and PSJ are the most popular exercises for strengthening lower limb muscles and are characterized as multi-joint exercises involving hip, knee, and ankle joint extension, which require the use of various lower limb muscles. We hypothesized that the recruitment of the individual muscles involved in an exercise differs between BS and PSJ, even when the difference in the developed joint torque is taken into consideration.

Materials and Methods

Ethics Statement

This study was approved by the Ethics Committee on Human Research of Waseda University, and all procedures were conducted in accordance with the Declaration of Helsinki. Prior to the experiments, all subjects were fully informed of the purpose and risks of the experiment and gave their written consent.

Subjects

Ten healthy men (age 28±4 years, height 173±5 cm, weight 69±6 kg, PSJ jump height 44±6 cm, mean ± SD) voluntarily participated in Experiment 1, and 8 healthy men (age 24±2 years, height 172±8 cm, weight 69±6 kg, PSJ jump height 43±6 cm) in Experiment 2. Seven of the subjects in Experiment 2 were also involved in Experiment 1, and they completed all procedures in both experiments. The subjects had practiced squat training for at least 1 year and were familiar with the proper technique for executing the BS and PSJ tasks, which was confirmed by a certified strength and conditioning coach.

Procedures

Experiment 1. Joint kinematics and the ground reaction forces were determined during BS and PSJ. Prior to the test, the subjects performed at least 5 min of warm-up exercises, including static and less intensive dynamic stretching. The subjects were allowed to perform warm-up exercises of their choice except that they were required to perform static and dynamic stretching exercises for the triceps surae, the quadriceps femoris, the Ham, and the gluteus muscles. At the end of the warm-up session, the subjects performed one or two repetitions of BS and PSJ with the same conditions as the test trials to get familiar with the tasks. Following at least 5 min of rest after the completion of the warm-up session, the subjects performed barbell BS with a load equivalent to their body weight, which was determined using 5 kg increments. PSJ was performed without an external load. The BS load corresponded to 60±6% of 1 RM. BS and PSJ were performed using the techniques proposed by the National Strength and Conditioning Association [9,21]. Specifically, in BS, the subjects stood erect, grasping the bar with a closed pronated grip and holding the barbell on the upper back and shoulders with their feet shoulder-width apart and parallel to each other (starting position). For the downward movement, they flexed their hips and knees until the posterior surface of the thigh was parallel to the floor. For the upward movement, they extended the hips and knees until they reached the starting position. Throughout the movement, they maintained a flat back, with their elbows high and chest up and out. The number of repetitions was set to three. The subjects performed each repetition every 4 s at a steady speed following a verbal cue from an examiner. In the PSJ trials, the subjects performed six rebound jumps preceded by a counter movement jump. In other words, the subjects jumped explosively from the squatting position (the posterior surface of the thigh was parallel to the floor) using a counter movement with their feet shoulder-width apart, landed in the squat position, and immediately repeated the rebound jump six times. The subjects were instructed to jump as fast and as high as possible. Throughout the movement, they maintained a flat back and placed their hands behind their head. In both exercises, the depth of the descent was confirmed by an examiner and with a high-speed video camera. The number of repetitions was selected as three and six for BS and PSJ, respectively, to minimize the chances of fatigue and to obtain data from stable repetitions of each exercise. The number of repetitions for PSJ was set to six because the jump height in PSJ reached a plateau after the third or fourth jump, which was confirmed in a pilot experiment. The order of the conditions was randomized for each subject. The subjects had a rest period of at least 5 min between the different conditions.

Experiment 2. T2 weighted cross-sectional MR images were obtained before and after the completion of BS and PSJ. The subjects performed BS and PSJ under the same conditions used in Experiment 1. The load for BS was set to 59±5% of 1 RM. The measurements for BS and PSJ were performed on separate days, with a minimum interval of 1 wk. The order of the conditions was randomized for each subject. The subjects performed three sets of 15 repetitions, with a 90 s rest interval between sets, for both the BS and PSJ tasks. Although it is recommended that power-training exercise should be performed without fatigue [9,22], the same number of repetitions and sets and rest intervals, as in BS, were adopted in PSJ to ensure T2 changed and reached a plateau [23].

Data collection and analysis

Experiment 1. The positions of reflective markers placed on six body landmarks (i.e., costa XII, the greater trochanter, the center of rotation of the knee joint, the lateral malleolus, the great toe, and the calcaneal tuber) on the right side were recorded using a high-speed video camera (EX-F1; Casio, Japan) with a sampling frequency of 300 fps. The camera was positioned perpendicular to the sagittal plane of motion at a distance of 15 m from the subject. Simultaneously, vertical and horizontal ground reaction forces on the right foot were recorded using a force platform (Model 6012–15; Bertec, USA). The reflective markers were digitized in each field using a motion analysis software (Frame-DIAS IV; DKH, Japan) to obtain the coordinates in the sagittal plane, and the data were smoothed using a fourth-order zero-lag Butterworth low pass filter with a cut-off of 8 Hz based on residual analysis [24]. The torques at the hip, knee, and ankle were determined from the body landmark coordinates and the ground reaction forces using two-dimensional inverse dynamics analysis [24]. The joint power was calculated by multiplying the joint torque by the joint angular velocity. Subsequently, the maximal and mean extension torques, extension and flexion angular velocity, and positive and negative joint power were calculated. The analyses were performed for the phase from the start to the end of lower limb joint movement for BS, and from touch-down to take-off for PSJ. Data processing was performed using the MATLAB software (MATLAB 7.10; MathWorks, USA). For BS, the average value of three repetitions, and for PSJ, the average value of the last three jumps was used as representative data.

Experiment 2. Before and after the execution of the exercise tasks, 15 consecutive 10-mm thick T2 weighted cross-sectional MR images were obtained at 20 mm intervals using an MR imaging system (Signa HDxt 1.5T; GE, USA) (Figure 1). The MR images were obtained in an order so that the position of the third slice corresponded with the greater trochanter. During imaging, the subject lay prone on the test bench of the MR imaging system and was fixed at the waist and knee with straps. The image sequence for T2 measurement was as follows: echo time, 25, 50, 75, and 100 ms; repetition time, 2500 ms; field of view, 48 cm; matrix, 256 × 192. The MR imaging started within 2 min from the completion of exercise.

The MR images were transferred to a computer, and the cross-sectional areas of the GM, the rectus femoris (RF), the vasti (Vas; including the vastus medialis, vastus lateralis, and vastus intermedius), the hip adductors (Add; including the adductor magnus, adductor brevis, and adductor longus), and the Ham of both legs were determined from each image using an open source image processing software (OsiriX v.2.4; Pixmeo, Switzerland). Care was taken to exclude non-contractile tissues such as intramuscular fat, nerves, and blood vessels. For each muscle, a T2 analysis was performed for the images with a cross-sectional area greater than 1000 mm^2 because the reproducibility of T2 measurement was poor in the images with a cross-sectional area less than 1000 mm^2, i.e., the coefficient of variance and intraclass correlation coefficient for repeated measures were more than 10% and less than 0.8, respectively. The number of slices used for the T2 measurements were 6, 6, 12, 7, and 6 for the GM, RF, Vas, Add, and Ham, respectively. For the pre-exercise images, the T2 for each pixel within each muscle was calculated, and the mean value was computed. In the post-exercise images, the pixels with a T2 value greater than the pre-exercise mean +1 SD were regarded as activated, and the proportion of the total number of pixels in the muscle cross-sectional area was expressed as a percent of the activated area (% activated area) [20,25]. The T2 measurement was performed on both sides, and the mean value was used.

Statistical Analyses

Descriptive data are expressed as mean ± SEM. For the data obtained in Experiment 1, a paired t-test was used to examine the differences between exercises. For the data obtained in Experiment 2, a repeated measures two-way ANOVA was used to test the interaction between the region and exercise for each muscle. Additionally, a repeated measures two-way ANOVA with Bonferroni post-hoc test was used to examine the main effects of muscle (5 muscles) and exercise (2 exercises), as well as their interaction. Cohen's *d* and the partial eta squared (η^2_p) were calculated to demonstrate the effect sizes. The Greenhouse-Geisser statistic was applied when the sphericity assumption was violated. For all statistics, the significance level was set at $p<0.05$.

Results

Experiment 1

Figure 2 shows an example of the time course of torques and angles of the ankle, knee, and hip joints during BS and PSJ. Descriptive data on the maximal and mean joint torques for each of the BS and PSJ are shown in Table 1. The plantar flexion

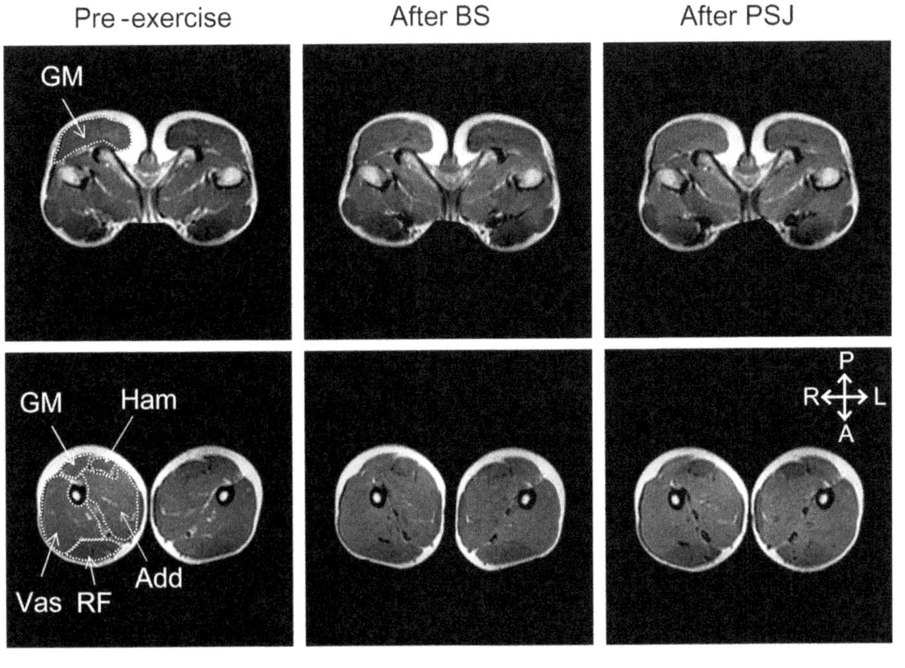

Figure 1. Examples of T2-weighted magnetic resonance images of hip (upper) and thigh (lower) regions at pre-exercise (left), after BS (middle), and after PSJ (right). GM, the gluteus maximus; Vas, the vasti muscles; RF, the rectus femoris muscle; Add, the hip adductors; Ham, the hamstrings. A, anterior; P, posterior; R, right; L, left.

torque in PSJ rapidly increased after foot contact and peaked at 33±8% contact time and decreased immediately before take-off, while that in BS was almost constant over the time course. The maximal and mean plantar flexion torques were significantly greater in PSJ than in BS ($p<0.01$). For the knee joint, an impulsive extension torque was found immediately after foot contact (4±0% contact time) and the torque was greater through the foot contact, especially in the downward phase, i.e., eccentric phase. The maximal and mean knee extension torques were significantly greater in PSJ than in BS ($p<0.01$). In contrast, there was no significant difference in the mean hip extension torque between the two tasks, while the maximal hip extension torque associated with an impulsive hip extension torque after foot contact (12±1% contact time) was significantly greater in PSJ than in BS ($p<0.01$). At all joints, the extension and flexion angular velocities (Table 2) and positive and negative power values (Table 3) were significantly ($p<0.01$) greater in PSJ than in BS.

Experiment 2

Figure 3 shows the % activated area of each muscle along its length. A two-way ANOVA revealed no significant interactions between the exercise and region for all muscles (GM, $F[5,35]=1.520$, $p=0.209$, $\eta^2_p=0.178$; RF, $F[5,35]=1.409$, $p=0.245$, $\eta^2_p=0.168$; Vas, $F[11, 77]=1.599$, $p=0.116$, $\eta^2_p=0.186$; Add, $F[2.3, 16.3]=0.264$, $p=0.802$, $\eta^2_p=0.036$; Ham, $F[5,35]=1.273$, $p=0.298$, $\eta^2_p=0.154$). On the other hand, a 2-way ANOVA for % activated area value averaged for all slices revealed a significant interaction between exercise and muscle ($F[4,28]=3.183$, $p=0.028$, $\eta^2_p=0.313$). Paired comparisons (Table 4) showed that the % activated areas of the GM and Add were significantly larger in PSJ than in BS ($p<0.05$). In addition, in both exercises, the % activated area of the Ham was smaller than that of other muscles except for the RF ($p<0.05$).

Discussion

The joint power output was much greater in PSJ than in BS, which confirms that the PSJ was an appropriate exercise for improving muscular power. The % activated areas of the Vas and RF were similar between BS and PSJ, while the maximal and mean knee extension torques were much greater during PSJ. In contrast, the % activated areas of the GM and Add were greater (16% and 18%, respectively) during PSJ, whereas the mean hip extension torque did not differ between the two exercises. The observed differences had a large effect size. According to Adams et al. [26], a 1% increase in an electrically evoked isometric knee extension torque corresponded with a 0.7% increase in the % activated area of the quadriceps femoris muscle, i.e., a 1% difference in the % activated area corresponded with a 1.4% difference in the joint torque. In addition, a previous study reported that a ~10% difference in the % activated area during a resistance training exercise induced a difference in the magnitude of hypertrophy after a long-term training period [20]. Thus, we may say that the observed differences in muscle recruitment have a practical significance in the designing of a training program that includes BS and PSJ. As noted earlier, it has been established that the changes in T2 reflect the recruitment of individual muscles [18,26]. Therefore, the present findings indicate that the individual muscle recruitment differs between BS and PSJ, which does not necessarily correspond with the joint kinetics. In other words, the current results imply that the lifting condition affects individual muscle recruitment and joint kinetics differently.

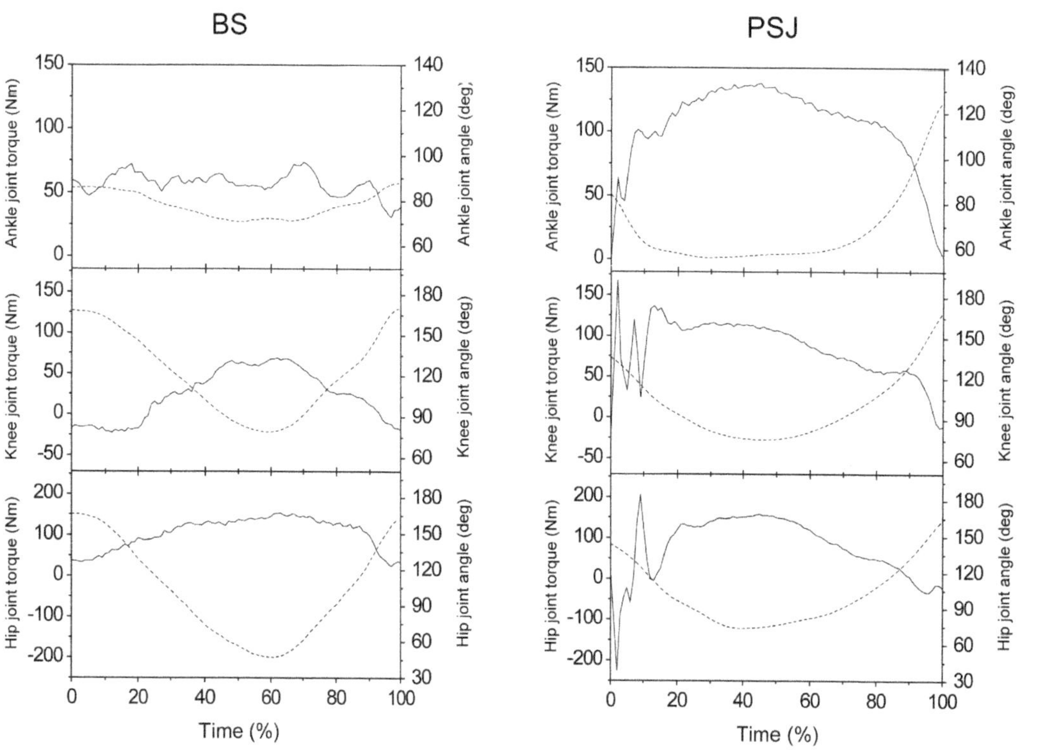

Figure 2. Time course of each joint torque and angle during back squat and plyometric squat jumping. BS, back squat; PSJ squat jumping. Data from 1 subject are presented. The solid and dashed lines indicate the torque and angle, respectively. Positive values indicate extension. Time is represented as percentage of analysis time, i.e., from start to end of repetition in BS and from touch down to take off in PSJ.

Table 1. Comparison of the joint torque between BS and PSJ (N · m).

		BS	PSJ	*d*
Plantar flexion	Maximum	78±3	125±8*	1.87
	Mean	48±2	81±6*	1.70
Knee extension	Maximum	82±3	186±21*	1.70
	Mean	55±2	76±5*	1.61
Hip extension	Maximum	149±5	272±32*	1.27
	Mean	95±4	97±7	0.09

Values are mean ± SEM. PSJ, plyometric squat jumping, BS, back squat.
*indicates that PSJ is greater than BS ($p<0.01$).

The results of the % activated area of the quadriceps femoris muscle (Table 4) indicate that the recruitment of this muscle group was similar between the two exercise tasks, although the maximal and mean knee extension torques were greater during PSJ than during BS (Table 1). This may be due to the difference in the type of muscle contraction between the two lifting conditions. It is well known that during a stretch-shortening cycle type of muscle action, the skeletal muscles can exert greater force than that during pure concentric muscle action [27]. Therefore, it seems that the quadriceps femoris muscle could generate greater knee extension torque during PSJ with the same recruitment level as BS. In addition, EMG studies have shown lower activation levels in isometric contractions compared to dynamic contractions [28]. Similarly, the change in the MR-based signal intensity has been shown to be less during isometric contraction than during dynamic contraction [29], indicating that the signal intensity depends on the type of contraction. During squat exercises with a stretch-shortening cycle, the vastus lateralis muscle fibers contract quasi-isometrically due to tendon elongation [30]. Based on these findings, it may be assumed that the quadriceps muscle fibers could generate a force with a smaller length change during PSJ, which might have contributed to a similar % activated area between PSJ and BS, in spite of the significant difference in the knee extension torque.

Another explanation for the knee extension torque being greater in PSJ with a similar recruitment of the quadriceps muscle is that the passive knee extension force of non-contractile elements such as tendon or connective tissue would be greater in PSJ. In PSJ, the hip was in a more extended position (Figure 2). Therefore, there is a possibility that the RF, which crosses the knee and hip joints, is longer, and consequently, the passive knee extension force would be greater in PSJ. This would result in a greater musculo-tendon force, or joint torque, which is the sum of the forces generated by contractile (active) and non-contractile (passive) elements.

The contraction levels of antagonist muscles can affect the net joint torque and should therefore be considered when discussing the discrepancy in the use of the knee joint and the quadriceps muscles between the two lifting conditions. The net joint torque is the sum of torques produced by the agonist and antagonist muscles. During knee extension, the Ham and gastrocnemius muscles operate as major antagonistic muscles. Thus, there is a possibility that the lower contraction levels of antagonist knee flexors could be associated with greater knee joint torque with the same recruitment level of the quadriceps muscles during PSJ than during BS. However, the % activated area of the Ham did not differ between the two conditions (Table 4). In addition, it is quite unlikely that the recruitment of gastrocnemius muscles was lower during PSJ than during BS because the plantar flexion torque was much greater during PSJ than during BS (Figure 2, Table 1).

Table 2. Comparison of the joint angular velocity between BS and PSJ (deg/s).

			BS	PSJ	*d*
Ankle	Plantar flexion	Maximum	51±5	743±29*	8.02
		Mean	19±2	246±14*	5.19
	Dorsiflexion	Maximum	42±3	679±36*	5.63
		Mean	15±1	208±22*	2.84
Knee	Extension	Maximum	153±13	828±25*	7.01
		Mean	74±5	348±13*	8.61
	Flexion	Maximum	113±7	522±28*	4.32
		Mean	54±3	264±11*	6.21
Hip	Extension	Maximum	150±11	504±25*	4.83
		Mean	74±5	248±10*	5.08
	Flexion	Maximum	117±5	461±34*	3.28
		Mean	60±4	260±22*	2.93

Values are mean ± SEM. PSJ, plyometric squat jumping, BS, back squat.
* indicates that PSJ is greater than BS ($p<0.01$).

Table 3. Comparison of the joint power between BS and PSJ (Watt).

			BS	PSJ	*d*
Plantar flexion	Positive	Maximum	44±6	940±81*	3.50
		Mean	18±3	314±36*	2.60
	Negative	Maximum	29±2	900±81*	3.38
		Mean	10±1	239±36*	2.03
Knee extension	Positive	Maximum	95±7	545±47*	3.00
		Mean	40±3	294±27*	3.14
	Negative	Maximum	97±10	1418±137*	3.05
		Mean	46±5	413±36*	3.29
Hip extension	Positive	Maximum	244±24	664±76*	1.65
		Mean	128±12	289±27*	1.69
	Negative	Maximum	184±15	1948±248*	2.28
		Mean	91±7	442±51*	2.22

Values are mean ± SEM. PSJ, plyometric squat jumping, BS, back squat.
* indicates that PSJ is greater than BS ($p<0.01$).

These aspects suggest that the recruitment of antagonists is unlikely to be the reason for the discrepancy between the knee joint kinetics and the recruitment of the quadriceps muscle.

The influence of the lifting conditions on the joint kinetics and recruitment of muscles at the hip joint differed from that at the knee joint. That is, the % activated area of the GM and Add was greater in PSJ than in BS (Table 4), although there was no significant difference in the mean hip extension torque between the two conditions (Table 1). This indicates that during PSJ, the recruitment of hip extensor was greater so as to generate the same mean joint torque as during BS. Four possibilities might explain these findings. First, the hip angular velocity in PSJ was much greater than that in BS (Table 2). In contrast to the quadriceps femoris muscle, GM and Add do not have long tendons [31], and thus, the contraction velocity of muscle fibers in PSJ would be greater than in BS. Based on the force-velocity characteristic of muscle fibers, the concentric force is greatly affected by the contraction velocity, while the eccentric force is less influenced by it [32]. Thus, it seems that, for GM and Add, force production during the upward (concentric) phase of PSJ would be performed in a disadvantageous condition as compared to that in BS. Second, there could be a difference in the contraction level of the antagonistic muscles between the two conditions. That is, the activities of the hip flexors and/or abductors could be greater during PSJ than during BS. Considering that the % activated area of the RF did not differ between the exercise conditions, it might be assumed that the activities of muscles such as the psoas major and gluteus medius, (a major hip flexor and a major hip abductor, respectively) could be greater during PSJ. For the Add muscles, it is also possible that a greater hip adduction torque would be exerted during PSJ, probably for stabilizing the pelvis during dynamic movement. Third, the difference in the hip joint angle between the two conditions might have affected the present results. During PSJ, the hip joint was in a more extended position than during BS (Figure 2). According to their joint angle and moment arm length relationships [33], the GM and Add can exert a greater hip extension torque in a more flexed position of the hip. Therefore, it seems that during PSJ, the GM and Add would be highly activated to generate the same hip extension torque as during BS. Lastly, a decreased hip flexion angle in PSJ would cause an increase in passive hip flexion force and a decrease in passive hip extension force resulting in increased muscular contribution for developing a given hip extension torque.

Previous studies have reported that during a squat, the EMG activity of the Ham is relatively high (30–80% maximal isometric contraction level) [34–36]. However, regardless of exercise conditions, the % activated area of the Ham was much lower than that of other muscles, except for the RF (Table 4). It seems that 60% of the 1 RM load or body weight was not large enough to elicit a strong co-contraction response of the Ham. However, Ploutz-Snyder et al. [37] reported that there was no MR contrast shift in the Ham following a 10 RM barbell squat. Enocson et al. [38] also reported that the change in the Ham MR signal intensity following the leg press exercise was negligible, regardless of the load. The present results support these findings and indicate that the change in the muscle MR signal intensity does not always correspond with the electromyographic activity. While EMG represents the neural input to a muscle, MR signal intensity is thought to reflect metabolites produced as a result of muscle contraction [19]. We therefore believe that the Ham were used lesser, in the presence of neural drive, during squat exercises, regardless of the load and/or speed conditions. This idea is supported by the evidence of lack of Ham hypertrophy after a 7-week, 3–25 RM BS training program, regardless of the load [39].

The lower % activated area of the Ham during a squat may also be due to the limited length change of these muscles during squat exercises. As described earlier, the change in the MR signal intensity is less during isometric contraction than during dynamic contraction [29]. The Ham cross the hip and knee joints, and flexion of these joints induces elongation and shortening of the Ham, respectively, and vice versa. Therefore, during squat exercises, there would be no change in the length of the Ham, and these muscles would contract almost isometrically resulting in a lower % activated area. In addition, it should be taken into consideration that the T2 change is more prominent in fast twitch fibers than in slow fibers [19]. The percentage of fast twitch fibers of the Ham (33.1% for the biceps femoris) has been reported to be relatively lower than those of the other muscles tested in the present study (GM, 47.6%; RF, 57.2–70.5%; Vas, 38.5–67.3%; Add, 36.7–46.5%) [40]. Therefore, we cannot rule out that the recruitment level of the Ham, assessed with the change in T2,

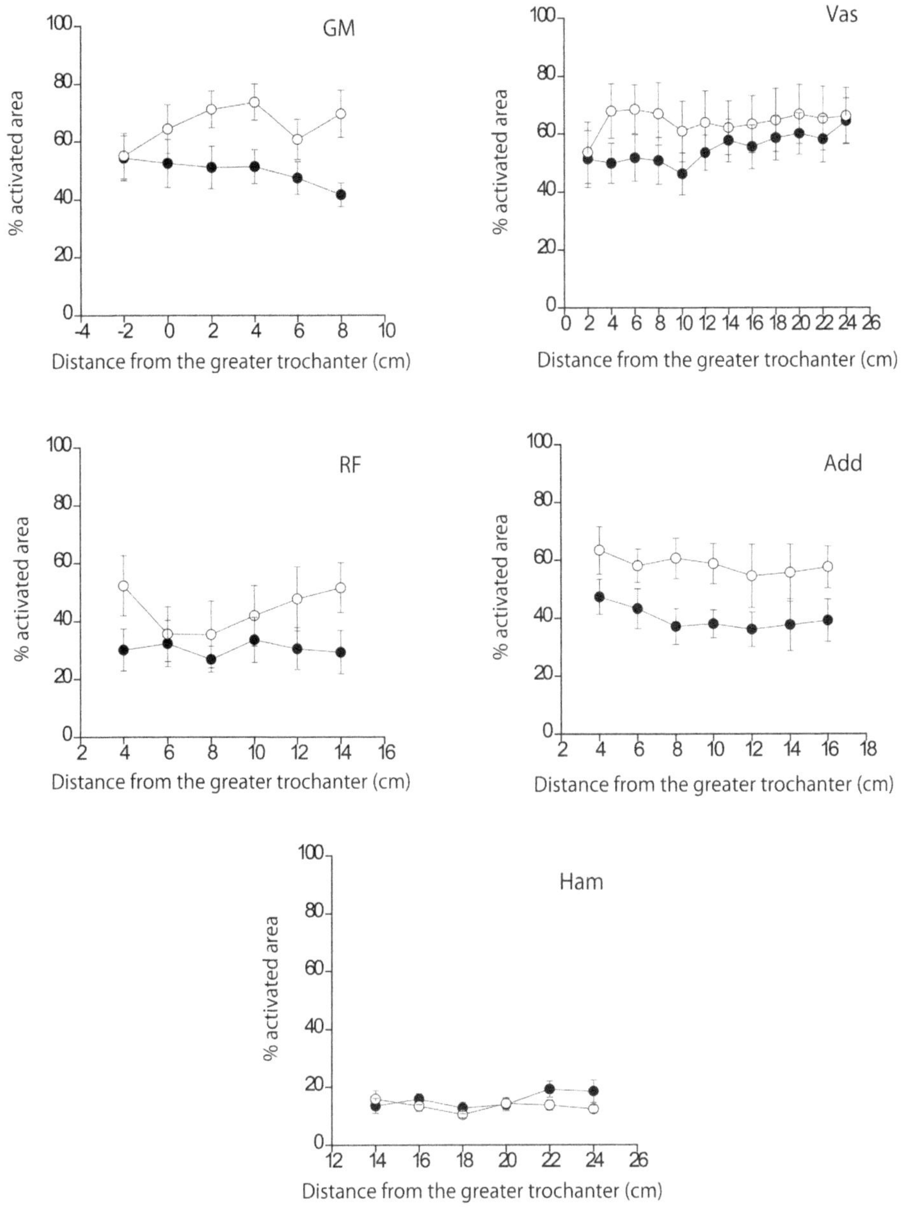

Figure 3. The % activated area of each muscle along its length as a function of the distance from the greater trochanter. The closed and open circles indicate back squat and plyometric squat jumping, respectively. GM, the gluteus maximus; Vas, the vasti muscles; RF, the rectus femoris muscle; Add, the hip adductors; Ham, the hamstrings. There was no significant interaction between the region and exercise condition.

Table 4. % activated area value averaged for all slices.

	BS	PSJ	*d*
Gluteus maximus	50±5	66±7*	0.92
Vasti	55±8	64±10	0.35
Rectus femoris	36±10	44±7	0.23
Adductors	40±6	58±7*	1.11
Hamstrings	16±2†	13±1†	0.40

Values are mean ± SEM. PSJ, plyometric squat jumping, BS, back squat.
*indicates that PSJ is greater than BS ($p<0.05$).
†indicates that Hamstrings was smaller than Gluteus maximus, and Adductors ($p<0.01$).

could be affected by the muscle fiber type and consequently might have been underestimated to some degree.

The present results indicated that in a multi-joint exercise, synergist muscle recruitment differs between the two lifting conditions, even though the exercises used are similar in terms of joints involved and their motions (i.e., hip and knee extension and flexion). For designing an effective and efficient training program, however, knowledge of how each of the load and speed conditions affects the synergist muscle use is essential. If the observed differences in individual muscle use between the lifting conditions were caused by differences in the type of muscle action, co-contraction levels, hip joint angular position, and/or velocity, as mentioned above, it seems that the speed of movement (slow constant speed vs. dynamic) rather than the load would be a major factor producing it; this should be clarified in future studies.

In addition, it should be noted that in the T2 measurement adopted here, the time course of muscle recruitment during an exercise cannot be determined. Therefore, we cannot identify the timing or phase of the exercise during which the difference in synergist muscle recruitment between BS and PSJ was yielded. When devising a training program on the basis of specificity (i.e., specific adaptation to imposed demand), information on the recruitment pattern during an exercise is important and should be investigated in future studies. The combined use of EMG and T2 MRI could provide more insight into this issue. Furthermore, the approach to this issue should include limiting the range of motion (i.e., depth of dip) or the phase (i.e., only the descending phase).

Lastly, we would like to comment on the accuracy and repeatability of T2 measurements. The present study used T2 measurements and compared two extremely different lifting conditions and revealed the differences in the synergist muscle use with a large effect size. However, more elaborate studies with higher accuracy and repeatability of T2 measurements would be needed for a more complete understanding of the effect of the lifting conditions on synergist muscle recruitment. It is therefore essential to improve the imaging resolution and examiner's skill required for identification of non-contractile tissue such as intramuscular fat, nerve, tendinous tissue, and blood vessels in MR images. In addition, the subjects should be highly skilled in the tasks used to examine whether muscular recruitment differs between the tasks in spite of the similarity in joints involved and action mode adopted. Furthermore, the observer of T2-weighted MR images in the present study was not blinded to the subjects and pre-/post-exercise images. The post-exercise T2-weighted MR images clearly differed from the pre-exercise images in that some of the muscles appeared lighter on the images. However, the fact that the observer of the images was not blind to the subjects and pre-/post-exercise images raises the possibility of an unintended bias on the observer's part that would affect the results. In future studies, these issues should be improved upon to take advantage of the T2 technique for identifying muscle recruitment during various resistance exercises.

In conclusion, the present study shows that the individual use of hip and knee muscles, assessed based on the T2 measurements from MR images, differs between BS as a muscular endurance training exercise and PSJ as a power training exercise. This difference did not necessarily correspond with the joint kinetics. The current results indicate that the difference in lifting conditions produces a different synergist muscle use, even when an exercise with similar movements of the body segments is adopted. Thus, not only the exercise type but also the lifting condition should be taken into consideration as a determinant of the major muscles trained in a resistance exercise.

Author Contributions

Conceived and designed the experiments: NS JO HK. Performed the experiments: NS. Analyzed the data: NS SK HK. Wrote the paper: NS SK JO HK.

References

1. Ratamess A (2011) Resistance training program design. In: Ratamess A, editor. ACSM's foundation of strength training and conditioning. Philadelphia, PA: Lippincott Williams &Wilkins. 192–228.
2. Wathen D, Baechle TR, Earle RW (2008) Periodization. In: Baechle TR, Earle RW, editors. Essentials of strength training and conditioning 3rd ed. Champaign, IL: Human Kinetics. 507–522.
3. Rhea MR, Phillips WT, Burkett LN, Stone WJ, Ball SD, et al. (2003) A comparison of linear and daily undulating periodized programs with equated volume and intensity for local muscular endurance. J Strength Cond Res 17: 82–87.
4. Smilios I, Hakkinen K, Tokmakidis SP (2010) Power output and electromyographic activity during and after a moderate load muscular endurance session. J Strength Cond Res 24: 2122–2131.
5. Willardson JM, Burkett LN (2006) The effect of rest interval length on the sustainability of squat and bench press repetitions. J Strength Cond Res 20: 400–403.
6. Baker D, Nance S, Moore M (2001) The load that maximizes the average mechanical power output during jump squats in power-trained athletes. J Strength Cond Res 15: 92–97.
7. Kaneko M, Fuchimoto T, Toji H, Suei K (1983) Training effect of different loads on the force-velocity relationship and mechanical power output in human muscle. Scandinavian Journal of Sports Sciences 5: 50–55.
8. Newton RU, Murphy AJ, Humphries BJ, Wilson GJ, Kraemer WJ, et al. (1997) Influence of load and stretch shortening cycle on the kinematics, kinetics and muscle activation that occurs during explosive upper-body movements. Eur J Appl Physiol Occup Physiol 75: 333–342.
9. Potach DH, Chu DA (2008) Plyometric training. In: Baechle TR, Earle RW, editors. Essentials of strength training and conditioning. 3rd ed. Champaign, IL: Human Kinetics. 413–456.
10. Sedano S, Marin PJ, Cuadrado G, Redondo JC (2013) Concurrent training in elite male runners: the influence of strength versus muscular endurance training on performance outcomes. J Strength Cond Res 27: 2433–2443.
11. Taipale RS, Mikkola J, Vesterinen V, Nummela A, Hakkinen K (2013) Neuromuscular adaptations during combined strength and endurance training in endurance runners: maximal versus explosive strength training or a mix of both. Eur J Appl Physiol 113: 325–335.
12. Earle RW, Baechle TR (2008) Resistance training and spotting techniques. In: Baechle TR, Earle RW, editors. Essentials of Strength Training and Conditioning. 3rd ed. Champaign, IL: Human Kinetics. 325–376.
13. Elder GC, Bradbury K, Roberts R (1982) Variability of fiber type distributions within human muscles. Journal of Applied Physiology 53: 1473–1480.
14. Kawakami Y, Abe T, Kanehisa H, Fukunaga T (2006) Human skeletal muscle size and architecture: variability and interdependence. Am J Hum Biol 18: 845–848.
15. Voigt M, Dyhre-Poulsen P, Simonsen EB (1998) Modulation of short latency stretch reflexes during human hopping. Acta Physiol Scand 163: 181–194.
16. Farina D, Merletti R, Enoka RM (2004) The extraction of neural strategies from the surface EMG. J Appl Physiol 96: 1486–1495.
17. Farina D (2006) Interpretation of the surface electromyogram in dynamic contractions. Exerc Sport Sci Rev 34: 121–127.
18. Fisher MJ, Meyer RA, Adams GR, Foley JM, Potchen EJ (1990) Direct relationship between proton T2 and exercise intensity in skeletal muscle MR images. Investigative Radiology 25: 480–485.
19. Prior BM, Ploutz-Snyder LL, Cooper TG, Meyer RA (2001) Fiber type and metabolic dependence of T2 increases in stimulated rat muscles. Journal of Applied Physiology 90: 615–623.
20. Wakahara T, Miyamoto N, Sugisaki N, Murata K, Kanehisa H, et al. (2012) Association between regional differences in muscle activation in one session of resistance exercise and in muscle hypertrophy after resistance training. Eur J Appl Physiol 112: 1569–1576.
21. Baechle TR, Earle RW, Wathen D (2008) Resistance training. In: Baechle TR, Earle RW, editors. Essentials of strength training and conditioning 3rd ed. Champaign, IL: Human Kinetics. 414–456.
22. Ratamess A (2011) Plyometric training. In: Ratamess A, editor. ACSM's foundation of strength training and conditioning. Philadelphia, PA: Lippincott Williams &Wilkins. 331–379.
23. Fleckenstein JL, Watumull D, McIntire DD, Bertocci LA, Chason DP, et al. (1993) Muscle proton T2 relaxation times and work during repetitive maximal voluntary exercise. Journal of Applied Physiology 74: 2855–2859.

24. Winter DA (2009) Biomechanics and motor control of human movement 4th ed. Hoboken, NJ: John Wiley & Sons. 370 p.
25. Adams GR, Harris RT, Woodard D, Dudley GA (1993) Mapping of electrical muscle stimulation using MRI. Journal of Applied Physiology 74: 532–537.
26. Adams GR, Duvoisin MR, Dudley GA (1992) Magnetic resonance imaging and electromyography as indexes of muscle function. Journal of Applied Physiology 73: 1578–1583.
27. Cavagna GA, Dusman B, Margaria R (1968) Positive work done by a previously stretched muscle. J Appl Physiol 24: 21–32.
28. Ball N, Scurr JC (2011) Efficacy of current and novel electromyographic normalization methods for lower limb high-speed muscle actions. European Journal of Sport Science 11: 447–456.
29. Price TB, Kennan RP, Gore JC (1998) Isometric and dynamic exercise studied with echo planar magnetic resonance imaging (MRI). Medicine and Science in Sports and Exercise 30: 1374–1380.
30. Ishikawa M, Finni T, Komi PV (2003) Behaviour of vastus lateralis muscle-tendon during high intensity SSC exercises in vivo. Acta Physiologica Scandinavica 178: 205–213.
31. Yamaguchi GT, Sawa AGU, Moran DW, Fessler MJ, Winters JM (1990) A survey of human musculotendon actuator parameters. In: Winters JM, Woo SL-Y, editors. Multiple muscle system: Biomechanics and movement organization. New York: Springer. 717–773.
32. Edman KA (1979) The velocity of unloaded shortening and its relation to sarcomere length and isometric force in vertebrate muscle fibres. J Physiol 291: 143–159.
33. Dostal WF, Soderberg GL, Andrews JG (1986) Actions of hip muscles. Physical Therapy 66: 351–361.
34. Escamilla RF, Fleisig GS, Zheng N, Barrentine SW, Wilk KE, et al. (1998) Biomechanics of the knee during closed kinetic chain and open kinetic chain exercises. Med Sci Sports Exerc 30: 556–569.
35. Escamilla RF, Fleisig GS, Zheng N, Lander JE, Barrentine SW, et al. (2001) Effects of technique variations on knee biomechanics during the squat and leg press. Med Sci Sports Exerc 33: 1552–1566.
36. Wilk KE, Escamilla RF, Fleisig GS, Barrentine SW, Andrews JR, et al. (1996) A comparison of tibiofemoral joint forces and electromyographic activity during open and closed kinetic chain exercises. Am J Sports Med 24: 518–527.
37. Ploutz-Snyder LL, Convertino VA, Dudley GA (1995) Resistance exercise-induced fluid shifts: change in active muscle size and plasma volume. Am J Physiol 269: R536–543.
38. Enocson AG, Berg HE, Vargas R, Jenner G, Tesch PA (2005) Signal intensity of MR-images of thigh muscles following acute open- and closed chain kinetic knee extensor exercise - index of muscle use. European Journal of Applied Physiology 94: 357–363.
39. Weiss LW, Coney HD, Clark FC (2000) Gross measures of exercise-induced muscular hypertrophy. J Orthop Sports Phys Ther 30: 143–148.
40. Johnson MA, Polgar J, Weightman D, Appleton D (1973) Data on the distribution of fibre types in thirty-six human muscles. An autopsy study. J Neurol Sci 18: 111–129.

15

Genetic Evaluation of the Nine Component Features of Hip Score in UK Labrador Retrievers

Thomas W. Lewis[1]*, John A. Woolliams[2], Sarah C. Blott[1]

1 Kennel Club Genetics Centre at the Animal Health Trust, Animal Health Trust, Newmarket, United Kingdom, 2 The Roslin Institute and Royal (Dick) School of Veterinary Studies, University of Edinburgh, Roslin, United Kingdom

Abstract

The aim of this study was to explore the genetic relationship between the nine component traits comprising the British Veterinary Association (BVA) total hip score in UK registered Labrador Retrievers. Data consisted of 11,928 single records of trait scores of dogs aged between one and four years (365–1459 days) old, from radiographs evaluated between 2000 and 2007. Pedigree information was provided by the UK Kennel Club. The distribution of trait scores showed only small numbers of dogs with visible malformation in the six traits that were scored according to the severity of osteoarthritis. Linear mixed models were fitted using ASREML. Estimates of heritability ranged from 0.15 to 0.38, and litter effects from 0.04 to 0.10. Genetic correlations between all nine traits were extremely high ranging from 0.71 to 1.0, implying considerable genetic similarity. The decomposition demonstrated that aggregate scores of only the 3 traits indicative of laxity in one year old dogs was predictive of the phenotype of the remaining six scored on osteoarthritic severity in dogs at 4+ years old. The application of selection index methodology in selecting against hip dysplasia using the trait scores was explored and potential improvements in accuracy (directly related to response to selection) of over 10% are reported compared to the current total hip score. This study demonstrates that traits descriptive of joint laxity are valuable early-age predictors of osteoarthritis and shows that there is scope for improvement in the way data from the UK hip score scheme are used for selection against hip dysplasia in Labradors. This was verified via use of selection indices, which identified substantial increases in accuracy, not only via optimum coefficients, but also through an easily applicable aggregate of scores of just two or three traits only compared with the current total hip score.

Editor: Amanda Ewart Toland, Ohio State University Medical Center, United States of America

Funding: This work was funded by the Kennel Club Charitable Trust. JAW is grateful to BBSRC for funding through an ISPG. The funders had no role in study design, data analysis, decision to publish, or preparation of the manuscript. Hip score and pedigree data is collated and provided by the Kennel Club.

Competing Interests: Hip score and pedigree data was collated and provided by the Kennel Club.

* E-mail: tom.lewis@aht.org.uk

Introduction

It has been demonstrated that progress against hip dysplasia in Labradors has been discernible but slow and that the rate of genetic improvement could be greatly enhanced through selection on estimated breeding values (EBVs) rather than phenotypic hip score [1,2,3,4]. However a major challenge remains: improvement in the design of recording schemes, through examination of the biological relevance of the recorded traits, to determine how response to selection against the debilitating effects of hip dysplasia may be improved.

Hip dysplasia is a developmental orthopaedic disorder characterised by the formation of a loose, ill-fitting coxofemoral (hip) joint [5]. Over time the malformation leads to abnormal wearing of bone surfaces and the appearance of the osteoarthritic signs of degenerative joint disease (DJD), such as exostosis (abnormal bone growth) and bone remodelling [6]. It has both genetic and environmental influences [1,7,8,9] and is often impossible to treat since the osteoarthritis that develops is irreversible. Therefore, reduction in the prevalence of hip dysplasia through genetic selection is the best method available to provide a lasting and widespread improvement in the welfare of susceptible breeds.

The British Veterinary Association (BVA)/Kennel Club (KC) hip score scheme is in operation in the UK, EIRE, Australia and New Zealand and examines nine aspects of a pelvic radiograph for signs of malformation and secondary osteoarthritic signs of DJD in each hip. Each of the nine traits is scored and the aggregate total score is reported as an indication of hip dysplasia. However, while the scores of some traits are descriptive of deviation from normal morphology and indicative of joint laxity, others describe the degree of osteoarthritis (OA) secondary to laxity of the hip joints. Thus, the total score appears to contain elements that are both prognostic and diagnostic of OA characteristic of hip dysplasia.

The rate of participation in the BVA/KC hip score scheme in the UK is relatively good with submission of radiographs for 8–10% of all annually registered Labrador Retrievers (the most popular breed in the UK), equating to 50–60% of all dogs of that breed used for breeding. However, dogs may only be scored once in their lifetime and over ninety percent of UK registered Labrador Retrievers are scored before four years of age. Thus, it appears that many breeders wish to consider hip condition prior to breeding but that practical constraints have limited consideration to phenotypes of prospective parents only. While selection using EBVs for hip score is more accurate than using phenotypes, the total hip score as it is currently measured and aggregated may not be the most efficient phenotypic indicator of hip dysplasia for use in selection against the disease. For example, inclusion of traits relating to the pathological response to joint laxity may dilute information pertaining to the innate hip morphology. Furthermore, it may be argued that there is a moral obligation in selecting against the cause of malformation rather than the severity of the consequences.

Selection index theory provides a method of using all available phenotypic information to determine individual trait selection coefficients that will result in optimal progress towards a specific selection objective. The selection objective can be adjusted via differential weighting of some or all traits. Although selection indices have most often been used in livestock breeding (where weights have been economically derived) it may be achievable to develop 'welfare' values and construct an index for optimal selection against inherited disease, of which canine hip dysplasia is a prime example. For the nine traits currently measured under the BVA/KC scheme this would involve: 1) being clear on the extent to which traits are definitive of disease and which are biomarkers or secondary consequences, 2) analysing the genetic contribution to prediction of disease, and 3) deriving how the traits may be best weighted to provide the most accurate predictions. Such an undertaking would reveal the selection coefficients of traits producing the maximum progress against hip dysplasia, but would require extensive debate on the precise calculation of 'welfare values' for each of the nine traits.

This study has the objectives of examining 1) the genetic parameters of all nine traits in the BVA/KC hip scoring scheme in 1–4 year old dogs using mixed model analyses, 2) the predictive ability of traits describing joint laxity and secondary osteoarthritic signs using EBVs, and 3) the advantages conferred by a selection index in the effective selection against inherited disease.

Results

Distributions of score for the nine traits

The distribution of scores for each of the nine traits (1 = Norberg Angle, NA; 2 = Subluxation, SUB; 3 = Cranial Acetabular Edge, CrAE; 4 = Dorsal Acetabular Edge, DAE; 5 = Cranial Effective Acetabular Rim, CrEAR; 6 = Acetabular Fossa, AF; 7 = Caudal Acetabular Edge, CAE; 8 = Femoral Head and Neck Exostosis, FHNE; and 9 = Femoral Head Recontouring, FHR) are shown in Figure 1 and statistics in Table 1. Over 91% of all records for AF, CAE, and FHR had been scored zero and 86%, 84% and 77% of all records were scored zero for DAE, FHNE and CrEAR respectively. Thus, the means of these six traits are smaller and coefficients of skew larger than for NA, SUB and CrAE (Table 1), with the important implication that there is very little phenotypic deviation from 'normal' morphology in these six features of the hip joint in UK registered Labradors evaluated between 1 and 4 years of age. The distribution of CrAE has a modal score of four (72% of records), rather than zero as was the

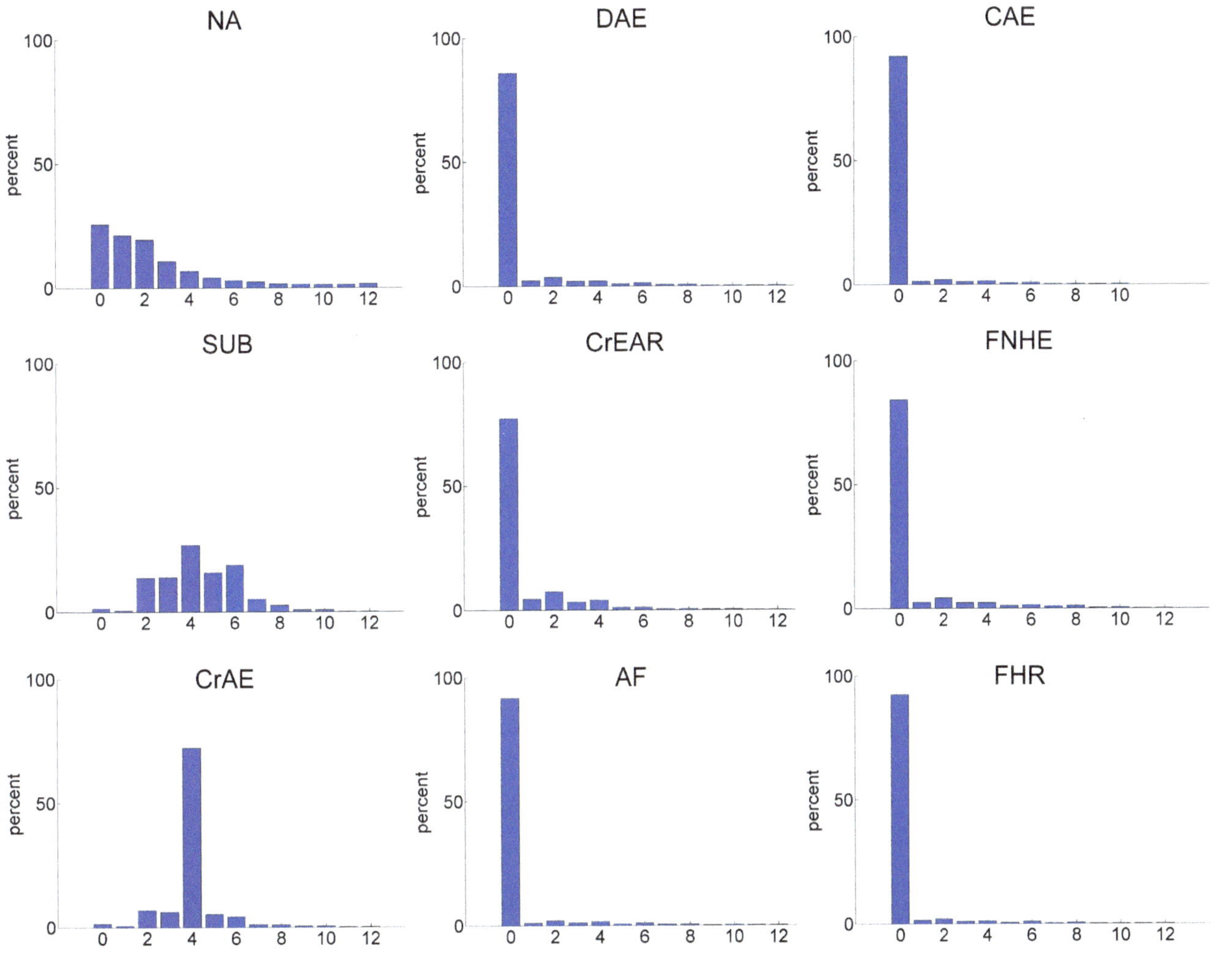

Figure 1. Distribution of total score. Left + right hip score for the 9 traits contributing to total hip score.

Table 1. Summary statistics for the 9 traits contributing to total hip score.

Component		Mean	S.D.	CV	Skew	Correlation L&R
1	NA	2.436	2.731	1.121	1.646	0.619
2	SUB	4.389	1.761	0.401	0.306	0.447
3	CrAE	3.984	1.193	0.299	1.002	0.757
4	DAE	0.547	1.692	3.093	3.856	0.768
5	CrEAR	0.692	1.570	2.269	2.862	0.799
6	AF	0.340	1.338	3.935	4.754	0.780
7	CAE	0.281	1.150	4.093	4.954	0.752
8	FHNE	0.610	1.712	2.807	3.335	0.755
9	FHR	0.266	1.119	4.207	5.108	0.760

Mean, standard deviation (S.D.), coefficient of variation (CV), coefficient of skew, and phenotypic correlation between left and right score for each of the 9 traits that sum to the total hip score according to the BVA/KC scheme (NA = Norberg angle, SUB = subluxation, CrAE = cranial acetabular edge, DAE = dorsal acetabular edge, CrEAR = cranial effective acetabular rim, AF = acetabular fossa, CAE = caudal acetabular edge, FHNE = femoral head and neck exostosis, FHR = femoral head recontouring).

case for traits 4–9, affording a lower coefficient of skew and a higher mean, but a standard deviation of comparable magnitude to that for traits 4–9. NA and SUB are more evenly distributed over scores and consequently showed greater phenotypic variation. The distribution of NA scores was positively skewed, reflecting the categorisation of abnormality in what would be expected to be a normally distributed, empirically measured trait.

Heritabilities and genetic correlations of the nine features of total hip score

An objective of this study was to estimate the genetic parameters of the nine traits and explore the genetic relationships between them. Estimates of heritability and litter variation of untransformed scores from univariate analysis are presented in Table 2. Heritability estimates were highest for SUB (0.38±0.026) and NA (0.37±0.027), with estimates for all seven remaining traits ranging from 0.15 (CAE and AF) to 0.24 (FHNE). The inclusion of litter in the model was significant ($P<0.05$) for all traits except FHR ($P<0.10$ using likelihood ratio test). For all traits the variation due to litter explained a much smaller fraction of total variation than the genetic variation, ranging from 0.04 (CAE) to 0.10 (SUB).

The genetic and phenotypic correlations between each pair of the nine traits (and standard errors in parentheses) are presented in Table 3. The genetic correlations range from 0.71 between SUB and FHR, up to 1.0 between DAE and AF, and FHR and AF. Overall, the genetic correlations were extremely high, with only three correlations at less than 0.8 (SUB with each of AF, CAE and FHR). The phenotypic correlations followed a similar pattern (ranging from 0.47 between SUB and FHR, to 0.88 between AF and CAE) but were lower in magnitude than the genetic correlations. Residual or environmental correlations showed a much wider range than the genetic correlations (from 0.37 between SUB and FHR, to 0.86 between AF and CAE) reflecting more differential environmental influences among traits.

Table 2. Variance components of hip score traits.

Component		Heritability (s.e.)		Litter effect (s.e.)	
1	NA	0.37	0.027	0.08	0.017
2	SUB	0.38	0.026	0.10	0.017
3	CrAE	0.21	0.023	0.06	0.017
4	DAE	0.18	0.024	0.06	0.018
5	CrEAR	0.21	0.024	0.09	0.018
6	AF	0.15	0.023	0.08	0.019
7	CAE	0.15	0.022	0.04	0.018
8	FHNE	0.24	0.026	0.07	0.018
9	FHR	0.19	0.025	0.04	0.019

Estimates of heritability and the fraction of phenotypic variance explained by litter on each of the nine traits that sum to the total hip score according to the BVA/KC scheme (NA = Norberg angle, SUB = subluxation, CrAE = cranial acetabular edge, DAE = dorsal acetabular edge, CrEAR = cranial effective acetabular rim, AF = acetabular fossa, CAE = caudal acetabular edge, FHNE = femoral head and neck exostosis, FHR = femoral head recontouring).

Genetic correlations between groups of aggregate scores

The relationship between groups of traits according to scoring criteria was subsequently explored. The genetic correlation between $SCORE_{4-9}$ (aggregate score of traits scored on the pathological signs of OA) and $SCORE_{1-3}$ (aggregate score of traits scored largely on signs of morphological malformation) was 0.89 (±0.023) when both were transformed using natural logarithm of aggregate score +1, and 0.92 (±0.020) when untransformed, indicating substantial genetic similarity between the two groups. Such high genetic correlations indicate that morphology will potentially act as a good predictor of damage due to OA. However on both scales genetic correlations were significantly smaller than one ($P<0.001$), implying that whilst $SCORE_{1-3}$ and $SCORE_{4-9}$ are genetically very similar traits, they are not genetically identical on these scales. The heritability estimates of $SCORE_{1-3}$ were 0.38 (±0.026) and 0.33 0(±0.025), and of $SCORE_{4-9}$ were 0.18 (±0.022) and 0.25 (±0.025), when untransformed and transformed respectively.

Prediction of $SCORE_{4-9}$ using $SCORE_{1-3}$

Having ascertained the magnitude of the genetic relationship between these two groups of traits, the predictive ability of morphological traits on the pathologically descriptive traits was assessed using EBVs calculated from dogs scored at a young age and using them as predictors of phenotypes of offspring scored at a late age (see Materials and Methods). The correlations of 'early age' EBVs for $SCORE_{1-3}$, $SCORE_{4-9}$ and total score ($SCORE_{1-9}$) with 'late age' phenotypes are shown in Table 4. All correlations were significantly greater than zero, except that for EBV_{4-9} with $SCORE_{1-3}$. EBV_{1-3} and EBV_{1-9} were each similarly correlated with the three score groups, but in each case the correlation with EBV_{1-3} was of greater magnitude representing greater predictive ability. The maximum correlation was of early score EBV_{1-3} on $SCORE_{1-9}$ at 4+ years old ($r=0.22$). Correlations of EBV_{1-3} and EBV_{1-9} with each score group were significantly higher than EBV_{4-9} for both $SCORE_{1-9}$ and $SCORE_{4-9}$. Thus, EBV_{1-3} calculated at birth using data from one year old dogs is a more accurate predictor of subsequent $SCORE_{4-9}$ at 4+ years old than the EBV_{4-9} of the same trait. Therefore selection on EBVs for $SCORE_{1-3}$ using data from young dogs will have no detrimental impact on the improvement of $SCORE_{4-9}$, and may rather be slightly more accurate than EBVs for total score at improving all component traits.

Table 3. Genetic and phenotypic correlations among traits contributing to total hip score.

	NA	SUB	CrAE	DAE	CrEAR	AF	CAE	FHNE	FHR
NA		0.75 (0.005)	0.66 (0.007)	0.71 (0.005)	0.74 (0.005)	0.63 (0.006)	0.60 (0.006)	0.70 (0.005)	0.58 (0.006)
SUB	0.85 (0.018)		0.66 (0.006)	0.57 (0.007)	0.61 (0.006)	0.51 (0.007)	0.48 (0.008)	0.57 (0.007)	0.47 (0.008)
CrAE	0.93 (0.018)	0.93 (0.018)		0.70 (0.005)	0.70 (0.005)	0.65 (0.006)	0.62 (0.006)	0.65 (0.006)	0.61 (0.006)
DAE	0.96 (0.019)	0.83 (0.033)	0.93 (0.022)		0.84 (0.002)	0.87 (0.002)	0.85 (0.003)	0.85 (0.003)	0.82 (0.003)
CrEAR	0.93 (0.017)	0.86 (0.026)	0.95 (0.016)	0.97 (0.011)		0.77 (0.004)	0.73 (0.004)	0.80 (0.004)	0.71 (0.005)
AF	0.90 (0.037)	0.78 (0.044)	0.89 (0.033)	1.00 (0.000)	0.91 (0.025)		0.88 (0.002)	0.83 (0.003)	0.84 (0.003)
CAE	0.91 (0.033)	0.78 (0.043)	0.89 (0.032)	0.97 (0.013)	0.93 (0.022)	0.99 (0.007)		0.82 (0.003)	0.83 (0.003)
FHNE	0.84 (0.027)	0.81 (0.032)	0.90 (0.026)	0.99 (0.006)	0.95 (0.014)	0.97 (0.012)	0.95 (0.014)		0.86 (0.003)
FHR	0.83 (0.040)	0.71 (0.046)	0.87 (0.034)	0.99 (0.011)	0.90 (0.028)	1.00 (0.006)	0.95 (0.016)	0.96 (0.013)	

Genetic (below diagonal) and phenotypic (above diagonal) correlations between each of the nine traits that sum to the total hip score according to the BVA/KC scheme (NA = Norberg angle, SUB = subluxation, CrAE = cranial acetabular edge, DAE = dorsal acetabular edge, CrEAR = cranial effective acetabular rim, AF = acetabular fossa, CAE = caudal acetabular edge, FHNE = femoral head and neck exostosis, FHR = femoral head recontouring). Standard errors in parentheses.

Demonstration of suitability of a selection index for hip dysplasia

An alternative approach to explore the potential improvements in response to selection is to combine them into an index I with 'index coefficients' for each of the traits 1–9 that are no longer constrained to 1 or 0. The coefficients are derived to provide the highest accuracy for an objective H which places relative values on the progress achieved in each of the traits. This is explained in more detail in Materials and Methods. The accuracies of optimised selection coefficients were, as expected, always highest when information on all nine traits was incorporated into the index I, whatever the selection objective (H). When all nine traits in H were equally valued after being scaled by their standardised phenotypic variation ($\mathbf{a}_1$), the selection coefficients were: 0.538 (NA), 0.546 (SUB), 0.121 (CrAE), −0.184 (DAE), −0.126 (CrEAR), −0.310 (AF), −0.186 (CAE), 0.371 (FHNE), 0.564 (FHR). This profile of index weights is quantitatively similar for the two other objective scenarios that were considered, the total score as calculated currently by BVA/KC ($\mathbf{a}_2$) or relative values based upon the impact of OA ($\mathbf{a}_3$). On a technical note, the negative values in the index coefficients do *not* imply that the index results in selection for features definitive of dysplasia, but rather signifies that due to the high phenotypic and genetic correlations some traits act as 'environmental corrections' to more informative traits that are richer in genetic information, allowing better prediction of genetic merit.

Table 5 displays the accuracies (directly related to rate of improvement) of the optimum selection coefficients determined by selection index theory for each of the three objectives considered, together with accuracies obtained by using index coefficients representing simplified aggregate scores of the nine traits. The results show that using aggregate total score is only between 88–90% as accurate as the optimum coefficients over all 3 scenarios for the relative values in the objective. Furthermore, selection with indices representative of aggregate scores of morphological traits (NA+SUB+CrAE and NA+SUB) were between 10–12% more accurate than total score for $\mathbf{a}_1$ and $\mathbf{a}_2$ and 6–7% more accurate for $\mathbf{a}_3$ where higher value is placed on improving the traits that are descriptive of pathological OA.

Table 4. Correlation of EBVs and phenotypes for 3 groupings of hip score traits.

	SCORE1–9	SCORE1–3	SCORE4–9
EBV_{1-9}	0.2086 (0.0003)	0.1958 (0.0006)	0.1811 (0.0018)
EBV_{1-3}	0.2165 (0.0002)	0.2065 (0.0003)	0.1831 (0.0014)
EBV_{4-9}	0.1276 (0.0272)	0.1024 (0.0765)	0.1453 (0.0117)

Correlations of 'early age scored' EBVs for SCORE1–3, SCORE4–9 and SCORE1–9 with phenotypes in 300 'late age' progeny at time of scoring. Standard errors in parentheses.

Discussion

The results from this study suggest that there is significant scope for improvement in the application of data from the UK hip score scheme to selection against hip dysplasia in Labradors. The aggregate score of just three of the trait scores that sum to the total hip score was demonstrated to be both substantially genetically related to, and adequately predictive of, the remaining six, as well as exhibiting marked variation in the malformation indicative of joint laxity at 1–4 years old. The results from analyses with selection indices further underline the genetic predictive value of the morphological traits on the pathology associated with hip dysplasia, with optimum selection coefficients yielding a 14% increase in accuracy (directly related to response to selection) over the current aggregate score at improving all nine traits. Furthermore an easily applicable aggregate of scores of morphological traits would only be marginally less accurate than the optimum.

The six traits indicative of pathology DAE, CrEAR, AF, CAE, FHNE and FHR showed no malformation in the vast majority of data from 1–4 year old dogs, the age at which >90% of dogs are scored. All these traits are graded on the degree of pathological OA in response to joint laxity and were subject to detrimental age affects. Conversely, NA, SUB and CrAE were scored >0 for the majority of dogs, indicative of sub-clinical malformation detectable at an early age and implying that the causal factors are effective at one year old. It therefore appears that in the many dogs displaying malformation in these three traits (for example 96% of animals had a bilateral SUB score of 2–8) either the development of osteoarthritic signs is rare; or more likely that in the large majority of cases insufficient time had passed at age of evaluation for such signs to develop. Breeders wishing to take hip score into account in their selections inevitably score dogs prior to breeding age; an age

Table 5. Accuracies of selection coefficients for optimum and derived indices over different welfare weights.

Weights (a)	Selection coefficients (b)				
	Optimum	$[111111111]^T$	$[111000000]^T$	$[110000000]^T$	$[000111111]^T$
$1/\sigma_{PI}$	0.616	0.545	0.598	0.602	0.456
$[111111111]^T$	0.619	0.545	0.603	0.608	0.454
$[00\frac{1}{2}111111]^T$	0.595	0.537	0.570	0.573	0.462

Accuracies from selection indices with different coefficients (***b***) (from left to right: the optimum, aggregate total hip score, aggregate NA+SUB+CrAE, aggregate NA+SUB, aggregate DAE+CrEAR+AF+CAE+FHNE+FHR), and at different welfare weights (***a***) (from top to bottom: scaled and equal, unscaled and equal, and weighted on impact on OA).

at which the pathological responses to joint laxity appear not to have had sufficient time to become manifest in all but the most extreme cases.

The heritability estimates of NA and SUB are substantially higher than those for the remaining seven traits, indicating that these traits concerning (near) innate morphology are richer in genetic information than those traits describing development and severity of OA. Coupled with the high genetic correlations of NA and SUB with traits indicative of the pathological signs associated with dysplasia this makes them of high value for selection against hip dysplasia. The heritability of NA could potentially be further increased if the angle measured was reported since categorisation simply adds measurement error and serves no predictive purpose. Whilst it has been suggested that differences in heritability estimates reflect the ease of categorisation according to the scoring criteria and therefore smaller diagnostic variation [10], an additional reason may be due to the low prevalence of abnormalities in traits 4–9 at the age of scoring. The scoring of these traits is dominated by the binary categorisation of 'normal' and 'abnormal' and for such binary traits in a liability model, heritability will increase with prevalence. One consequence of this is that as the prevalence increases with age the heritabilities may become higher as they begin to express a more complete spectrum of liabilities, however this is of only academic interest since delay in hip scoring will drastically reduce the genetic progress through fewer prospective parents scored by breeding age and/or longer generation intervals. Nevertheless, these six traits do appear heritable to a modest degree (0.15–0.24) in 1–4 year old dogs suggesting they can contribute useful genetic information on the pathological response to joint laxity, although the magnitude of the heritabilities limit their usefulness.

The large and positive genetic correlations between the traits are advantageous, indicating that selection for improvement in any one trait would result in improvement in them all. However, because scoring of six of the traits is dependent on osteoarthritic signs, they may act as repeat indicators of the severity of the pathological response to joint laxity. This may partly explain some of the extremely high genetic correlations, particularly between DAE, CrEAR, AF, CAE and FHNE, all of which are graded according to the severity of exostosis observed. Furthermore, DAE, CrEAR, AF, CAE, FHNE and FHR appear to be conditional on NA, SUB and CrAE. For example it is very unlikely that dogs with an aggregate score of zero for NA, SUB and CrAE would have high scores for the other six traits. Therefore selection for improvement in NA, SUB and CrAE will improve the other trait scores partly by easing the predicate. However, although large the genetic correlation between the two groups of traits was significantly less than one indicating non-identicality, possibly due to genetic variation in the pathological response to laxity of the coxofemoral joint. Selection for improvement in DAE, CrEAR, AF, CAE, FHNE and FHR would therefore not only result in less efficient selection against the predictive traits (NA, SUB and CrAE) but a reduction in propensity to display a biologically normal pathological response to laxity as well. Similarly, while the traits examined are one step away from the clinical manifestation of hip dysplasia as pain and lameness, selection against the symptom risks the response being a reduction in normal expression of such symptom, even when the underlying cause remains.

This study has also demonstrated that EBVs of NA, SUB and CrAE derived from scoring of one year old dogs are better predictors of OA in the other six traits in later life than are EBVs for these six traits themselves. This result strengthens the case of causality of NA, SUB and CrAE on the other six traits, implied by the scoring criteria and supported by the high genetic correlations. Although this might lead to the proposal of simply dropping traits 4–9 from consideration in selection against hip dysplasia, results from the selection index demonstrated that the inclusion of all information always results in higher accuracy of selection coefficients, no matter what the selection objective. Thus their continued presence in the BVA/KC scheme is justified. The presence of negative coefficients for four of the traits descriptive of pathological OA indicates that they serve a purpose as 'environmental corrections'. To give a simple illustration, consider two traits, and assume merit is positively related to each trait: the first has heritability 0.5, with a phenotype obtained by summing two numbers drawn from N(0,1), the first representing the breeding value, the second representing the environmental deviation; the second trait consists of only the second number, i.e. environmental deviation. It is clear that the optimum predictor of genetic merit is the first trait minus the second, even though both traits increase as merit increases. The second trait which is richer in environmental variation is acting to correct the first so as to better predict genetic merit. The same phenomena will occur with the nine traits here but the relationships are obviously more complex.

The results from analyses of selection indices have not only quantitatively endorsed the conclusions of the predictive ability of the morphological traits on those describing pathology, but have also quantified the improvement achievable by use of either optimum coefficients derived from index theory, or aggregate scores of traits describing hip morphology only. Such improvement initially seems counter-intuitive since it appears that information is being discarded, but in fact may be explained due to the relative increase in environmental variation that occurs when the scores of pathology traits are included. Heuristically, the index $\boldsymbol{b} = [111000000]^T$ is 'closer' to the optimum coefficients than the total score ($\boldsymbol{b} = [111111111]^T$). Results from this study indicate that improvements in selective efficacy of >10% are available simply by re-weighting the information already collected.

The study described decomposes of the genetic and phenotypic variances of the current hip score as observed into it the components arising from the 9 traits contributing to it, although this brings with it difficulties of distribution with ordinal data, most notably in traits 4–9. For these traits we have maintained the differentiation among positive scores with the supposition that the use of the scale by the BVA/KC panel of experts embodies confidence in diagnosis as well as degree and that ignoring scoring categories may 'coarsen' the scale of analysis. Nevertheless, we replicated the analyses described and calculated optimum selection coefficients considering traits 4–9 as scaled binomial traits (0 = unaffected, $a>0$ = affected), where a is chosen to maintain the same mean value, but the changes in optimum selection coefficients from those reported were negligible. Furthermore, the objectives of this study rely on a seamless framework that encompasses the individual trait scores and their total sum, which is the current reported total hip score. Clarity of results for 'end users' relies in part on the maintenance of the framework of linearity; otherwise the transformed sum is no longer the sum of the transformed. Further analysis of individual trait transformation to address distributional issues more directly might be more advantageous once the total hip score is no longer seen as the widespread and accepted evaluation of hip condition, for example once EBVs are publically available.

The demonstration of how selection index theory can improve the efficacy of selection against hip dysplasia has far reaching implications illustrating that substantial increases in response to selection are easily achievable. Such methods could be extended to breeding for health in breeds where there are many inherited diseases. The principles involved are easily transferable from their traditional use in livestock production, although the economic values must be replaced with values derived from the welfare impact of each disease or feature of disease. Hip dysplasia is probably unique among companion animals in the provision of such a large quantity of data on so many of the features of disease, but the disease and the screening data is complex, reflecting underlying genetics, environmental effects and the debilitating developmental consequences of innate malformation. Although more detailed exploration of the assignment of welfare values and investigation into the effect of transformation of scores of the features considered to describe hip dysplasia is desirable, as the one of the most prominent canine inherited diseases the increases in selective accuracy identified in this study emphasize easily applicable changes to the ways data is used that will result in a greater response to selection.

Materials and Methods

Data

In the BVA/KC hip score scheme, radiographs of the pelvic area in the "extended hip" position are taken by a general practice vet according to standardised protocols and are voluntarily submitted to the BVA for evaluation by three members of a panel of certified radiologists or small animal surgeons. The anatomical features of the canine pelvis involved in evaluation are represented in Figure 2 and a précis of scoring criteria for the nine features that comprise the total hip score are given in supplementary material (File S1 and Figure S1). Score data on the nine traits of both (left and right) hips was generated by the BVA/KC scheme (computerized records kindly provided by Dr Malcolm Willis). 11,928 records of dogs with individual trait scores directly corresponded to records in the larger data set described in a previous study [11], which was limited to animals ≥1 and <4 years old (365–1459 days inclusive) at the time of radiograph, and evaluated between 2000 and 2007. Initial analysis utilised these data, and feature scores of left and right hips were summed to give a total score for each of the nine traits. The data were in similar proportions according to class of sex and coat colour as those previously reported [11]. Records were distributed over years of evaluation as shown in table 6.

The pedigree used in the analyses was identical to the one described previously [11], unless stated otherwise.

Statistical Analysis

Statistical analyses of the data had the objectives of fitting mixed linear models using ASREML [12] to estimate the genetic parameters of the nine traits. It was previously ascertained that a logarithmic transformation was appropriate given the skewed nature of the total hip score [11]. However score distribution was not consistent across the nine traits and analysis of one trait (SUB) with the family of power transformations [13] determined that in this case logarithm was not the optimal scale for analysis. Furthermore, aggregate total score relates to a simple, equal weighting of trait scores and maintaining this format would simplify evaluation with selection index models. Therefore analyses of the nine individual traits were conducted on untransformed scores.

Substantial genetic similarity in log-transformed aggregate score of left and right hips, with near perfect genetic correlation and near identical genetic and environmental variances was reported previously [11], inferring that a sum of scores of left and right hips was a reasonable simplification. Furthermore, preliminary investigations of this study determined that the genetic correlation between the untransformed scores of left and right hips for two of the nine traits was very close to one (0.996±0.007 for CrAE and 0.998±0.006 for FHNE) and therefore the phenotypes used in all analyses were sums of scores from both hips for each of the nine traits.

Small but significant unique litter effect on total hip score were previously reported [11], having failed to detect significant maternal and litter specific effects, and so litter effects only were included in this analysis.

Initially, nine univariate analyses were conducted (one for each trait) to determine variance components. Subsequently, thirty six ($\sum_{k=1}^{n-1} k$, where n = 9) pair-wise bivariate analyses were conducted to estimate the genetic correlations between every pair of the nine traits comprising the BVA/KC total hip score. The general form of the linear model was as follows:

$$\mathbf{Y} = \mathbf{Xb} + \mathbf{Za} + \mathbf{Wc} + \mathbf{e}$$

where $\mathbf{Y}$ is the vector of observations; $\mathbf{X}$, $\mathbf{W}$ and $\mathbf{Z}$ are known incidence matrices, $\mathbf{b}$ is the vector of fixed effects, $\mathbf{a}$ is the vector of random additive genetic effects with the distribution assumed to be multivariate normal (MVN), with parameters $(0, \sigma^2_a \mathbf{A})$; $\mathbf{c}$ is the vector of random litter effects with the distribution assumed to be MVN, with parameters $(0, \sigma^2_c\mathbf{I})$; and $\mathbf{e}$ is the vector of residuals distributed MVN with parameters $(0, \sigma^2_e\mathbf{I})$; and where $\mathbf{I}$ denotes an identity matrix of the appropriate size, $\mathbf{A}$ is the numerator relationship matrix, and σ^2 is a scalar denoting variance. In the case of bivariate analyses σ^2 was replaced by the appropriate covariance matrix for traits, $\mathbf{\Sigma}$, with the direct product operator. The fixed effects included in the model were: sex, age, season of birth (winter = January – March, spring = April – June, summer = July – September, autumn = October – December) and year of evaluation. Age in days was centred and scaled according to the

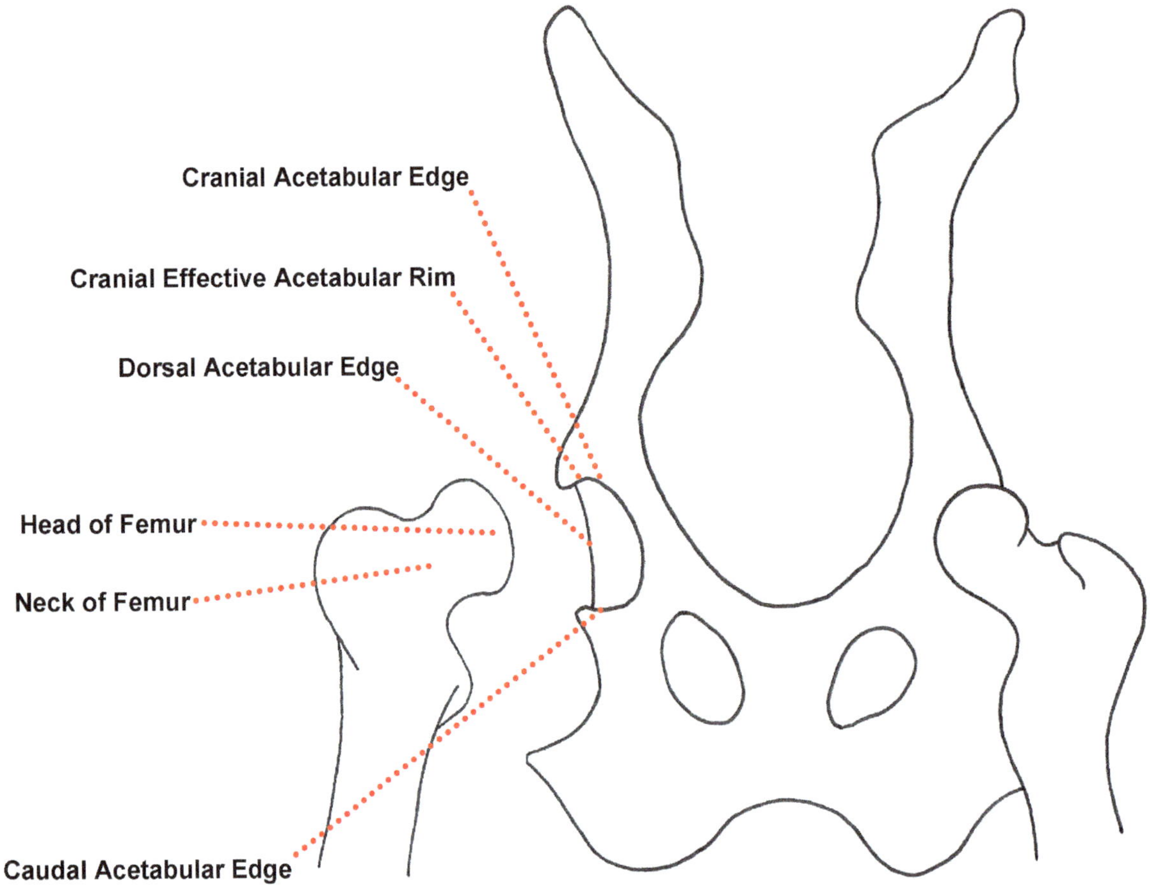

Figure 2. Diagrammatical representation of the skeletal features of the hip joint. Features pertinent to those graded by the BVA/KC hip score scheme.

mean and SD of the data used (for reference, mean = 709.60, SD = 291.10 for data currently described; n = 11,928) and a polynomial regression was fitted. These fixed effects are a simpler form to those fitted previously [11], and therefore more tractable in a computationally more intensive series of models. However they are adequate to describe the effects on score.

Component score group relationships

The genetic correlation between two groups of traits was calculated to determine the likely effect that selection on fewer traits would have on the others. Scores for NA, SUB and CrAE ($SCORE_{1-3}$) were summed (out of a maximum of 36) since these features are scored largely on the detection of morphological malformation (i.e. independent of OA). Scores for DAE, CrEAR, AF, CAE, FHNE and FHR ($SCORE_{4-9}$) were summed (with a maximum of 70) since the scoring of these traits is entirely dependent on the severity of observed pathological malformation (i.e. signs of OA). Pairwise bivariate analyses were conducted using 1) the raw scores and 2) $\log_e$(score+1) transformation of each of the aggregate groups ($SCORE_{4-9}$ and $SCORE_{1-3}$), as described previously. This logarithmic transformation was shown to normalise the skewed distribution of aggregate total hip score [11].

Table 6. Distribution of data over year of evaluation.

Evaluation year	Count	Percent
2000	1963	16.46%
2001	1804	15.12%
2002	2039	17.09%
2003	2483	20.82%
2004	2543	21.32%
2005	1035	8.68%
2006	61	0.51%

Predictive power of groups of component scores

The predictive power of EBVs derived from $SCORE_{1-3}$, $SCORE_{4-9}$ and total score ($SCORE_{1-9}$) on each of the phenotypic groups of scores was assessed. Data from a cohort of dogs scored at one year (365–729 days) old (n = 3,912) and born before 1995 were isolated. The data were restricted to records where sex was explicitly stated as male or female, coat colour stated as one of the 3 'permitted' colours (black, chocolate and yellow) and scores were within the prescribed ranges. A linear mixed model was fitted as previously described to calculate EBVs for $\log_e(1+ SCORE_{1-3})$, $\log_e(1+ SCORE_{4-9})$ and $\log_e(1+ SCORE_{1-9})$ of all animals with data and in the pedigree. The fixed effects included in the model were as previously described. Pedigree of up to a maximum of four generations of ancestors of dogs with data was used in the analysis (n = 30,527). The pedigree was augmented with the 300 progeny of animals with 'early score' data that were themselves 'late scored' at over 4 years (1460+ days) old and born after 1995, in order to obtain 'early score' EBVs for dogs with a 'late score' phenotype. Correlation of EBV_{1-3}, EBV_{4-9} and EBV_{1-9} with transformed phenotypes $SCORE_{1-3}$, $SCORE_{4-9}$ and $SCORE_{1-9}$ in the 300 dogs scored at >4 years old illustrated the predictive power of traits in 1 year old dogs on traits in older dogs (>4 years old) when the clinical signs of joint disease have had more time to become manifest.

Demonstration of a selection index for hip dysplasia

The construction of a selection index was undertaken to demonstrate simple improvements in selective efficacy that are available via the use of optimally weighted EBVs of the BVA/KC hip score data. A more detailed description of the methodology of selection indices is given by Cameron [14]. Optimum selection indices for selection objectives (*H*) using selection criteria (*I*) were obtained with coefficients (*b*) calculated:

$$\mathbf{b} = \mathbf{P}_{II} - 1\mathbf{G}_{IH}\mathbf{a}$$

where **P** is the phenotypic variance/covariance matrix and **G** is the additive genetic covariance matrix derived from the individual pairwise bivariate analysis of each of the 9 traits scored. **G** was made positive definite by the substitution of two small, negative eigenvalues by small, positive values; this correction amounted to a change of 0.4% of the sum of the magnitudes of the original eigenvalues. This procedure minimises the Frobenius distance of the corrected matrix from the original estimate. Subscripts *I* and *H* define the relevant sub-matrices of **P** and **G** for traits in *I* and *H*. **a** represents the vector of relative values for traits in the selection objective (*H*) defining the aggregate breeding value and may be adjusted to reflect the welfare values implicit in each scored trait. Welfare values would need to be derived from consideration of the impact on welfare of malformation of each trait considered. In this study, optimum indices were considered using: 1) $\mathbf{a} = 1/\sigma_{P_i}$ for trait *i*, attaching equal welfare value to the traits when standardised phenotypically; 2) $\mathbf{a} = [1,1,1,1,1,1,1,1,1]^T$, representing an equal welfare value of all nine traits and therefore aggregate breeding value equal to breeding value for the total hip score; 3) $\mathbf{a} = [0, 0, ½, 1, 1, 1, 1, 1, 1]^T$ where the aggregate breeding value is a measure of propensity for pathological damage, which might be considered to better reflect welfare. For each value of **a**, the accuracy of the optimum index was compared to: 1) current selection practice which uses the total hip score, as represented by $\mathbf{b}^T = [1\ 1\ 1\ 1\ 1\ 1\ 1\ 1\ 1]$; 2) the aggregate score of traits scored wholly or partially on morphological malformation only, represented by $\mathbf{b}^T = [1\ 1\ 1\ 0\ 0\ 0\ 0\ 0\ 0]$ (NA+SUB+CrAE) or $\mathbf{b}^T = [1\ 1\ 0\ 0\ 0\ 0\ 0\ 0\ 0]$ (NA+SUB); and 3) the aggregate score of traits scored wholly on pathological malformation, represented by $\mathbf{b}^T = [0\ 0\ 0\ 1\ 1\ 1\ 1\ 1\ 1]$ (DAE+CrEAR+AF+CAE+FHNE+FHR). The accuracy of the selection index was determined as the correlation of the aggregate breeding value with the index value.

Supporting Information

File S1 A précis of scoring criteria for the nine features that comprise the total hip score.

Figure S1 Three examples of progressively deteriorating Norberg Angle. The left is a radiograph of a hip joint showing a positive angle indicating good acetabular depth. The middle radiograph is an example of a small negative Norberg Angle, and the right radiograph an example of a large negative angle. Other signs of joint malformation and osteoarthritic effects may also be seen. Images courtesy of Ruth Dennis.

Acknowledgments

The authors are grateful to Dr Malcolm Willis for collating and kindly providing score data on the individual traits comprising total hip score and to the BVA hip scoring panellists for data provided by their ongoing work.

Author Contributions

Conceived and designed the experiments: JAW SCB. Performed the experiments: TWL. Analyzed the data: TWL. Contributed reagents/materials/analysis tools: JAW SCB. Wrote the paper: TWL JAW.

References

1. Malm S, Fikse WF, Danell B, Strandberg E (2008) Genetic variation and genetic trends in hip and elbow dysplasia in Swedish Rottweiler and Bernese Mountain Dog. J Anim Breed Genet 125: 403–412.
2. Willis MB (1997) A review of the progress in canine hip dysplasia control in Britain. J Am Vet Med Assoc 210: 1480–1482.
3. Hou Y, Wang Y, Lust G, Zhu L, Zhang Z, et al. (2010) Retrospective analysis for genetic improvement of hip joints of cohort labrador retrievers in the United States: 1970–2007. PLoS One 5: e9410.
4. Leppanen M, Saloniemi H (1999) Controlling canine hip dysplasia in Finland. Prev Vet Med 42: 121–131.
5. Brass W (1989) Hip dysplasia in dogs. Journal of small animal practice 30: 166–170.
6. Maki K (2004) Breeding against hip and elbow dysplasia in dogs [PhD Thesis]: University of Helsinki. 27 p.
7. Ohlerth S, Busato A, Gaillard C, Fluckiger M, Lang J (1998) [Epidemiologic and genetic studies of canine hip dysplasia in a population of Labrador retrievers: a study over 25 years]. Dtsch Tierarztl Wochenschr 105: 378–383.
8. Silvestre AM, Ginja MM, Ferreira AJ, Colaco J (2007) Comparison of estimates of hip dysplasia genetic parameters in Estrela Mountain Dog using linear and threshold models. J Anim Sci 85: 1880–1884.
9. Wood JL, Lakhani KH, Rogers K (2002) Heritability and epidemiology of canine hip-dysplasia score and its components in Labrador retrievers in the United Kingdom. Prev Vet Med 55: 95–108.
10. Gibbs C (1997) The BVA/KC scoring scheme for control of hip dysplasia: interpretation of criteria. Vet Rec 141: 275–284.
11. Lewis TW, Blott SC, Woolliams JA (2010) Genetic evaluation of hip score in UK Labrador Retrievers. PLoS One. In press.
12. Gilmour AR, Gogel BJ, Cullis BR, Thompson R, eds (2006) ASReml user guide release 2.0: VSN International Ltd, Hemel Hempstead, HP1 1ES, UK. 372 p.
13. Box GEP, Cox DR (1964) An analysis of transformations. Journal of the Royal Statistical Society B 26: 211–252.
14. Cameron ND (1997) Selection Indices and Prediction of Genetic Merit in Animal Breeding: CAB International. 203 p.

16

Knee Arthroplasty: Disabilities in Comparison to the General Population and to Hip Arthroplasty Using a French National Longitudinal Survey

Agnes Dechartres[1,2,3], Isabelle Boutron[1,2,3]*, Remy Nizard[4,5], Serge Poiraudeau[6,7,9], Carine Roy[1,2,3], Gabriel Baron[1,2,3], Philippe Ravaud[1,2,3], Jean-François Ravaud[8,9]

1 INSERM, U738, Paris, France, **2** Université Paris 7, UFR de Médecine, Paris, France, **3** AP-HP, Hôpital Bichat, Département d'Epidémiologie, Biostatistique et Recherche Clinique, Paris, France, **4** Assistance Publique-Hôpitaux de Paris (AP-HP), Hôpital Lariboisière, Service d'Orthopédie, Paris, France, **5** Université Paris VII, Paris, France, **6** Assistance Publique-Hôpitaux de Paris (AP-HP), Hôpital Cochin, Service de Médecine Physique et de Réadaptation, Paris, France, **7** Université Paris V, Paris, France, **8** INSERM, U750-CERMES, Paris, France, **9** Institut Fédératif de Recherche sur le Handicap, Paris, France

Abstract

Background: Knee arthroplasty is increasing exponentially due to the aging of the population and to the broadening of indications. We aimed to compare physical disability and its evolution over two years in people with knee arthroplasty to that in the general population. A secondary objective was to compare the level of disabilities of people with knee to people with hip arthroplasty.

Methodology/Principal Findings: 16,945 people representative of the French population were selected in 1999 from the French census and interviewed about their level of disability. This sample included 815 people with lower limb arthroplasty. In 2001, 608 of them were re-interviewed, among whom 134 had knee arthroplasty. Among the other participants re-interviewed, we identified 68 who had undergone knee arthroplasty and 145 hip arthroplasty within the last two years (recent arthroplasty). People with knee arthroplasty reported significantly greater difficulties than the general population with bending forward (odds ratio [OR] = 4.7; 95% confidence interval [CI]: 1.7, 12.6), walking more than 500 meters (OR = 6.0; 95% CI: 1.5, 24.7) and carrying 5 kg kilograms for 10 meters (OR = 4.6; 95% CI: 1.3, 16.4). However, the two years evolution in disability was similar to that in the general population for most activities. The level of mobility was similar between people with recent knee arthroplasty and those with recent hip arthroplasty. Nevertheless, people with recent knee arthroplasty reported a lower level of disability than the other group for washing and bending forward (OR = 0.3; 95% CI: 0.1, 0.6 and OR = 0.4; 95% CI: 0.1, 0.9, respectively).

Conclusions/Significance: People with knee arthroplasty reported a higher risk of disability than the general population for common activities of daily living but a similar evolution. There was no relevant difference between recent knee and hip arthroplasties for mobility.

Editor: Ewout W. Steyerberg, University Medical Center Rotterdam, Netherlands

Funding: This study was supported by a grant from INSERM to IFR 25 for the RRC-SP "endoprothèses". The funders had a role in study design and data collection but not in analysis, decision to publish, or preparation of the manuscript.

Competing Interests: The authors have declared that no competing interests exist.

* E-mail: isabelle.boutron@bch.aphp.fr

Introduction

The prevalence of knee replacement is increasing exponentially because of the aging of the population but also due to the broadening of indications [1]. The projections between 1996 and 2030, based on changes expected in the population's age profile, foresee an increase of about 85% in total knee replacements in United States [2]. Data on the level of disability and evolution over time of this increasing population are needed for health service planning and budgeting resources and for better informing patients about their potential difficulties after the surgery. Cohort studies have confirmed that mobility and relief of pain are improved after knee arthroplasty [3–7], but no study has compared the remaining level of disability after the replacement to that in the general population. Results of a French longitudinal community-based study, the "Handicap, Incapacité, Dépendance" (Handicap, Disability and Dependence) or HID survey, showed that people with hip arthroplasty had a higher level of disability than the general population [8]. Most published results suggest that improvement after knee arthroplasty is lower than after hip arthroplasty [3–5,9–14]. Actually, many prospective studies [3–5,9–14] reported that postoperative improvement in pain relief and physical function were greater for subjects with hip arthroplasty than for those with knee arthroplasty. Fitzgerald et al. [15] compared data on physical activities of people with hip and knee arthroplasty to normative data and showed physical function to be remarkably similar at 6 and 12 months postoperatively between patients undergoing either hip or knee arthroplasty. However, to our knowledge no published data has provided a comparison of activity limitations and evolution of disability between people with knee arthroplasty and those with hip arthroplasty in a national representative sample.

Methods

Objectives

The primary objective of our study was to compare physical disabilities and their evolution over two years between people with knee arthroplasty and the general population with use of the two-year follow-up data of the HID survey. A secondary objective was to compare activity limitations and their evolution over two years between subjects with recent (less than two years) knee arthroplasty and those with similarly recent hip arthroplasty.

Participants

The data constituting the basis of this report were collected from the HID survey, a national longitudinal community-based survey undertaken by the French National Institute of Statistics and Economic Studies (INSEE) to describe disability and handicap in France. The target population included residents in all French households (n = 57.4 million) including children. This survey methodology is described in detail elsewhere [8,16,17].

Briefly, a two-stage method was used according to United Nations recommendations [18] to set up the cohort in 1999. For the first stage, a representative sample of census districts (approximately 600 inhabitants per district) was selected. During the census taking, enumerators gave these households the standard forms of the 1999 French population census and an additional questionnaire concerning daily life and health. This screening questionnaire allowed for classifying people into 6 groups of increasing probability of presumed disability. This first 1999 phase concerned approximately 417,500 people and had an 86% response rate.

For the second stage, we selected the population by randomization, using disproportional sampling, with a high sampling rate for the most severely disabled group and a minimum sampling rate for people without daily living restrictions (the largest group). Each of the resulting groups was allocated a specific sampling coefficient that increased with the probability or severity of the presumed handicap. The sample design allowed for weighting the data to estimate representative results at a national level[8]. This cohort included 16,945 subjects representative of the French population living at home, 815 of whom reported having undergone lower-limb arthroplasty (i.e., estimated 691,000 people in the French noninstitutionalised population consistent with the result of another French study[19]). For the two year follow-up survey, 12,530 people were re-interviewed, among whom were 608 of the 815 subjects with lower-limb arthroplasty and 11,922 of the 16,130 other participants. Reasons for no interview are shown in figure 1. Characteristics of nonrespondents are described elsewhere and show that they were significantly older and more disabled for walking and bending forward than respondents [8].

The questionnaire included several items to identify people with hip and knee arthroplasty. There were both open-ended questions concerning health problems and 2 specific questions concerning lower limb arthroplasty "Do you have hip arthroplasty" and "Do you have knee arthroplasty". Among the 608 subjects with lower-limb arthroplasty identified in 1999, 134 (i.e., estimated 147,000 people in the French noninstitutionalised population) had received knee arthroplasty (older knee arthroplasty), 382 hip arthroplasty, 30 both hip and knee arthroplasty and 62 had uncertain data. Among the general population re-interviewed, 68 and 145 (i.e., estimated 49,000 and 121,000 people, respectively, in the French noninstitutionalised population) declared having undergone knee and hip arthroplasty since 1999 (recent knee and hip arthroplasty).

To validate the quality of our data and particularly to avoid the possibility that recent arthroplasty was misclassified as older arthroplasty, one member of our team systematically assessed the chronic diseases reported during the 1999 survey and the 2001 survey by the people identified as having recent arthroplasty. Consequently, 202 people with knee arthroplasty (i.e., estimated 196,000 people in the French noninstitutionalised population) were selected.

Data collection

Two computer-assisted personal interviews were conducted according to a standardized protocol from November 1999 to January 2000 by 442 trained interviewers for the 1999 survey and from October 2001 to January 2002 by 408 trained interviewers for the 2001 survey. During each interview, respondents were asked about their impairment, disability, social participation and help. For the current study, we used data related to participants' disability. Respondents were asked to indicate the degree of difficulty or the need for help in five defined areas: activities involving personal care, mobility, housekeeping, and cognitive and sensorial abilities. Answers were presented as a 5-point Likert scale, ordered by growing probability of disability, from "no disability" to "impossible without help". Respondents also indicated their walking distance: no more than 100 meters, 300 meters, 500 meters and 1000 meters. For the 2001 survey, conditions were considered improved for each task if the answer decreased by at least one category and worse if the answer increased by at least one category. If the answers did not differ between 1999 and 2001, we considered that there was no change in disability for the studied task. The complete questionnaire will be available at the following address: http://ifr-handicap.inserm.fr/HID/ACCUEIL_HID_NEW.HTM

Ethics

This study was planned as a research project. This study was performed in an intense collaboration with the French National Institute of Statistics. This study was declared of public interest by the CNIS ("Conseil National d'Information Statistique") and was approved by the CNIL ("Commission Nationale de l'Informatique et des Libertés", French law number 78-17). According to the French law, written inform consent was not required for this type of study.

Statistical methods

The study design allowed for weighting the data to estimate representative results at a national level. To calculate statistical parameters and their 95% confidence intervals [CI], we used SAS procedures specific for handling complex sample designs to obtain correct variance estimates (SAS version 9.1, PROC SURVEYFREQ, PROC SURVEYMEAN, PROC SURVEYREG and PROC SURVEYLOGISTIC [20].

To take into account attrition bias, we built a propensity score to assess the probability of nonresponse. To do so, we performed a logistic regression with the 2001 responses to the survey used as the dependent variable. The covariates were the 1999 demographic, economic, and educational variables as well as the level of disability in performing common activities of daily living from the 1999 survey. The logistic regression analysis was used to determine the probability of nonresponse (from 0 to 1), the propensity score, for each patient in the data set. Then, multiple logistic regression models adjusted for age, sex, education, number of chronic conditions and probability of 2001 nonresponse allowed for estimating odds ratios [ORs] and their 95% confidence interval [CI] for 1) the level of disability in all subjects with knee

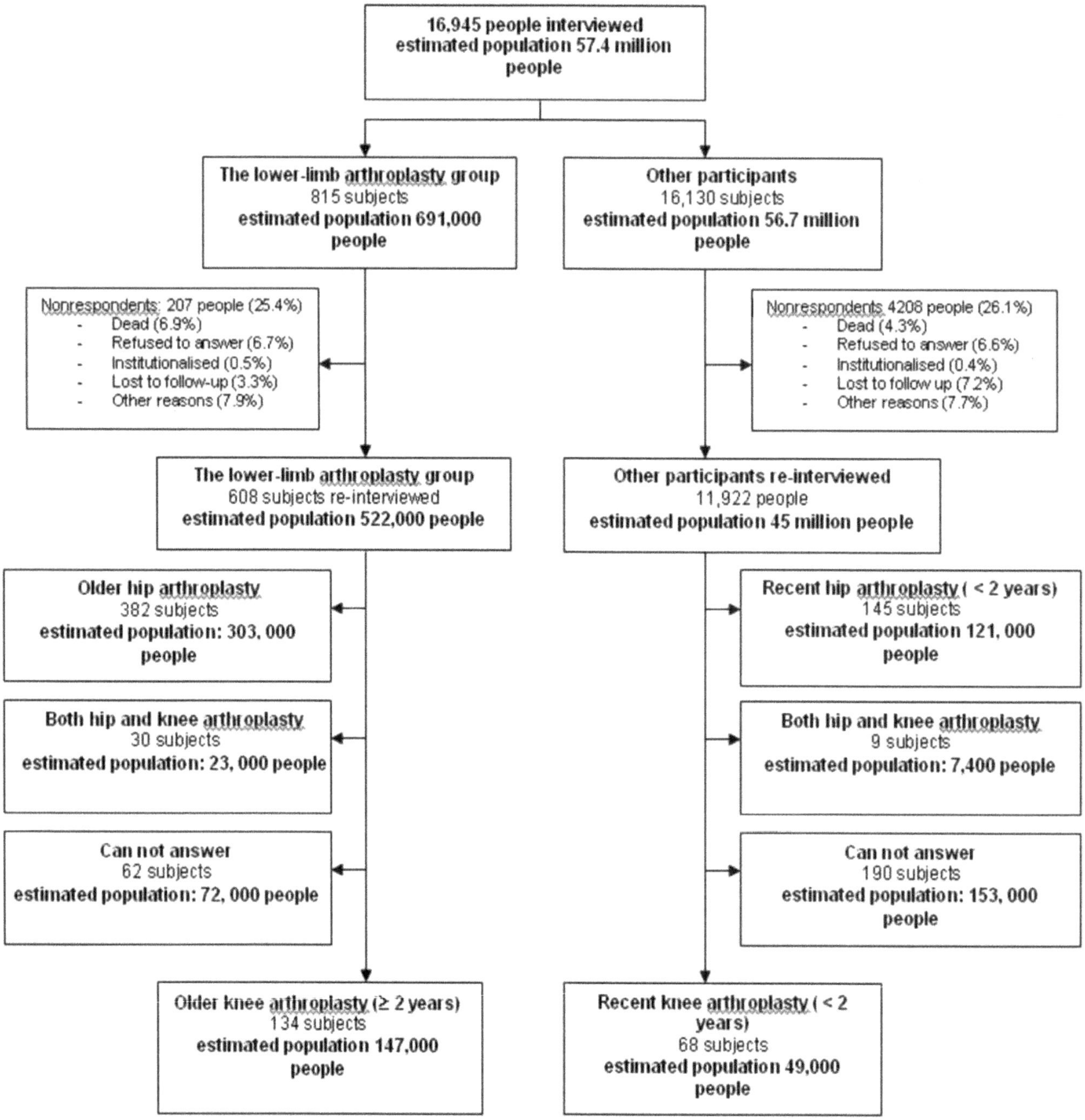

Figure 1. Study population of the HID survey.

arthroplasty compared to the general population in 2001; 2) the evolution of disability (i.e., worsening) in subjects with knee arthroplasty identified in 1999 compared to the general population; and 3) the comparison of disability and its evolution over two years (i.e., worsening) between subjects with recent knee arthroplasty and those with recent hip arthroplasty. To compare the level of disability, the dependent variable was 'reporting at least some difficulties for each activity of daily living'. To compare the evolution of disability, we decided to focus on the worsening of disability as defined above. This choice was based on the descriptive analysis of recent hip and knee arthroplasty, which showed a higher rate of worsening disability than improved condition. Because the delay since the procedure is not known, evolution of disability in our analysis does not reflect evolution since surgery. Thus, analysis of evolution refers to worsening disability for all analysis. Separate models were created for each activity of daily living. All data analyses involved use of the SAS statistical software (version 9.1, SAS Institute).

Results

Demographic characteristics

The knee arthroplasty population comprised 202 subjects, for an estimated 196,000 people in the French noninstitutionalised population (95% CI: 124,000, 269,000). The overall prevalence of knee arthroplasty in France is, consequently, estimated at 0.43%

(95% CI 0.27, 0.59). The annual incidence of knee arthroplasty in France is estimated at 0.05% (95% CI: 0.04%, 0.06%).

The mean age of subjects with knee arthroplasty was 70.2 years (95% CI: 64.8, 75.6; minimum 20, maximum 96); 40.8% of subjects were 75 years or older (95% CI: 24.2, 57.4). Most people were retired: 66.5% (95% CI: 38.3, 94.7). Women represented 52.7% of the study population (95% CI: 32.1, 73.3). Primary school was the highest level of education for 83.2% of people with knee arthroplasty (95% CI: 72.7, 93.7).

Disability and self-reported health status for all people with knee arthroplasty

Subjects with knee arthroplasty claimed 3.6 chronic conditions, on average (95% CI: 3.3, 3.9; minimum 0, maximum 11). Activity limitations concerned mainly the areas of mobility: 52.2% (95% CI: 32.1, 72.3) could not walk more than 500 meters; 73.6% (95% CI: 61.9, 85.4) reported at least some difficulties in bending forward and picking up something; 53.3% (95% CI: 31.5, 75.0) had at least some difficulties climbing up and down stairs; and 70.1% (95% CI: 57.0, 83.2) at least some difficulties carrying 5 kilograms for 10 meters. Self-reported health was poor or very poor for 37.2% of subjects (95% CI: 6.6, 74.9).

After adjustment for age, sex, education, chronic conditions and probability of nonresponse, subjects with knee arthroplasty reported significantly greater difficulties than the general population for bending forward and picking up something (OR = 4.7; 95% CI: 1.7, 12.6), walking more than 500 meters (OR = 6.0; 95% CI: 1.5, 24.7), carrying 5 kilograms for 10 meters (OR = 4.6; 95% CI: 1.3, 16.4) and cutting toenails (OR = 4.1; 95% CI: 1.2, 13.8) (table 1). They also more often reported the use of technical devices to walk (OR = 3.6; 95% CI: 1.7, 7.2). There was a tendency for self-reported health probability to be worse than in the general population (OR = 2.0; 95% CI: 0.9, 4.7).

Table 1. Disability according to domains of disability, for all subjects with knee arthroplasty (202 subjects) compared to the other participants (11,510 subjects) in 2001, after adjustment for age, sex, education, number of chronic conditions and probability of nonresponse. Adjusted Odds ratio [Adj-OR] and 95% confidence interval [CI].

Domains of disability	Subcategory	Adj-OR*	95% CI
Self-care	Washing	0.7	[0.3–1.4]
	Dressing	0.6	[0.3–1.4]
	Cutting toenails	**4.1**	**[1.2–13.8]**
	Using the toilet	0.9	[0.4–2.0]
Mobility	Getting in and out of a bed	1.1	[0.6–2.2]
	Getting in and out of a chair	**2.1**	**[1.05–4.4]**
	Climbing up and down stairs	1.7	[0.7–4.8]
	Bending forward and picking up something	**4.7**	**[1.7–12.6]**
Walking-distance limitation	≤100 meters	1.5	[0.7–3.3]
	≤300 meters	1.3	[0.6–2.6]
	≤500 meters	**6.0**	**[1.5–24.7]**
	≤1000 meters	**5.9**	**[1.6–21.9]**
Shopping		3.3	[0.9–12.9]
Carrying 5 kilograms for 10 meters		**4.6**	**[1.3–16.4]**
Heath status	Having fair, poor or very poor self-reported health	2.0	[0.9–4.7]
Use of technical devices to walk		**3.6**	**[1.7–7.2]**

*Adj-OR, adjusted OR.
Significant ORs are in bold.
The dependent variable is «reporting at least some difficulties for each activity of daily living».

Evolution of disability declared by people with knee arthroplasty for more than 2 years

Worsening disability was mainly declared for mobility: of subjects with knee arthroplasty identified in 1999, 49.3% (95% CI: 19.9, 78.7) declared worsening disability for bending forward and picking up something, 47.1% (95% CI: 19.4, 74.8) for cutting toenails, 21.4% (95% CI: 7.4, 35.4) for shopping, 17.9% (95% CI: 5.5, 30.3) for climbing up and down stairs and 17.7% (95% CI: 5.6, 29.9) for walking-distance limitation.

After adjustment for age, sex, education, chronic conditions and probability of nonresponse, the evolution was similar between subjects with knee arthroplasty for more than 2 years and the general population, except for bending forward and picking up something (OR = 6.4, 95% CI: 1.1, 38.3), cutting toenails (OR = 6.4, 95% CI: 1.1, 37.6) and using the toilet (OR = 0.2, 95% CI: 0.05, 0.9) (Table 2).

Comparison between subjects with recent knee arthroplasty and those with recent hip arthroplasty

For this comparison, we focused only on recent arthroplasty. Subjects with recent knee arthroplasty tended to be younger than people with recent hip arthroplasty (69.8 years *vs.* 73.1 years, p = 0.07). The number of chronic conditions and proportion of women were not significantly different between the 2 groups. Figure 2 provides a description of the level of difficulties for the 2 groups for four common activities of daily living. For walking-distance limitation and climbing stairs, overall, people with recent knee or hip arthroplasty reported the same level of difficulties. However, people with knee arthroplasty reported less difficulties for washing and bending forward than those with hip arthroplasty.

Evolution over two years was largely characterized by no change for both people with recent knee or hip arthroplasty (table 3).

After adjustment for age, sex, education, chronic conditions and probability of nonresponse, subjects with recent knee arthroplasty reported significantly less difficulties than those with recent hip arthroplasty for washing (OR = 0.3; 95% CI: 0.1, 0.6), dressing (OR = 0.3; 95% CI: 0.1, 0.5), bending forward (OR = 0.4; 95% CI: 0.1, 0.9) and cutting toenails (OR = 0.2; 95% CI: 0.1, 0.5) (table 4). After adjustment, worsening disability was less often reported by subjects with recent knee arthroplasty for washing (OR = 0.4; 95% CI: 0.1, 0.9) and dressing (OR = 0.3 95% CI: 0.1, 0.9) than by subjects with recent hip arthroplasty (table 4).

Discussion

This study compared the disabilities of people with knee arthroplasty and their evolution over two years to the general population and to people with hip arthroplasty, on a national representative sample. Our results showed that, despite a higher level of disability for several activities of daily living reported by people with knee arthroplasty, the evolution in disability over two years was similar to that in the general population for most tasks.

Table 2. Disability worsening over two years according to domains of disability, for subjects with knee arthroplasty identified in 1999 (134 subjects) compared to the other participants (11,510 subjects), after adjustment for age, sex, education, chronic conditions and probability of nonresponse.

Domains of disability	Subcategory	Adj-OR	95% CI
Self-care	Washing	0.6	[0.2–1.6]
	Dressing	0.7	[0.3–1.9]
	Cutting toenails	**6.4**	**[1.1–37.6]**
	Using the toilet	**0.2**	**[0.05–0.9]**
Mobility	Getting in and out of a bed	0.6	[0.2–1.7]
	Getting in and out of a chair	1.7	[0.7–4.2]
	Climbing up and down stairs	0.9	[0.4–2.1]
	Bending forward and picking up something	**6.4**	**[1.1–38.3]**
Walking-distance limitation*		1.3	[0.5–3.1]
Shopping		1.2	[0.6–2.4]
Carrying 5 kilograms for 10 meters		0.8	[0.4–1.8]
Heath status		0.4	[0.2–1.2]
Use of technical devices to walk		1.5	[0.5–4.3]

Adjusted Odds ratio [Adj-OR] and 95% confidence interval [CI].
Significant ORs are in bold.
*Worsening walking-distance limitation was defined by the decrease of a class (i.e., <100, 100–300, 300–500, 500–1000) to another.

Moreover, people with recent knee arthroplasty did not report more disabilities or worsening of these disabilities than people with recent hip arthroplasty for activities involving mobility; they reported an even lower level of disability and less worsening of disability for self-care activities.

Many studies have reported significant improvements in ability after knee arthroplasty [3–5,7,21–24]. Only a few have described activity limitations for people with knee arthroplasty [9,23,25,26]: Hawker *et al.* [23] showed, in a community-based survey that 70.2% of subjects with knee arthroplasty had difficulties going upstairs, 66.3% bending to the floor, and 56.9% shopping, and only 38.8% could walk more than 10 blocks; Weiss *et al.* [25] reported that 72% could not kneel and 40% had difficulties carrying heavy objects; and Rissanen *et al.* [9] reported that only 34.7% and 16.7% had no problem with walking and negotiating stairs, respectively, at 24 months. Our results support these studies showing that people with knee arthroplasty do not reach the level of mobility reported by the general population. Evolution of these disabilities over 2 years was not different from the general population except for bending forward and cutting toenails that had a higher risk of worsening. People with knee arthroplasty have less risk of worsening disability for using the toilet than the general population. This result is surprising and unexplained; it could only be related to multiple testing. Our results suggest that mean age at surgery seems to increase since people with recent and older knee arthroplasty have nearly the same mean age during the follow-up visit. This result may be related to the selection of older people for knee replacement.

Results of surveys comparing hip and knee arthroplasty are inconsistent. Many studies report larger pain relief and improvement in physical function for people with hip arthroplasty than for people with knee arthroplasty [3–5,9–14]; others did not find differences between the 2 groups [15,22]. These studies were mainly performed in a few specialized centers by highly qualified surgeons, and their results should not be generalizable to the entire arthroplasty population [27–29]. Our survey, involving a national representative sample, found that subjects with recent knee or hip arthroplasty did not differ in level of disability in mobility activities and evolution over two years. This finding confirms the results of Fitzgerald *et al.* [15] and Ritter *et al.* [22], who showed no difference in physical functioning between people with hip arthroplasty and those with knee arthroplasty 12 months postoperatively and two years later, respectively. A possible explanation concerning the lack of difference in mobility between people with knee arthroplasty and those with hip arthroplasty may be that knee replacements are performed for a lower level of disability than are hip replacements, which implies better outcomes for the former patients [21,30]. The higher risk of disability reported by people with hip arthroplasty for self-care activities and bending forward than for people with knee arthroplasty could be related to the recommendations given to patients after hip arthroplasty to limit activities to reduce the risk of dislocation. These recommendations concern mainly movements to avoid when washing, dressing and bending forward.

Limitations

Our study has some limitations. First, the design of this study is based on self-reported conditions. Self reporting is important to assess disabilities [31,32] but could imply possible under-reporting of arthroplasty by the participants interviewed. We also missed other important information about the different indications for surgery, the timing of procedures, the surgical procedures (total or partial knee replacement), the rehabilitation programmes, the postoperative complications and the revision rates. Second, nonrespondents in the general population could have undergone an arthroplasty within the two years, which would also contribute to possible underestimation of arthroplasty prevalence. Third, our study concerned only French noninstitutionalised people, which would lead to both underestimation of arthroplasty prevalence and disability, because, typically, disabled people tend to live in institutions. Moreover, we can hypothesize that the more disabled and health-impaired people are not undergoing arthroplasty. Although France has no register of knee arthroplasty, our results of prevalence are consistent with those of another survey performed in France in 1999 [19] that identified an estimated 270,000 people with knee arthroplasty. The comparison between people with recent hip arthroplasty and those with recent knee arthroplasty should be interpreted carefully since these results may differ for a longer follow-up. As already studied, the delay before optimal improvement could be between 6 months [33] and 2 years after the procedure [10,12,13,15] and may be different for hip and knee arthroplasty. In this study, assuming a normal distribution of procedure, about one-quarter of patients may be in the period before optimal improvement. Moreover, recent hip arthroplasty may comprise cases of hip fracture. Inclusion of this sub-group in the analysis may contribute to a higher reporting of disability for the recent hip arthroplasty group. Testing 4 different categories of walking distance may be inappropriate because tests are not independent. However, we found interesting to report these 4 categories to better inform clinicians and patients. We did not develop any strategies to take into account multiple testing; some of our results may have occurred by chance. All these limitations are counterbalanced by the fact that this national survey provides both a detailed description of disabilities over time for the entire knee arthroplasty population, which consequently reflects functional

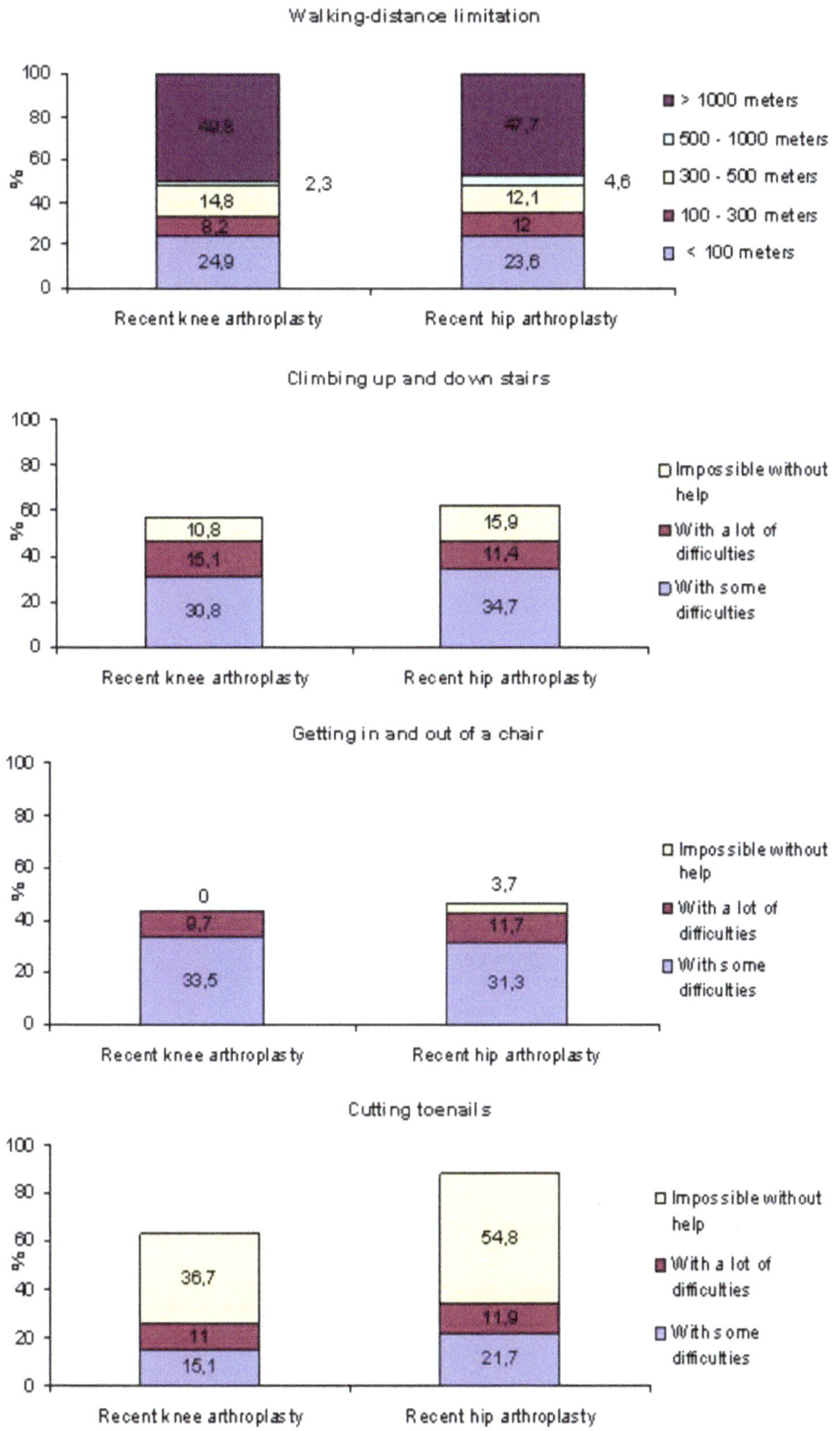

Figure 2. Disability level for people with recent knee arthroplasty and those with recent hip arthroplasty for some activities of daily living in 2001.

Table 3. Evolution of disability for people with recent (less than 2 years) knee arthroplasty (68 subjects) and for those with recent hip arthroplasty (145 subjects).

Domain	Subcategory	Worsening: % [95% CI]		No Change: % [95% CI]		Improvement: % [95% CI]	
		Knee	Hip	Knee	Hip	Knee	Hip
Self-care	Washing	18.8[7.9–29.7]	35.2[25.2–45.2]	73.8[61.4–86.2]	52.0[41.7–62.3]	7.4[0–14.8]	12.8[6.3–19.3]
	Dressing	18.1[7.7–28.5]	34.6[24.7–44.6]	69.5[56.7–82.3]	47.5[37.2–57.8]	12.4[3.2–21.6]	17.9[10.5–25]
	Cutting toenails	30.5[18.0–43.0]	31.3[22.1–40.5]	53.0[38.9–67.2]	55.2[45.0–65.3]	16.4[6.1–26.8]	13.5[6.6–20.4]
	Using the toilet	8.8[0.9–16.8]	16.4[9.4–23.4]	87.8[78.6–96.9]	77.0[69.2–84.8]	3.4[0–8.4]	6.6[2.7–10.5]
Mobility	Getting in/out of a bed	20.6[10.1–31.1]	29.6[19.8–39.3]	58.8[45.2–72.5]	59.2[49.2–69.3]	20.6[9.6–31.5]	11.2[6.3–16.2]
	Getting in/out of a chair	26.1[13.7–38.5]	27.8[18.7–36.9]	54.4[40.2–68.5]	58.6[48.7–68.5]	19.5[8.8–30.2]	13.6[7.8–19.4]
	Bending forward	36.8[22.3–51.3]	32.3[22.6–41.9]	53.0[38.1–67.8]	48.8[37.8–59.7]	10.2[2.2–18.3]	18.9[11–26.7]
	Climbing stairs	23.7[11.4–36.1]	28.3[19.4–37.2]	45.2[30.0–60.3]	49.8[39.1–60.5]	31.1[17–45.2]	21.9[13–30.7]
Walking		39.6[25.2–53.9]	29.6[18.9–40.2]	42.0[27.5–56.5]	51.6[40.1–63.1]	18.4[8.2–28.7]	18.8[8.9–28.6]
Shopping		28.0[15.3–40.6]	21.9[13.7–30.0]	53.4[39.0–67.9]	64.7[54.8–74.6]	18.6[8.1–29.0]	13.5[7.1–19.8]
Carrying 5 kg for 10 m		33.3[19.9–46.7]	33.4[23.6–43.1]	49.8[35.5–64.1]	51.1[40.7–61.4]	16.9[7.0–26.8]	15.6[8.1–23.0]
Health status		21.0[9.3–32.8]	20.3[12.6–28.1]	45.9[31.0–60.8]	57.5[47.3–67.7]	33.0[18–47.9]	22.2[14–30.2]
Use devices to walk		15.9[5.3–26.4]	21.6[12.2–31.0]	73.6[61.2–86.0]	72.7[62.9–82.5]	10.5[2.4–18.6]	5.8[1.2–10.3]

Percentages and 95% confidence interval [CI].

status, and a comparison of activity limitations for people with recent knee arthroplasty and those with recent hip arthroplasty.

People with knee arthroplasty reported a higher risk of disability than the general population for common activities of daily living but a similar evolution. There was no relevant difference between recent knee and hip arthroplasties for mobility. This national longitudinal survey may help clinicians and other clinical practitioners such as occupational therapists, physical therapists

Table 4. Disability and evolution (i.e., worsening) over two years according to domains of disability, for subjects with recent knee arthroplasty (68 subjects) compared to those with recent hip arthroplasty (145 subjects) adjusted for age, sex, education, chronic conditions and probability of nonresponse.

Domains of disability	Subcategory	Disability$		Worsening	
		Adj-OR	95% CI	Adj-OR	95% CI
Self-care	Washing	**0.3**	**[0.1–0.6]**	**0.4**	**[0.1–0.9]**
	Dressing	**0.3**	**[0.1–0.5]**	**0.3**	**[0.1–0.9]**
	Cutting toenails	**0.2**	**[0.1–0.5]**	0.7	[0.3–1.7]
	Using the toilet	0.4	[0.1–1.5]	0.4	[0.1–1.7]
Mobility	Getting in and out of a bed	0.6	[0.2–1.4]	0.5	[0.2–1.5]
	Getting in and out of a chair	0.9	[0.4–2.1]	1.3	[0.5–3.3]
	Climbing up and down stairs	0.9	[0.3–2.3]	0.7	[0.3–1.9]
	Bending forward and picking up something	**0.4**	**[0.1–0.9]**	1.0	[0.4–2.4]
Walking-distance limitation	≤100 meters	1.1	[0.4–3.0]		
	≤300 meters	0.9	[0.3–2.2]		
	≤500 meters	1.4	[0.5–3.6]		
	≤1000 meters	1.1	[0.4–2.9]		
	Worsening*			1.3	[0.5–3.3]
Shopping		0.5	[0.2–1.3]	0.9	[0.4–2.2]
Carrying 5 kg for 10 m		0.6	[0.2–1.8]	0.9	[0.4–2.1]
Heath status	Having fair, poor or very poor self-reported health	0.9	[0.3–2.6]	1.5	[0.5–4.4]
Devices to walk	Use of technical devices to walk	0.5	[0.2–1.2]	0.7	[0.2–2.1]

Adjusted Odds ratio [Adj-OR] and 95% confidence interval [CI].
$The dependent variable is «reporting at least some difficulties» for each activity of daily living.
*The term worsening was used to assess overall worsening of walking-distance limitation.
Significant ORs are in bold.

and service planners think about specific rehabilitation programs to reduce disability according to the type of arthroplasty, hip or knee.

Acknowledgments

The study design is the result of an intense cooperation between INSEE and leading research institutes in the field, including INSERM and particularly the "Institut Fédératif de Recherche sur le Handicap".

The authors thank the INSEE division " Enquêtes et études démographiques" and especially Pierre Mormiche, who is responsible for the "Handicap, Incapacité, Dépendance" (HID) project task force.

Author Contributions

Conceived and designed the experiments: IB JR. Analyzed the data: PR SP GB AD IB CR RN. Contributed reagents/materials/analysis tools: PR AD IB JR. Wrote the paper: PR SP AD RN JR.

References

1. Jain NB, Higgins LD, Ozumba D, Guller U, Cronin M, et al. (2005) Trends in epidemiology of knee arthroplasty in the United States, 1990–2000. Arthritis Rheum 52: 3928–3933.
2. Praemer AFS, Rice DP (1999) Arthroplasty and total joint procedures. In: Praemer A, Furner S, Rice DP, eds. Musculoskeletal conditions in the United States USA American Academy of Orthopedic Surgeons. pp 119–138.
3. Jones CA, Voaklander DC, Johnston DW, Suarez-Almazor ME (2000) Health related quality of life outcomes after total hip and knee arthroplasties in a community based population. J Rheumatol 27: 1745–1752.
4. Rissanen P, Aro S, Slatis P, Sintonen H, Paavolainen P (1995) Health and quality of life before and after hip or knee arthroplasty. J Arthroplasty 10: 169–175.
5. Salmon P, Hall GM, Peerbhoy D, Shenkin A, Parker C (2001) Recovery from hip and knee arthroplasty: Patients' perspective on pain, function, quality of life, and well-being up to 6 months postoperatively. Arch Phys Med Rehabil 82: 360–366.
6. Forrest GP, Roque JM, Dawodu ST (1999) Decreasing length of stay after total joint arthroplasty: effect on referrals to rehabilitation units. Arch Phys Med Rehabil 80: 192–194.
7. March LM, Cross MJ, Lapsley H, Brnabic AJ, Tribe KL, et al. (1999) Outcomes after hip or knee replacement surgery for osteoarthritis. A prospective cohort study comparing patients' quality of life before and after surgery with age-related population norms. Med J Aust 171: 235–238.
8. Dechartres A, Boutron I, Nizard R, Poiraudeau S, Roy C, et al. (2007) Evolution of disability in adults with hip arthroplasty: a national longitudinal study. Arthritis Rheum 57: 364–371.
9. Rissanen P, Aro S, Sintonen H, Slatis P, Paavolainen P (1996) Quality of life and functional ability in hip and knee replacements: a prospective study. Qual Life Res 5: 56–64.
10. Kirwan JR, Currey HL, Freeman MA, Snow S, Young PJ (1994) Overall long-term impact of total hip and knee joint replacement surgery on patients with osteoarthritis and rheumatoid arthritis. Br J Rheumatol 33: 357–360.
11. Kiebzak GM, Vain PA, Gregory AM, Mokris JG, Mauerhan DR (1997) SF-36 general health status survey to determine patient satisfaction at short-term follow-up after total hip and knee arthroplasty. J South Orthop Assoc 6: 169–172.
12. Kiebzak GM, Campbell M, Mauerhan DR (2002) The SF-36 general health status survey documents the burden of osteoarthritis and the benefits of total joint arthroplasty: but why should we use it? Am J Manag Care 8: 463–474.
13. Bachmeier CJ, March LM, Cross MJ, Lapsley HM, Tribe KL, et al. (2001) A comparison of outcomes in osteoarthritis patients undergoing total hip and knee replacement surgery. Osteoarthritis Cartilage 9: 137–146.
14. Mainard D, Guillemin F, Cuny C, Mejat-Adler E, Galois L, et al. (2000) [Quality of life assessment one year after total hip or knee arthroplasty]. Rev Chir Orthop Reparatrice Appar Mot 86: 464–473.
15. Fitzgerald JD, Orav EJ, Lee TH, Marcantonio ER, Poss R, et al. (2004) Patient quality of life during the 12 months following joint replacement surgery. Arthritis Rheum 51: 100–109.
16. Leclerc A, Chastang JF, Ozguler A, Ravaud JF (2006) Chronic back problems among persons 30 to 64 years old in France. Spine 31: 479–484.
17. Mormiche (1998) L'enquête HID de l'INSEE. Objectifs et schéma organisationnel. Courrier des statistiques.
18. United Nations SD (1996) Manual for the development of statistical information for disability programs and policies. New York: UN publications.
19. Courpied JP, Caton J, Bouee S, Charpak Y, Thomine JM (2001) [Osteoarticular disease in adults in France. A survey of 2000 persons]. Rev Chir Orthop Reparatrice Appar Mot 87: 424–436.
20. Zhenyi XEL, Daftary M. Wutoh A Building Logistic Regression Models to Analyze Survey Data with Complex Sampling Design. **http://www.nesug.org/html/Proceedings/nesug04/an/an08.pdf**.
21. Fortin PR, Clarke AE, Joseph L, Liang MH, Tanzer M, et al. (1999) Outcomes of total hip and knee replacement: preoperative functional status predicts outcomes at six months after surgery. Arthritis Rheum 42: 1722–1728.
22. Ritter MA, Albohm MJ, Keating EM, Faris PM, Meding JB (1995) Comparative outcomes of total joint arthroplasty. J Arthroplasty 10: 737–741.
23. Hawker G, Wright J, Coyte P, Paul J, Dittus R, et al. (1998) Health-related quality of life after knee replacement. J Bone Joint Surg Am 80: 163–173.
24. Walker DJ, Heslop PS, Chandler C, Pinder IM (2002) Measured ambulation and self-reported health status following total joint replacement for the osteoarthritic knee. Rheumatology (Oxford) 41: 755–758.
25. Weiss JM, Noble PC, Conditt MA, Kohl HW, Roberts S, et al. (2002) What functional activities are important to patients with knee replacements? Clin Orthop Relat Res. pp 172–188.
26. Noble PC, Gordon MJ, Weiss JM, Reddix RN, Conditt MA, et al. (2005) Does total knee replacement restore normal knee function? Clin Orthop Relat Res. pp 157–165.
27. Lavernia CJ, Guzman JF (1995) Relationship of surgical volume to short-term mortality, morbidity, and hospital charges in arthroplasty. J Arthroplasty 10: 133–140.
28. Kreder HJ, Deyo RA, Koepsell T, Swiontkowski MF, Kreuter W (1997) Relationship between the volume of total hip replacements performed by providers and the rates of postoperative complications in the state of Washington. J Bone Joint Surg Am 79: 485–494.
29. Field RE, Cronin MD, Singh PJ (2005) The Oxford hip scores for primary and revision hip replacement. J Bone Joint Surg Br 87: 618–622.
30. Fortin PR, Penrod JR, Clarke AE, St-Pierre Y, Joseph L, et al. (2002) Timing of total joint replacement affects clinical outcomes among patients with osteoarthritis of the hip or knee. Arthritis Rheum 46: 3327–3330.
31. Amadio PC (1993) Outcomes measurements. J Bone Joint Surg Am 75: 1583–1584.
32. Fitzpatrick R, Fletcher A, Gore S, Jones D, Spiegelhalter D, et al. (1992) Quality of life measures in health care. I: Applications and issues in assessment. Bmj 305: 1074–1077.
33. Shields RK, Enloe LJ, Leo KC (1999) Health related quality of life in patients with total hip or knee replacement. Arch Phys Med Rehabil 80: 572–579.

17

The Impact of Preoperative Hip Heterotopic Ossification Extent on Recurrence in Patients with Head and Spinal Cord Injury

François Genêt[1]*, Claire Jourdan[1], Christine Lautridou[2], Clément Chehensse[1], Kambiz Minooee[3], Philippe Denormandie[2], Alexis Schnitzler[1]

1 Service de Médecine Physique et de Réadaptation, CHU R.Poincaré, Garches, France, **2** Service de chirurgie Orthopédique, CHU R.Poincaré, Garches, France, **3** Service de Rhumatologie et de Médecine Physique, CHU Erasme, Bruxelles, Belgique

Abstract

Background: The preoperative Heterotopic Ossification (HO) extent is usually one of the main used criteria to predict the recurrence before excision. Brooker et al built a radiologic scale to assess this pre operative extent around the hip. The aim of this study is to investigate the relationship between the recurrence risk after hip HO excision in Traumatic Brain Injury (TBI) and Spinal Cord Injury (SCI) patients and the preoperative extent of HO.

Methodology/Principal Findings: A case control study including TBI or SCI patients following surgery for troublesome hip HO with (case, n = 19) or without (control, n = 76) recurrence. Matching criteria were: sex, pathology (SCI or TBI) and age at the time of surgery (+/−4.5 years). For each etiology (TBI and SCI), the residual cognitive and functional status (Garland classification), the preoperative extent (Brooker status), the modified radiological and functional status (GCG-BD classification), HO localization, side, mean age at the CNS damage, mean delay for the first HO surgery, and for the case series, the mean operative delay for recurrence after the first surgical intervention were noted.

Conclusions/Significance: The median delay for first HO surgery was 38.6 months (range 4.5 to 414.5;) for the case subgroup and 17.6 months (range 5.7 to 339.6) for the control group. No significant link was found between recurrence and operative delay (p = 0.51); the location around the joint (0.07); the Brooker (p = 0.52) or GCG-BD status (p = 0.79). Including all the matching factors, no significant relationship was found between the recurrence HO risk and the preoperative extent of troublesome hip HO using Brooker status (OR = 1.56(95% CI: 0.47–5.19)) or GCG-BD status (OR class 3 versus 2 = 0.67(95% CI: 0.11–4.24) and OR class 4 versus 2 = 0.79(95%CI: 0.09–6.91)). Until the pathophysiology of HO development is understood, it will be difficult to create tools which can predict HO recurrence.

Editor: Mel B. Feany, Brigham and Women's Hospital, Harvard Medical School, United States of America

Funding: The authors have no support or funding to report.

Competing Interests: The authors have declared that no competing interests exist.

* E-mail: francois.genet@rpc.aphp.fr

Introduction

Secondary orthopaedic complications after central nervous system lesion are common, mainly after Traumatic Brain Injury (TBI), but also after Spinal Cord Injury (SCI) and in a smaller proportion after stroke or cerebral anoxia [1]. Among them, Heterotopic Ossifications (HO) are frequent (from 11 to 76%) and induce pain and limit range of motion until complete ankylosis or vessel and nerve compression [1,2,3]. Nowadays, the predisposing factors to HO are well described for TBI and SCI patients: associated bone fracture, sepsis, prolonged immobilization, neuro-vegetative disorders, etc. [4,5,6,7,8,9,10,11,12].

The only effective treatment is still surgery for excision [1,2, 3,13]. Complications of these interventions are obviously hematoma, fractures and sepsis which depend on surgical and perioperative procedures. Indeed this patient group is complex, often with several co-morbid factors. Recurrence appears to depend not only on the surgical procedure but equally the etiology and the HO features [13,14,15,16]. However, postoperative recurrence rate is rarely assessed for several reasons: there is no generally accepted definition (clinical or X-Ray diagnosis of recurrence); follow up is not standardised; surgical techniques change, mainly regarding peri operative and medical management. The delay of recurrence after surgery seems to be the same as that for the initial occurrence: within the first 3 months according to Gacon and Ippolito [17,18] and between 3 and 6 weeks according to Stover [15]. Several studies have attempted to report the incidence of recurrence after HO excision [18,19,20,21,22,23,24,25,26,27,28, 29,30,31]. However, in most cases, these studies were descriptive (without statistical analysis) and involved a small sample of patients, frequently heterogeneous. The results of a meta analysis including 16 studies and 255 patients [32] suggested that there is no relationship between recurrence and operative delay, however, the average operative delay from neurological damage or HO diagnosis to surgery was widely dispersed in the studies included (13 to 30 months). The mean recurrence rate was estimated at

19.8% (IC 95%: 14,4–26,1%) but outcome measures were disparate (recurrence of decreased range of motion, ankylosis, X-Ray recurrence and surgical indications). In a previous study including a large sample of patients (357 patients, 539 surgeries) suffering surgery for troublesome HO after CNS lesion we found a mean recurrence rate of 5.8% (31 surgeries) [1].

Brooker et al., in 1973, proposed a method to classify the degree of ectopic bone formation about the hip following total hip arthroplasty [33]. They defined 4 classes (Class I: island of bone within the soft tissues about the hip, Class II: bone spurs from the pelvis or proximal end of the femur leaving at least one centimeter between opposing bone surfaces, Class III: bone spurs from the pelvis or proximal end of the femur, reducing the space between opposing bone surfaces to less than one centimeter, Class IV: apparent bone ankylosis of the hip, figures 1 and 2). Later, Stover et al. suggested that the extent of the initial HO is the most important factor in predicting postoperative recurrence in SCI patients [15]. Several teams have tried to find a link between the risk of recurrence and the pre operative extent of the HO however, their results were based on clinical observations and not a real scientific assessment [14]. The aim of this study was to assess if there is a relationship between the recurrence risk and the pre operative extent of hip HO in two large, homogenous samples of TBI and SCI patients undergoing surgery for troublesome HO in a single center and operated on by a single surgeon.

Materials and Methods

Ethics statement

The study was approved by the institutional review board, Comité de Protection des Personnes XI, Ile de France. It was a non-interventional study in which usual procedures were carried out and without any additional procedures (diagnosis or medical supervision). In France, patient consent is not needed for such an anonymous retrospective data analysis. We confirm that our named institutional review board specifically waived the need for consent for this study [Comité de Protection des Personnes Ile de France XI Pavillon Jacques Courtois - 2ème étage 20, rue Armagis 78105 Saint Germain en Laye Cedex. tél: 01.39.27.42.58 - fax: 01.39.27.49.01 mail: cppidf11@chi-poissy-st-germain.fr"].

Study design

Case control study comparing clinical features, extent of hip HO and medical history of patients with troublesome HO requiring surgery after TBI or SCI with or without recurrence. Files of patients containing complete details of the pathology and HO were selected from a database of patients with central neurological system damage who had undergone surgery for troublesome HO in a single center specialized in this kind of treatment. Each patient in whom recurrence had occurred was matched with 4 control patients (no recurrence after 3 months of follow up) who were randomly selected by the manager of the Medical Information Department in files of patients with a follow up ensured in our physicians' network. Each TBI patient was matched with TBI controls and similarly for SCI patients. Matching criteria were: sex, pathology (TBI or SCI), and age at the time of surgery (+/−4.5 years). The residual cognitive and functional status (only for TBI patients, Garland classification [24]), the Brooker status [33], the modified radiological and functional GCG-BD classification of HO [14], the HO localization (around the joint), the side (right or left), the age at the time of CNS damage (months), the delay for the first HO surgery (months), the diagnosis delay for recurrence from the first surgery (surgeon consultation even if the diagnosis was certainly done before by the physicians who followed the patients after surgery)) (months) and the operative delay for recurrence from the first surgery (months) were recorded for each patient. The Brooker status was found in the surgical file. The GCG-BD was assessed retrospectively by another surgeon and a physician (Physical Medicine and Rehabilitation) who were blinded to the Brooker status, using preoperative X-Rays and reports.

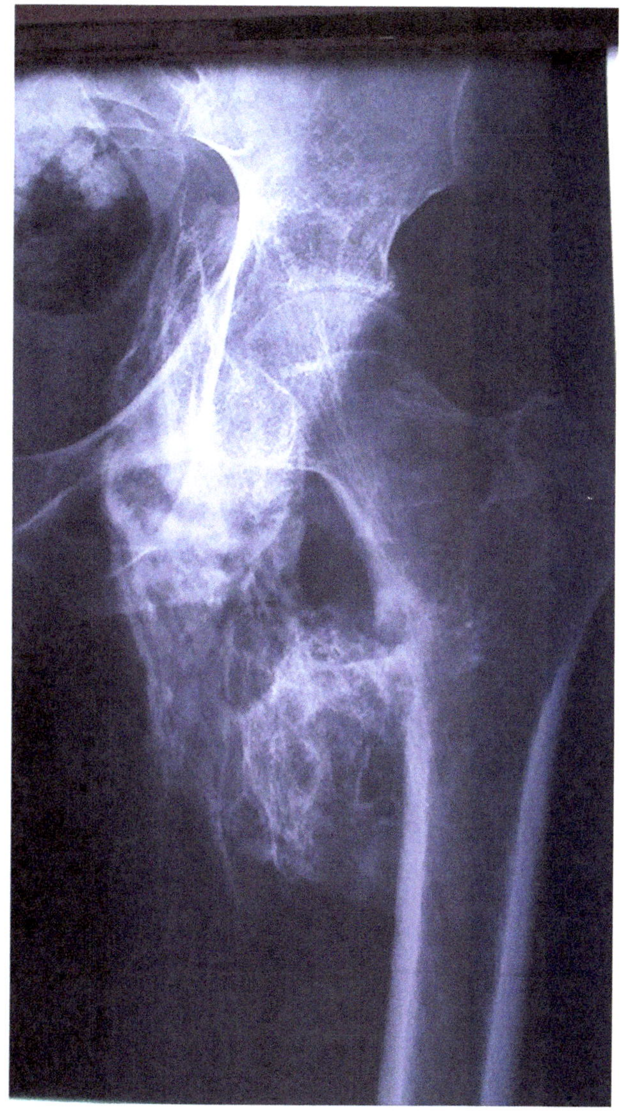

Figure 1. Hip Medial Heterotopic Ossification (Brooker Class IV).

Constitution of the case database [1]

This single-centre study concerned a period between May 1993 and November 2009. Patients had been referred for a specialized neuro-orthopedic consultation for troublesome HO following CNS damage. Indications for surgery were loss of ROM with functional repercussions, ankylosed joint, and nerve or vessel compression. The surgical and immediate post-operative assessments were performed by the same surgeon.

Pre-operative investigations did not include serum alkaline phosphatase levels, Tc99 bone scanning or positivity for human leukocyte antigen B27 [32]. Several patients had received

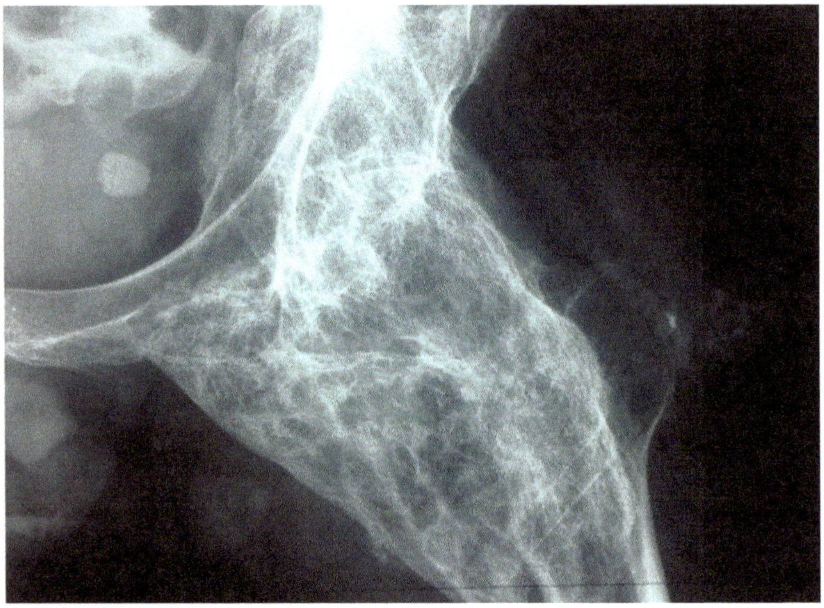

Figure 2. Encircling Hip Heterotopic Ossification.

prophylactic treatment for HO, such as nonsteroidal anti-inflammatory drugs (for pain) or radiation therapy between 1993 and 2002 (this treatment was discontinued, probably due to lack of effectiveness).

A standardised surgical approach was used for each HO location. The surgical goal was resection of the amount of bone necessary to allow restoration of motion in all planes. Each patient underwent regular clinical examinations and x-rays; they were hospitalized in a surgical care unit for about 1 week, and then received regular consultations in rehabilitation units (inpatient care followed by outpatient care for a minimum of 1 year).

Patients were followed up in the rehabilitation unit of the same institution if they lived locally or by out-patient surgical consultation if they lived far away for about 3 months. For those patients, the prolonged supervision was organized by the physician of PMR over several months or years after these surgeries. The majority of these cases and controls are always followed by our colleagues. Therefore, all the troublesome recurrences had been diagnosed this especially as we work with a network agreement with these units: the surgeon would have been alerted.

Statistical analysis

Statistical analysis was carried out with "R" Software® version 2.10.1 (Copyright (C) 2009. The R Foundation for Statistical Computing). Data are reported as numbers and percentages for categorical variables; median, minima, maxima and interquartile range for quantitative variables. Distributions of operative delays for first HO excision in the control and case samples were further described in a box plot.. Univariate tests used Kruskal-Wallis for quantitative variables, and Fisher tests for qualitative variables. All tests were two tailed, and a p value <0.05 was considered statistically significant. Correlation between Brooker and GCG-BD classification in the general sample of patients was assessed by Kendall's Tau.

The association between the Brooker or the GCG-BD status and the recurrence of HO was tested by a Fisher test.,Then two multivariate logistic models were carried out, to adjust for variables used for pairing The dependent variable was the presence of recurrence. Independent variables were gender and age, and either Brooker or GCG-BD(reference category was status 2 for GCG-BD). Adjusted odds ratios were calculated with 95% confidence intervals.

Results

We found 19 cases of recurrence in our series of 539 surgeries since 1993 after TBI (9/19) and SCI (10/19). Following the matching criteria, we randomly selected 76 control files of TBI (36/76) and SCI (40/76) patients without recurrence after 3 months after surgery into the surgical database.

Total population (Table 1)

95 patients with hip HO were included (85 men; SR: 81.3%). Median age was 30.2 (range 15.0 to 56.0, IQR 24.8; 37.7). Median operative delay for first HO excision was 17.9, (range 4.5 to 415.5; IQR: 10.9; 49.7, figure 3). Locations around the joint were anterior (43; 45.3%), posterior (14; 14.7%), medial (9; 9.5%), lateral (25; 26.3%) and encircling (4; 4.2%). The median follow-up by the surgeon was 10.3months (range 0.7 to 159.4; , IQR: 5.7; 30.0).

Based on Surgeon's files, the Brooker status on preoperative X-Ray was 61 (64.2%) patients with status 3 and 34 (35.8%) with status 4.

Based on preoperative X-Rays and functional abilities, the distribution of the GCG-BD status was class 2: 8 patients (8.4%), class 3: 54 patients (56.8%) and class 4: 33 patients (34.7%).

Case series (Table 1)

There were 19 cases of recurrence (17 men, SR: 89.5%), 19 hips (7 left side). Median age at CNS damage was 30.7 years (range 16.4 to 53.0; IQR: 25.8–39.1). Median delay for the recurrence diagnosis from the first surgery by the surgeon was 2.57 months (range 1.1 to 62.4; IQR 1.6–3.9). Median delay for first HO surgery was 38.6 months (range 4.5 to 414.5; IQR 9.5–63.6) and

Table 1. Demographic data and univariate analysis.

			Demographic data		Univariate analysis
			Case (n = 19) **10 SCI** **9 TBI**	**Control (n = 76)** **40 SCI** **36 TBI**	**p**
Sex ratio	Total		17 men (89.5%)	68 men (89.5%)	
	TBI		7 men (77.8%)	28 men (77.8%)	
	SCI		10 men (100.0%)	40 men (100.0%)	
Location	Hip		19 (100.0%)	76 (100.0%)	
Location around the joint	ANT		9 (47.4%)	34 (44.7%)	0.07
	POST		2 (10.5%)	12 (15.8%)	
	MEDIAL		5 (26.4%)	20 (26.3%)	
	LATERAL		0 (0.0%)	9 (11.8%)	
	ENCIRCLING		3 (15.8%)	1 (1.3%)	
Side (left/right)			7/12	32/44	0.75
Age at surgery median : IQR (min-max) (years)	Total		30.7 ; 25.8–39.1 (16.4–53.0)	30.0 ; 24.9–37.0 (15.0–56.0)	0.71
	TBI		29.8 ; 24.5–30.7 (16.4–38.6)	29.2 ; 23.7–31.2 (15.0–38.7)	0.84
	SCI		36.0 ; 28.4–42.5 (21.9–53.0)	35.7 ; 26.8–42.5 (18.5–56.0)	
Time from CNS damage to first surgery – median : IQR (min-max) (months)	Total		38.6; 9.5–63.6 (4.5–414.5)	17.6; 11.1–43.7 (5.7–339.6)	0.53
	TBI		10.0 ; 8.8–38.9 (5.6–50.1)	13.0 ; 9.3–26.7 (5.7–116.5)	0.50
	SCI		63.5 ; 32.5–202.2 (4.5–414.5)	24.5 ; 14.3–60.2 (7.2–339.6)	0.07
Brooker Status	Total	1	0/19 (0.0)	0/76 (0.0)	0.59
		2	0/19 (0.0)	0/76 (0.0)	
		3	11/19 (57.9)	50/76 (65.8)	
		4	8/19 (42.1)	26/76 (34.2)	
	TBI	1	0/9 (0.0)	0/36 (0.0)	1
		2	0/9 (0.0)	0/36 (0.0)	
		3	8/9 (88.9)	32/36 (88.9)	
		4	1/9 (11.1)	4/36 (11.1)	
	SCI	1	0/10 (0.0)	0/40 (0.0)	0.49
		2	0/10 (0.0)	0/40 (0.0)	
		3	3/10 (30.0)	18/40 (45.0)	
		4	7/10 (70.0)	22/40 (55.0)	
GCG-BD Status	Total	1	0/19 (0.0)	0/76 (0.0)	0.79
		2	2/19 (10.6)	6/76 (7.9)	
		3	10/19 (52.6)	44/76 (57.9)	
		4	7/19 (36.8)	26/76 (34.2)	
	TBI	1	0/9 (0.0)	0/36 (0.0)	0.71
		2	2/9 (22.2)	6/36 (16.7)	
		3	7/9 (77.8)	26/36 (72.2)	
		4	0/9 (0.0)	4/36 (11.1)	
	SCI	1	0/10 (0.0)	0/40 (0.0)	0.49
		2	0/10 (0.0)	0/40 (0.0)	
		3	3/10 (30.0)	18/40 (45.0)	
		4	7/10 (70.0)	22/40 (55.0)	
Garland Status For TBI	1		0/9 (0.0)	1/36 (2.8)	0.28
	2		2/9 (22.2)	5/36 (13.9)	
	3		1/9 (11.1)	1/36 (2.8)	
	4		1/9 (11.1)	15/36 (41.6)	
	5		5/9 (55.6)	14/36 (38.9)	

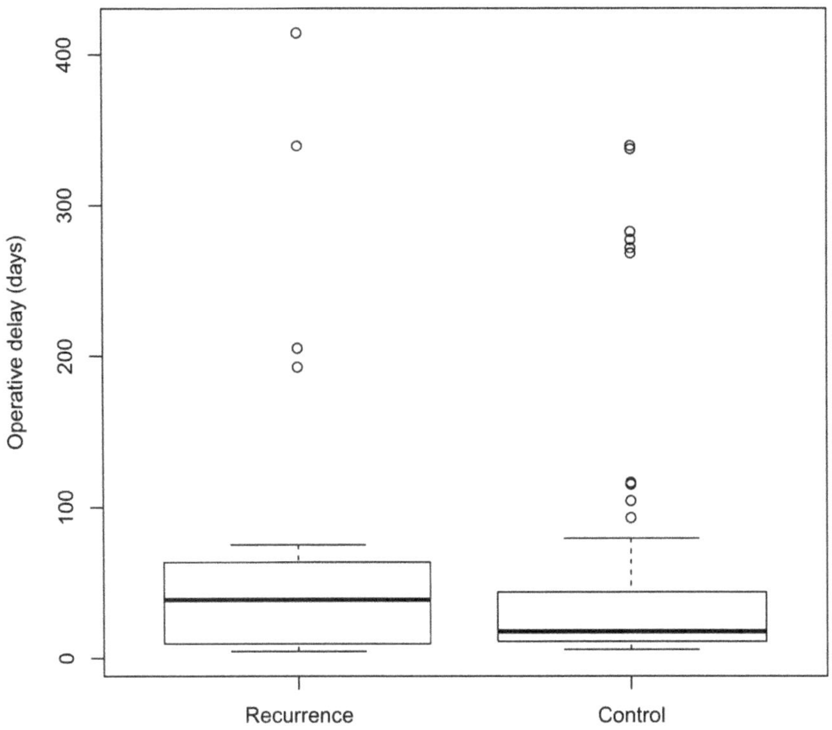

Figure 3. Operative delay for first HO excision in the case sample ('recurrence") and in the control sample. The upper and lower hinges indicate the 25th and 75th percentiles, the line in the box indicates the median.

the median follow-up by the surgeon was 20.1 months (range 2.5 to 95.3; IQR: 6.4–69.9).

Control series (Table 1)

76 patients had no recurrence following surgical intervention for troublesome HO (68 men, SR: 89.5%), 76 hips (32 left side). Median age at CNS damage was 30.0 years (range 15.0 to 56.0; IQR: 24.9–37.0). The median delay for first HO surgery was 17.6 months (range 5.7 to 339.6; IQR: 11.1–43.7) and the median follow-up by the surgeon was 7.44 months (range 2.7 to 78.5; IQR: 5.6–27.7).

Univariate analysis (Table 1)

No relationship was found between recurrence and operative delay ($p = 0.51$), HO side ($p = 0.75$), location around the joint ($p = 0.07$); Brooker status ($p = 0.52$) or GCG-BD status ($p = 0.79$).

A strong correlation was found between Brooker status and GCG-BD status (Kendall's Tau = 0.88, $p < 0.00001$). When the TBI and SCI subgroups were dichotomized, no link between Brooker status and recurrence was found for either group ($p = 0.74$ for TBI; $p = 0.48$ for SCI), nor between GCG-BD status and recurrence ($p = 0.71$ for TBI; $p = 0.49$ for SCI) despite the significant difference in operative delay between these two subgroups.

Logistic regression

When all the matching factors were taken into account, no significant relationship between Brooker status and HO recurrence risk was found (OR = 1.56 (95% CI: 0.47–5.19) nor between GCG-BD status and HO recurrence risk (OR for GCG-BD class 3 versus class 2 = 0.67 (95% CI: 0.11–4.24); OR for GCG-BD class 4 versus class 2 = 0.79 (95% CI: 0.09–6.91)).

Comparability between the two groups: TBI versus SCI (Table 2)

There was a significant difference between the two groups for sex ($p < 0.01$, no women in the SCI sub group), age at first surgery

Table 2. Comparability between the two groups: TBI versus SCI.

		TBI (%)	SCI (%)	p
Age at first surgery				p<0.01
Mean +/− SD		27.6+/−SD	35.5+/−SD	
Range		15.0 to 38.7	18.5 to 56.0	
Time from accident to first surgery				p<0.01
Mean +/− SD		24.2+/−SD	81.1+/−SD	
Range		5.5 to 114.6	4.4 to 407.5	
Location around the joint	ANTERIOR	14 (31.1)	29(58.0)	p = 0.03
	POSTERIOR	6 (13.3)	8 (16.0)	
	MEDIAL	16 (35.6)	9 (18.0)	
	LATERAL	7 (15.6)	2 (4.0)	
	ENCIRCLING	2 (4.4)	2 (4.0)	
Brooker status	3	40 (65.6)	21 (34.4)	p<0.01
	4	5 (14.7)	29 (85.3)	
GCG-BD	2	8 (100.0)	0 (0.0)	p<0.01
	3	33 (61.1)	21(38.9)	
	4	4 (12.1)	29 (87.9)	

($p<0.01$), operative delay from accident to first surgery ($p<0.01$), location around the joint ($p=0.03$), Brooker status ($p<0.01$) and GCG-BD status ($p<0.01$).

Discussion

Main results

No significant relationship was found between the preoperative extent of hip HO and recurrence risk after surgical excision. The two subgroups, TBI and SCI, were significantly different in terms of sex, age at first surgery, operative delay, location around the joint and the both classifications of HO extent. A strong relationship was found between the scores of the two classifications (Brooker and GCG-BD).

Preoperative HO extent and recurrence risk

Preoperative extent of HO has previously been suggested as being the main risk factor for recurrence after excision [14,15,33,34]. Stover et al. followed 38 HO excisions of 18 patients with SCI [15]. The mean operative delay after the accident was about 26 months (range: 11 months to 17 years). They found 13 recurrences with severe limitation of range of motion and all had a Brooker status above 3. Ebinger et al. found a significant link between the Glasgow coma scale score and the Brooker status for the hip HO ($r=-0.83$) [13]. They carried out a prospective study of 64 patients with HO (3 groups, I = severe TBI and local hip trauma (25 patients); II: isolated head injury (18 patients) and III: isolated local hip trauma (21 patients)) and their results revealed a tendency for a higher Brooker status score for group I than respectively for classes II and III. However, they did not find a difference for the Brooker status of the HO recurrence between the 3 classes at one and five years of follow up. They did not assess if the Brooker status was a predictive factor for recurrence. Garland et al. found a significant link between HO volume and maturity and recurrence risk after SCI (24 patients, 31 hips) [34]. However, they did not use the Brooker status, the severity of preoperative HO was assessed by a subjective X-Ray grading system: 1 = minimal, 2 = mild, 3 = moderate, 4 = severe, 5 = ankylosed. For TBI patients, they found a link between the HO score for a single patient (≥ 3) and the recurrence risk [24].

Seegenschmiedt et al. in a review [14], evoked some limitations of the Brooker classification. Firstly, the x-Ray incidence is estimated only in the frontal plane which could lead to underestimation of anterior and posterior HO development by superimposition, notably with the femor (Figure 1). Moreover, we can add that in our sample of patients (troublesome HO with surgical indications), the majority of patients had a status of III or IV which corresponds to voluminous HOs and a three-dimensional analysis seems to be more precise (Figure 1 and 2). Patients in class I are rarely symptomatic. The other limit, also highlighted by Seegenschmiedt et al., is that this classification cannot be transferred to other joints [14]. Since HO after CNS damage develops around joints of different sizes (hip, knee, shoulder elbow), the transposition of an assessment using the extent of HO in centimeters is difficult. This is why Hastings and Graham proposed a radiological and functional classification of HO about the elbow and forearm joint [14]. There were three classes, from non-symptomatic (Class 1) to ankylosis (Class 3). The second class is interesting because it includes range of motion decrease in different planes (sub class A: flexion/extension for the elbow and sub class B: pronation/supination for the forearm and Sub class C for both). This classification was not assessed by means of a clinical study. The German patterns-of-care study (PCS) proposed a general classification system (named GCG-BD) for HO development which could be used for any joint and based on X-Ray or CT scan. Their classification is based on the Brooker status with the addition of functional components (no, minor, major or complete functional deficit or symptoms of the involved joint or body segment).

The results of the present study found that Brooker and GCG-BD statuses were significantly higher for SCI than TBI patients. This is likely to be related to operative delay [1]. Because surgery is often proposed for TBI patients earlier than SCI patients, functional outcomes improve sooner since they have more ability to stand or walk. Furthermore, SCI patients frequently have a loss of sensation which can lead to a longer delay for diagnosis because of the absence of pain.

Even if the Brooker and GCG-BD classifications do not seem to be good markers for the recurrence risk, it would be interesting to assess if these classifications can predict other post operative complications such as fractures, hematoma or sepsis.

Correlations between the two classifications

The results of this study showed a strong, significant correlation ($k=0.81$) between the two classifications of preoperative HO extent, even if they were obtained by different means. This is probably due to the fact that most patients had quite severe neurological sequelae. Secondly, the score for pre operative HO extent was quite similar for all patients (III or IV). This is probably because Seegenschmiedt et al. were inspirited by the Brooker classification for the radiologic extent when they created their scale [14]. It seems likely that the degree of neurological sequelae has a smaller impact on Brooker status than the pre operative extent of HO. Moreover, functional ability depends on many factors such as the severity of cognitive and motor deficits, behavioral modifications, co-morbid factors (neurological, orthopaedic...) and pre injury status. This could make this classification insensitive for the assessment of risk factors for HO development or recurrence. Until the pathophysiology of HO development is understood, it will be difficult to create tools which can predict HO recurrence.

Limits of the study

This study may lack power especially for the separate analysis of each etiology (TBI and SCI) because of the small size of each sample. However, to our knowledge no other study has assessed the impact of preoperative extent of HO on recurrence risk, particularly in such a large group of patients. The lack of comparability between the two groups (TBI and SCI) has previously been found [1]. The functional prognosis of gait recovery and the presence of sensory deficits are two of the major explanations for these differences. The matching strategy which respected the same etiology between case and control patients tends to reduce the impact of this limit. Finally, although inclusion of controls was random in our series, the sample only included the two more extended Brooker classes (3 and 4) which can entail a selection bias. This could be related to the specific recruitement in our institution of patients who are most bothered by their HO, as Brooker classes 1 or 2 POA require less often surgical treatment.

Conclusion

No relationship was found between the preoperative extent of the troublesome hip HO and recurrence risk for patients with TBI or SCI. Surgery should be undertaken as soon as the co-morbid factors are under control.

Author Contributions

Conceived and designed the experiments: FG CJ AS. Performed the experiments: FG CJ CL PD. Analyzed the data: FG CJ CC. Wrote the paper: FG CJ. Updated database: KM.

References

1. Genet F, Jourdan C, Schnitzler A, Lautridou C, Guillemot D, et al. (2011) Troublesome heterotopic ossification after central nervous system damage: a survey of 570 surgeries. PLoS One 6: e16632.
2. Cipriano CA, Pill SG, Keenan MA (2009) Heterotopic ossification following traumatic brain injury and spinal cord injury. J Am Acad Orthop Surg 17: 689–697.
3. Vanden Bossche L, Vanderstraeten G (2005) Heterotopic ossification: a review. J Rehabil Med 37: 129–136.
4. Garland DE, Alday B, Venos KG (1984) Heterotopic ossification and HLA antigens. Arch Phys Med Rehabil 65: 531–532.
5. Garland DE, Blum CE, Waters RL (1980) Periarticular heterotopic ossification in head-injured adults. Incidence and location. J Bone Joint Surg Am 62: 1143–1146.
6. Hajek VE (1987) Heterotopic ossification in hemiplegia following stroke. Arch Phys Med Rehabil 68: 313–314.
7. Minaire P, Betuel H, Girard R, Pilonchery G (1980) Neurologic injuries, paraosteoarthropathies, and human leukocyte antigens. Arch Phys Med Rehabil 61: 214–215.
8. Rosin AJ (1975) Ectopic calcification around joints of paralysed limbs in hemiplegia, diffuse brain damage, and other neurological diseases. Ann Rheum Dis 34: 499–505.
9. Sazbon L, Najenson T, Tartakovsky M, Becker E, Grosswasser Z (1981) Widespread periarticular new-bone formation in long-term comatose patients. J Bone Joint Surg Br 63-B: 120–125.
10. Simonsen LL, Sonne-Holm S, Krasheninnikoff M, Engberg AW (2007) Symptomatic heterotopic ossification after very severe traumatic brain injury in 114 patients: incidence and risk factors. Injury 38: 1146–1150.
11. Tsur A, Sazbon L, Lotem M (1996) Relationship between muscular tone, movement and periarticular new bone formation in postcoma-unaware (PC-U) patients. Brain Inj 10: 259–262.
12. Hendricks HT, Heeren AH, Vos PE (2010) Dysautonomia after severe traumatic brain injury. Eur J Neurol 17: 1172–1177.
13. Ebinger T, Roesch M, Kiefer H, Kinzl L, Schulte M (2000) Influence of etiology in heterotopic bone formation of the hip. J Trauma 48: 1058–1062.
14. Seegenschmiedt MM, O. Heyd R (2008) Heterotopic ossifications: general survey for all sites.. Medical Radiology, Radiotherapy for Non-Malignant Disorders 3: 333–335.
15. Stover SL, Niemann KM, Tulloss JR (1991) Experience with surgical resection of heterotopic bone in spinal cord injury patients. Clin Orthop Relat Res. pp 71–77.
16. Chalidis B, Stengel D, Giannoudis PV (2007) Early excision and late excision of heterotopic ossifications after traumatic brain injury are equivalent: a systematic review of the literature. J Neurotrauma 24: 1675–1686.
17. Gacon G, Deidier C, Rhenter JL, Minaire P (1978) [Ectopic bone formation in neurological lesions (author's transl)]. Rev Chir Orthop Reparatrice Appar Mot 64: 375–390.
18. Ippolito E, Formisano R, Caterini R, Farsetti P, Penta F (1999) Operative treatment of heterotopic hip ossification in patients with coma after brain injury. Clin Orthop Relat Res. pp 130–138.
19. Carlier RY, Safa DM, Parva P, Mompoint D, Judet T, et al. (2005) Ankylosing neurogenic myositis ossificans of the hip. An enhanced volumetric CT study. J Bone Joint Surg Br 87: 301–305.
20. Charnley G, Judet T, Garreau de Loubresse C, Mollaret O (1996) Excision of heterotopic ossification around the knee following brain injury. Injury 27: 125–128.
21. Denormandie P, Viguie G, Denys P, Dizien O, Carlier R (1999) Results of excision of heterotopic new bone around the elbow in patients with head injuries. A series of 25 cases. Chir Main 18: 99–107.
22. Frischhut B, Stockhammer G, Saltuari L, Kadletz R, Bramanti P (1993) Early removal of periarticular ossifications in patients with head injury. Acta Neurol (Napoli) 15: 114–122.
23. Fuller DA, Mark A, Keenan MA (2005) Excision of heterotopic ossification from the knee: a functional outcome study. Clin Orthop Relat Res 438: 197–203.
24. Garland DE, Hanscom DA, Keenan MA, Smith C, Moore T (1985) Resection of heterotopic ossification in the adult with head trauma. J Bone Joint Surg Am 67: 1261–1269.
25. Ippolito E, Formisano R, Caterini R, Farsetti P, Penta F (1999) Resection of elbow ossification and continuous passive motion in postcomatose patients. J Hand Surg Am 24: 546–553.
26. Lazarus M, Guttmann D, Rich C, Keenan M (1999) Heterotopic ossification resection about the elbow. Neurorehabilitation 12: 145–153.
27. McAuliffe JA, Wolfson AH (1997) Early excision of heterotopic ossification about the elbow followed by radiation therapy. J Bone Joint Surg Am 79: 749–755.
28. Moore TJ (1993) Functional outcome following surgical excision of heterotopic ossification in patients with traumatic brain injury. J Orthop Trauma 7: 11–14.
29. Roberts JB, Pankratz DG (1979) The surgical treatment of heterotopic ossification at the elbow following long-term coma. J Bone Joint Surg Am 61: 760–763.
30. Sarafis KA, Karatzas GD, Yotis CL (1999) Ankylosed hips caused by heterotopic ossification after traumatic brain injury: a difficult problem. J Trauma 46: 104–109.
31. Sorriaux G, Denormandie P, Martin JN, Kiefer C, Judet T (2005) [Excision of heterotopic new bone around the elbow in patients with head injury: 51 cases]. Rev Chir Orthop Reparatrice Appar Mot 91: 415–422.
32. Chalidis B, Stengel D, Giannoudis PV (2007) Early excision and late excision of heterotopic ossification after traumatic brain injury are equivalent: a systematic review of the literature. J Neurotrauma 24: 1675–1686.
33. Brooker AF, Bowerman JW, Robinson RA, Riley LH, Jr. (1973) Ectopic ossification following total hip replacement. Incidence and a method of classification. J Bone Joint Surg Am 55: 1629–1632.
34. Garland DE, Orwin JF (1989) Resection of heterotopic ossification in patients with spinal cord injuries. Clin Orthop Relat Res. pp 169–176.

Heritability and Phenotypic Variation of Canine Hip Dysplasia Radiographic Traits in a Cohort of Australian German Shepherd Dogs

Bethany J. Wilson*, Frank W. Nicholas, John W. James, Claire M. Wade, Imke Tammen, Herman W. Raadsma, Kao Castle, Peter C. Thomson

Faculty of Veterinary Science, The University of Sydney, Sydney, New South Wales, Australia

Abstract

Canine Hip Dysplasia (CHD) is a common, painful and debilitating orthopaedic disorder of dogs with a partly genetic, multifactorial aetiology. Worldwide, potential breeding dogs are evaluated for CHD using radiographically based screening schemes such as the nine ordinally-scored British Veterinary Association Hip Traits (BVAHTs). The effectiveness of selective breeding based on screening results requires that a significant proportion of the phenotypic variation is caused by the presence of favourable alleles segregating in the population. This proportion, heritability, was measured in a cohort of 13,124 Australian German Shepherd Dogs born between 1976 and 2005, displaying phenotypic variation for BVAHTs, using ordinal, linear and binary mixed models fitted by a Restricted Maximum Likelihood method. Heritability estimates for the nine BVAHTs ranged from 0.14–0.24 (ordinal models), 0.14–0.25 (linear models) and 0.12–0.40 (binary models). Heritability for the summed BVAHT phenotype was 0.30±0.02. The presence of heritable variation demonstrates that selection based on BVAHTs has the potential to improve BVAHT scores in the population. Assuming a genetic correlation between BVAHT scores and CHD-related pain and dysfunction, the welfare of Australian German Shepherds can be improved by continuing to consider BVAHT scores in the selection of breeding dogs, but that as heritability values are only moderate in magnitude the accuracy, and effectiveness, of selection could be improved by the use of Estimated Breeding Values in preference to solely phenotype based selection of breeding animals.

Editor: Henry Harpending, University of Utah, United States of America

Funding: The authors have no support or funding to report. This work was completed as part of a PhD candidacy.

Competing Interests: The authors have declared that no competing interests exist.

* E-mail: bethany.wilson@sydney.edu.au

Introduction

Canine Hip Dysplasia (CHD) has been considered the most common musculoskeletal disease affecting both purebred dogs and their crossbreds. It is a multifactorial disease, with occurrence and severity modulated by many non-genetic factors and the action of genes at multiple loci in the dog genome, potentially including some major genes [1–5]. While hip structures develop to be grossly normal prenatally, in some dogs an intrinsic excess laxity or "looseness" in the joint causes abnormal joint forces once weight-bearing begins, resulting in misshaping of the cartilaginous matrix of the developing hip and repetitive microdamage to joint structures. Over time, this leads to the development of potentially severe osteoarthrtits [6–8]. CHD is a significant welfare problem, can result in significant disability and can lead to euthanasia on humane grounds.

Given the overwhelming evidence of additive genetic variation for liability to CHD, many selection schemes have been established worldwide to reduce the incidence (if dogs are classified as either affected or normal) or average severity of CHD in dog populations using various phenotypic assessments of hip laxity and morphology, mostly obtained by various radiographic techniques [9]. One such set of traits which has been used by the British Veterinary Association/Kennel Club Scheme (BVA/KC scheme) and later by the Australian Veterinary Association/Australian National Kennel Council (AVA/ANKC scheme), as well as the German Shepherd Dog Council of Australia Hip Dysplasia Breed Scheme (GSDCA scheme) and other schemes, is based on a set of hip phenotypes referred to here as the BVA hip traits (BVAHTs).

The BVAHTs are a collection of nine radiographic traits of a hip, collected from a radiograph of a skeletally mature dog, taken in an "extended hip" position, where the dog is placed in dorsal recumbency and hips are extended with legs held in parallel to each other and to the radiographic plate, with a slight internal rotation rendering the patellae directly above the stifle joint. The nature of these nine traits has been reported previously [10–12].The traits are all scored on a subjective seven-point ordinal scale (labelled 0–6) except Norberg angle (NORB), which is an objective quantitative trait (an angle measurement) that is collapsed into seven ordinal categories (with lower scores indicating higher angles); and Caudal Acetabular Edge (CaAE), which is scored on a subjective ordinal six-point scale (labelled 0–5). For each of these traits, 0 indicates a sound hip, and higher scores indicate increasing degrees of deterioration. Previous research on the genetic correlation between the BVAHTs of the right and left hip has provided estimates very close to 1.0, indicating that, in essence, the same genes modulate the formation and development of both hips and that variation between them is a result of non-genetic (environmental) variation experienced differently by each hip [12–15].

The effectiveness of phenotype-based selection schemes for a multifactorial disease is dependent upon the nature and extent of the variation that is seen in the population for this phenotype. The variation of the phenotype must be at least partly heritable and must also be genetically correlated to the selection goal, in this case improved health, function and welfare with respect to Canine Hip Dysplasia. In other words, dogs with better hip scores must both tend to have offspring with better hip scores (to some degree) and also to have better health, function and welfare (to some degree) than dogs with worse hip scores. If this is the case, it may be presumed that dogs with better hip scores will tend to have alleles which confer a health, function and welfare advantage, and that by transmitting these alleles to offspring they will similarly confer some degree of health, function and welfare advantage on their offspring. Preferentially selecting such dogs for breeding will tend to cause an increase in the frequency of advantageous alleles (and a decrease in the frequency of disadvantageous alleles), resulting in a favourable genetic trend and improvement in the hip dysplasia status of the population over generations. The other factor determining response to selection is the extent of variability in the trait undergoing selection. It is thus important to estimate the extent of variation and the heritability of the chosen phenotype in the population under selection, and to show that the chosen phenotype correlates to some extent with health, function and welfare.

Despite the operation of a hip dysplasia evaluation scheme in Australia for several decades, there is a disappointing paucity of studies evaluating the suitability and effectiveness of genetic control of hip dysplasia in Australian dog populations. Ideally, the extent of the additive genetic variation in hip dysplasia traits would be assessed and tracked temporally in all breed populations under selection in Australia, to ensure that favourable genetic trends are emerging over time and to monitor variation. Recent work by Lewis *et al.* [13], and earlier work by Wood *et al.* [16], Wood *et al.* [17] and Wood *et al.* [18], demonstrates substantial heritability and substantial phenotypic variation of BVAHTs in dog populations in the United Kingdom. Other studies [13,15–24] have shown substantial heritability of different radiographic hip dysplasia phenotypes in various German Shepherd Dog populations (Table 1). While these results are encouraging, estimates of phenotypic variation and heritability should be obtained in Australian populations, as allele frequencies might be expected to vary between breed populations, and certainly between breeds, and over time. The correspondence between hip dysplasia phenotypes and hip dysplasia-related health, function and welfare is considerably more challenging to study, and perhaps because of this, there are regrettably few studies assessing this question. An important recent study [25] does demonstrate a relationship between insurance claims related to hip dysplasia and a hip dysplasia phenotype assessing similar features to the BVAHTs from a similar radiograph (although the phenotype is quantified quite differently).

An Estimated Breeding Value (EBV) is the weighted combination of the scores of an individual and its relatives for the trait in question, for correlated traits and for molecular information; providing the best available prediction of the average performance of the offspring of that animal. Unless the heritability of the trait is very high (virtually all phenotypic variation arises from variation in genetic merit), EBVs will represent a better assessment of genetic merit than phenotypic scores alone. Therefore, if we determine BVAHTs to be heritable (but not of very high heritability), as has been reported in studies from other dog populations, this will be strong evidence that selection using EBVs should replace phenotype-based selection in this population.

In this paper we estimate the extent of phenotypic variation and the heritability of BVAHTs in a cohort of Australian-born German Shepherd Dogs. Given that BVAHTs are ordinal phenotypes, we report the use of a mixed-model multi-threshold ordinal logistic regression technique to estimate heritability. Further, we also fit models to the BVAHTs ignoring the ordinal nature of the data, using standard Restricted Maximum Likelihood (REML)/linear mixed model techniques, which is the typical strategy used in other studies. This dual approach allows us to investigate the extent to which ignoring the ordinal nature of the BVAHT data may affect such estimates.

Materials and Methods

Data

Sources of data were 1) data accumulated by Dr Malcolm Willis in the United Kingdom from records collected within the Australian Veterinary Association/Australian National Kennel Council (AVA/ANKC) scheme and the records of radiologists sent to him privately (kindly provided by the ANKC); 2) Data supplied by the German Shepherd Dog Council of Australia (GSDCA) hip dysplasia breed scheme; and 3) Pedigree information regarding Australian German Shepherd Dogs (GSDs) held by the ANKC and supplied to us with permission of the GSDCA by Dogs NSW. All data sets included all data available electronically at the time at which the records were obtained.

Australian records obtained from Dr Willis included records from about 10020 dogs, born between 1976 and 2005. Records obtained from the GSDCA scheme included records from approximately 6065 animals born between 1977 and 2006. There was considerable overlap between the two sets of data with respect to the dogs represented. Where more than one record was available for any unique dog, any identical duplicated records were deleted. Of the remaining **rare cases**, where phenotypes had been obtained at different times, only the record taken closest to the average age of radiography was retained. The data set included the animal's name, pedigree information, year of birth, age at radiographic study, sex and scores for each of the eighteen BVAHTs. Any record that lacked any information was removed from the data set, unless this information could be inferred from the pedigree file. In the pedigree file, duplicate records were removed. Dogs were matched to the pedigree file using their registered names, date of birth and available pedigree information. Animals that were born overseas (as evidenced by an overseas-type registration number and lack of an Australian kennel prefix) were excluded from the phenotype file but were retained in the pedigree file.

The final data set comprised records from 13,124 (8,793 female, 4,331 male) GSDs born in Australia between 1976 and 2006. Completeness of the data set was investigated by matching scores against the pedigree file for Australian-born GSDs.

Models

Three different types of single-trait models were used, namely (1) a "full" ordinal logistic model that treats the BVAHT data in a multi-threshold approach, with each threshold corresponding to a point on the ordinal scale; (2) a series of binary logistic models in which each model involves a single threshold at a different BVAHT ordinal point; and (3) a standard linear mixed model fitted to each of the 18 BVAHTs and to the summed BVAHT data, ignoring the ordinal nature of the data. Only single-trait models were conducted because the software used was not able to run multi-trait models assuming ordinal data. A previous paper

Table 1. A sample of heritability estimates for British Veterinary Association Hip Traits in various breeds and heritability of other Canine Hip Dysplasia Phenotypes in German Shepherd Dogs.

Phenotype	Breed	Heritability	Standard Error	Method	Reference
BVAHT-NORB	Labrador Retriever	0.29	0.05	Regression	[16]
BVAHT-NORB	Gordon Setter	0.19	0.08	Regression	[18]
BVAHT-NORB	Labrador Retriever	0.37	0.03	REML LMM	[15]
BVAHT-SUBL	Labrador Retriever	0.26	0.04	Regression	[16]
BVAHT-SUBL	Gordon Setter	0.24	0.08	Regression	[18]
BVAHT-SUBL	Labrador Retriever	0.38	0.03	REML LMM	[15]
BVAHT-CrAE	Labrador Retriever	0.17	0.04	Regression	[16]
BVAHT-CrAE	Labrador Retriever	0.21	0.02	REML LMM	[15]
BVAHT-DAE	Labrador Retriever	0.16	0.06	Regression	[16]
BVAHT-DAE	Labrador Retriever	0.18	0.02	REML LMM	[15]
BVAHT-CrEAR	Labrador Retriever	0.07	0.05	Regression	[16]
BVAHT-CrEAR	Labrador Retriever	0.21	0.02	REML LMM	[15]
BVAHT-AF	Labrador Retriever	0.17	0.06	Regression	[16]
BVAHT-AF	Labrador Retriever	0.15	0.02	REML LMM	[15]
BVAHT- CaAE	Labrador Retriever	0.08	0.06	Regression	[16]
BVAHT-CaAE	Labrador Retriever	0.15	0.02	REML LMM	[15]
BVAHT-FHNE	Labrador Retriever	0.14	0.05	Regression	[16]
BVAHT-FHNE	Labrador Retriever	0.24	0.03	REML LMM	[15]
BVAHT-FHR	Labrador Retriever	0.15	0.05	Regression	[16]
BVAHT-FHR	Labrador Retriever	0.19	0.03	REML LMM	[15]
BVAHT-Total	Flat Coated Retriever	0.74	0.25	Regression	[17]
BVAHT-Total	Newfoundland	0.49	0.08	Regression	[17]
BVAHT-Total	Gordon Setter	0.20	0.10	Regression	[18]
BVAHT-Total	Labrador Retriever	0.34	0.02	Regression	[16]
BVAHT-Total	Labrador Retriever	0.35	0.02	REML LMM	[13]
I-VI grading	German Shepherd Dog	0.43–0.43	0.08	Least squares ANOVA	[20]
1-5 (A-E)	German Shepherd Dog	0.24–0.26	0.02–0.04	Bayesian LMM with animal model	[19]
A-E	German Shepherd Dog	0.31–0.35		REML LMM with animal model	[22]
A-E	German Shepherd Dog	0.15	0.02	Binary GLMM	[23]
1–5	German Shepherd Dog	0.56	0.011	REML LMM	[21]
A-E	German Shepherd Dog	0.254	0.013	Bayesian LMM with animal model	[24]

NORB = Norberg Angle, SUBL = Subluxation, CrAE = Cranial Acetabular Edge, DAE = Dorsal Acetabular Edge, CrEAR = Cranial Effective Acetabular Rim, AF = Acetabular Fossa, CaAE = Caudal Acetabular Edge, FHNE = Femoral Head and Neck Exostosis, FHR = Femoral Head Remodelling.

[12] offered evidence which suggests that right and left scores for each BVAHT in Australian GSDs are two expressions of the same set of genes, with differences arising due to non-additive genetic and non-genetic causes, and could therefore be considered repeated measures. The alternatives to this approach are to select only a single hip from each dog (either systematically, such as taking the worst hip, or selecting a record at random) or to employ some measure of central tendency of the two measurements. The former approach needlessly halves the data set by removing meaningful information about each animal's likely genetic merit. The latter approach, employing a measure of central tendency, requires finding a methodologically sound method of doing so. Taking the mean or median of the scores assumes linearity of scores that are truly ordinal, which is not readily methodologically justified. Given the evidence that right and left hip scores have a genetic correlation near one, the assumptions behind the repeatability model appear to be better supported by the available evidence and this method was therefore used in the present analysis. Modelling was undertaken using the "stand alone" version of ASReml 3 (VSN Intl., Hemel Hempstead UK).

1) Ordinal (Multi-threshold) analysis. This model considers two scores (left and right) from each of n dogs. For a single observation in the data set, the model has the following form:

$$\log_e\left(\frac{P(Y_{ij}\leq k)}{P(Y_{ij}>k)}\right)=\theta_k+x_{ij}'\hat{\mathbf{a}}+u_{i1}+u_{i2}+u_{i3},\ k=0,\ 1,\ \ldots,\ C-2 \qquad (1)$$

where Y_{ij} is the BVAHT score of the ith dog (i = 1, …, n) on the jth side (j = 1, 2), C is the number of points on the ordinal scale (C= 7 for all BVAHT except CaAE where C= 6). For each cut point, there is a separate "intercept" (θ_k), with the constraint that $\theta_0<\theta_1<\ldots<\theta_{C-2}$. $\boldsymbol{\beta}$ is a vector of p levels of fixed effects related to the vector of explanatory variables, $\mathbf{x}_{ij}$. The random effects for this model are u_{i1}, a term for the dog's breeding value; u_{i2}, a term for the permanent environment effect of the dog linking left and right hand scores together; and u_{i3}, a litter effect. This form of ordinal logistic regression is known as the proportional odds model [26].

When considered as a model for the vector of all $2n$ observations, the model can be expressed in matrix notation as

$$\text{logit}(\boldsymbol{\gamma}) = \mathbf{T}\boldsymbol{\theta} + \mathbf{X}\boldsymbol{\beta} + \mathbf{Z}_1\mathbf{u}_1 + \mathbf{Z}_2\mathbf{u}_2 + \mathbf{Z}_3\mathbf{u}_3 \qquad (2)$$

where $\boldsymbol{\gamma} = \{\gamma_{ij}\}$ with $\gamma_{ij} = P(Y_{ij} \leq k)$, $\mathbf{T}$ is a $2n\times(C-1)$ matrix with elements in column k taking values 1 if the score $Y_{ij} \leq k$ and 0 otherwise, $\mathbf{X} = (\mathbf{x}'_{11}, \mathbf{x}'_{12}, \ldots, \mathbf{x}'_{n1}, \mathbf{x}'_{n2})'$ is a $2n\times p$ matrix of predictor variables, the indicator matrices $\mathbf{Z}_1 = \mathbf{Z}_2 = \mathbf{I}_n \otimes (1,1)'$ are of dimension $2n\times n$, and $\mathbf{Z}_3$ is of size $2n\times L$ where L is the number of litters. The logit(·) function is defined as $\text{logit}(\gamma) = \log_e[\gamma/(1-\gamma)]$.

Fixed effects incorporating $\boldsymbol{\beta}$ include the sex of the dog (male or female), the age of the dog in months at the time of radiographic study, the year in which the dog was born, and left vs right hip. The random effects $\mathbf{u}_1$ are "animal model" additive genetic effects. The animal model is fitted by calculation of the numerator relationship matrix (NRM), a matrix of additive genetic relationships which contains information about the flow of genes through the population and information allowing for inbreeding. The permanent environmental effect associated with each dog is $\mathbf{u}_2$ and the effect associated with being from each litter is $\mathbf{u}_3$. The model also assumes that $\mathbf{u}_1 \sim N(0, \sigma_A^2\mathbf{A})$ where σ_A^2 is the additive genetic variance, $\mathbf{A}$ is the NRM; and also that $\mathbf{u}_2 \sim N(0, \sigma_2^2\mathbf{I}_n)$ and $\mathbf{u}_3 \sim N(0, \sigma_3^2\mathbf{I}_L)$.

This model is advantageous over linear methods as it recognises the ordinal nature of the data, rather than assuming that each cut point is evenly spaced along an underlying scale, and is advantageous over individual binary models as it does not require loss of information above and below a cut point. Therefore, for comparison among the different EBVs generated from the different models in this study, we treat these ordinal EBVs as the "gold standard" EBVs to which the others, either less methodologically correct, or calculated using less information, are compared. Due to the manner in which ASReml parameterises the ordinal model, it was necessary to multiply effects from the ASReml output by -1 to maintain correct associations and a scale in which a number above zero corresponds to an increase in average expected score of offspring (the undesirable direction) and a negative number corresponds to a favourable breeding value.

2) Binary (Logistic) analysis. In addition to the multi-threshold ordinal analysis of the nine BVAHTs, modelling using the same fixed and random effects as described above was undertaken at each possible cut point, i.e. at each interval (on the ordinal scale) at which a threshold can be used to divide dogs into two classes: normal and affected. To accommodate the binary nature of these data, a logistic generalised linear mixed model (GLMM) was fitted to the data.

The seven-point scale of most of the traits offered a maximum of six possible cut points at which a hip could be classified as normal (0) or affected (1). For CaAE there were five possible cut points. Logistic regression analysis was attempted at each cut point. Each analysis makes fewer unsupported assumptions than the conventional linear mixed model LMM (see below) but involves loss of information consequential upon the pooling of all scores above and all scores below the cut point, e.g. at a cut point between 1 and 2, a score of 2 is awarded the same phenotype (1) as a score of 3, 4, 5 or 6. The form of the GLMM is

$$\text{logit}(\boldsymbol{\pi}) = \mathbf{X}\boldsymbol{\beta} + \mathbf{Z}_1\mathbf{u}_1 + \mathbf{Z}_2\mathbf{u}_2 + \mathbf{Z}_3\mathbf{u}_3 \qquad (3)$$

where $\text{logit}(\pi_i) = \log_e[\pi_i/(1-\pi_i)]$, and π_i is the probability that dog i has a score at or below the cut point. All the other terms in the model are as specified in [EQ2]. A separate logistic GLMM was fitted for each BVAHT× cut-point combination.

3) Linear mixed models (LMM). In this analysis, each of the nine BVAHTs was modelled by an LMM using the score as the phenotype. This strategy, which ignores the ordinal nature of the scoring system, was undertaken to compare EBVs with those obtained taking the ordinal nature into account, and to enable direct comparison with most other comparable studies. Scores were transformed logarithmically to attempt to correct positive skew in the distribution of the scores. While reduced, substantial skew remained for many traits. As the main role of this analysis was to compare results from a more correct ordinal analysis with a simpler analysis, more powerful transformations, while possible, were not attempted. Lewis *et al.* [15] performed analyses on untransformed scores after not finding a single transformation which was optimal for all nine BVAHTs and in order to simplify their analysis. For this study, the authors felt that the log-transformation for all traits to correct some, but not all, of the positive skew of each trait was the best compromise between methodological correctness and clarity. The model was of the form

$$\mathbf{y} = \mathbf{X}\boldsymbol{\beta} + \mathbf{Z}_1\mathbf{u}_1 + \mathbf{Z}_2\mathbf{u}_2 + \mathbf{Z}_3\mathbf{u}_3 + \boldsymbol{\varepsilon} \qquad (4)$$

where $\mathbf{y}$ is a vector of $2n = 26{,}248$ hips, and $\boldsymbol{\varepsilon}$ is a $2n\times 1$ vector of random residual effects, where $\boldsymbol{\varepsilon} \sim N(\mathbf{0}, \sigma^2_\varepsilon\mathbf{I}_{2n})$. All other terms are as defined in [EQ2] and [EQ3].

In addition to the analysis of individual BVAHTs, total hip scores (THS) were obtained by addition of the 18 BVAHT scores for each dog. This has been the standard trait used for selection in the GSDCA scheme and in all other schemes using BVAHTs. The scores were again logarithmically transformed. A linear mixed model was then fitted to the THS data of the form

$$\mathbf{y} = \mathbf{X}\boldsymbol{\beta} + \mathbf{Z}_1\mathbf{u}_1 + \mathbf{Z}_3\mathbf{u}_3 + \boldsymbol{\varepsilon} \qquad (5)$$

where $\mathbf{y}$ now is a vector of $n = 13{,}124$ THS observations, and $\mathbf{X}$ does not include a term for left versus right hip. The model does not include a permanent environment effect for the dog because there is now only one record for each dog in the data set, but does include a litter effect ($\mathbf{u}_3$).

4) Heritability estimates. Heritability estimates were obtained by calculation of the proportion of the total variance explained by additive genetic variance. Heritability estimates were obtained for all analyses of all BVAHTs.

For ordinal and binary models, heritability for the trait on the underlying scale was calculated as $\sigma^2_A / (\sigma^2_A + \sigma^2_2 + \sigma^2_3 + \pi^2/3)$, using the REML-like estimate of σ^2_A, with $\pi^2/3$ being the variance of a standard logistic distribution, taking on the role of the environmental variance on the underlying liability scale. For the linear mixed model, heritabilities are estimated as $\sigma_A^2/(\sigma_A^2 + \sigma_2^2 + \sigma_3^2 + \sigma_\varepsilon^2)$ (model [EQ4]) or as $\sigma_A^2/(\sigma_A^2 + \sigma_3^2 + \sigma_\varepsilon^2)$ (Model [EQ5]). Using ASReml "pin" files, delta method estimates (i.e. first order Taylor series approximation) of the standard errors of the heritability estimates were also calculated.

5) Maternal models. Maternal heritabilities and maternal environmental effects are estimates of the proportion of phenotypic variation due to the genetic and environmental developmental conditions which a dam provides for her offspring. They were examined in a separate ordinal (multi-threshold) analysis model which added additional random effects to the model above, a dam effect linked to a pedigree structure and a dam effect divorced from the pedigree structure, which modelled a maternal additive genetic component and a maternal environmental effect, respectively. However, the litter effect had to be removed from the models due to failure of convergence. This may be due to the increasing complexity and (partial) confounding of the litter effects and a combination of the maternal environmental effects and year effects which were also in the model, given that a dam only had one litter in a year.

Results

Completeness of Data Set

The completeness of the data set, expressed as the percentages of dogs for which scores were available, is presented in Table 2. The data set provides good coverage of dogs born in recent years, with scores available for the sires of 87.8% of puppies born in 2000–2005 and scores for the dams of 90.6% of puppies born in these years. Percentage coverage declines for dogs born earlier, although it is reasonable (greater than 50%) since 1991 and appears to be increasing. Care needs to be taken in making inferences about the use of hip dysplasia scoring by GSD breeders based on this table (although these numbers may be considered minimum values). Relative paucity of coverage in older date ranges could indicate fewer assessments for hip dysplasia but could equally reflect poorer submission rates or the possibility that older data have either been mislaid or were never made available electronically.

In the most recent year-of-birth range (2001–2005), usage of the scheme appears to have been good for parents of Australian-born GSDs, with scores missing from only between 10–15% of parents. It is also worth noting that percentages worked out on a per-puppy basis have tended to be higher than when treating all sires and dams as equal regardless of the number of registered puppies that are produced. This suggests there is no evidence that unscored parents are being used more frequently than scored parents and may, indeed, be suggestive of the opposite. It is also possible that some of the sires and dams for which hip score data were not available have been assessed for hip dysplasia using other methods, or their scores were calculated but not recorded in either of the available data sets. The proportion of Australian-born-and-registered GSDs for which hip scores are available generally increased over time and is around 11% in the most recent year-of-birth ranges.

Phenotypic Variation in BVAHTs

The distribution of scores is illustrated in Figure 1. It is evident that the BVAHTs may be divided into two groups based upon their score distribution: Group 1 consisting of Norberg Angle (NORB), Subluxation (SUBL) and Cranial Actebular Edge (CrAE), in which there is substantial variation; and Group 2 consisting of Dorsal Acetabular Edge (DAE), Cranial Effective Acetabular Rim (CrEAR), Acetabular Fossa (AF), Caudal Acetabular Edge (CaAE), Femoral Head and Neck Exostosis (FHNE) and Femoral Head Remodelling (FHR) in which there is appreciably less variation. A similar finding was noted in a study of Gordon Setters from the United Kingdom where NORB, SUBL and CrAE accounted for 60% of the summed BVAHT [18]. Interestingly, Group 1 BVAHTs could be said to roughly correspond to traits most concerned with joint laxity and acetabular shallowing during development, whereas Group 2 BVAHTs roughly correspond to osteoarthritic changes. Given that the natural course of the disease is to worsen with respect to osteoarthritis over time, it would be expected for there to be fewer more-severe scores in the BVAHTs more associated with osteoarthritis, if animals were mostly scored at a relatively young age, before osteoarthritis has progressed to severe phenotypes. Figure 2 demonstrates that the age at which dogs in the sample were scored was young, on average, with a median (19 months) substantially less than the 24 months required for evaluation by some other organisations.

Heritability

Heritability estimates for the BVAHTs obtained using ordinal models and LMMs for single BVAHTs are presented in Table 3. Generally, there was reasonable agreement between the LMM method and the more desirable ordinal method for most of the BVAHTs. While the point estimates varied between the methods, they were generally within one standard error, although CaAE estimates differed more substantially. All estimates represent an additive variation of sufficient proportion of the phenotypic variation to lead to a substantial response in a well designed selection program, indicating that selection using EBVs for these BVAHTs is likely to be successful in reducing BVAHT scores, given sufficient selection pressure. The LMM heritability estimate for the summed BVAHT was 0.30 ± 0.02.

Heritability estimates from binary models are presented in Figure 3. Standard errors associated with the higher cut-points tended to be larger due to a smaller proportion of dogs having increasingly higher scores (See Figure 1). For many of the BVAHTs there seems to be a trend toward increasing heritability

Table 2. Availability of British Veterinary Association Hip Trait scores for registered Australian German Shepherd Dogs.

	Year of birth					
	1976–1980	1981–1985	1986–1990	1991–1995	1996–2000	2001–2005
% of born Puppies						
with score available	0.2	2.2	5.7	8.8	11.2	10.7
with sire's score available	1.3	6.5	28.4	50.8	61.4	87.8
with dam's score available	0.4	4.8	24.2	53.1	65.2	90.6
Sires						
% unique sires with scores	0.4	3.8	16.7	34.6	54.5	85.6
Dams						
% unique dams with scores	0.3	4.5	21.0	47.3	62.6	87.9

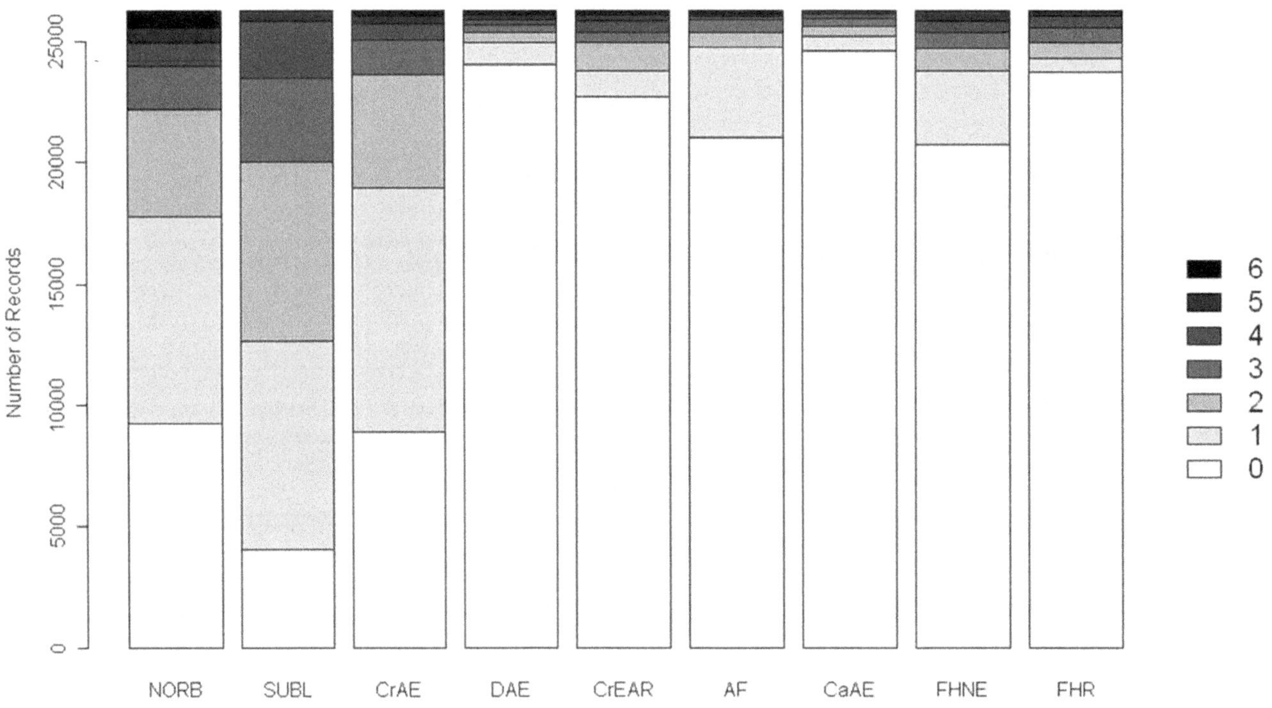

Figure 1. Distribution of British Veterinary Association Hip Trait scores in Australian German Shepherd Dogs.

as the cut-point increases. This could suggest either that non-genetic/environmental factors are more important in dogs with lower scores (and therefore that the additive heritable proportion of the variation is less) or possibly that the radiographic scoring is more repeatable for higher scores. Ultimately, the reason for this pattern is not understood and warrants further study.

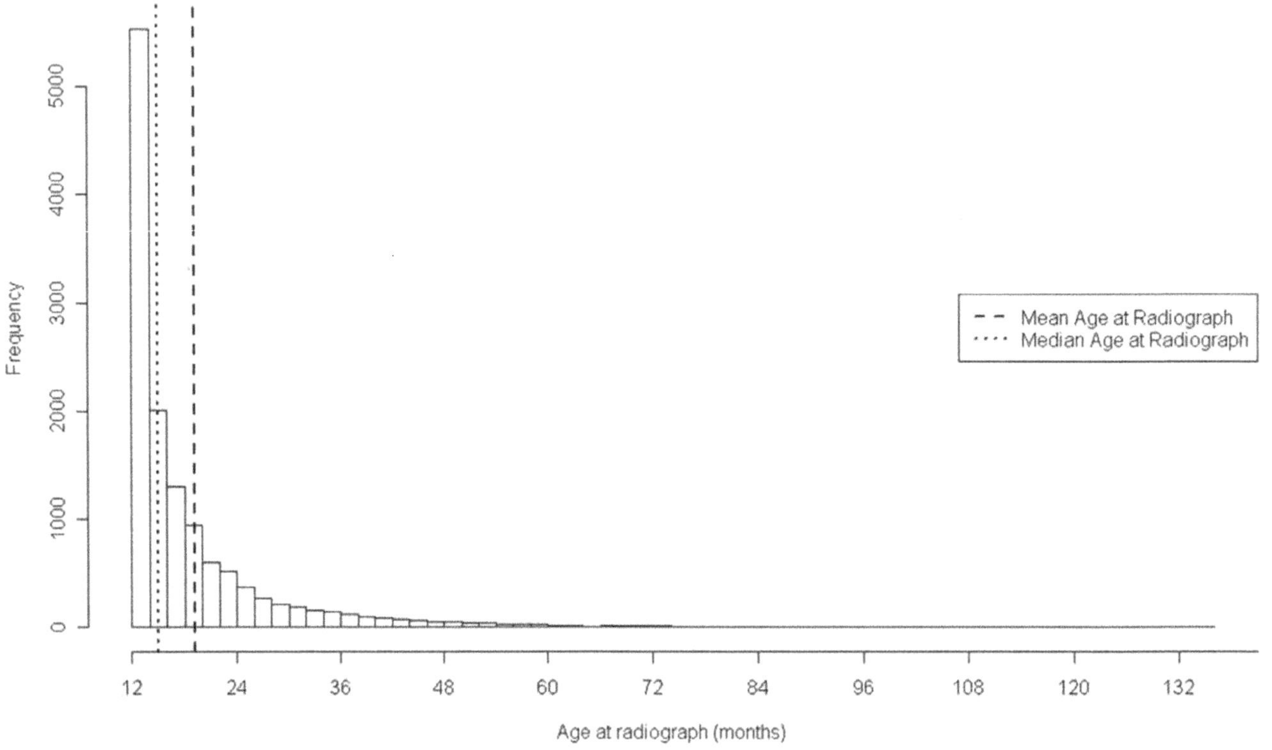

Figure 2. Reported age at time of radiograph for all 13,124 German Shepherd Dogs used in the present analyses.

Table 3. Heritability estimates (h^2), with standard errors (SE), of British Veterinary Association hip traits (BVAHTs) in Australian German Shepherd Dogs.

	Multi-threshold ordinal analysis		Log-transformed linear analysis (LMM)	
BVAHT	h^2	**SE**	h^2	**SE**
Norberg Angle (NORB)	0.23	0.02	0.23	0.02
Subluxation (SUBL)	0.23	0.02	0.18	0.01
Cranial Acetabular Edge (CRAE)	0.24	0.02	0.22	0.02
Dorsal Acetabular Edge (DAE)	0.14	0.02	0.14	0.02
Cranial Effective Acetabular Rim (CrEAR)	0.20	0.02	0.19	0.02
Acetabular Fossa (AF)	0.22	0.02	0.18	0.02
Caudal Acetabular Edge (CAAE)	0.20	0.03	0.25	0.02
Femoral Head and Neck Exostosis (FHNE)	0.21	0.02	0.22	0.02
Femoral Head Remodelling (FHR)	0.17	0.03	0.17	0.02
Sum of BVAHTs	NA	NA	0.30	0.02

Age Effect

Age at scoring in months (see Figure 2) was included as a variable in the ordinal models. Based on Wald z-tests, increasing age resulted in significantly increasing scores for SUBL and all Group 2 traits (all $P<0.05$). While increases in osteoarthritis (Group 2) traits with age is not surprising, the increase in SUBL is somewhat surprising, given that remodelling may act to reduce laxity over time. It is possible that this effect is due to an apparent increase in the appearance of subluxation with age due to changes in the shape and relative position of other joint landmarks.

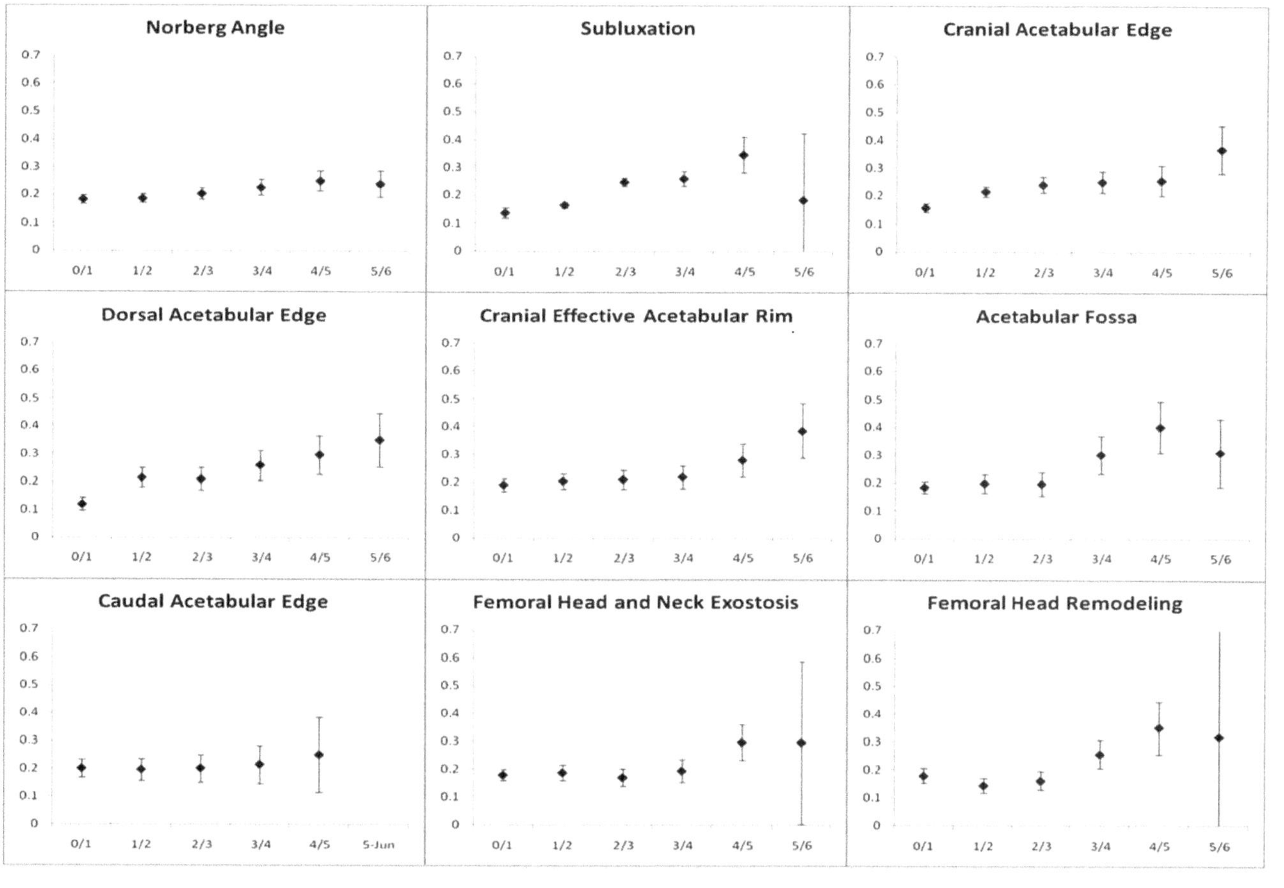

Figure 3. Heritability estimates of British Veterinary Association Canine Hip Dysplasia Phenotypes in a cohort of Australian German Shepherd Dogs when the ordinal phenotypes are expressed as binary outcomes.

Changes in NORB and CrAE over time were not statistically significant. The pattern observed in the LMM single-trait analysis was similar.

Hip Effect

A previous paper [12] demonstrated that the genetic correlation between left and right hips for the BVAHTs is very high, but all traits except for AF and CaAE displayed marginal asymmetry, indicating a significant environmental hip effect. The left hip effects (compared to a reference right hip effect of zero) are presented in Table 4, along with standard errors. The left hip is associated with higher scores for all traits except NORB, and was significantly so for SUBL, CrAE, CrEAR, FHNE and FHR. The right hip was associated with significantly higher scores for NORB. As explained in the previous paper [12], these hip effects are not inconsistent with a high genetic correlation between hips.

Sex Effect

Sex was also included as a fixed effect. Approximately 67% of records were from female dogs and 33% from male dogs. The size of the effects (male effect compared with a reference female effect of zero) and their standard errors are also presented in Table 4. For all of the BVAHTs, male sex was associated with significantly lower scores.

Year-of-birth Effect

The year-of-birth effects were fitted as a factor (categorical term) rather than as a trend over time. These effects demonstrate differences in the sum total of all non-genetic effects from year to year. For many of the BVAHTs, the combined non-genetic effects appear to show a declining (favourable) trend over time (see Figure 4); for some, there is an apparent rise in the late 1980s and early 1990s. Overall, no particular trend in the combined non-genetic factors is observable across BVAHTs. For the majority of Group 2 (osteoarthritic) traits, the combined effect of non-genetic effects appears to demonstrate either a plateau or a slight fall, suggesting either no change, or a slight improvement in the combined non-genetic factors influencing these traits. It is worth noting that the majority of animals were scored when they were quite young and that more improvement from environmental management may become evident later in life.

For NORB and CRAE (Group 1 BHAHTs), the combined non-genetic factors follow a similar pattern, showing improvement up to the early 1980s, a worsening over the next decade, followed by improvement since. The trend in non-genetic effects for AF and SUBL is somewhat atypical. Given that these traits could be considered one of the better measures of joint laxity, which is suspected as the underlying lesion in hip dysplasia, it is pleasing to see an improvement in the combined effect of non-genetic factors since 2000. With the exception of AF, movements in the combined non-genetic effects have been in a favourable direction in recent times, suggesting that, overall, the present management strategies by breeders, owners and veterinarians are producing favourable results with regard to hip dysplasia.

Litter Variance Component

Litter variance components from the ordinal (multi-threshold) trait analyses are shown in Table 5. All components-to-standard-error ratios exceeded 2 (range 2.86–7.65). NORB, SUBL and CrAE appear to have higher ratios than all the remaining traits. The percentage of the variance for which the litter effect accounted ranged between 5.82 and 8.70% and no pattern is evident.

Maternal Effect

As shown in Table 6, models including terms for a maternal mode of inheritance and a maternal environmental effect returned positive variance components for all traits except FHNE and FHR for which the maternal additive component was negative and of very small magnitude not significantly different from 0. Maternal environmental components were positive for all BVAHTs, and mostly in excess of twice their standard errors.

Discussion

This study was undertaken to investigate the presence of meaningful phenotypic variation in this population and to determine if this variation is sufficiently heritable to be amenable to selection pressure. While the ordinal models can give an estimate of model variance components relative to the residual variance ($\pi^2/3$) they cannot provide any information about the phenotypic variance on the underlying scale (variation in the precise quantitative amount of joint disease present). While linear models do provide an estimate of phenotypic variance on the observed scale (not shown), the phenotypes cannot be mapped onto the underlying scale, as it is not proven that the units of the observed scale (the BVAHT category numbers) are spaced equidistantly over the underlying scale. On the contrary, the units on the observed scale are arbitrary. A hypothetical observed scale

Table 4. Hip and sex effects in British Veterinary Association Hip Trait (BVAHTs) scores in Australian German Shepherd Dogs for the multi-threshold ordinal analysis.

BVAHT	Left Hip Effect	(SE)	Male Sex Effect	(SE)
Norberg Angle (NORB)	−0.29	0.02	−0.58	0.04
Subluxation (SUBL)	0.10	0.02	−0.39	0.04
Cranial Acetabular Edge (CRAE)	0.12	0.02	−0.63	0.04
Dorsal Acetabular Edge (DAE)	0.09	0.05	−0.40	0.07
Cranial Effective Acetabular Rim (CREAR)	0.19	0.04	−0.62	0.06
Acetabular Fossa (AF)	0.03	0.04	−0.38	0.06
Caudal Acetabular Edge (CAAE)	0.06	0.05	−0.50	0.08
Femoral Head and Neck Exostosis (FHNE)	0.07	0.03	−0.34	0.05
Femoral Head Remodelling (FHR)	0.16	0.05	−0.44	0.07

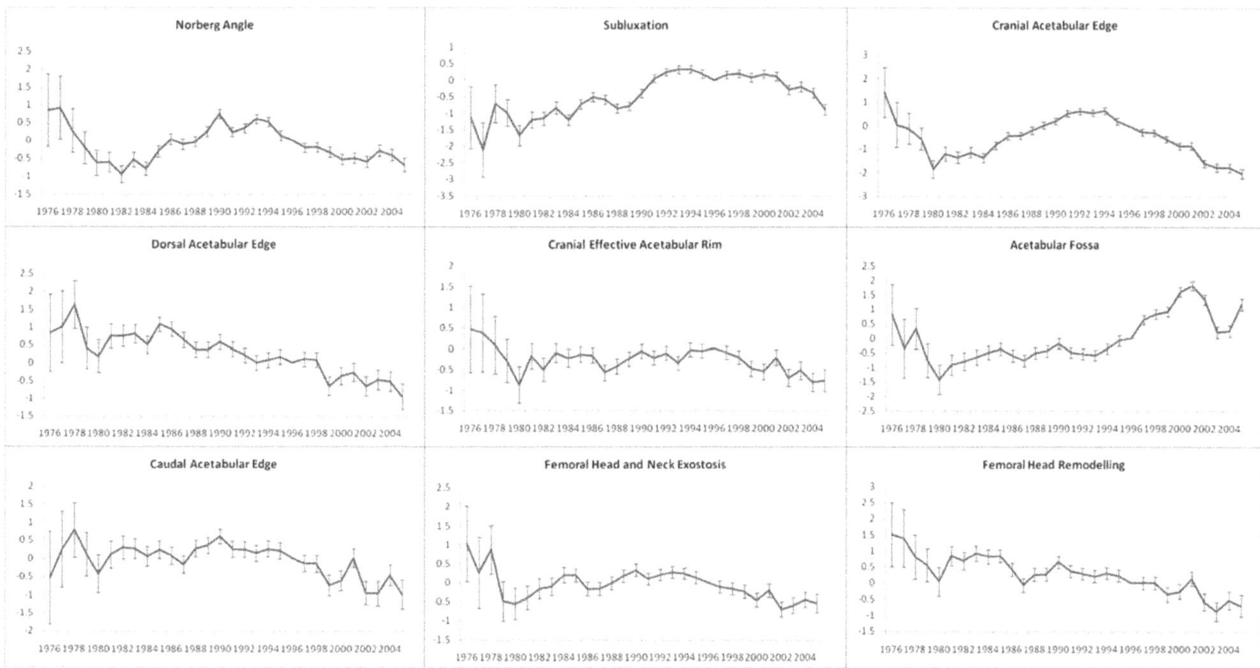

Figure 4. Non Genetic Year-of-Birth effects for British Veterinary Association Hip Trait Phenotypes in a population of Australian German Shepherd Dogs.

with a different number or spacing of category numbers could give vastly different (and no more valid) phenotypic variance estimates to data which was identical on the underlying scale. However, although phenotypic variation cannot be quantified, Figure 1 clearly demonstrates that phenotypic variation is present and allows a comparison between the BVAHTs.

Although heritability estimates for CHD phenotypes are relatively abundant in the literature (see Table 1), heritability estimates of the BVAHTs are rarer [13,15–18]. The presence of meaningful, heritable phenotypic variation in the BVAHTs demonstrates that BVA scores are amenable to improvement through selection. Selection refers, in effect, to identifying animals with superior alleles for a trait and breeding preferentially from these animals. This selective breeding aims to increase the frequency with which the superior alleles are found in the population (with a concomitant decrease in the frequency of less desirable alleles). The change in allele frequency leads to a change in BVA scores. The extent to which the change in allele frequency improves CHD-related welfare depends on the extent to which the alleles which determine a favourable BVA score also determine desirable welfare outcomes. Even setting aside the dog's internal experience of CHD-related welfare, the relationship between BVA phenotypes and clinical hip dysplasia is virtually unstudied. However, Malm *et al.* [25] demonstrated an association between insurance claims for clinical hip dysplasia and a similar hip phenotype providing evidence of a genetic correlation between BVA -like phenotypes and clinical outcomes, and therefore a potential for selection for such phenotypes to modify the likelihood of clinical outcomes.

This paper presents heritability estimates of BVA hip traits in Australian German Shepherd Dogs obtained by taking into account the ordinal nature of the traits, using an ordinal logistic

Table 5. Litter variance component in British Veterinary Association Hip Trait (BVAHTs) scores in Australian German Shepherd Dogs for the multi-threshold ordinal analysis.

BVAHT	Litter Variance Component/Standard Error	% variance due to Litter Effect
Norberg Angle (NORB)	7.46	7.47
Subluxation (SUBL)	7.65	7.08
Cranial Acetabular Edge (CRAE)	6.26	6.57
Dorsal Acetabular Edge (DAE)	3.23	7.35
Cranial Effective Acetabular Rim (CREAR)	4.46	7.71
Acetabular Fossa (AF)	3.87	6.14
Caudal Acetabular Edge (CAAE)	3.31	8.70
Femoral Head and Neck Exostosis (FHNE)	4.06	5.82
Femoral Head Remodelling (FHR)	2.86	6.24

Table 6. Maternal genetic and environmental effects on British Veterinary Association Hip Trait (BVAHTs) scores in a cohort of Australian German Shepherd Dogs.

BVAHT	Maternal Additive Comp/SE	Maternal heritability	Maternal Environ. Comp/SE	% variance due to Maternal Env Comp
Norberg Angle (NORB)	2.44	0.03	3.08	2.64
Subluxation (SUBL)	2.57	0.03	3.63	3.13
Cranial Acetabular Edge (CRAE)	0.3	0.00	5.00	4.26
Dorsal Acetabular Edge (DAE)	0.47	0.01	1.45	2.56
Cranial Effective Acetabular Rim (CREAR)	1.07	0.01	3.38	4.47
Acetabular Fossa (AF)	0.71	0.01	3.78	4.93
Caudal Acetabular Edge (CAAE)	0.08	0.00	2.23	4.76
Femoral Head and Neck Exostosis (FHNE)	–	–	4.62	4.43
Femoral Head Remodelling (FHR)	–	–	2.09	2.86

regression based REML-like mixed model. The models fitted also enabled evaluation of the importance of several fixed effects relating to right and left hip effects, year of the animal's birth, its age at the time of radiography for scoring and its sex. Unfortunately data were not available for several other fixed effects which have been suggested as potential sources of variation for BVAHTs, including extent of sedation at the time of radiography [27] and identity of the radiograph evaluator. Had data on these effects been available, we would have been able to investigate the effect of these factors on BVAHT scores and, if necessary, adjust for any tendency for related animals to be more similar for these factors than unrelated animals which could result in over-estimation of heritability. Similarly, it would have been useful to be able to include the identity of the veterinarian taking the radiograph, or the veterinary practice in which the radiograph was taken, as a random effect, given that positioning has been reported in the literature [10] as a potentially significant source of variation. All CHD scoring protocols should include the recording of this information.

This study included nearly twice as many records from female dogs as from males, and for all nine BVAHTs female dogs tended to score more poorly. An effect of sex on BVAHT has been noted previously, but the more affected sex has been inconsistent across breeds [17–18]. In studies of other hip dysplasia phenotypes in the German Shepherd Dog, sex effects have been variable, with one study noting males were less affected [23] and another finding no significant difference between males and females [21]. The reason for male animals exhibiting lower BVAHT scores than females in this study is unclear. It is likely that a greater breeding selection pressure is placed upon males prior to submission of radiographs and that part of this selection pressure is toward a trait which is correlated with BVAHTs in some fashion, potentially related to the gait or ease of movement of the young dog. The pedigree file showing relationships between dogs for which there were data had similar sex proportions to those in the phenotype dataset, in that 31.3% of unique parents were male and 68.7% were female. If this pattern is consistent with the whole breeding population (i.e. individual sires father more than twice as many puppies as individual mothers), then there is no real indication of a sex-related submission bias. On the other hand, there may be a biological basis for this finding, given that the human analogue (developmental hip dysplasia) is substantially more common in female infants [28] and the potential for hormones to modulate CHD phenotypes has been postulated [29].

All nine BVAHTs are clearly heritable in our studied population: eight of the nine BVAHTs have a substantial heritability in the range 0.17–0.24; and the heritability of the other trait (DAE) is 0.14. Heritability estimates of the individual BVAHTs have been obtained from United Kingdom populations of Gordon Setters and Labrador Retrievers (Table 1) [15,16,18]. For both breeds the authors noted higher heritability estimates for NORB and SUBL than for other traits. Our results are somewhat similar, with the heritability of these two traits ranking equal second. Different breeds from different countries are not expected to have exactly the same heritability for a phenotype, as they are not expected to have exactly the same allele frequencies or the same set of non-genetic factors. The differences between the estimates from our studies and other studies are likely due to both the use of ordinal logistic regression in this study and to innate differences in the population. The heritability of the summed BVAHT scores was 0.30 in this study which is comparable to findings in UK Labradors, 0.34 (by a regression-based method) [16], and 0.35 (by a linear REML-based method) [13]. Heritability estimates for the summed scores in other breeds have varied from 0.20 to 0.75 (See Table 1).

Differences in heritability estimates between threshold and linear models for canine hip dysplasia have been compared previously, in a cohort of Estrela Mountain Dogs. Silvestre *et al.* [30] compared the use of a threshold model using a Bayesian approach, and an LMM using REML, in modelling a five-point ordinal categorical scale of hip dysplasia severity in use in Europe under the criteria of the Fédération Cynologie Internationale (FCI). The estimates of heritability obtained by the two methods were similar, which is consistent with the findings of this study [30]. Despite the similarity of the estimates from the two methods, there is no compelling reason to use an LMM for the analysis of data which are truly ordinal, now that an appropriate REML-like method is available for fitting ordinal models.

The accuracy of selection based on phenotypic selection is the square root of the heritability. Based on the ordinal model estimates, the accuracy for phenotypic ("performance") selection based upon the BVAHT scores is between 0.40–0.52. This range is similar to the range of accuracies for the major dairy-cattle production traits, which have been improved so markedly by selection in recent decades.

Unlike the direct heritability estimates, the maternal heritability was very small in all cases. The relevant component divided by its standard error suggested statistical significance for only NORB and SUBL, and the absolute magnitude of the heritability for even these two traits was very small, suggesting there would be no great advantage in selecting for maternal protective traits for hip dysplasia within this population. Dietsche *et al.* [31] similarly reported only a small maternal heritability of a hip dysplasia trait, once a permanent maternal environmental effect was included.

The maternal environmental effect accounted for between 2.6% and 4.9% of the variance, and the relative size of the standard error suggested this may be statistically significant for all but one trait (DAE). A kennel effect was not included in the present analysis as there was no direct information about the environments in which dogs were raised and produced litters, having only the kennel prefix which reflects only into which kennel the dog was born. Therefore it is possible that identified maternal effects are in fact a proxy for an effect for some other non-genetic effect, rather than one specifically related to the mothering of the dam. Dietsche *et al.* [31] found maternal environmental effect accounting for around 10% of the phenotypic variation for another hip dysplasia trait. No additional variation was explained when they added a kennel effect to a model already including a maternal environmental effect.

Submission of radiographs radiographs for evaluation is voluntary, which creates a potential concern regarding submission bias among offspring. Additionally, obviously symptomatic animals may not be selected as potential parents, which could potentially create an evaluation bias among offspring. In later time-periods covered by the study, the proportion of hip scores among parents is high (see Table 2), but in earlier time-periods there is some potential for submission and evaluation biases among parents compared to all dogs scored, and there may be an additional bias against high scores in animals selected for radiography initially. Such selection would be expected to lower the phenotypic variation but also lower the variation in differences between families. Additionally, it appears that higher hip scores may be more heritable than lower hip scores (see Figure 3). From consideration of all these issues, the effect on heritability estimates of any submission or evaluation bias is not definitively predictable in sign or in magnitude. However, if there is a bias, its effect is likely to be small. The main purpose of this study was to evaluate whether heritability is sufficiently large to warrant selection in this population, and whether the use of EBVs is advisable. Particularly as the estimates reported in this paper are in broad agreement with other estimates in the literature, any bias (if present) has not compromised the conclusions reached.

Estimates of variation and of direct heritability by all methods were in the range that indicates that firstly, selection based upon these phenotypes can be effective and secondly, that development of EBVs which would allow the inclusion of phenotypic data from related animals could result in substantial improvements in accuracy of selection. The response to selection which can be expected from a genetic control scheme of this type depends on the phenotypic variation and heritability of the phenotype in the population, whether EBVs are used, the selection pressure which is applied by the end users of the scheme and how well the selection criterion (BVAHT scores) genetically correlates to the goal phenotype (also called breeding objective). Wilson *et al.* [32] argued that the goal phenotype is improved animal welfare. Consequently, the extent to which any phenotype used in a CHD control scheme genetically correlates to improved animal welfare is a key question. Our analysis suggests that with adequate selection pressure, BVAHT phenotype scores should improve over time, and would do so at a considerably faster rate if selection on EBVs replaces phenotype selection. The extent to which this improvement in BVAHT phenotypes would result in improved welfare is unfortunately unknown, but should be at least positive. Other types of radiographic evaluation may potentially have higher genetic correlations with welfare, and promising phenotypes should be evaluated in this population for variation, heritability and genetic correlation with welfare. Detailed discussion regarding the response to the selection which this population underwent over the time of the study is beyond the scope of this paper, but will be addressed in future work.

While selection based on BVAHT scores continues, the complex construction of the BVA phenotypes complicates the analysis. Assuming that the summed phenotypes are truly linear, as was probably the intention when the phenotypes were devised, simplifies the analysis by allowing the use of linear models. However, this approach makes several assumptions (discussed in the materials and methods) which may not be justified. We recommend that estimated breeding values for BVA hip traits be developed and implemented to increase the effectiveness of selection and that where possible, ordinal methods of analysis are utilised. Future papers will further explore the optimal methods for calculating EBVs for selection in this population.

Acknowledgments

The authors would like to acknowledge the German Shepherd Dog Council of Australia, the Australian National Kennel Council, the Australian Veterinary Association and Doctor Malcolm Willis for their kind contribution of the data for this study.

Author Contributions

Conceived and designed the experiments: BJW FWN JWJ CMW IT HWR KC PCT. Performed the experiments: BJW PCT. Analyzed the data: BJW FWN JJ PCT. Contributed reagents/materials/analysis tools: PCT. Wrote the paper: BJW.

References

1. Janutta V, Hamann H, Distl O (2006) Complex segregation analysis of canine hip dysplasia in German shepherd dogs. Journal of Heredity 97: 13–20.
2. Leighton EA (1997) Genetics of canine hip dysplasia. Journal of the American Veterinary Medical Association 210: 1474–1479.
3. Maki K, Janss LLG, Groen AF, Liinamo AE, Ojala M (2004) An indication of major genes affecting hip and elbow dysplasia in four Finnish dog populations. Heredity 92: 402–408.
4. Marschall Y, Distl O (2007) Mapping quantitative trait loci for canine hip dysplasia in German Shepherd dogs. Mammalian Genome 18: 861–870.
5. Todhunter RJ, Bliss SP, Casella G, Wu R, Lust G, et al. (2003) Genetic structure of susceptibility traits for hip dysplasia and microsatellite informativeness of an outcrossed canine pedigree. Journal of Heredity 94: 39–48.
6. Demko J, McLaughlin R (2005) Developmental Orthopedic Disease. Veterinary Clinics Small Animal Practice 35: 1111–1135.
7. Everts RE, Hazewinkel HAW, Rothuizen J, van Oost BA (2000) Bone disorders in the dog: A review of modern genetic strategies to find the underlying causes. Veterinary Quarterly 22: 63–70.
8. Ginja MMD, Silvestre AM, Gonzalo-Orden JM, Ferreira AJA (2010) Diagnosis, genetic control and preventive management of canine hip dysplasia: A review. The Veterinary Journal 184: 269–276.
9. Flückiger M (2007) Scoring radiographs for canine hip dysplasia - the big three organizations in the world. European Journal of Companion Animal Practice 17: 135–140.
10. Gibbs C (1997) The BVA/KC scoring scheme for control of hip dysplasia: interpretation of criteria. Veterinary Record 141: 275–284.
11. Lawson DD (2000) Hip Dysplasia and its control in Great Britain. In: Morgan JP, Wind A, Davidson AP, editors. Hereditary Bone and Joint Diseases in the Dog. Hannover, Germany: Shlütersche. pp 267–283.
12. Wilson BJ, Nicholas FW, James JW, Wade CM, Tammen I, et al. (2011) Symmetry of hip dysplasia traits in the German Shepherd Dog in Australia. Journal of Animal Breeding and Genetics 128: 230–243.
13. Lewis TW, Blott SC, Woolliams JA (2010) Genetic Evaluation of Hip Score in UK Labrador Retrievers. PLoS ONE 5: e12797.
14. Woolliams JA, Lewis TW, Blott SC (2011) Canine hip and elbow dysplasia in UK Labrador retrievers. The Veterinary Journal In Press, Corrected Proof.

15. Lewis TW, Woolliams JA, Blott SC (2010) Genetic Evaluation of the Nine Component Features of Hip Score in UK Labrador Retrievers. PLoS ONE 5: e13610.
16. Wood JLN, Lakhani KH, Rogers K (2002) Heritability and epidemiology of canine hip-dysplasia score and its components in Labrador retrievers in the United Kingdom. Preventative Veterinary Medicine 55: 95–108.
17. Wood JLN, Lakhani KH, Dennis R (2000) Heritability and epidemiology of canine hip-dysplasia score in flat-coated retrievers and Newfoundlands in the United Kingdom. Preventative Veterinary Medicine 46: 75–86.
18. Wood JLN, Lakhani KH, Dennis R (2000) Heritability of canine hip-dysplasia score and its components in Gordon Setters. Preventative Veterinary Medicine 46: 87–97.
19. Hamann H, Kirchhoff T, Distl O (2003) Bayesian analysis of heritability of canine hip dysplasia in German Shepherd Dogs. Journal of Animal Breeding and Genetics 120: 258–268.
20. Hedhammar Å, Olsson S-E, Andersson S-Å, Persson L, Pettersson L, et al. (1979) Canine Hip Dysplasia: Study of Heritability in 401 Litters of German Shepherd Dogs. Journal of the American Veterinary Medical Association 174: 1012–1016.
21. Karsada R, Mészáros G, Kadleík O, Bluecea JJ (2007) Impact of inbreeding and heritability of Canine Hip Dysplasia in German Shepherd population. Folia Veterinaria 51: 142–145.
22. Leppänen M, Mäki K, Juga J, Saloniemi H (2000) Estimation of heritability for hip dysplasia in German Shepherd Dogs in Finland. Journal of Animal Breeding and Genetics 117: 97–103.
23. Sturaro E, Menegazzo L, Piccinini P, Bittante G, Carnier P, et al. (2006) Prevalence and genetic parameters for hip dysplasia in Italian population of purebred dogs. Italian Journal of Animal Science 5: 107–116.
24. Stock KF, Klein S, Tellhelm B, Distl O (2011) Genetic analyses of elbow and hip dysplasia in the German shepherd dog. Journal of Animal Breeding and Genetics 128: 219–229.
25. Malm S, Fikse F, Egenvall A, Bonnett BN, Gunnarsson L, et al. (2010) Association between radiographic assessment of hip status and subsequent incidence of veterinary care and mortality related to hip dysplasia in insured Swedish dogs. Preventive Veterinary Medicine 93: 222–232.
26. Agresti A (2002) Categorical Data Analysis. Hoboken, New Jersey, USA: John Wiley & Sons, Inc.
27. Malm S, Strandberg E, Danell B, Audell L, Swenson L, et al. (2007) Impact of sedation method on the diagnosis of hip and elbow dysplasia in Swedish dogs. Preventive Veterinary Medicine 78: 196–209.
28. Sewell MD, Rosendahl K, Eastwood DM (2009) Developmental dysplasia of the hip. British Medical Journal 339: 12.
29. Steinetz BG, Williams AJ, Lust G, Schwabe C, Bullesbach EE, et al. (2008) Transmission of relaxin and estrogens to suckling canine pups via milk and possible association with hip joint laxity. American Journal of Veterinary Research 69: 59–67.
30. Silvestre AM, Ginja MMD, Ferreira AJA, Colaco J (2007) Comparison of estimates of hip dysplasia genetic parameters in Estrela Mountain Dog using linear and threshold models. J Anim Sci 85: 1880–1884.
31. Dietschi E, Schawalder P, Gaillard C (2003) Estimation of genetic parameters for canine hip dysplasia in the Swiss Newfoundland population. Journal of Animal Breeding and Genetics 120: 150–161.
32. Wilson B, Nicholas FW, Thomson PC (2011) Selection against canine hip dysplasia: Success or failure? The Veterinary Journal 189: 160–168.

Comparison of Patient and Surgeon Expectations of Total Hip Arthroplasty

Claire Jourdan[1,5]*, Serge Poiraudeau[4], Stéphane Descamps[2], Rémy Nizard[3], Moussa Hamadouche[4], Philippe Anract[4], Stéphane Boisgard[2], Myriam Galvin[2], Philippe Ravaud[5]

1 AP-HP, Hôpital R. Poincaré, Service de Médecine Physique et Réadaptation, Garches, France, 2 CHU Clermont-Ferrand, Hôpital Gabriel Montpied, Service d'Orthopédie, Traumatologie, Chirurgie plastique et reconstructive, Université Claude Monnet, Clermont-Ferrand, France, 3 AP-HP, Hôpital Lariboisière, Service de Chirurgie Orthopédique et Traumatologique, Université Paris 7, Paris, France, 4 AP-HP, Hôpital Cochin, Service d'Orthopédie, Université Paris Descartes, Paris, France, 5 Institut National de la Santé et de la Recherche Médicale (INSERM) E 0738, Centre d'Epidémiologie Clinique, Université Paris Descartes, Paris, France

Abstract

Objectives: Analysis of discrepancies between patient and surgeon expectations before total hip arthroplasty (THA) should enable a better understanding of motives of dissatisfaction about surgery, but this question has been seldom studied. Our objectives were to compare surgeons' and patients' expectations before THA, and to study factors which affected surgeon-patient agreement.

Methods: 132 adults (mean age 62.8+/−13.7 years, 52% men) on waiting list for THA in three tertiary care centres and their 16 surgeons were interviewed to assess their expectations using the Hospital for Special Surgery Total Hip Replacement Expectations Survey (range 0–100). Patients' and surgeons' answers were compared, for the total score and for the score of each item. Univariate analyses tested the effect of patients' characteristics on surgeons' and patients' expectations separately, and on surgeon-patient differences.

Results: Surgeon and patient expectations' mean scores were high (respectively 90.9+/−11.1 and 90.0+/−11.6 over 100). Surgeons' and patients' expectations showed no systematic difference, but there was little agreement on Bland and Altman graph and correlation coefficient was low. Patients had higher expectations than surgeons for sports. Patients rated their expectations according to trust in physician and mental quality of life, surgeons considered disability. More disabled patients and patients from a low-income professional category were often "more optimistic" than their surgeons.

Conclusion: Surgeons and patients often do not agree on what to expect from THA. More disabled patients expect better outcomes than their surgeons.

Editor: Joel Joseph Gagnier, University of Michigan, United States of America

Funding: The research of the first author was supported by a grant from the Institut Fédératif de Recherche sur le Handicap (IFRH) - IFR 25. No additional external funding was received for this study. The funders had no role in study design, data collection and analysis, decision to publish, or preparation of the manuscript.

Competing Interests: The authors have declared that no competing interests exist.

* E-mail: claire.jourdan@rpc.aphp.fr

Introduction

Total hip arthroplasty (THA) is the most effective treatment for disabling hip osteoarthritis [1]. Main goals of THA are to reduce pain and increase patients' functional abilities. Patient's preferences play a pivotal role in surgery decision making, and the assessment of patients expectations regarding the functional benefits of THA is recommended [2].

Expectations in this domain can be understood as "expectancies" (or "probability expectations"), meaning patients' judgments about the benefits of surgery, or "value expectations", meaning patients' desires, hopes, or wishes concerning outcome. This last approach is close to "importance", which refers to patients' priorities concerning function post-surgery [3].

Patient's expectations about THA have been shown to depend on several demographic, clinical, psychological and socioeconomic factors [4–6]. Patients ethnical origins, employment status, and trust in surgeon have a significant effect on expectations about THA [5]. Patients with worse disease severity have been shown to have higher expectations scores than those with less severe disease [6]. Expectations can also vary from one country to another, as shown in total knee arthroplasty [7].

The relationship between pre-operative expectations and later satisfaction with surgery is complex. Optimistic expectations can be an independent predictor of better joint arthroplasty outcome [4,8]. However, satisfaction with surgery is also associated with the proportion of fulfilled expectation [9], and unmet expectations can cause dissatisfaction [10,11].

Moreover, patients with low expectations might decline surgery although they would benefit from it, as expectations determine willingness to undergo surgery [12–14]. It is therefore important to determine which patients have high or low expectations about THA compared to their surgeons, in order to maximize THA indication and outcomes. One way to address this question is to better understand the differences between patients' and surgeons' views on the expected results of THA.

While it is established that patients suffering from osteoarthritis and their physicians might differ in their assessment of important health and symptom status [15], and of surgical outcome [16,17], the difference between patients' and surgeons' expectations before THA has seldom been studied. Moran and colleagues [18], found that surgeons had better expectations of predicted postoperative functional scores than patients. Street and colleagues [19] showed that patient-surgeon concordance regarding the expected benefits of surgery was poor, and differed with quality of communication, especially surgeon's information giving. These studies used different means of evaluating patient's expectations: functional "expected" scale or close-ended questions. Assessments of expectations have used various methods until recently, when patient-derived scales have been validated for patients' "probability" expectations [6,20] or for patients' concerns and "value" expectations [21].

This study aimed to compare surgeons' and patients' "probability expectations" of THA using a validated patient-derived questionnaire. Its first objective was to assess how much, in which direction, and for which items these could differ. Its second objective was to study which parameters explained patient-surgeon differences in expectations.

Methods

This cross-sectional survey was approved by the ethical committee of the Institutional Review Board of APHP Bichat Hospital, Paris. Participants gave oral informed consent before telephone interview, followed by written informed consent through post.

Population

Patients and surgeons were recruited from three French tertiary care orthopaedic centres (APHP Hospital Lariboisière, Paris, APHP Hospital Cochin, Paris, and Hospital Gabriel Montpied, Clermont-Ferrand) between January and July 2009. Surgeons participating in the study included consecutive adult patients on waiting list for hip replacement surgery. Exclusion criteria were tumoral, infectious or inflammatory disease of the hip, revision THA surgery, and patient's refusal or inability to answer the questionnaire.

Evaluation

Expected benefits of hip surgery were assessed using the Hospital for Special Surgery Total Hip Replacement Expectations Survey (THR Survey) [6,20], adapted to French by back translation [22]. In this patient-derived questionnaire, patients are asked the following question: "How much relief or improvement do you expect in the following areas as a result of hip replacement surgery?" The scale contains 18 items addressing symptoms, daily function, exercise, employment, and psychological well-being, and the answers range from "patient does not have this expectation, or this expectation does not apply" (scoring 0) to "complete improvement or back to normal" (scoring 4). We chose to separate the answer "patient does not have this expectation" (scoring 0) from the answer "this expectation does not apply" ("not applicable item").

The same questionnaire was used by the patient's surgeon, with a question modified as follows: "How much relief or improvement seems realistic to you in the following areas as a result of hip replacement surgery for this specific patient?" The 18 items and their answers were identical.

Patients' and surgeons' expectation scores were calculated by summing the scores of all the applicable items, higher scores indicating higher expectations. Scores were transformed by the formula: (sum/number of applicable items for the patient$\times$4)$\times$100, to obtain scores ranging from 0 to 100, as described before [23]. In order to compare patients' and surgeons' scores, the items considered "not applicable" by a patient were considered "not applicable" in the surgeon's assessment also. Differences in expectations were defined as: surgeon's score - patient's score (a positive difference suggested that the surgeon had higher expectations than his patient and *vice versa*).

Demographic characteristics included gender, retirement status, professional category (liberal or senior officer versus employee or worker), marital status (married or in couple versus single), educational level (pre-secondary level versus post-secondary level), and the physical activity that the patient wished to resume after surgery (recommended or not after hip arthroplasty, according to The Hip Society and the American Association of Hip and Knee Surgeons [24]).

Health status evaluation included age, Body Mass Index (inferred from patients' reports of height and weight), and average hip pain during the last four weeks on a numeric rating scale (0–10). Co-morbidities were measured using the Charlson Comorbidity Index [25], dichotomized as zero (no relevant comorbidity) versus one or more co-morbidities. A history of ipsilateral hip arthroplasty was recorded.

Functional evaluation used the short 8-item Western Ontario and Mac Master Universities (Womac) function subscale [26,27], which ranges from 0 (no disability) to 32 (extreme disability). Quality of life was assessed by the Medical Outcome Study Short Form-12 (SF-12) [28,29], for which higher scores indicate better quality of life.

To measure patient-surgeon communication during the clinical visit, patient self-report measures were used, with previously described questions [19]: five questions measured patient's perception of their own involvement during visit, three questions measured patient's perception of the surgeon's partnership building, and five questions measured patient's perception of information given by the surgeon. Each question allowed three answers: "disagree", "neither agree nor disagree", "agree". Scores (1–3) were summed for each dimension of communication. Patients' trust in their surgeon was measured by a numeric rating scale (0–10).

Patients were recruited consecutively after their clinical visit with their surgeons and before surgery. Visits did not differ from usual, no specific questions were asked. They were interviewed by phone by a unique independent assessor, using a standardized questionnaire, to assess their expectations of surgery, and sociodemographic and health status characteristics. The attending surgeon for each patient was asked to fill in the THR Survey, to assess the benefit which their patient could reasonably expect. Surgeons' completed the survey a few days after clinical visit, using their own clinical record. The patient and the assessor were unaware of the surgeon's responses and *vice versa*. Clinical reports were reviewed to collect medical data.

Statistical analysis

Description of the sample characteristics and expectation scores used mean and standard deviation (SD) for continuous variables, and counts and percentages for categorical variables.

Considering that expectations of results of THA had been evaluated by two judges, the patient and his surgeon, concordance between surgeons' and patients' total expectations was judged using an intra-class correlation coefficient and the Bland and Altman method [30], and correlation between surgeons' and patients' expectations was assessed by the Pearson correlation coefficient. An aggregated score of surgeon-patient discrepancies was computed for each patient, using the sum of the absolute values of surgeon-patient differences for each item, corrected for the number of applicable items.

Differences (mean, 95% confidence interval (CI)) between surgeon's and patient's rating of expectations for each separate item were described.

We studied which parameters, among the variables previously stated, were associated with either patient expectations' scores or with surgeon expectations' scores separately. Spearman correlation coefficients were used for continuous variables, and ANOVAs (or Kruskal Wallis tests if necessary) for categorical variables. Alpha error limit was set at 5%.

To study surgeon-patient discrepancies in expectations, we used surgeon-patient difference in total expectation score, as defined above. We described patients according to the tertiles of this difference, thus dividing the population into three groups of equal size (n = 44). The group of patients with lowest (negative) surgeon-patient differences was classified as "more optimistic", the group with highest differences was classified as "more pessimistic", while the middle group had low surgeon/patient discrepancies. We compared the two extreme groups of patients ("optimistic" vs. "pessimistic") using chi square tests for categorical variables, and ANOVAs for continuous variables.

Surgeons' effect on differences in expectation was described using a box plot. To account for surgeons' effect, the same variables were tested through mixed effect logistic regression models, with "optimistic" vs. "pessimistic" as the dependant variable, the patient being analysed as nested within his surgeon (fixed effect were patients characteristics, random effects were surgeons).

Table 1. Characteristics of study population (n = 132).*

Socio-demographic characteristics		**Number (%)**
History of ipsilateral THA		19 (14.4%)
Charlson Comorbidity Index : score = 0		72 (54.5%)
Retired		85 (64.4%)
Profession : liberal or senior officer		75 (56.8%)
Education : post secondary level		63 (47.7%)
Married or in couple		82 (62.1%)
Sport : not recommended after THA		16 (12.1%)
Health status and survey scores		**Mean ± standard deviation**
Body Mass Index (kg/m^2)		25.6±4.1
Trust (NS, max = 10)		9.2±1.0
Communication	Patient participation (max = 15)	8.0±2.7
	Partnership building (max = 9)	5.6±2.1
	Information (max = 15)	11.1±3.0
Pain (NS, max = 10)		6.8±1.9
WOMAC (max = 32)		18.7±5.4
SF-12 : PCS (max = 100)		32.2±7.9
SF-12 : MCS (max = 100)		48.6±11.4

*THA = Total Hip Arthroplasty; NS = Numeric Scale; WOMAC = Western Ontario and McMaster Universities Osteoarthritis Index; SF-12 = Medical Outcome Study Short Form-12; PCS = Physical Component Summary; MCS = Medical Component Summary.

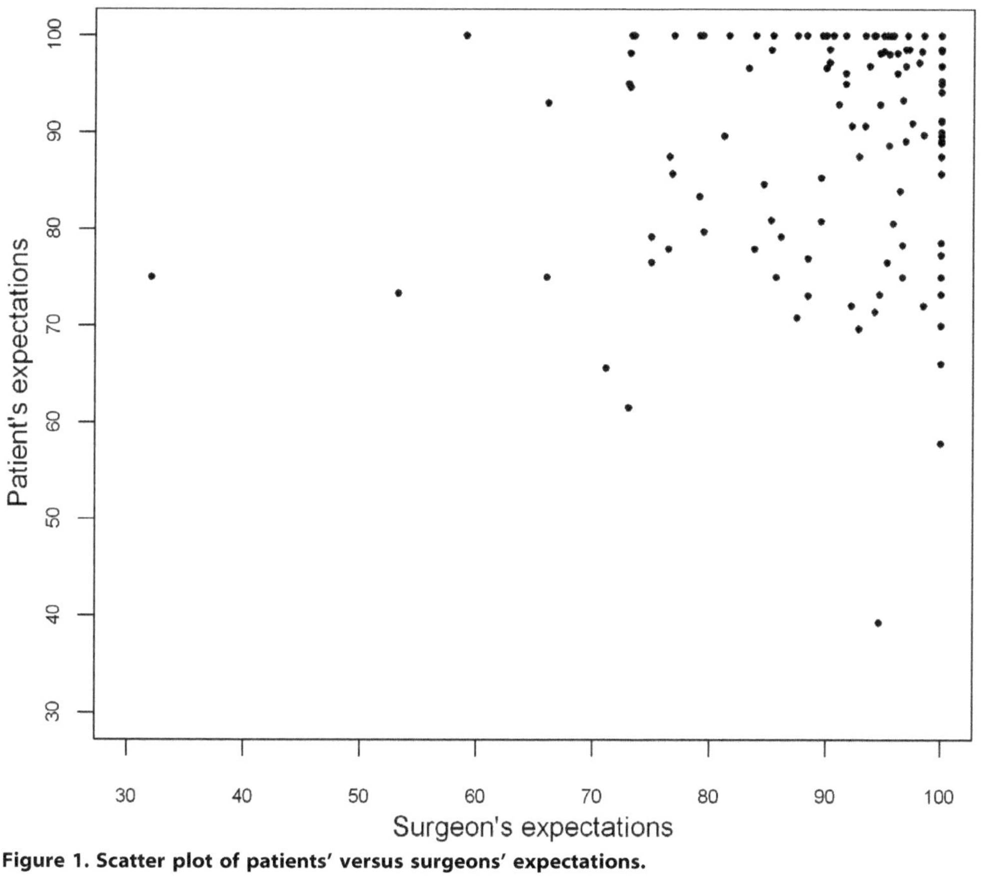

Figure 1. Scatter plot of patients' versus surgeons' expectations.

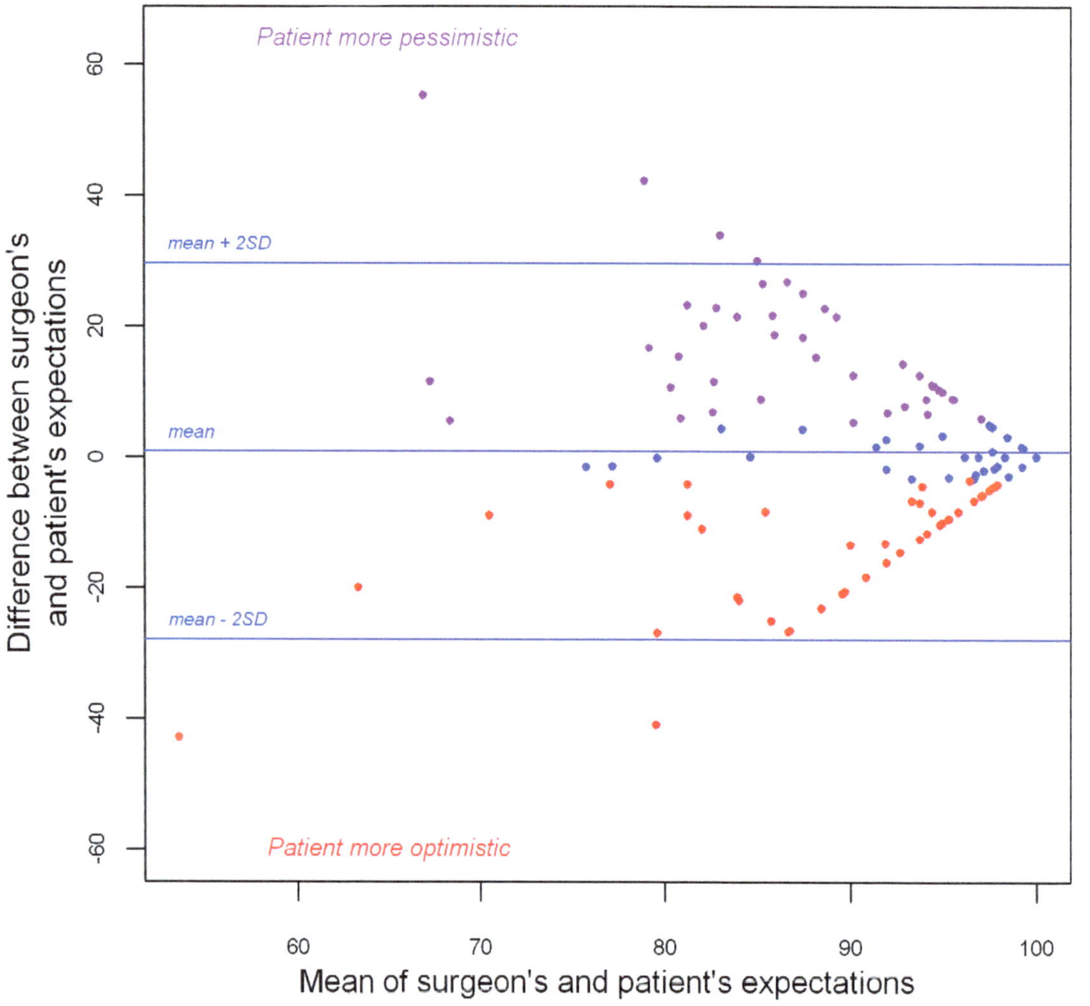

Figure 2. Bland and Altman graph of differences in expectations (surgeon's score - patient's score). For each patient, X-axis represents mean (½×(surgeon's score+patient's score)), Y-axis represents difference. The three tertiles-defined groups of patients are represented by three colors (red = "more optimistic patients"; blue = middle group, purple = "more pessimistic patients").

As missing data were scarce (0 to 4%), analyses were realized on complete data. The statistical software SAS® version 9.1 (SAS Institute, Cary, North Carolina) and R® version 2.8.1 were used.

Results

Population characteristics

A total of 16 surgeons agreed to participate and screened 202 patients. Seventy were not included: 22 patients were undergoing revision surgery, 6 had inflammatory or infectious disease of the hip, 9 patients declined to participate, 5 were unable to answer, 26 were impossible to contact before the surgery, and 2 had their surgery cancelled before the interview. The final sample consisted of 132 patients: respectively 63 (48%), 50 (38%) and 19 (14%) from each centre.

Mean +/− SD age was 62.8±13.7 years, ages ranging from 19 to 87 years. Patients were male in 52%. Indications for surgery were mostly primary or secondary hip osteoarthritis (82%) and avascular necrosis (12%). Patients were interviewed on average 37 days before surgery. Patients' characteristics and survey scores are shown in table 1. Patients' characteristics did not significantly differ according to centres or surgeons (data not shown).

Patients' and surgeons' expectations

Surgeons' and patients' expectations scores were both high, respectively 90.9±11.1 and 90.0±11.6. No systematic bias, but marked discrepancies between surgeons' and patient's expectations in both directions were found (figures 1 and 2), and mean aggregated score of surgeon-patient discrepancy was 9.3±7.3 (range = [0–39.9]). Intra-class correlation coefficient was low (0.16; $CI_{95\%} = [-0.03; 0.33]$), and Pearson's coefficient revealed no significant correlation (rho = 0.17, p = 0.06). On the Bland & Altman graph (figure 2), the differences in expectations (surgeon's score – patient's score) were distributed around zero and ranged from −42.9 to 55.4. Greatest absolute value of surgeon-patient differences were observed for lowest mean expectation scores, while patients with high expectations showed less surgeon-patient differences.

Surgeon-patient differences for each item are shown in figure 3. Greatest divergences were found for item 14 ("Improve ability to exercise or participate in sports"), patients being there more optimistic than surgeons.

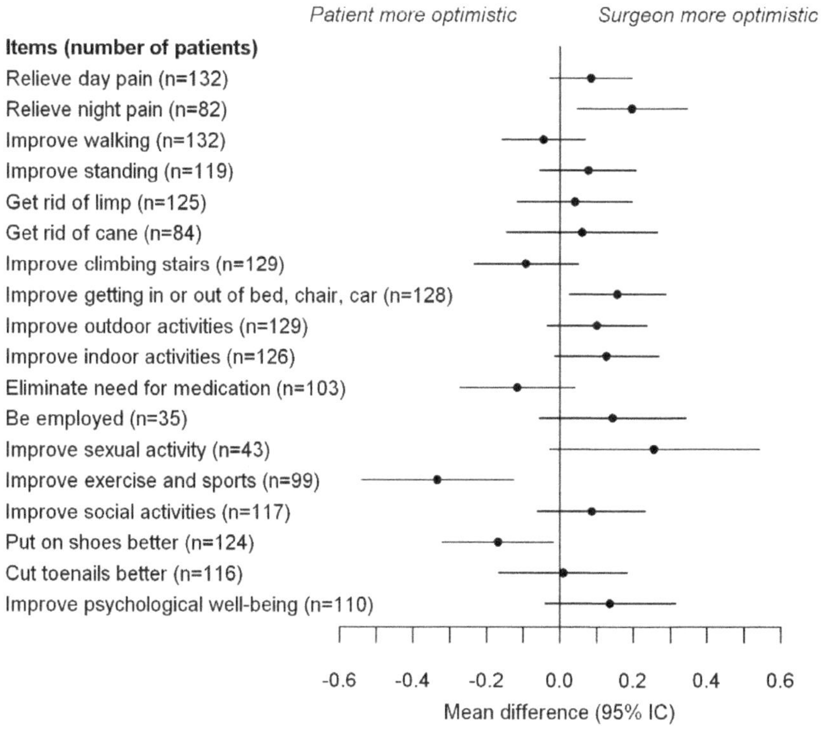

Figure 3. Mean (95% CI) surgeon – patient differences for each item of the THR Survey. Scores for each item range from 0 to 4. N = number of patients who stated this item as "applicable".

Factors affecting patient's or surgeons' expectations separately (table 2)

Patients' and surgeons' scores in expectations were both significantly associated with age (both p value<0.05), expectations being lower for older patients. Trust in surgeon (p<0.05), SF-12's mental component (p<0.05), and comorbidity index (p<0.01) significantly influenced patients' expectations. Surgeons' scores were associated with Womac (p<0.05), SF-12's physical component (p<0.01), marital and professional status (p<0.05 and <0.01, respectively). Surgeons' expectations were lower concerning more disabled patients (p<0.05).

Surgeons' expectations were significantly different amongst different recruitment sites (p<0.01) or amongst surgeons themselves (p<0.001 for Kruskal-Wallis test). Patients' expectations did not show any significant difference between surgeons or sites. Surgeons' effect was also significant on surgeon-patient differences in expectations (see figure 4, p = 0.003 for Kruskal-Wallis test).

Factors affecting surgeon-patient agreement: comparison between patients markedly more optimistic and patients markedly more pessimistic (table 3)

A significant effect of study site (p value = 0.003) was found.

Womac and physical quality of life yielded significant effects (both p values<0.01). "More optimistic" patients had a mean SF-12 physical component score of 29.4±1.1 while "more pessimistic" patients scored 34.6±1.3. A similar significant effect was found for Womac score, confirming that more disabled patients had higher expectations than their surgeons.

The other characteristic which differed between the two groups was professional category (p value = 0.02). Two thirds of patients who had "more pessimistic" expectations were from a liberal or senior officer professional category (62%), while two third of the "more optimistic" patients were employees or workers (66%).

Discussion

To our knowledge, this is the first study to compare expectations of THA of patients and of their surgeons with a validated multidimensional expectations questionnaire.

Surgeons and patients expectations were both high as previously reported [23], reflecting the favourable outcomes usually observed after THA. Although it has been reported that surgeons could expect better outcomes than patients [18], we did not observe such a bias between surgeons' and patients' mean scores.

However, concordance was poor, as differences in expectations (surgeon's score – patients' score) showed high variability and poor correlation. Marked discrepancies could be seen in both directions, and were especially important for patients with lower expectations. Moreover, the methods of this study, which included solely patients for which both patients and surgeons had agreed for surgery, could have understated the discrepancy that really existed: if a patient has great expectations for surgery and the doctor does not, or vice versa, it is unlikely the operation will be scheduled. A study including all patients for which THA is discussed would thus be likely to find higher surgeon-patient discrepancies.

As shown on figure 1 and 2, the sample could be roughly divided into three groups explaining the peculiar structure of the Bland and Altman graph: one middle group of patients with high expectations and high surgeon-patient concordance, and two other groups, with patients who had "more optimistic" expectations than their surgeons on one side, and patients who had "more pessimistic" expectations on the other. Dividing the population into three tertiles-defined groups thus enabled us to compare patients in these two extreme groups.

Table 2. Determinants of patients' or surgeons' expectation (total THR Survey score, max = 100).*

Socio-demographic characteristics		Patients' expectations		Surgeons' expectations	
		mean ± standard error	***p***	**mean ± standard error**	***p***
Recrutement site	Cochin	89.9±1.4	ns	**94.5±0.9**	**<0.01**
	Lariboisière	89.8±2.8		**86.5±1.8**	
	Gabriel Montpied	91.0±2.4		**90.4±2.8**	
Gender	Male	88.5±1.5	ns	91.2±1.5	ns
	Female	91.6±1.3		90.5±1.2	
Ipsilateral THA	Yes	90.5±2.4	ns	89.8±2.3	ns
	No	90.0±1.1		91.1±1.1	
Comorbidities	Score = 0	**92.4±1.2**	**<0.01**	92.1±1.1	ns
	Score > 0	**87.0±1.7**		89.3±1.7	
Retirement	Yes	89.6±1.3	ns	92.2±1.5	ns
	No	90.7±1.6		90.2±1.3	
Profession	Liberal, senior officer	89.9±1.2	ns	**92.5±1.3**	**<0.01**
	Employee, worker	90.1±1.7		**88.7±1.5**	
Education	Post secondary	89.3±1.4	ns	91.0±1.5	ns
	Pre secondary	90.7±1.4		90.8±1.3	
Marital status	Married/in couple	89.9±1.4	ns	**92.4±1.1**	**<0.05**
	Single	90.3±1.5		**88.4±1.8**	
Sport	Recommended	90.0±1.1	ns	94.6±3.0	ns
	Not recommended	90.4±2.4		98.4±1.0	
Health status and survey scores		**Patients' expectations**		**Surgeons' expectations**	
		Spearman correlation	***p***	**Spearman correlation**	***p***
Age		**−0.17**	**<0.05**	**−0.18**	**<0.05**
Body Mass Index (kg/m^2)		−0.07	ns	0.04	ns
Trust in surgeon (NS, max = 10)		**0.19**	**<0.05**	−0.08	ns
Communication	Patient participation	0.07	ns	−0.10	ns
	Partnership building	0.06	ns	−0.02	ns
	Information	0.06	ns	−0.15	ns
Pain (NS, max = 10)		0.12	ns	−0.06	ns
WOMAC (max = 32)		0.13	ns	**−0.20**	**<0.05**
SF-12 : PCS (max = 100)		−0.10	ns	**0.25**	**<0.01**
SF-12 : MCS (max = 100)		**0.21**	**<0.05**	0.01	ns

*Bold characters indicate significative tests; NS = Numeric Scale; WOMAC = Western Ontario and McMaster Universities Osteoarthritis Index; SF-12 = Medical Outcome Study Short Form-12; PCS = Physical Component Summary; MCS = Medical Component Summary.

The specific study of each item of the scale suggested that patients had higher expectations than their surgeons for the item "exercise and sports". We also found that 12% of the sample wished to resume a sport which was not recommended after THA (table 1). It has been recently suggested that expectations regarding exercise and sports was one of the less frequently fulfilled [9]. Our study thus shows that this could be due to a mismatch in pre-operative expectations. This question of sports after THA might then be a cause of post-operative disappointment, and should be a matter of careful pre-operative discussion.

The study of factors affecting surgeons' and patients' expectations separately enabled us to highlight interesting differences in surgeons' and patients' point of views. Surgeons' ratings of expectations seemed to be significantly associated with hip-related clinical data (Womac, SF-12's physical component). On the other side, patients seemed to rate their expectations on criteria that were mainly psychological and non-hip-related: SF-12's mental component, trust in surgeon, and comorbidities. Patients with higher scores on trust in surgeon and higher scores on SF-12's mental component were likely to have higher expectations.

Age significantly affected both patients' and surgeons' expectations in the same direction, so that no effect of age on differences in expectations was seen. The evidence on the role of age on disability and quality of life after THA is conflicting, but a large number of studies show that post-THA improvement is comparable in older and younger patients [1]. In our study, both patients and surgeons seemed to agree on being more prudent on the

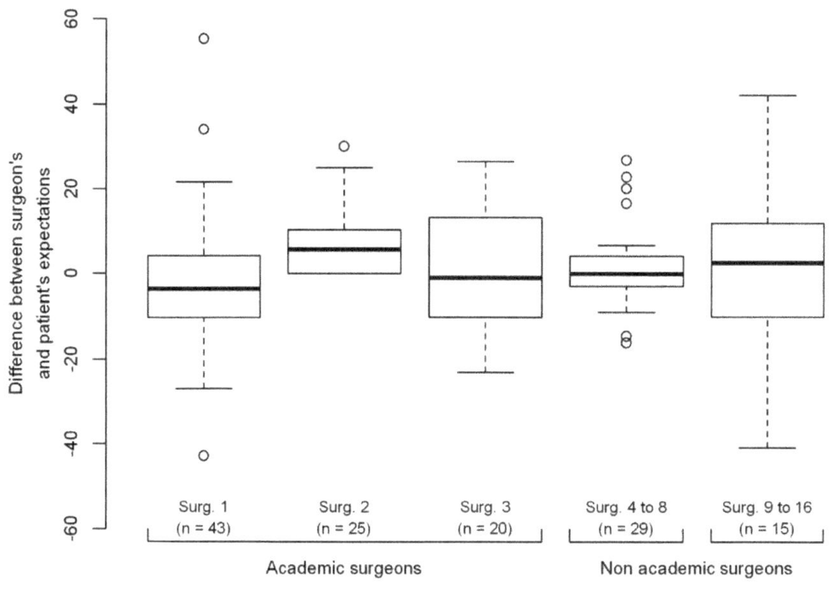

Figure 4. Box plots comparing surgeon-patient differences between surgeons. Boxes include the first quartile, the median and the third quartile. Surgeons 4 to 8, who recruited 5–11 patients each, and surgeons 9 to 16, who recruited 1–3 patients each, were aggregated.

estimated outcome of surgery for older patients, having thus somewhat more pessimistic views than the literature.

When studying surgeon-patient differences in total expectations scores, we found that several parameters were associated with disagreements. First, patients with low functional status and physical quality of life tended to be "more optimistic" than their surgeons. It has been shown that patients with poor functional status have high expectations for THA [6], and are at high risk of having unfulfilled expectations [9]. This study confirms that more disabled patients have higher expectations than surgeons before THA, which could mean unrealistic expectations, and that special attention should be given when informing these patients about their expected outcome.

Professional category significantly affected surgeon-patient agreement. Patients who were from a lower income category were often in the "more optimistic" group. The role of such socio-demographic variables on patients expectations has already been noted by other authors [5,6], and should probably be also taken into account when delivering pre-operative information to patients.

We found significant effects of centres and surgeons on surgeons' ratings of expectations, which in turn influenced surgeon-patient differences in expectations. In contrast, neither patients' general characteristics nor patients' expectations were significantly different according to surgeons or centres. This is an interesting finding, as expectations of surgeons have not to our knowledge been described or compared by this kind of scale before, and further study on this subject could be of interest, as this effect might be related, at least partly, to the psychological profiles of each care providers. We chose not to standardize surgeons' evaluations, as the objective of this work was to study surgeon-patient concordance and communication for each surgeon–patient pair, rather than the appropriateness of patients' expectations in reference to a standard. It is unlikely that this surgeon effect on difference in expectations affected results of comparison tests between "more optimistic" and "more pessimistic" patients, as statistical analyses using mixed effect models and taking into account the clustered structure of the data, gave similar results.

Surprisingly, the three subscales evaluating surgeon-patient communication during clinical visits did not have any significant effect on surgeon-patient agreement in our study. A previous study noted that these scales, and especially information given by surgeons during clinical visit, predicted surgeon-patient concordance in expectations about THA [19]. An explanation could be that in our study, information was delivered not only during visits to surgeons, but also during structured information meetings with physiotherapists or by information leaflets and web sites. As our patients' interviews could take place at different times during this process, patients' assessments of provided information could vary.

This study has several strengths. The scarcity of missing data, due to the study protocol, which used telephone interviews to collect data, lowered the risks of bias. A unique evaluator performed all interviews, to ensure that questionnaires were understood and answered the same way by patients. Precautions were taken during our study to ensure that patients' and surgeons' assessments were done independently of each other.

As the aim of the study was to compare patients' and surgeons' judgments of the likely benefit from surgery, we chose to study "probability expectations". We thus used a slightly modified question format, asking patients how much improvement they expected in each domain rather than how important each domain was for them. This modified question has been used before and validated for this questionnaire [5,23]. The assessor ascertained during interviews that the question and its underlying concept were clearly understood by patients. The study of "value expectations" and relative importance of different domains for patients is a complementary approach in understanding patients' point of view and has been addressed by several authors [6,31].

Several items of the questionnaire were often considered "not applicable" by patients, mostly because patients never found themselves in such situations. When calculating the total score, scoring zero for such items could have made total scores lower, even when patients had high expectations on all applicable items. We chose to calculate total scores by omitting items which were considered inapplicable by patients and dividing scores by the

Table 3. Comparison between patients more optimistic than his surgeon and patients more pessimistic.

Patients characteristics		More optimistic patients (n = 44)	More pessimistic patients (n = 44)	p-value (univariate tests)[1]	p-value (adjusted for surgeon effect)[2]
Socio-demographic characteristics					
Recrutement site	Cochin	**12 (31%)**	**27 (69%)**	**0.003**	-
	Lariboisière	**27 (69%)**	**12 (31%)**		
	Gabriel Montpied	**5 (50%)**	**5 (50%)**		
Gender	Male	19 (43%)	25 (57%)	0.3	0.2
	Female	25 (57%)	19 (43%)		
Ipsilateral THA	Yes	7 (47%)	8 (53%)	1	0.6
	No	37 (51%)	36 (49%)		
Comorbidity Index	Score = 0	24 (59%)	17 (42%)	0.2	0.07
	Score>0	19 (41%)	27 (59%)		
Retirement	Yes	33 (53%)	29 (47%)	0.5	0.2
	No	11 (42%)	15 (58%)		
Profession	Liberal, senior officer	**19 (38%)**	**31 (62%)**	**0.02**	**0.03**
	Employee, worker	**25 (66%)**	**13 (34%)**		
Education	Post secondary	18 (44%)	23 (56%)	0.4	0.4
	Pre secondary	26 (55%)	21 (45%)		
Marital status	Married/in couple	22 (45%)	27 (55%)	0.4	0.2
	Single	22 (56%)	17 (44%)		
Sport	Recommended	41 (52%)	38 (48%)	0.5	0.1
	Not recommended	3 (33%)	6 (67%)		
Health status and survey scores					
Age		65.3±2.2	64.4±2.0	0.8	0.4
Body Mass Index (kg/m^2)		25.2±0.8	25.9±0.5	0.4	0.9
Trust in surgeon (NS, max = 10)		9.4±0.1	9.1±0.2	0.2	0.1
Communication	Patient participation	8.3±0.5	7.6±0.4	0.3	0.7
	Partnership building	5.7±0.3	5.7±0.3	0.9	0.8
	Information	11.7±0.5	10.8±0.5	0.2	0.8
Pain (NS, max = 10)		7.0±0.3	6.4±0.3	0.2	0.1
WOMAC (max = 32)		**20.4±0.8**	**17.2±0.8**	**0.006**	**0.006**
SF-12 : PCS (max = 100)		**29.4±1.1**	**34.6±1.3**	**0.003**	**0.005**
SF-12 : MCS (max = 100)		50.7±1.7	47.8±1.8	0.3	0.4

Bold characters indicate significative tests; NS = Numeric Scale; WOMAC = Western Ontario and McMaster Universities Osteoarthritis Index; SF-12 = Medical Outcome Study Short Form 12; PCS = Physical Component Summary; MCS = Medical Component Summary.
[1] = comparisons using chi-square tests and ANOVAs.
[2] = comparisons using mixed effect logistic models (random effects = surgeon).

number of applicable items. The two different methods of scoring gave very different scores (data not shown), and this question should be raised when using this questionnaire.

This study has several limitations. Telephone interviews were performed at different times before surgery, and it has been shown that patients' expectations can change over time [32], although it is not clear how patients expectations are built and modified during the pre-surgical period. We believe that these variations were small in our study, as delay before surgery did not significantly affect surgeon-patient agreement.

Another limitation lies in the lack of calibration of measures between surgeons and patients before the study. Although the same evaluator delivered questionnaires to surgeons and assessed patients, it is not sure that surgeons and patients assessed their expectations in the same manner. However, the comparability of surgeons' and patients' scores on this specific scale was shown in a previous study [23], where patients' evaluations through telephone interviews were compared to a reference rating from surgeons. Comparison showed that 49% of patients had scores that were within 6 points of surgeons' values before, and 54% after a specific educative intervention.

Patients were classified as more optimistic or more pessimistic in comparison to their surgeons' expectations, which could be a matter of discussion, as surgeons' expectations do not seem to be a good predictor of patient satisfaction after total knee arthroplasty [33]. It is not known which of both assessments best predicts patient outcome and satisfaction after THA, and this will be a topic for further research.

In conclusion, surgeons and patients often did not agree on what to expect from THA, but there was no systematic bias between both evaluations. Patients had higher expectations than surgeons on post-operative sports. Patients rated their expectations according to trust in surgeon and mental quality of life, whereas surgeons considered disability and physical quality of life. Patients with higher disability expected higher outcome than their surgeons.

Acknowledgments

We thank the Institut Fédératif de Recherche sur le Handicap (IFRH) - IFR 25 for their technical and logistic support. The data collected and analysed in this study will be available through the corresponding author (claire.jourdan@rpc.aphp.fr).

Author Contributions

Conceived and designed the experiments: CJ SP SD RN MH PA SB PR. Performed the experiments: CJ SD RN MH PA SB MG. Analyzed the data: CJ SP PR. Contributed reagents/materials/analysis tools: CJ MG SD. Wrote the paper: CJ SP PR.

References

1. Ethgen O, Bruyère O, Richy F, Dardennes C, Reginster J (2004) Health-related quality of life in total hip and total knee arthroplasty. A qualitative and systematic review of the literature. J Bone Joint Surg Am 86-A: 963–974.
2. (1995) NIH consensus conference: Total hip replacement. NIH Consensus Development Panel on Total Hip Replacement. Jun.. pp 1950–1956.
3. Kravitz RL (1996) Patients' expectations for medical care: an expanded formulation based on review of the literature. Med Care Res Rev 53: 3–27.
4. Mahomed NN, Liang MH, Cook EF, Daltroy LH, Fortin PR, et al. (2002) The importance of patient expectations in predicting functional outcomes after total joint arthroplasty. J Rheumatol 29: 1273–1279.
5. Groeneveld P, Kwoh C, Mor M, Appelt C, Geng M, et al. (2008) Racial differences in expectations of joint replacement surgery outcomes. Arthritis Rheum 59: 730–737.
6. Mancuso CA, Sculco TP, Salvati EA (2003) Patients with poor preoperative functional status have high expectations of total hip arthroplasty. J Arthroplasty 18: 872–878.
7. Lingard EA, Sledge CB, Learmonth ID, Kinemax Outcomes G (2006) Patient expectations regarding total knee arthroplasty: differences among the United States, United kingdom, and Australia. J Bone Joint Surg Am 88: 1201–1207.
8. Gandhi R, Davey JR, Mahomed N (2008) Patient Expectations Predict Greater Pain Relief with Joint Arthroplasty. J Arthroplasty.
9. Mancuso C, Jout J, Salvati E, Sculco T (2009) Fulfillment of patients' expectations for total hip arthroplasty. J Bone Joint Surg Am 91: 2073–2078.
10. Noble PC, Conditt MA, Cook KF, Mathis KB (2006) The John Insall Award: Patient expectations affect satisfaction with total knee arthroplasty. Clin Orthop Relat Res 452: 35–43.
11. Marcinkowski K, Wong V, Dignam D (2005) Getting back to the future: a grounded theory study of the patient perspective of total knee joint arthroplasty. Orthop Nurs 24: 202–209.
12. Ibrahim SA, Siminoff LA, Burant CJ, Kwoh CK (2002) Understanding ethnic differences in the utilization of joint replacement for osteoarthritis: the role of patient-level factors. Med Care 40: I44–51.
13. Suarez-Almazor ME, Souchek J, Kelly PA, O'Malley K, Byrne M, et al. (2005) Ethnic variation in knee replacement: patient preferences or uninformed disparity? Arch Intern Med 165: 1117–1124.
14. Toye FM, Barlow J, Wright C, Lamb SE (2006) Personal meanings in the construction of need for total knee replacement surgery. Soc Sci Med 63: 43–53.
15. Kwoh C, Ibrahim S (2001) Rheumatology patient and physician concordance with respect to important health and symptom status outcomes. Arthritis Rheum 45: 372–377.
16. Brokelman R, van Loon C, van Susante J, van Kampen A, Veth R (2008) Patients are more satisfied than they expected after joint arthroplasty. Acta Orthop Belg 74: 59–63.
17. Lieberman J, Dorey F, Shekelle P, Schumacher L, Thomas B, et al. (1996) Differences between patients' and physicians' evaluations of outcome after total hip arthroplasty. J Bone Joint Surg Am 78: 835–838.
18. Moran M, Khan A, Sochart DH, Andrew G (2003) Expect the best, prepare for the worst: surgeon and patient expectation of the outcome of primary total hip and knee replacement. Ann R Coll Surg Engl 85: 204–206.
19. Street RL, Jr., Richardson MN, Cox V, Suarez-Almazor ME (2009) (Mis)understanding in patient-health care provider communication about total knee replacement. Arthritis Rheum 61: 100–107.
20. Mancuso CA, Salvati EA, Johanson NA, Peterson MG, Charlson ME (1997) Patients' expectations and satisfaction with total hip arthroplasty. J Arthroplasty 12: 387–396.
21. Wright JG, Young NL, Waddell JP (2000) The reliability and validity of the self-reported patient-specific index for total hip arthroplasty. J Bone Joint Surg Am 82: 829–837.
22. Beaton D, Bombardier C, Guillemin F, Ferraz M (2000) Guidelines for the process of cross-cultural adaptation of self-report measures. Spine 25: 3186–3191.
23. Mancuso CA, Graziano S, Briskie LM, Peterson MG, Pellicci PM, et al. (2008) Randomized trials to modify patients' preoperative expectations of hip and knee arthroplasties. Clin Orthop Relat Res 466: 424–431.
24. Klein GR, Levine BR, Hozack WJ, Strauss EJ, D'Antonio JA, et al. (2007) Return to athletic activity after total hip arthroplasty. Consensus guidelines based on a survey of the Hip Society and American Association of Hip and Knee Surgeons. J Arthroplasty 22: 171–175.
25. Charlson M, Pompei P, Ales K, MacKenzie C (1987) A new method of classifying prognostic comorbidity in longitudinal studies: development and validation. J Chronic Dis 40: 373–383.
26. Bellamy N, Buchanan W, Goldsmith C, Campbell J, Stitt L (1988) Validation study of WOMAC: a health status instrument for measuring clinically important patient relevant outcomes to antirheumatic drug therapy in patients with osteoarthritis of the hip or knee. J Rheumatol 15: 1833–1840.
27. Tubach F, Baron G, Falissard B, Logeart I, Dougados M, et al. (2005) Using patients' and rheumatologists' opinions to specify a short form of the WOMAC function subscale. Ann Rheum Dis 64: 75–79.
28. Stucki G, Liang MH, Phillips C, Katz JN (1995) The Short Form-36 is preferable to the SIP as a generic health status measure in patients undergoing elective total hip arthroplasty. Arthritis Care Res 8: 174–181.
29. Ware JJ, Kosinski M, Keller S (1996) A 12-Item Short-Form Health Survey: construction of scales and preliminary tests of reliability and validity. Med Care 34: 220–233.
30. Bland J, Altman D (1986) Statistical methods for assessing agreement between two methods of clinical measurement. Lancet 1: 307–310.
31. Wright JG, Young NL (1997) The patient-specific index: asking patients what they want. J Bone Joint Surg Am 79: 974–983.
32. Lieberman JR, Thomas BJ, Finerman GA, Dorey F (2003) Patients' reasons for undergoing total hip arthroplasty can change over time. J Arthroplasty 18: 63–68.
33. Meijerink HJ, Brokelman RB, van Loon CJ, van Kampen A, de Waal Malefijt MC (2008) Surgeon's expectations do not predict the outcome of a total knee arthroplasty. Arch Orthop Trauma Surg.

20

From the Trenches: A Cross-Sectional Study Applying the GRADE Tool in Systematic Reviews of Healthcare Interventions

Lisa Hartling[1,2]*, Ricardo M. Fernandes[3], Jennifer Seida[1], Ben Vandermeer[1], Donna M. Dryden[1]

1 Department of Pediatrics, Alberta Research Centre for Health Evidence, University of Alberta, Edmonton, Canada, **2** Department of Pediatrics, Cochrane Child Health Field, University of Alberta, Edmonton, Alberta, Canada, **3** Gulbenkian Programme for Advanced Medical Education; Departamento da Criança e da Família (Child and Family Department), Hospital de Santa Maria; Laboratório de Farmacologia Clínica e Terapêutica (Clinical Pharmacology and Therapeutics), Instituto de Medicina Molecular, Lisboa, Portugal

Abstract

Background: GRADE was developed to address shortcomings of tools to rate the quality of a body of evidence. While much has been published about GRADE, there are few empirical and systematic evaluations.

Objective: To assess GRADE for systematic reviews (SRs) in terms of inter-rater agreement and identify areas of uncertainty.

Design: Cross-sectional, descriptive study.

Methods: We applied GRADE to three SRs (n = 48, 66, and 75 studies, respectively) with 29 comparisons and 12 outcomes overall. Two reviewers graded evidence independently for outcomes deemed clinically important a priori. Inter-rater reliability was assessed using kappas for four main domains (risk of bias, consistency, directness, and precision) and overall quality of evidence.

Results: For the first review, reliability was: $\kappa = 0.41$ for risk of bias; 0.84 consistency; 0.18 precision; and 0.44 overall quality. Kappa could not be calculated for directness as one rater assessed all items as direct; assessors agreed in 41% of cases. For the second review reliability was: 0.37 consistency and 0.19 precision. Kappa could not be assessed for other items; assessors agreed in 33% of cases for risk of bias; 100% directness; and 58% overall quality. For the third review, reliability was: 0.06 risk of bias; 0.79 consistency; 0.21 precision; and 0.18 overall quality. Assessors agreed in 100% of cases for directness. Precision created the most uncertainty due to difficulties in identifying "optimal" information size and "clinical decision threshold", as well as making assessments when there was no meta-analysis. The risk of bias domain created uncertainty, particularly for nonrandomized studies.

Conclusions: As researchers with varied levels of training and experience use GRADE, there is risk for variability in interpretation and application. This study shows variable agreement across the GRADE domains, reflecting areas where further guidance is required.

Editor: German Malaga, Universidad Peruana Cayetano Heredia, Peru

Funding: The authors have no support or funding to report.

* E-mail: hartling@ualberta.ca

Introduction

The GRADE tool (Grading of Recommendations Assessment, Development and Evaluation) has been developed and refined over recent years by an international working group (www.gradeworkinggroup.org). One of the motivations for developing the tool was to address shortcomings of other approaches to rating the strength or quality of a body of evidence. The GRADE tool offers a "common, sensible, and transparent approach to grading quality of evidence and strength of recommendations". It represents an important tool for decision-makers as it provides a mechanism to bridge the gap from evidence synthesis to application of the evidence for informed decision-making.

Much has been published about the GRADE tool (www.gradeworkinggroup.org/publications/index.htm). One of the first citations regarding the GRADE tool appeared in the *Canadian Medical Association Journal* in 2003 [1] with a second in the *British Medical Journal* soon after [2]. Recently, a series of publications about the GRADE tool was published in the *Journal of Clinical Epidemiology* [3–12]. These reports provide details about the development of the tool and general instructions on how the tool should be applied. GRADEPro software is available which offers a structured format to present the information, with an accompanying handbook that contains instructions and examples (www.ims.cochrane.org/revman/gradepro) [13].

In brief, reviewers assess the body of evidence available for a given question and outcome with respect to several key domains. These include risk of bias, consistency, precision, directness, and publication bias. Additional domains that can be considered are magnitude of effect, confounding, and dose-response relationship. In general, evidence from randomized trials may start at high quality while evidence from observational studies starts at low quality. The evidence can be upgraded or downgraded based on the remaining domains. This results in a final assessment of quality of the evidence into one of four categories: high, moderate, low, or very low. These categories reflect the confidence the assessors have that the evidence represents the true effect and is unlikely to change with future research. Assessors are encouraged to document the reasons for their decisions for transparency.

Use of the GRADE tool has recently been adopted by The Cochrane Collaboration, and grading the evidence is now a recommended step within Cochrane systematic reviews [14]. Summary of Findings tables can be developed using GRADEPro software and integrated into Cochrane reviews. These tables show effect estimates for key outcomes as well as assessments of the quality of evidence based on the GRADE tool. This provides an effective summary of the evidence for the reader. By providing a quality of evidence assessment alongside the effect estimates, the reader has some indication of how much confidence they can place in the findings. Moreover, the reader has a sense of whether "the evidence reflects the true effect" and whether additional research would likely change the effect estimate or the reader's confidence in the estimate [15].

Despite numerous publications about the GRADE tool (including some criticisms [16]), there have been few empirical and systematic evaluations of applying the tool in practice [17]. As grading the evidence is now a recommended step in Cochrane systematic reviews and in other evidence synthesis initiatives outside The Cochrane Collaboration [15,18], new users with variable levels of training are likely to be applying the tool. The widespread use of the tool by users with variable training has implications for interpretation and application of the tool.

The objectives of this study were to apply GRADE in systematic reviews in order to assess inter-rater reliability and identify areas of uncertainty. Our focus was on use of the tool to rate quality of evidence, not the strength of recommendations. The goal was to identify areas that require further guidance in order to provide clarity for users, particularly systematic reviewers.

Methods

We applied the GRADE tool to three systematic reviews that we conducted at our research centre [19–21]. The systematic reviews were broad in scope and each included several interventions and comparisons. They were on varied clinical topics and involved different types of interventions (e.g., pharmacological and non-pharmacological) and outcomes. Further, one included only randomized controlled trials (RCTs) while the other two also included select nonrandomized study (NRS) designs. The topics of the systematic reviews were: 1) steroids and bronchodilators for bronchiolitis; 2) operative and nonoperative interventions for rotator cuff tears; and, 3) pain management interventions for hip fracture (Table 1).

For each review, two reviewers independently graded the evidence for key outcomes. The outcomes were selected a priori by the team of investigators associated with each review based on clinical importance. In general the team of investigators for each review included at least two clinicians with expertise in the area and at least one methodologist with expertise in research methods and systematic reviews. Assessments were made for the four main domains (risk of bias, consistency, directness, and precision), as well as overall quality of evidence (high, moderate, low, very low [or insufficient]) (Table 2). The GRADE tool includes a fifth main domain (publication bias); however, we followed guidance set out by the Agency for Healthcare Research and Quality Evidence-based Practice Center Program which considers publication bias an optional domain [15]. Further, the GRADE tool has additional domains, including dose-response association, possible confounding, and strength of association (magnitude of effect); we chose to focus on the main domains for this study.

Four individuals were involved in assessing the quality of evidence. All individuals had substantial experience and/or training in systematic review methods. LH has doctoral level training in research methods, more than 10 years of SR experience, and clinical training and experience in rehabilitation medicine. DD has doctoral level training in epidemiology and more than 5 years of SR experience. RF is a practicing pediatrician currently completing a doctoral degree with 4 years of SR experience. AA-S is a physician with specialty training, a doctoral degree in research methods, and 6 years of SR experience. The reviews were assessed by LH and RF (bronchiolitis), LH and DD (rotator cuff), and DD and AA-S (hip fracture). All reviewers read and were familiar with guidance on applying the GRADE tool [13,15].

Within reviews, we calculated inter-rater reliability between reviewers for each domain and overall quality of evidence using kappa statistics. Agreement was categorized as poor (0.00), slight (0.01–0.20), fair (0.21–0.40), moderate (0.41–0.60), substantial (0.61–0.80), or almost perfect (0.81–1.00) using one of the standard approaches [22]. We were unable to calculate kappa if one or both reviewers in the pair always gave the same assessment for the domain (e.g., directness always assessed as direct). In this case, we calculated the percent of assessments within the domain for which the two reviewers agreed. For each domain, we identified items that may have led to discrepancies between reviewers. We have presented this information in a narrative summary.

Results

Overall results are presented in Table 3 and are described by review and by domain below.

Case 1: Steroids and bronchodilators for bronchiolitis [19]

We included 48 RCTs in this review. We graded the evidence for six comparisons and four outcomes (Table 1). Further, we pooled and graded the evidence separately for inpatient and outpatient populations. There were a total of 51 assessments. Inter-rater reliability ranged from slight for precision ($\kappa = 0.18$) to almost perfect for consistency ($\kappa = 0.84$). Reliability for overall quality of evidence was moderate ($\kappa = 0.44$).

Case 2: Operative and nonoperative interventions for rotator cuff tears [20]

This review included 27 trials (21 RCTs and 6 controlled clinical trials) and 39 cohort studies. We graded evidence for 11 comparisons and four outcomes (Table 1). There were a total of 24 assessments. Inter-rater reliability was calculated for two domains and was slight for precision ($\kappa = 0.19$) and fair for consistency ($\kappa = 0.37$). Reliability could not be assessed for the other domains or overall strength of evidence, as one rater assessed all the same.

Table 1. Comparisons and outcomes examined in the systematic reviews.

Review	Comparisons	Outcomes
Case 1: Steroids and bronchodilators for bronchiolitis [19]	• steroid vs. placebo	• admissions
	• epinephrine vs. placebo	• length of stay
	• salbutamol vs. placebo	• clinical score
	• epinephrine vs. salbutamol	• adverse events
	• epinephrine and dexamethasone combined vs. placebo	
	• epinephrine and dexamethasone combined vs. salbutamol	
Case 2: Operative and nonoperative interventions for rotator cuff tears [20]	• early vs. late surgical RCR	• health-related quality of life
	• open vs. mini-open RCR	• function
	• mini-open vs. arthroscopic RCR	• time to return to work
	• open RCR vs. arthroscopic RCR	• cuff integrity
	• open or mini-open RCR vs. arthroscopic RCR	
	• open RCR vs. open or arthroscopic debridement	
	•	
	•	
	• arthroscopic RCR vs. RCR plus acromioplasty	
	• arthroscopic RCR vs. acromioplasty alone	
	• single-row vs. double-row suture anchor repairs	
	• mattress vs. simple stitch	
	• continuous passive motion with physical therapy vs. physical therapy alone	
Case 3: Pain management interventions for hip fracture [21]	• analgesia vs. other	• acute pain
	• spinal vs. general anesthesia	• chronic pain
	• continuous vs. single administration of spinal anesthesia	• mortality
	• addition of fentanyl to spinal anesthesia	• incidence of serious adverse events
	• addition of morphine to spinal anesthesia	
	• addition of sulfentanil to spinal anesthesia	
	• comparative alternative medicine	
	• nerve blocks vs. no block	
	• nerve blocks vs. regional anesthesia	
	• neurostimulation	
	• rehabilitation	
	• traction	

RCR = rotator cuff repair.

Table 2. GRADE domains and assessment options*.

Risk of bias	Consistency	Directness	Precision	Overall Strength of Evidence
• High	• Consistent	• Direct	• Precise	• High
• Medium	• Inconsistent	• Indirect	• Imprecise	• Moderate
• Low	• Unknown or not applicable			• Low
				• Insufficient (very low)

*Based on Owens et al. [15].

Table 3. Inter-rater reliability and agreement for GRADE domains and overall strength of evidence.

Domain	Case 1 [19]		Case 2 [20]		Case 3 [21]	
	Kappa or percent agreement	Level of agreement based on kappa	Kappa or percent agreement	Level of agreement based on kappa	Kappa or percent agreement	Level of agreement based on kappa
Risk of bias	0.41	Moderate	33%	n/a	0.06	Slight
Consistency	0.84	Almost perfect	0.37	Fair	0.79	Substantial
Directness	41%	n/a	100%	n/a	100%	n/a
Precision	0.18	Slight	0.19	Slight	0.21	Fair
Overall strength of evidence	0.44	Moderate	58%	n/a	0.18	Slight

Agreement for these domains was 33% for risk of bias, 100% for directness, and 58% for overall quality of evidence.

Case 3: Pain management interventions for hip fracture [21]

This review included 65 RCTs and 10 cohort studies. We graded evidence for 12 comparisons and four outcomes (Table 1) for a total of 36 assessments. Inter-rater reliability ranged from slight ($\kappa = 0.06$) for risk of bias to substantial ($\kappa = 0.79$) for consistency. Reliability for overall quality of evidence was slight ($\kappa = 0.18$). There was 100% agreement between reviewers for directness.

Sources of disagreement by domain

Risk of bias. One of the key challenges that arose during assessment of this domain was how to integrate risk of bias or quality assessments of the individual studies. This was more straightforward for RCTs than NRS. For instance, if the majority of evidence came from RCTs assessed as low risk of bias based on the Cochrane Risk of Bias tool [14], then we assessed the overall body of evidence for the comparison and outcome of interest as low risk of bias. That is, there was room for a fairly direct translation from assessments using the Risk of Bias tool to the risk of bias domain. However, there was more discrepancy when other quality assessment tools were used, particularly for NRS. For example, questions arose regarding how to translate a range of scores for cohort studies on the Newcastle Ottawa Scale [23] (from 0 to 9) into one of three risk of bias classifications. Moreover, the move away from overall quality scores or summaries towards a component approach for individual studies [14] was found to be incongruous with forcing an overall assessment of the risk of bias for a group of studies.

Another question that arose was whether there should be pre-specified starting points for different study designs. For instance, it was questioned whether RCTs should always start out as low risk of bias overall whereas all NRS start out as high risk of bias overall. One restriction that we noted within the GRADE recommendations is that NRS are considered as a homogeneous body and start at high risk of bias. Moreover, they are all referred to as "observational studies." This does not distinguish between studies that may be more or less prone to bias based on design features, such as prospective comparative studies versus a single sample before-after study. We questioned whether there should be a distinction among "observational studies" where some would start at high risk of bias because of key design limitations whereas others would start at moderate risk of bias based on more rigorous methodological approaches. For example, in the review of operative and nonoperative interventions for rotator cuff injuries, we considered prospective cohort studies that controlled for confounding to be less prone to bias and graded these higher than retrospective studies that failed to control for key confounders.

A final key question that arose for the risk of bias domain was whether there should be different thresholds for different study designs. For instance, should RCTs always be higher in terms of risk of bias compared with NRS. Further, should the minimum threshold for RCTs be moderate risk of bias because the use of an appropriate randomized design always ensures less risk of bias compared with NRS. Alternatively, is it ever appropriate to rate NRS as low risk of bias given that they do not employ randomization and are always prone to bias due to potential imbalance between groups being compared, even when rigorous design or analytic methods are used to attempt to control for confounding.

Consistency. When a meta-analysis was available for the comparison of interest, we relied heavily on the I^2 statistic, which provides an indication of the extent of statistical heterogeneity across a set of studies [14]. As a general guideline if I^2 was greater than 50%, the results were considered inconsistent. Similarly if I^2 was less than 20%, the results were considered consistent. However, these were general guides and were not consistently applied; there were also areas where judgment was required. More disagreement arose when there was no meta-analysis. In general, the reviewers took a qualitative approach to assessing consistency across studies. For example, they considered whether the estimates were similar in terms of magnitude and direction of effect, as well as statistical significance. The somewhat different approach with and without meta-analysis raises the issue of whether assessments are made with differential standards depending on whether a meta-analysis is done. Often the reason for not conducting a meta-analysis, or pooling data, is due to heterogeneity across studies; hence, one option is that the default is "inconsistent" or "unknown" when there is no meta-analysis.

Directness. The two main criteria we used to assess this domain were whether the outcomes were intermediate or surrogate rather than the final health outcome, and whether the evidence came from direct head-to-head comparisons. We found that determining whether an outcome was intermediate or surrogate was somewhat context-specific and dependent on the research question posed in the review. For example, pain may be considered a surrogate or an intermediate outcome related to function. In the hip fracture review, pain itself was a primary outcome of interest, whereas in the rotator cuff review, pain was intermediate and function was among the primary outcomes of interest. We felt that directness with respect to whether the outcome is intermediate or surrogate could be determined at the outset of the review, thus eliminating disagreement at the stage of grading the evidence.

We did not assess for applicability within this domain as there are discrepancies in current published guidance for grading evidence. One approach restricts the assessment to the two main criteria above [15], whereas the other approach includes considerations of generalizability or applicability of the findings [13]. The first approach considers generalizability outside the context of grading the evidence and within the context of making recommendations for application of the evidence, whereas the second would consider an indirect population as a possible source of indirectness.

Precision. This domain consistently had low reliability. Assessments were particularly problematic when no meta-analysis had been conducted as there was no confidence interval around a single estimate to determine the inclusion or exclusion of no effect or important benefit/harm. Similarly, assessment of precision was difficult when multiple meta-analyses were available for a given outcome due to differences in how an outcome was measured across studies. For instance, precision may have varied between a meta-analysis of pain measured on a continuous scale and a meta-analysis reporting the proportion of patients experiencing pain. In these cases, we relied heavily on the minimum thresholds for number of events (dichotomous outcomes) or subjects (continuous outcomes) that are specified in the GRADEPro Handbook [13].

We found it critical to set, a priori, a clinical decision threshold [12] for each outcome. This is not currently a standard step within systematic reviews. Furthermore, in some clinical areas there is not a well-defined or generally accepted threshold; in other cases these are based on expert opinion or consensus statements and have not been validated in patient-oriented outcomes. There is a need to develop this information for different clinical areas and guidance is needed for how this should be done.

Much of the guidance in the GRADEPro Handbook is directed toward assessing precision around evidence of effect [13]. There was, however, a lack of clarity around whether the same rules apply regarding evidence of no effect. Figure 1 illustrates a finding of no difference between treatment and placebo with a narrow confidence interval that does not include an important difference. Further, the total sample size exceeded the stipulated threshold of 400. However, we were unclear whether the same thresholds applied in order to rate the finding as precise or whether different sample size thresholds were needed akin to differences in sample sizes for trials with different hypotheses (e.g., superiority, inferiority, non-inferiority, equivalence).

Overall quality of evidence. We found inconsistencies in our approach to upgrading and downgrading as well as the extent of upgrading and downgrading. For the most part, we used study design as our starting point and downgraded by one step for each domain that was not met; this approach appears to be consistent with the GRADE recommendation [13]. There were discrepancies between reviewers in the bottom threshold of overall quality: some reviewers felt that if there was some evidence (even from one study), the overall quality should be rated "low", while "very low" (alternatively referred to as "insufficient" [15]) should be reserved for cases where there was no evidence at all.

Other general observations

As we gained experience with applying GRADE for various review topics which had different questions and different types of evidence, we questioned whether we should aim for consistency across different bodies of evidence. For instance, should the evidence for the rotator cuff project, which was generally based on weak study designs with high risk of bias, ever be rated the same or higher than topics where the evidence comes only from RCTs. For instance, in the bronchiolitis review, some of the evidence was graded as low because it was based on a single trial, therefore the consistency was unknown and the confidence interval just crossed the null. However, the trial was at low risk of bias and was adequately powered to detect differences in the outcome of interest. Moreover, it was the largest trial conducted to date in the field, in some cases exceeding the sample size of all the other trials combined. Yet, the grade of evidence was comparable or in some cases lower than the body of evidence for the rotator cuff review which was driven by NRS.

Two additional points were raised during the course of our work. First, we questioned whether we should develop strict rules for application of the GRADE tool in the work at our centre with the intent of increasing agreement between reviewers and across reviews; or, alternatively provide general guidance and reach consensus within the different reviews or clinical/topic areas. The latter approach may yield more inconsistency across reviews although this may provide important information for the end-user. For instance, if the reviewers report their agreement, the reader can judge the extent to which the specific issue is open to judgment and interpret the evidence more or less cautiously based on this information.

The second additional point was challenges with terminology. We found it confusing for the risk of bias domain to use the same terminology as the process of assessing risk of bias of individual

	Steroid			Placebo				Mean Difference
Study or Subgroup	Mean	SD	Total	Mean	SD	Total	Weight	IV, Random, 95% CI
Bentur 2005	5.469	7.87	29	6.288	8.778	32	0.3%	-0.82 [-5.00, 3.36]
Cade 2000	2	1.48	82	2	2.22	79	11.7%	0.00 [-0.59, 0.59]
De Boeck 1997	6	2.619	14	6.6	1.162	15	2.1%	-0.60 [-2.09, 0.89]
Gomez 2007	0.654	0.192	24	0.779	0.223	25	58.4%	-0.13 [-0.24, -0.01]
Klassen 1997	2.375	2.39	35	2	0.722	32	6.3%	0.38 [-0.46, 1.21]
Richter 1997	2	2.647	21	3	1.626	19	2.5%	-1.00 [-2.35, 0.35]
Teeratakulpisarn 2007	2.258	1.246	89	2.817	1.742	85	17.6%	-0.56 [-1.01, -0.11]
Zhang 2003	6	4.05	28	5	3.34	24	1.2%	1.00 [-1.01, 3.01]
Total (95% CI)			**322**			**311**	**100.0%**	**-0.18 [-0.39, 0.04]**

Heterogeneity: Tau² = 0.02; Chi² = 8.33, df = 7 (P = 0.30); I² = 16%
Test for overall effect: Z = 1.58 (P = 0.12)

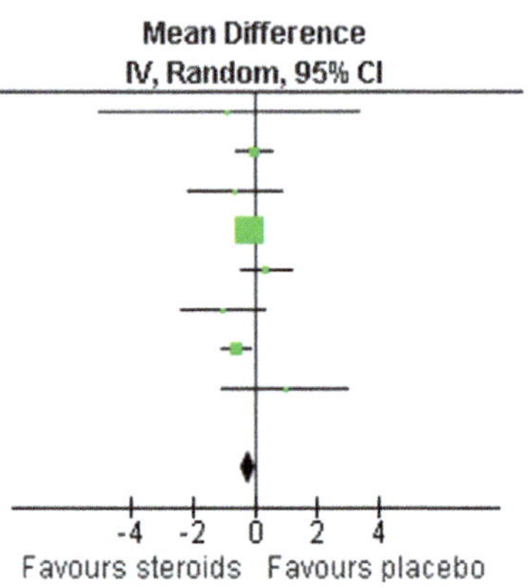

Figure 1. Example of meta-graph showing no difference in length of stay between treatments.

studies. Similarly, the overall quality of evidence was at times confused with quality of studies. Moreover, guidance documents differentially referred to the same overall assessment as quality of evidence [13] and strength of evidence [15].

Discussion

Rating a body of evidence using the GRADE tool is becoming an important and recommended step in systematic reviews and other evidence synthesis initiatives. Rating the quality of a body of evidence is valuable for the end-users of evidence syntheses as it provides an indication of the confidence they can place in the results. Moreover, it is a key step in translating the body of evidence into clinical practice guidelines. We undertook this study to identify areas of uncertainty in applying the GRADE tool in order to inform the evidence synthesis efforts at our centre. Our research identified key areas where further guidance is needed to inform the application of the tool. Specifically, the domains of precision and risk of bias created the most inconsistency and challenges, whereas directness and consistency were more straightforward (although still had substantial disagreement at times). Further, we encountered challenges when there were no meta-analyses upon which to base assessments, when outcomes were measured in different ways, and when evidence included nonrandomized studies.

Application of the GRADE tool is complex as evidenced by the series of 20 articles that are currently being published in the *Journal of Clinical Epidemiology* [11]. It is clear that both methodological and clinical expertise is required when applying the GRADE tool. Further, we believe the GRADE developers would agree that specific training in use of the GRADE tool is recommended. Our concern is that with widespread adoption of the GRADE tool in Cochrane systematic reviews and non-Cochrane synthesis efforts, there will be inconsistent application of the tool and context-specific decision rules that emerge. Moreover, different organizations or researchers may adapt the GRADE approach for their specific interests, as has already occurred [15,24]. This has the potential to yield discordant assessments, which will ultimately affect those using this information to make decisions and recommendations for clinical care. To alleviate some of these concerns, all reviews using tools such as GRADE should have a minimum of two reviewers independently apply the tool, their agreement should be reported, and the basis for their decisions should be transparent.

Strengths and limitations

This is one of the first systematic and empirical evaluations of applying the GRADE tool in systematic reviews. We recognize that the tool is not meant to eliminate disagreements nor the need for judgments [11]. Our intent in measuring agreement was to identify areas of greatest uncertainty and explore reasons for the discrepancies. We graded the evidence for three systematic reviews; while the number of reviews was small, there were numerous comparisons and outcomes within each review (29 comparisons and 12 outcomes overall). The reviews also represented a variety of clinical topics and types of evidence. The reviewers who applied the GRADE tool had not undergone formal training in the use of the tool; however, the reviewers all had extensive experience and training in research methods and specifically systematic reviews. We expect that many individuals who apply the GRADE tool may also do so without formal training. Hence, our experience reflects what we are likely to see in practice. Finally, we did not assess the domain of publication bias. This is specified as one of the main domains in the GRADEPro Handbook but not by other guidance documents, and specifically the guidance offered by the stakeholder group for two of our three reviews [15]. Nevertheless, in most cases, we did not have sufficient numbers of studies within outcomes and comparisons to formally test for publication bias.

Conclusions

As the GRADE developers acknowledge, "refinements are inevitable" for new and innovative tools such as GRADE [11]. The intent of our research was to describe our experience applying to GRADE tool and to document the areas that created uncertainty and where clarity and guidance are needed. We trust that our results will serve to optimize the utility of GRADE as a tool for evidence synthesis and practice recommendations.

Acknowledgments

We acknowledge Dr. Ahmed Abou-Setta for assessing the strength of evidence for one of the systematic reviews.

Author Contributions

Conceived and designed the experiments: LH RF JS BV DD. Performed the experiments: LH RF JS DD. Analyzed the data: LH RF JS BV DD. Contributed reagents/materials/analysis tools: BV. Wrote the paper: LH RF JS BV DD.

References

1. Schunemann HJ, Best D, Vist G, Oxman AD (2003) Letters, numbers, symbols and words: how to communicate grades of evidence and recommendations. Can Med Assoc J 169: 677–680.
2. Atkins D, Best D, Briss PA, Eccles M, Falck-Ytter Y, et al. (2004) Grading quality of evidence and strength of recommendations. Brit Med J 328: 1490.
3. Guyatt G, Oxman A, Akl E, Kunz R, Vist G, et al. (2011) GRADE guidelines: 1. Introduction-GRADE evidence profiles and summary of findings tables. J Clin Epidemiol 64(4): 383–394.
4. Guyatt G, Oxman A, Kunz R, Atkins D, Brozek J, et al. (2011) GRADE guidelines: 2. Framing the question and deciding on important outcomes. J Clin Epidemiol 64: 395–400.
5. Balshem H, Helfand M, Schuenemann H, Oxman A, Kunz RJ, et al. (2011) GRADE guidelines: 3. Rating the quality of evidence. J Clin Epidemiol 64: 401–406.
6. Guyatt GH, Oxman AD, Vist G, Kunz R, Brozek J, et al. (2011) GRADE guidelines: 4. Rating the quality of evidence–study limitations (risk of bias). J Clin Epidemiol 64: 407–415.
7. Guyatt GH, Oxman AD, Montori V, Vist G, Kunz R, et al. (2011) GRADE guidelines: 5. Rating the quality of evidence-publication bias. J Clin Epidemiol 64: 1277–1282.
8. Guyatt GH, Oxman AD, Kunz R, Woodcock J, Brozek J, et al. (2011) GRADE guidelines: 7. Rating the quality of evidence-inconsistency. J Clin Epidemiol 64: 1294–1302.
9. Guyatt GH, Oxman AD, Kunz R, Woodcock J, Brozek J, et al. (2011) GRADE guidelines: 8. Rating the quality of evidence-indirectness. J Clin Epidemiol 64: 1303–1310.
10. Guyatt GH, Oxman AD, Sultan S, Glasziou P, Akl EA, et al. (2011) GRADE guidelines: 9. Rating up the quality of evidence. J Clin Epidemiol 64: 1311–1316.
11. Guyatt GH, Oxman AD, Schunemann HJ, Tugwell P, Knottnerus A (2011) GRADE guidelines: a new series of articles in the Journal of Clinical Epidemiology. J Clin Epidemiol 64: 380–382.
12. Guyatt G, Oxman AD, Kunz R, Brozek J, onso-Coello P, et al. (2011) GRADE guidelines 6. Rating the quality of evidence-imprecision. J Clin Epidemiol 64: 1283–1293.
13. Schunemann H, Brozek J, Oxman A (2009) GRADE handbook for grading quality of evidence and strength of recommendation. Version 3.2 [update March 2009]. The Grade Working Group.
14. Higgins JPT, Green S, eds. (2011) Cochrane handbook for systematic reviews of interventions Version 5.1.0 [updated March 2011]. The Cochrane Collaboration, available from www.cochrane-handbook.org.
15. Owens D, Lohr K, Atkins D, Treadwell J, Reston J, et al. (2010) AHRQ series paper 5: grading the strength of a body of evidence when comparing medical interventions - agency for healthcare research and quality and the effective health-care program. J Clin Epidemiol 63: 513–523.

16. Kavanagh BP (2009) The GRADE system for rating clinical guidelines. PLoS Med 6(9): e1000094.
17. Atkins D, Briss PA, Eccles M, Flottorp S, Guyatt GH, et al. (2005) Systems for grading the quality of evidence and the strength of recommendations II: pilot study of a new system. BMC Health Serv Res 5: 25.
18. IOM (Institute of Medicine) (2011) Finding What Works in Health Care. Standards for Systematic Reviews. Washington, DC: The National Academies Press.
19. Hartling L, Fernandes R, Bialy L, Milne S, Johnson D, et al. (2011) A systematic review and meta-analysis of steroids and bronchodilators for acute bronchiolitis. Brit Med J 342: d1714.
20. Seida J, LeBlanc C, Schouten J, Mousavi S, Hartling L, et al. (2011) Systematic review: nonoperative and operative treatments for rotator cuff tears. Ann Intern Med 153(4): 246–255.
21. Abou-Setta A, Beaupre L, Rashiq S, Dryden D, Hamm M, et al. (2011) Comparative effectiveness of pain management interventions for hip fracture: a systematic review. Ann Intern Med 155: 234–245.
22. Landis JR, Koch GG (1977) The measurement of observer agreement for categorical data. Biometrics 33: 159–174.
23. Wells G, Brodsky L, O'Connell D, Shea B, Henry D, Mayank S, Tugwell P (2003) An Evaluation of the Newcastle-Ottawa Scale (NOS): an assessment tool for evaluating the quality of non-randomized studies [abstract]. XI Cochrane Colloquium: Evidence, Health Care and Culture; 2003 Oct 26–31; Barcelona, Spain.
24. Jamtvedt G, Dahm KT, Christie A, Moe RH, Haavardsholm E, et al. (2008) Physical therapy interventions for patients with osteoarthritis of the knee: an overview of systematic reviews. Phys Ther 88: 123–136.

Comparison between Bipolar Hemiarthroplasty and Total Hip Arthroplasty for Unstable Intertrochanteric Fractures in Elderly Osteoporotic Patients

Lihong Fan, Xiaoqian Dang, Kunzheng Wang*

Department of Orthopaedic Surgery, Second Affiliated Hospital, Medical School of Xi'an Jiaotong University, Xi'an, Shaanxi Province, People's Republic of China

Abstract

The present study was conducted to compare bipolar hemiarthroplasty (BA) with total hip arthroplasty (THA) in treatment of unstable intertrochanteric fractures in elderly osteoporotic patients. The THA group included 14 males and 26 females with a mean age of 73.4 years, and the BA group included 27 males and 45 females with a mean age of 76.5 years. Significant difference existed between the two groups in operation time, blood loss, transfusion volume and cost of hospitalization, while no remarkable difference was identified in hospitalization period, general complications, joint function, pain, rate of revision and mortality. No dislocation was observed in BA group while 3 occurred in THA group. The results indicated that for unstable intertrochanteric fractures in elderly osteoporotic patients, BA seems to be a better or more reasonable choice compared with THA for the reason of less blood loss, shorter operation time, lower cost and no dislocation.

Editor: Chi Zhang, University of Texas Southwestern Medical Center, United States of America

Funding: This study was supported by the National Natural Science Foundation of China (Grant No. 81101363). The funders had no role in study design, data collection and analysis, decision to publish, or preparation of the manuscript.

Competing Interests: The authors have declared that no competing interests exist.

* E-mail: drwangkz@eyou.com

Introduction

Intertrochanteric fractures of the femur often occur in elderly people. Their incidence has increased due to the increased life expectancy and osteoporosis [1]. Rigid internal fixation and early mobilization are the key points of the treatment. Stable intertrochanteric fractures can be easily treated by osteosynthesis with predictable good results [2,3], whereas the management of unstable intertrochantric fractures is challenging because of poor bone quality, osteoporosis and other underlying diseases [4,5]. Although there are some fixation methods such as fixed nail plate, sliding hip screw and intramedullary interlocking devices, no one guarantees absolute fracture stability and complete bone union in elderly patients [6–8]. Osteoporosis and instability are two of the most important factors leading to unsatisfactory results of treatment [9,10], and in the elderly the coexistence of unstable, comminuted fractures with osteoporosis worsens the prognosis [11].

Due to high failure rate and complications associated with internal fixation, prosthetic replacement has been recommended by some authors as primary treatment for unstable intertrochanteric fractures [12–14]. There have been various reports of successful outcomes after the use of hemiarthroplasty and total hip arthroplasty (THA) [15–17]. Stappaerts et al., in a prospective randomized study, concluded that primary cemented endoprosthesis brought better results than compression hip screw in unstable intertrochanteric fractures in elderly osteoporotic patients who were eligible for early mobilization [16]. Parvjeet found in his study that the patients treated with bipolar prosthesis had earlier rehabilitation than those treated with internal fixation, which decreased the overall morbidity, and he therefore concluded that bipolar prosthesis might be favored in old-aged patients even though there was no major difference in the choice of either implant [17]. After hip arthroplasty, patients can bear weight immediately and are encouraged to move and exercise the involved limbs, and thus reduce the period of bed rest and the rate of complications.

Bipolar hemiarthroplasty (BA) is a less complicated and more expensive surgery compared with THA [18]. However, no study is available that compares the effects and outcomes of the two treatments in intertrochanteric fractures. In order to get a clearer picture about the difference in their performance, we conducted the present study to compare the clinical effects of BA and THA in elderly osteoporotic patients with unstable intertrochanteric fractures, in terms of operation time, blood loss and transfusion, duration and cost of hospitalization, hip joint function, pain relief, general complications, and the rate of dislocation, revision and mortality.

Methods

All the patients with intertrochanteric fractures admitted to the hospital between March 2003 and September 2009 were evaluated. This study was a retrospective study of prospectively collected data. We used Singh's classification of the trabecular bone structure in the proximal femur as a measure of osteoporosis based on the anteroposterior (AP) radiograph of the contralateral hip. The inclusion criteria were: unstable intertrochanteric fractures (three or more part intertrochanteric fractures with a loss of posteromedial cortical buttress and reverse obliquity fractures), age over 70 years, severe osteoporosis (Singh index ≤3), no contraindication to anaesthesia, and pre-injury independent walking with or without aids. The exclusion criteria were: suspected pathological fracture, significant senile dementia, and osteoarthritis or rheumatoid arthritis in the fractured hip.

All patients were treated operatively with prosthetic replacement by the same surgery team. Follow-up evaluations were performed at 6 weeks, 3, 6, 9 and 12 months, and every year thereafter. THA was performed on the patients admitted in the hospital before December 31, 2005, but it was substituted by BA later in 2006 after the occurrence of three dislocations and for the sake of reducing dislocation rate and cost. The data of the patients' hospital courses were collected by chart abstracting.

All the patients underwent surgery with a standard posterior approach in lateral position under spinal or general anesthesia within 48 hours of admission. The fibres of the gluteus maximus were split and then the gluteus medius was retracted to expose the short external rotator muscles of the hip. These were divided close to their insertion and an inverted T shaped incision was made on the joint capsule. To avoid a further displacement of the fragments, with the limb maintained in traction by the surgical assistant, osteotomy of the femoral neck was performed prior to the dislocation of the hip joint. The femoral head was removed. The fragments of the greater trochanter were repositioned and temporarily fixed by using one or two bone forceps. The femoral canal was carefully detected with a long spoon and then was prepared by graduated reaming using rasps. Anteversion-retroversion of the prosthesis was determined using the lesser trochanter as a guide after the lesser trochanter was temporarily reduced. The height of the prosthesis was determined by temporarily fixing the greater trochanter in its anatomical position. In severely comminuted fractures, it was difficult to determine the prosthesis height properly only by anatomical landmarks of trochanters. Trial stem was used to decide the appropriate length of the extramedullary portion of the femoral component. The trial stem was assembled with a trial cup, and reduction test was performed to determine the exact length of the prosthesis that would achieve equal limb length.

The second-generation cementing technique was utilized. Thorough bony bed cleaning was performed by high speed pulsatile lavage. An intramedullary cement plug was placed, and the cement in a doughy state was delivered using a cement gun in a retrograde fashion. The Centrament® stem (Aesculap, Tuttlingen, Germany), with a length of 180 to 220 mm, was inserted inside the femoral canal and positioned at an anteversion angle of 15°. No obvious cardiopulmonary complications were observed. The fractured greater trochanter was attached to the prosthesis with two to four 16-gauge stainless steel wires. Isolated displaced fragments of the lesser trochanter were not reduced and fixed. In the THA group, the acetabulum was prepared and a cementless cobalt-chromium cup (Aesculap) with a UHMWPE liner inside was implanted, and then a 28-mm metal head was attached to the femoral stem. The optimal socket position was 40° to 45° of abduction and 10° to 25° of anteversion. Higher range of anteversion was preferred in order to reduce the risk of posterior instability. In the BA group, the acetabulum was not replaced, and a bipolar cup (Aesculap) was implanted instead. After the femoral head was removed, the diameter of the head was measured to determine the approximate size of the outer head of the chosen prosthesis. Range of motion and stability were checked after reduction. The capsule was repaired followed by reattachment of the short external rotators to the femur. Routine closure was performed and vacuum drainage was placed in both groups.

All patients underwent a routine postoperative physiotherapy protocol. The vacuum drains remained in place for 48 hours and were then removed. A pillow between the thighs was used for the first 2 weeks to prevent excessive adduction when the patients lied on the unoperated side. The patients, according to their conditions, were made to sit or stand with support from the first to the third postoperative day, and ambulated with support within the third to the fifth postoperative day. The rehabilitation progressed based on the toleration of the patients. Prophylaxis against deep venous thrombosis using Low-molecular-weight heparin (Lovenox 40 mg) was started 12 hours prior to the operation and continued for 35 days postoperatively.

At the final follow-up, the functional outcome was evaluated using Harris Hip Score (HHS) and the degree of pain was measured by visual analogue scale (VAS). Anteroposterior radiographs of the hip were taken at each follow-up for the evidence of subsidence of the stem, migration of acetabular component, erosion of acetabulum, and heterotopic ossification. The operation and medical records were reviewed to get the information of operation time, blood loss, blood transfusion volume, duration and cost of hospitalization.

All procedures used for this study were reviewed and approved by the Institutional Review Board of the Second Affiliated Hospital of Xi'an Jiaotong University, China. Written informed consent was obtained from participants after adequate explanation of the procedures of the study. Approval by the Institutional Review Board was documented.

The results were compared between the two groups for statistical significance either by a Student's t-test or a Mann-Whitney U test. Dichotomous variables, such as rates of revision and displacement, were analysed using a *chi*-squared test or Fisher's exact test. The p-value less than 0.05 was considered statistically significant.

Results

Between March 1, 2003 and September 30, 2009, a total number of 156 patients were admitted with a diagnosis of intertrochanteric fractures. Among the patients, 20 had severe hip arthritis, 16 had significant dementia, and 8 were excluded for pathological fractures. As a result, 112 patients that met the selection criteria were included. For these patients, 40 received THA and 72 underwent BA. The BA group had a mean follow-up period of 39.7 months (24 to 62 months) and the THA group had 48.8 months (32 to 75 months). The difference in the follow-up period between the two groups was statistically significant ($p<0.01$).

The demograghic characteristics of the 112 patients are summarized in Table 1. The THA group included 14 males and 26 females with a mean age of 73.4 years (range 70–80 years), and the BA group included 27 males and 45 females with a mean age of 76.5 years (range 71–85 years). Most patients had comorbidities that could adversely affect the functional outcomes, such as cardiovaslular problems, diabetes mellitus, pulmonary diseases and other associated diseases, but there was no significant difference in the number of comorbidities between the two groups. The data including age, sex, BMI, fracture type and Singh index of patients in the two groups also showed no significant difference.

The detailed surgery information of the patients is given in Table 2. The mean operation time in the THA group was 74.5 min, much longer than 53.4 min in the BA group. The average blood loss of the THA patients was 475.3 ml, two times

Table 1. Patient demographics.

	THA	BA
men:woman	14:26	27:45
Age (year)	73.4±5.8	76.5±8.3
BMI	22.3±4.7	25.1±5.2
Fracture type(IIIa)	12	23
Fracture type(IIIb)	22	33
Fracture type(IV)	6	16
Singh index	2.9±0.7	2.8±0.5
Follow-up (mon)	48.8±15.2	39.7±13.3
No. of Comorbid conditions	0.8±0.4	0.9±0.3

THA: total hip arthroplasty; BA: Bipolar hemiarthroplasty: Fracture type: Evans/Jensen classification system.

of the blood loss of 252.8 ml of the BA patients, and the average blood transfusion volume in the THA group was even more than two times that in the other group. The differences between the two groups in operation time, blood loss and transfusion volume were significant ($P<0.05$). It can be also seen that although the patients stayed in hospital for similar length of duration, the costs of hospitalization in the two groups were remarkably different. The THA patients spent a lot more than the BA patients did.

The mean HHS was 76.8 in the THA group and 74.6 in the BA group, and the mean VAS was 1.6 in the former and 1.8 in the latter group. Nine patients in the THA group (22.5%) and 16 patients in the BA group (22.2%) had two or more general complications. No significant difference was found between the two groups in HHS, VAS and general complications. For local complications, three dislocations occurred in the THA group while none was observed in the BA group, and this difference was statistically significant ($p<0.05$). One dislocation was treated by revision while the other two were closely reduced, and no recurrence was observed in the follow-up. During follow-up, two patients (4.4%) in the THA group and three patients (4.2%) in the BA group underwent a revision operation, eleven patients (27.5%) in the THA group and nineteen patients (26.3%) in the BA group died. The difference between the two groups in revision rate and mortality rate was not significant ($p>0.05$) (Table 3).

Radiography at the last available follow-up showed that all greater trochanter fractures had healed (Figure 1 and 2). The cerclage wire used for the greater trochanter was found broken in two patients in each group. Only one patient in the BA group developed osteoarthritis of the acetabulum and required a revision

Table 2. Operative records of patients.

	THA	BA	p-value
Operation time (minute)	74.5±15.2	53.4±12.5	<0.001
Blood loss (ml)	475.3±122.4	252.8±82.6	<0.001
Blood transfusion volume (unit)	3.5±1.2	1.5±0.8	<0.001
Hospitalization duration (day)	18.7±4.9	18.2±5.1	0.615
Hospitalization cost (thousand Yuan)	47.2±13.5	35.4±11.2	<0.001

THA: total hip arthroplasty; BA: Bipolar hemiarthroplasty.

Table 3. Outcome at the end of follow-up.

	THA	BA	p-value
Mean HHS	76.8±17.1	74.6±15.3	0.486
Mean VAS	1.6±0.6	1.8±0.5	0.062
Complications (%)	9(22.5)	16(22.2)	0.973
Dislocation (%)	3(7.5)	0(0)	0.018
Revision operation (%)	2(5.0)	3(4.2)	0.838
Mortality (%)	11(27.5)	19(26.3)	0.899

THA: total hip arthroplasty; BA: Bipolar hemiarthroplasty; The total modified Harris Hip score (HHS) was converted to a maximum of 100 points; HHS, VAS: students t-test; mortality: chi-squared test; revision operation, dislocation: Fisher's exact test.

to THA because of pain in the groin. The evidence of loosening of femoral component was seen in two BA patients and one THA patient, and revision was performed. There was no sign of heterotopic bone formation in any of the patients.

Discussion

The incidence of all hip fractures is approximately 80 per 100,000 persons and is expected to double over the next fifty years as the population ages [19]. According to the criteria of the modified Evans-Jensen classification, the two-part fractures are considered stable fractures and the rest of the fractures are unstable. About 35%–40% of all intertrochanteric hip fractures are unstable three- and/or four-part configurations with displacement of the posterior-medial cortex [20]. The failure rate of unstable intertrochanteric fractures with osteoporosis has been reported to be between 4% and 16.5% [21,22].

The dynamic hip screw and proximal femoral nail have been commonly used for internal fixation of intertrochanteric fractures. Elderly osteoporotic patients with unstable intertrochanteric fractures usually have a high prevalence of unsatisfactory outcome, with shortening and external rotation deformity of the limb following the treatment with a sliding screw. The failure rate of the dynamic hip screw in unstable fractures is up to 14% [23,24]. The use of intramedullary nail is associated with complications such as screw migration, femoral shaft fracture and implant failure. The failure rate of the proximal femoral nail is between 7.1% and 12.5% [8,25].

The incidence of general complications such as pulmonary embolism, deep venous thrombosis and pneumonia ranges from 22% to 50% when internal fixation was adopted [26,27]. Complications are also related to postsurgery rehabilitation, such as duration of bed rest and starting time of weight bearing [28]. Comminution, osteoporosis and instability often preclude the early resumption of full weight-bearing and worsen the prognosis. Mortality rate in hospital ranges from 0.03 to 10.5% [29], while one-year mortality reaches 22% [30].

Primary THA and hemiarthroplasty have been used to treat unstable intertrochanteric fractures in an effort to mobilize the patients more rapidly and avoid complications of hip screw migration [31–34], and they are found to have many merits against other fixation techniques. In a recent study, Faldini et al. reports the use of hemiarthroplasty and THA in 54 patients [15] and the finding that hip replacement permits a more rapid recovery with immediate weight-bearing and facilitates nursing care better than other fixation techniques. Sidhu et al also proved in their study on 53 patients that THA may be a valid treatment in

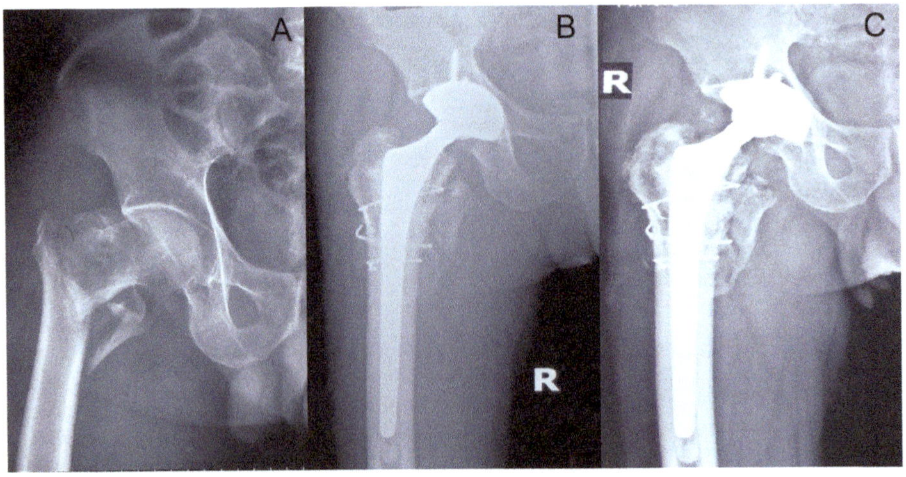

Figure 1. AP hip radiographs of a 76-year-old man with severe osteoporosis and unstable intertrochanteric fracture treated with cement THA using a long stem. A: Preoperative; B: At 6 months postoperatively, the fractured fragment has healed; C: Four years postoperative, the prosthesis was well fixed and his Harris hip score was excellent.

mentally healthy elderly patients with intertrochanteric hip fractures [12]. Hemiarthroplasty and THA, as two possible treatment options for unstable intertrochanteric fractures, may offer the potential for quick recovery with little risk of mechanical failure, avoid the risks often associated with internal fixation, and enable patients to maintain a good level of function immediately after surgery. Meanwhile, they do not result in nonunion or malunion of the fracture site or complications associated with avascular necrosis of the femoral head.

We have noticed that in treating femoral neck fractures, BA, compared with THA, has the advantages of less complexity, shorter operation time and a lower probability of dislocation. However, it may introduce concerns regarding groin and thigh pain due to acetabular erosion which reduces long-term survival and increases the likelihood of a second operation. For deciding whether BA or THA is a better choice for patients with intertrochanteric fractures, four factors should be taken into consideration: operation wound, surgery outcome, complications associated with procedures such as dislocation and acetabular erosion, and operation cost.

In our study, no significant difference has been identified between the group of patients treated by THA the patients treated by BA in surgery outcome, revision rate, mortality rate and general complications. However, the operation time of THA is evidently longer, and the blood loss and blood transfusion volume in the THA patients are significantly higher. The estimated cost of the components in THA is higher than that in BA, and the additional acetabular component in THA requires extra expense. In addition, the increased blood transfusion and longer operation time also increase the hospital cost. In resource-poor countries like China, cost is one of the major factors in patients' selection of treatments.

Haentjens [35] et al reviewed the literature and summarized the reports regarding prosthetic replacement for the treatment of intertrochanteric fractures and their complications. They concluded that elderly patients with severe osteoporosis may benefit from

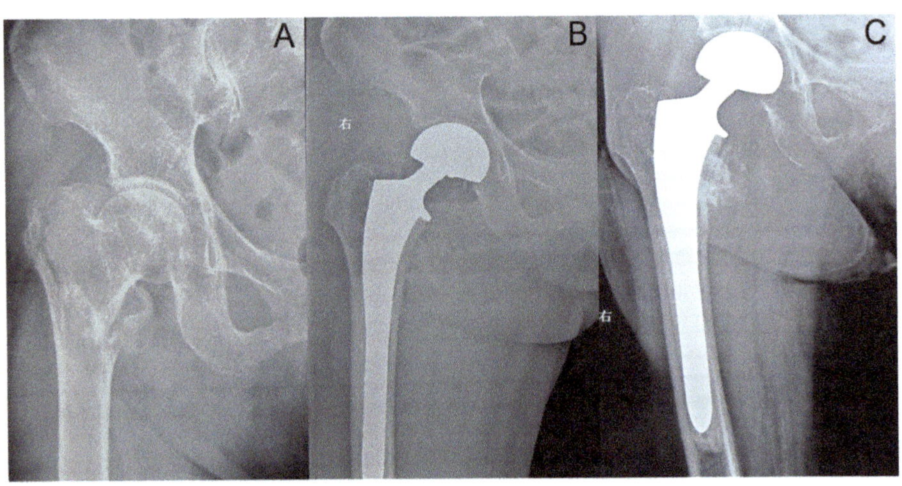

Figure 2. AP hip radiographs of a 78-year-old woman with severe osteoporosis and unstable intertrochanteric fracture treated with cement bipolar hemiarthroplasty using a long stem. A: Preoperative; B: At 6 months postoperatively, the fractured fragment has healed; C: radiographs obtained three years postoperatively, Femoral component was stable with no protrusion of cup.

prosthetic replacement for comminuted intertrochanteric fractures and non-unions. Few serious orthopaedic complications are associated with the procedure and most patients have good pain relief. The major concern post THA is dislocation, which increases the rate of pulmonary complications and bed sores [36]. The reported rate of dislocation in patients with intertrochanteric fractures after THA is up to 44.5% [34]. Despite that larger heads may give better stability, a larger bearing alone cannot prevent dislocation [37]. The standard metal ball with a diameter of 28 mm and the polyethylene cup have been in use since early 1960s and have been the most used till now. It is also the least expensive bearing. In our series, no dislocation occurred in the BA patients during follow-up, while three of the THA patients suffered dislocations. One patient with mal-positioning of the stem and acetabular component underwent revision after the failure of closed reduction. The other two patients received closed reduction under general anesthesia, and were protected with an abduction brace for two months. No recurrence was then observed. Bracing was not routinely practiced after THA surgery but only after closed reduction of dislocation, because it would immobilize the hip joints, which was poorly tolerated by elderly patients, and was a considerable expense.

The main concern with BA is the possibility of occurrence of protrusion acetabuli and groin pain from the acetabular erosion [38,39]. Cartilage damage and erosion of the acetabular surface are highly correlated with groin pain [40]. Compromised articular cartilage in the hips of normal elderly patients puts them at a greater risk. In our study, although VAS was slightly higher in the BA group, there was no statistically significant difference between the two groups. Patients with intertrochanteric fractures caused by osteoporosis often have coexisting medical problems and limited life expectancy, which means that the daily demands placed on prostheses are low [41]. It is also found in our study that more than 25% of the patients (19 out of 72) expired within 5 years post surgery, long before severe protrusion would occur. Obvious acetabular erosion was observed in only one BA patient, who underwent THA as a revision since the pain in the groin was not relieved by oral administration of NSAIDs.

This is a retrospective study, which bears some limitations. The number of cases included may not be large enough, and the follow-up period is relatively short. A further prospective, randomized study is necessary to compare the arthroplasty procedures in more cases with longer follow-up.

The present study reveals that the functional results and pain relief in patients undergoing THA and BA are similar, and there is no evident difference in hospitalization period, general complications, and rate of revision and mortality during follow-up. Both THA and BA are reliable treatment methods for unstable intertrochanteric fractures in elderly osteoporotic patients. However, the higher intra-operative blood loss, longer duration of surgery, higher incidence of dislocations, and greater costs of THA suggest that BA might be a better or more reasonable choice.

Author Contributions

Conceived and designed the experiments: KW LF. Performed the experiments: LF XD. Analyzed the data: LF XD. Contributed reagents/materials/analysis tools: XD. Wrote the paper: LF KW.

References

1. Koval KJ, Zuckerman JD (1998) Hip fractures are an increasingly important public health problem. Clin Orthop Relat Res 348:2.
2. Sancheti Kh, Sancheti P, Shyam A, Patil S, Dhariwal Q, et al (2010) Primary hemiarthroplasty or unstable osteoporotic intertrochanteric fractures in the elderly: A retrospective case series. Indian J Orthop 44(4): 428–434.
3. Lindskog DM, Baumgaertner MR (2004) Unstable intertrochanteric hip fractures in the elderly. J Am Acad Orthop Surg 12(3): 179–190.
4. Marsh JL, Slongo TF, Agel J, Broderick JS, Creevey W, et al. (2007) Fracture and dislocation classification compendium: Orthopaedic Trauma Association classification, database and outcomes committee. J Orthop Trauma 21: S1–133.
5. Larsson S (2002) Treatment of osteoporotic fractures. Scand J Surg 91: 140–146.
6. Kim SY, Kim YG, Hwang JK (2005) Cementless calcar-replacement hemiarthroplasty compared with intramedullary Wxation ofunstable intertrochanteric fractures: a prospective, randomized study. J Bone Joint Surg Am 87: 2186–2192.
7. Habernek H, Wallner T, Aschauer E, Schmid L (2000) Comparison of ender nails, dynamic hip screws, and gamma nails in the treatment of peritrochanteric femoral fractures. Orthopedics 23: 121–127.
8. Papasimos S, Koutsojannis CM, Panagopoulos A, Megas P, Lambiris E (2005) A randomised comparison of AMBI, TGN and PFN for treatment of unstable trochanteric fractures.Arch Orthop Trauma Surg 125(7): 462–468.
9. Kim WY, Han CH, Park JI, Kim JY (2001) Failure of intertrochanteric fracture fixation with a dynamic hip screw in relation to pre-operative fracture stability and osteoporosis. Int Orthop 25: 360–362.
10. Mariani EM, Rand JA (1987) Nonunion of intertrochanteric fractures of the femur following open reduction and internal fixation. Results of second attempts to gain union. Clin Orthop 218: 81–89.
11. Davis TR, Sher JL, Horsman A, Simpson M, Porter BB, et al (1990) Intertrochanteric femoral fractures: Mechanical failure after internal fixation. J Bone Joint Surg Br 72: 26–31.
12. Sidhu AS, Singh AP, Singh AP, Singh S (2010) Total hip replacement as primary treatment of unstable intertrochanteric fractures in elderly patients. Int Orthop. 34(6): 789–792.
13. Rodop O, Kiral A, Kaplan H, Akmaz I (2002) Primary bipolar hemiprosthesis for unstable intertrochanteric fractures.Int Orthop 26(4): 233–237.
14. Harwin SF, Stern RE, Kulick RG (1990) Primary Bateman-Leinbach bipolar prosthetic replacement of the hip in the treatment of unstable intertrochanteric fractures in the elderly. Orthopedics 13(10): 1131–1136.
15. C Faldini,G Grandi,M Romagnoli,S Pagkrati,V Digennaro,O., et al (2006) Surgical treatment of unstable intertrochanteric fractures by bipolar hip replacement or total hip replacement in elderly osteoporotic patients. J Orthopaed Traumatol 7: 117–121.
16. Stappaerts KH, Deldycke J, Broos PL, Staes FF, Rommens PM, et al (1995) Treatment of unstable peritrochanteric fractures in elderly patients with a compression hip screw or with a Vandeputte (VDP) endoprosthesis: a prospective randomised study. Journal of Orthopaedic Trauma 9(4): 292–297.
17. Parvjeet Singh Gulati, Rakesh Sharma, RPS Boparai, Rajesh Kapila, Aarti Deewan (2009) Comparative study of treatment of intertrochanteric fractures of femur with long-stem bipolar prosthetic replacement versus dynamic hip screw fixation. Pb Journal of Orthopaedics Vol-XI, No.1
18. Narayan KK, George T (2006) Functional outcome of fracture neck of femur treated with total hip replacement versus bipolar arthroplasty in a South Asian population.Arch Orthop Trauma Surg 126(8): 545–548.
19. Zuckerman JD (1996) Hip fractures. N Engl J Med 334: 1519.
20. Mariani EM, Rand JA (1987) Nonunion of intertrochanteric fractures of the femur following open reduction and internal fixation. Clin Orthop Relat Res 218: 81.
21. Haidukewych GJ, Berry DJ (2003) Hip arthroplasty for salvage of failed treatment of intertrochanteric hip fractures. J Bone Joint Surg Am 85(5): 899–904.
22. Cho CH, Yoon SH, Kim SY (2010) Better Functional Outcome of Salvage THA Than Bipolar Hemiarthroplasty for Failed Intertrochanteric Femur Fracture Fixation. Orthopedics 11; 33(10).
23. Watson JT, Moed BR, Cramer KE, Karges DE (1998) Comparison of the compression hip screw with the Medoff sliding plate for intertrochanteric fractures. Clin Orthop Relat Res 348: 79–86.
24. Adams CI, Robinson CM, Court-Brown CM, McQueen MM (2001) Prospective randomized controlled trial of an intramedullary nail versus dynamic screw and plate for intertrochanteric fractures of the femur. J Orthop Trauma 15(6): 394–400.
25. Boldin C, Seibert FJ, Fankhauser F, Peicha G, Grechenig W, et al. (2003) The proximal femoral nail (PFN)–a minimal invasive treatment of unstable proximal femoral fractures: a prospective study of 55 patients with a follow-up of 15 months. Acta Orthop Scand 74(1): 53–58.
26. Kenzora JE, McCarthy RE, Lowell JD, Sledge CB (1984) Hip fracture mortality. Relation to age, treatment, preoperative illness, time of surgery, and complications. Clin Orthop 186: 45–56.
27. Baumgaertner MR, Curtin SL, Lindskog DM (1998) Intramedullary versus extramedullary fixation for the treatment of intertrochanteric hip fractures. Clin Orthop 348: 87–94.
28. Brostrom LA, Barrios C, Kronberg M, Stark A, Walheim G (1992) Clinical features and walking ability in the early postoperative period after treatment of trochanteric hip fractures. Results with special reference to fracture type and surgical treatment. Ann Chir Gynaecol 81: 66–71.

29. Albareda J, Ladcriga A, Palanca D (1996) Complications and technical problems with the gamma nail. Int Orthop 20: 47–50.
30. Aprin H, Kilfoyle RM (1980) Treatment of trochanteric fractures with Ender rods. J Trauma 20: 32–42.
31. Chan KC, Gill GS (2000) Cemented hemiarthroplasties for elderly patients with intertrochanteric fractures. Clin Orthop Relat Res 371: 206.
32. Green S, Moore T, Proano F (1987) Bipolar prosthetic replacement for the management of unstable intertrochanteric intertrochanteric hip fractures in the elderly. Clin Orthop Relat Res 224: 169.
33. Stern MB, Angerman A (1987) Comminuted intertrochanteric fractures treated with a Leinbach prosthesis. Clin Orthop Relat Res 218: 75.
34. Haentjens P, Casteleyn PP, De Boeck H, Handelberg F, Opdecam P (1989) Treatment of unstable intertrochanteric and subtrochanteric fractures in elderly patients. Primary bipolar arthroplasty compared with internal fixation,J Bone Joint Surg Am 71(8): 1214–25.
35. Haentjens P, Lamraski G (2005) Endoprosthetic replacement of unstable, comminuted intertrochanteric fracture of the femur in the elderly, osteoporotic patient. Disabil Rehabil 27(18–19): 1167–1180.
36. Haentjens P, Casteleyn PP, Opdecam P (1994) Primary bipolar arthroplasty or total hip arthroplasty for the treatment of unstable intertrochanteric and subtrochanteric fractures in elderly patients. Acta Orthop Belg 60: 124–128.
37. Hummel MT, Malkani AL, Yakkanti MR, Baker DL (2009) Decreased dislocation after revision total hip arthroplasty using larger femoral head size and posterior capsular repair. J Arthroplasty 24(6): 73–76.
38. Phillips TW (1989) Thompson hemiarthroplasty and acetabular erosion. J Bone Joint Surg Am 71(6): 913–917.
39. Sierra RJ, Cabanela ME (2002) Conversion of failed hip arthroplasties after femoral neck fractures. Clin Orthop Relat Res 399: 129–139.
40. Gebhard JS, Amstutz HC, Zinar DM, Dorey FJ (1992) A comparison of total hip arthroplasty and hemiarthroplasty for treatment of acute fracture of the femoral neck. Clin Orthop Relat Res 282: 123–131.
41. Jamal Sepah Y, Umer M, Khan A, Ullah Khan Niazi A (2010) Functional outcome, mortality and in-hospital complications of operative treatment in elderly patients with hip fractures in the developing world. Int Orthop 34(3): 431–435.

22

Association between Several Clinical and Radiological Determinants with Long-Term Clinical Progression and Good Prognosis of Lower Limb Osteoarthritis

Erlangga Yusuf[1]*, Jessica Bijsterbosch[1], P. Eline Slagboom[2], Herman M. Kroon[3], Frits R. Rosendaal[4], Tom W. J. Huizinga[1], Margreet Kloppenburg[1,4]

1 Department of Rheumatology, Leiden University Medical Center, Leiden, The Netherlands, **2** Department of Molecular Epidemiology, Leiden University Medical Center, Leiden, The Netherlands, **3** Department of Radiology, Leiden University Medical Center, Leiden, The Netherlands, **4** Department of Clinical Epidemiology, Leiden University Medical Center, Leiden, The Netherlands

Abstract

Objective: To investigate the factors associated with clinical progression and good prognosis in patients with lower limb osteoarthritis (OA).

Methods: Cohort study of 145 patients with OA in either knee, hip or both. Progression was defined as 1) new joint prosthesis or 2) increase in WOMAC pain or function score during 6-years follow-up above pre-defined thresholds. Patients without progression with decrease in WOMAC pain or function score lower than pre-defined thresholds were categorized as good prognosis. Relative risks (RRs) for progression and good prognosis with 95% confidence interval (95% CI) were calculated by comparing the highest tertile or category to the lowest tertile, for baseline determinants (age, sex, BMI, WOMAC pain and function scores, pain on physical examination, total range of motion (tROM), osteophytes and joint space narrowing (JSN) scores), and for worsening in WOMAC pain and function score in 1-year. Adjustments were performed for age, sex, and BMI.

Results: Follow-up was completed by 117 patients (81%, median age 60 years, 84% female); 62 (53%) and 31 patients (26%) showed progression and good prognosis, respectively. These following determinants were associated with progression: pain on physical examination (RR 1.2 (1.0 to 1.5)); tROM (1.4 (1.1 to 1.6); worsening in WOMAC pain (1.9 (1.2 to 2.3)); worsening in WOMAC function (2.4 (1.7 to 2.6)); osteophytes 1.5 (1.0 to 1.8); and JSN scores (2.3 (1.5 to 2.7)). Worsening in WOMAC pain (0.1 (0.1 to 0.8)) and function score (0.1 (0.1 to 0.7)), were negatively associated with good prognosis.

Conclusion: Worsening of self-reported pain and function in one year, limited tROM and higher osteophytes and JSN scores were associated with clinical progression. Worsening in WOMAC pain and function score in 1- year were associated with lower risk to have good prognosis. These findings help to inform patients with regard to their OA prognosis.

Editor: German Malaga, Universidad Peruana Cayetano Heredia, Peru

Funding: This study was financially supported by Pfizer (Groton, CT, USA), the Dutch Arthritis Association, and TI-Pharma. The funders had no role in study design, data collection and analysis, decision to publish, or preparation of the manuscript.

Competing Interests: The authors have read the journal's policy and have the following conflicts: This study was financially supported by Pfizer (Groton, CT, United States of America) and TI-Pharma.

* E-mail: angga.yusuf@gmail.com

Introduction

Osteoarthritis (OA) of the lower limbs accounts for problems in performing lower extremities tasks such as walking and stair climbing.[1] Some of the patients with lower limb OA show progression of their OA with some progressing to total joint failure needing joint replacement.[2] Knowing those who will progress is important because it will improve patient information on the prognosis of OA.

Several studies have investigated determinants of the progression of knee and hip OA [3]–[5] and several remarks could be made on these studies. Firstly, none of the studies investigated knee and hip together. Investigating knee and hip separately is easy to understand but it does not reflect the clinical practice. In more than 30% of knee OA patients, hip OA is present at the same time [6] and up to 78% of patients have bilateral OA in knees or hips.[7] Concomitant presence of OA in lower limb joints will affect the experience of pain and influence disability in all lower limb joints. Arguably, it is difficult for a patient to allocate complaints to a particular knee or hip joint. The questionnaires used in OA, such as Western Ontario and McMaster Universities Osteoarthritis Index (WOMAC) asked questions on daily life activities such as climbing the stairs, where knee and hip joints are simultaneously needed.[8] Secondly, in most studies, progression was defined as joint deterioration on a radiograph while from the patient's perspective clinical progression is more important.[2], [9] Thirdly, almost exclusively baseline determinants of progression were investigated. However, OA patients are included in cohort studies at varying stages of the OA disease course, which make changes in determinants over a short time period of interest as prognostic factors on the long term.

Clinical progression is relevant for patients, but it is difficult to define. Probably this is one of the reasons why data on clinical progression are lacking compared to data on radiological progression. At this moment, there is no consensus on how to define clinical progression of knee and hip OA progression.[10],[11] Obviously, total joint replacement should be considered as OA disease progression. However, not all patients with worsening of their OA will receive joint replacement because of factors such as patient's comorbidity and surgeon's preference. Self-reported pain or disability could be used to define clinical progression, yet at present no standardized 'cut-off' for progression on self-reported outcome measures exists.

To deal with the abovementioned issues, we propose in the present study a composite outcome which combines total joint replacement and increase in self-reported pain and function during 6-years follow-up above a clinically relevant cut-off [8] as clinical progression. We sought to identify determinants associated with clinical progression and determinants associated with good prognosis of lower limb OA (knee and hip OA together). We assessed baseline determinants and determinants which were measured repeatedly over time.

Materials and Methods

Study design and patient population

This study is part of the Genetic ARthrosis and Progression (GARP) study, a cohort study aimed at identifying determinants of OA susceptibility and progression.[12] In this cohort, 192 Caucasian sib-pairs (384 patients), aged 40 to 70 years were included. To be included, patient should have symptomatic OA at multiple joint sites in the hands or OA in two or more of the following joint sites: hand, spine (cervical or lumbar), knee, or hip. Patients were recruited from the rheumatologic, orthopedic and general practice clinics around Leiden, The Netherlands. Patients with secondary OA, familial syndromes with a clear Mendelian inheritance, and a shortened life expectancy (<1 yr) were excluded. Patients underwent baseline assessment between August 2000 and March 2003 and filled-in questionnaires one year after this baseline visit. From April 2007 to June 2008 patients who consented for a follow-up evaluation (mean follow-up 6.1 years (range 5.1–7.5 years) were assessed.

To be eligible for the present study, patients needed to have OA in either knee or hip, or both. Knee OA was defined according to American College of Rheumatology (ACR) criteria as pain or stiffness in the knee on most days of the prior month and the presence of osteophytes in the tibiofemoral joints.[13] Hip OA was also defined according to ACR criteria as pain or stiffness in the groin and hip region on most days of prior month together with femoral or acetabular osteophytes or joint space narrowing on the radiograph.[14] There were 168 patients with knee or hip OA in the GARP cohort. Of these patients, 23 patients with prosthesis at baseline were excluded leaving 145 patients eligible for the follow-up. Patients with prosthesis at baseline were excluded because these patients could be considered as already having progressive disease at baseline and because having first prosthesis could influence the decision in having another prosthesis (confounder). This study was approved by the Medical Ethics Committee of the Leiden University Medical Center. Written informed consents form were obtained from all participants.

Clinical assessment

Demographic data at baseline were recorded using standardized questionnaires. Self-reported pain (five items) and functional limitations (17 items) were evaluated by using the Dutch version of the WOMAC in 100 mm visual analogue scale format at baseline, at 1-year and at 6-year follow-up. It considered both knees and hips in the last 48 hours. Total scores on the pain and function subscales range from 0–100, higher scores indicated worse outcome.

Physical health at baseline was assessed with the summary component scales for physical health (PCS) of the Dutch validated Medical Outcomes Study Short Form-36 (SF-36) derived from norm based data from the Dutch population (mean 50, standard deviation (SD) 10). [15,16] Higher scores indicate better physical health.

Physical examinations were performed at baseline. Pain on passive movement of the knee and hip joint was assessed using the modified articular index described by Doyle et al [17] (range 0 to 3; 0: no pain, 1: patient expressed tenderness, 2: patient expressed tenderness and winced, 3: patient expressed tenderness, winced and withdrew the joint). The total pain score ranged from 0 to 12. Flexion and extension of the knee and flexion and endorotation of the hip were measured using a goniometer and summed up as total range of motion (tROM).

Radiographs

Radiographs of the knees (posterior-anterior (PA); weight-bearing, non-fluoroscopic fixed-flexion protocol) and hips (PA; weight-bearing) at baseline were taken by a single experienced radiographer using a standard protocol with a fixed film focus distance (1.30 m). These analogue films were digitized using a film digitizer at a resolution corresponding to a pixel size of 100 mu. Using the OARSI atlas [18], two readers (EY, JB) scored the radiographs by consensus opinion. Osteophytes were graded 0 to 3 in the hip, on the medial and lateral femur and in the medial and lateral tibia. Joint space narrowing (JSN) was graded 0 to 3 in the hip, and in medial and lateral tibiofemoral compartments of the knees. Total scores for osteophytes ranged from 0–24 in the knees and 0–6 in the hips. Total scores for JSN ranged from 0–12 in the knees and 0–6 in the hips. Intra-reader reproducibility based on 25 randomly selected pairs of radiographs was excellent, with intra-class correlation coefficient (ICC) of 0.99 for osteophytes and 0.98 for JSN.

Definition of progression and good prognosis

Clinical progression was defined as: 1) the acquirement of joint replacement during follow-up or 2) an increase in self-reported (WOMAC) pain or function from baseline to 6-years follow-up above the predefined MPCI (minimum perceptible clinical improvement). The joint replacement should be due to OA and not due to other forms of arthritis or trauma. MPCI was originally developed as threshold value to define treatment response in OA. The threshold values were 9.7 for WOMAC pain and 9.3 for WOMAC function.[8]

These threshold values with negative sign, were used to define good prognosis. Patients without progression who had decrease in WOMAC pain or function score in 6-years lower than −9.7 or −9.3, respectively, were defined as having good prognosis.

Statistical analysis

Data were analyzed using PASW Statistics 17 (SPSS Inc., Chicago, Ill, USA). Mean changes (SD and 95% confidence interval (95% CI)) for WOMAC pain and function, PCS and pain on examination scores were calculated by subtracting baseline scores from follow-up scores. Mean changes of scores with the 95% CI that did not cross 0 was considered as significant. The self-reported pain and function change scores of every patient were plotted in cumulative probability plot.

Determinants of clinical progression were assessed using logistic regression analysis. We assessed the following baseline determinants age, sex, BMI, WOMAC pain and function scores, pain on physical examination, total range of motion (tROM) and radiographic scores. We also assessed the determinants worsening in WOMAC pain and function score in 1-year.

The following baseline determinants were categorized in tertiles: BMI, WOMAC pain and function, tROM, osteophytes, and JSN. Also categorized in tertiles were worsening in WOMAC pain and function in 1-year. Pain on physical examination was categorized into presence or absence of pain. In the logistic regression analysis, the odds ratios (ORs) were calculated by using the lowest category or the lowest tertile as reference except for tROM where the highest tertile was used as reference. The ORs were transformed to risk ratio (RRs) using the approximation formula of Zhang because ORs of common outcomes in a fixed cohort are not a good approximation of RRs.[19] Since the population of this study consists of sib pairs, intrafamily effect were taken into account by computing robust standard errors using Stata version 8 (Stata, College Station, Tx, USA). In the analyses, adjustments were made for age, sex, and BMI. A significant determinant of progression was defined as a determinant that the 95% CI of its RR did not cross 1.

The significant determinants were included in a multivariate model to investigate whether these determinants could independently predict the clinical progression. To get an impression on how good these determinants predict clinical progression when they presented together, the R^2 of this model was determined. Additionally, to investigate the discriminative ability of the multivariate model, we fitted a receiver operating characteristics curve (ROC) and calculated the area under the curve (AUC). We compared the predicted risk of progression with the observed clinical progression and good prognosis with the observed clinical progression and good prognosis.

Results

Population description

Of 145 patients eligible for the follow-up, 117 (81%) gave consent for follow-up assessment. The reasons for non-consent were: no interest in the follow-up study (n = 8), unavailability of transport (n = 8) health problems not associated with OA (n = 4), emigration (n = 1), and unknown (n = 2). Five patients died during follow-up.

Baseline characteristics of patients with and without follow-up and excluded patients due to joint prosthesis at baseline are presented in Table 1. No difference was found between baseline characteristics of patients with and without follow-up (Table 1).

Clinical course of lower limb osteoarthritis

The mean changes (95%CI) of self-reported (WOMAC) pain and function scores of all patients were −2.6 (−8.9 to 3.7) and 0.5 (−5.9 to 6.9), respectively (Table 2).

During follow-up, 36 patients (31%) received at least one joint replacement; 15 for the hip, 16 for the knee, and five for both knee and hip. In these patients with new joint replacements, the mean WOMAC pain score (95% CI) decreased over the six years of follow-up (−8.5 (−17.8 to −0.1). In the patients without new prosthesis (n = 81), WOMAC pain and WOMAC function scores did not change significantly over time: −0.1 (−8.3 to 8.1) and 1.9 (−6.3 to 10.1), respectively.

Cumulative probability plots show the variation in natural course of self-reported pain and function in the sub-group of patients without prosthesis (n = 81) (Figures 1a and 1b). Fifteen and 22 patients showed progression of WOMAC pain and WOMAC function based on changes above the MCPI, respectively. In total, 26 patients (19.7%) showed clinical deterioration. Together with the 36 patients receiving joint replacement during follow-up, 62 of 117 patients (53.0%) showed clinical progression. Thirty-one patients showed good prognosis, based on change in WOMAC pain or WOMAC function score change lower than −9.7 (n = 23) or −9.3 (n = 22), respectively.

In the total study sample, in the subgroup of patients with new prosthesis, and in patients without new prosthesis, physical health summary measures using SF-36 did not change during follow-up (Table 2). Compared to the general population (mean of 50 with SD of 10), physical health of lower limb OA patients was consistently shown to be worse at baseline and follow-up.

Pain during physical examination was worsened in the total population (Table 2). In the sub-group with new prosthesis, pain did not worsen.

Determinants of clinical progression of lower limb osteoarthritis

Determinants of clinical progression of lower limb OA are shown in Table 3. Age, female sex, and BMI, were not associated with clinical progression. Worsening of WOMAC pain and function scores in the first year were associated with 6-year progression while WOMAC pain and function score at baseline were not. Subjects in the highest tertile of WOMAC pain and function worsening in 1 year had a RR (95% CI) of 1.9 (1.2 to 2.3) and 2.4 (1.7 to 2.7), respectively, for clinical progression. The presence of pain on physical examination at baseline was associated with clinical progression (1.2 (1.0 to 1.5)). Patients in the lowest tertile of tROM had a higher risk for clinical progression RRs of 1.4 (1.1 to 1.6)). Osteophytes and JSN at baseline were associated with clinical progression, RR for being in the highest tertile of osteophytes and JSN scores were 1.5 (1.0 to 1.8) and 2.3 (1.5 to 2.6), respectively. In a multivariate regression model, WOMAC function worsening in 1 year, limited t ROM, and JSN scores were found as independent determinants of clinical progression (Table 3). With these variables, explained variance (R^2) was 48.6%. The AUCs of the ROC curves were 0.85 (95% CI 0.76 to 0.94).

Determinants of good prognosis of lower limb osteoarthritis

Worsening in WOMAC pain and function score in 1 year were negatively associated with good prognosis, i.e. patients in highest tertile of 1-year increase in WOMAC pain and function scores had lower risk to have good prognosis. (Table 4). Patients in the highest tertile of worsening of WOMAC pain and function in 1 year, had RR of 0.1 (95% CI 0.1 to 0.8) and 0.1 (0.1 to 0.7), respectively to have good prognosis of their lower limb OA compared to patients with WOMAC pain and function change in the lowest tertile. When these significant determinants were analyzed in one model, only worsening in WOMAC function in 1- year was negatively associated with good prognosis. The R^2 of this model was 43.3% and the AUCs of the ROC curves were 0.78 (0.68 to 0.89).

Table 1. Baseline characteristics of 168 patients with knee and/or hip OA stratified by availability of follow-up.

	Follow-up (n = 117)	*No follow-up (n = 28)*	*Joint prosthesis at baseline (n = 23)*
Age, yrs, median (IQR)			
	60 (55–66)	62 (53–58)	64 (61–68)
Female, no (%)			
	98 (84)	24 (74)	13 (72)
BMI, kg/m^2, mean (range)			
	28.0 (20 to 47)	27.3 (20 to 38)	29.3 (22 to 43)
Patients with OA, no (%)			
Knee	74 (63)	18 (55)	3 (17)
Hip	31 (27)	6 (18)	6 (33)
Knee and hip	11 (10)	9 (27)	9 (50)
Total range of motion, °, mean (range)			
	258 (133 to 389)	257 (219 to 441)	251 (48 to 360)
Knee flexion	86 (1 to 155)	86 (0 to 155)	85 (16 to 135)
Knee extension.	−4 (−30 to 10)	−3 (−30 to 16)	−2 (−15 to 16)
Hip flexion	134 (100 to 176)	134 (8 to 166)	133 (8 to 175)
Hip extension	41 (0 to 80)	39 (0 to 80)	26 (8 to 49)
Joint prosthesis, no.			
	n/a	n/a	23
Hip			16
Knee			6
Knee and hip			1
Presence of pain on physical examination, no (%)*			
	85 (73)	20 (71)	17 (74)
Hip	30 (26)	9 (32)	14 (61)
Knee	64 (55)	16 (57)	11 (48)

*Patients may have OA at multiple joints at one time and can have pain in the knee and hip joint simultaneously. Abbreviation: IQR: interquartile range; BMI: Body Mass Index.

Table 2. Mean (standard deviation (SD)) baseline, follow-up (FU), and change scores on self-reported pain and function (WOMAC), physical health (PCS), and pain on physical examination (PE) for the total population and sub-groups.

		Baseline	*Follow-up*	*Change (95% CI)*
All patients (n = 117)	WOMAC pain	36.2 (23.5)	33.6 (25.7)	−2.6 (−8.9 to 3.7)
	WOMAC function	33.1 (24.3)	33.6 (24.8)	0.5 (−5.9 to 6.9)
	PCS	41.8 (9.8)‡	42.0 (10.1)‡	0.2 (−2.4 to 2.8)
	Pain on PE	1.7 (1.7)	2.4 (2.4)	0.7 (0.2 to 1.2)‡
Patients receiving prosthesis during FU (n = 36)	WOMAC pain	36.5 (18.2)	28.0 (21.0)	−8.5 (−17.8 to−0.1)‡
	WOMAC function	32.4 (20.1)	30.0 (20.6)	−2.4 (−12.0 to 7.2)
	PCS	40.8 (9.1)‡	40.7 (10.0)‡	−0.1 (−4.6 to 4.4)
	Pain on PE	1.8 (1.6)	2.8 (3.1)	1.0 (−0.2 to 2.2)
Patient not receiving prosthesis during FU (n = 81)	WOMAC pain	36.1 (25.6)	36.0 (27.2)	−0.1 (−8.3 to 8.1)
	WOMAC function	33.4 (26.1)	35.3 (26.4)	1.9 (−6.3 to 10.1)
	PCS	42.3 (10.1)‡	42.6 (10.0)‡	0.3 (−2.8 to 3.4)
	Pain on PE	1.7 (1.8)	2.3 (2.1)	0.6 (−0.01 to 1.2)

‡: statistically significant; the significance of physical health summary were tested by comparing the study sample with the norm based population (mean = 50, SD = 10).

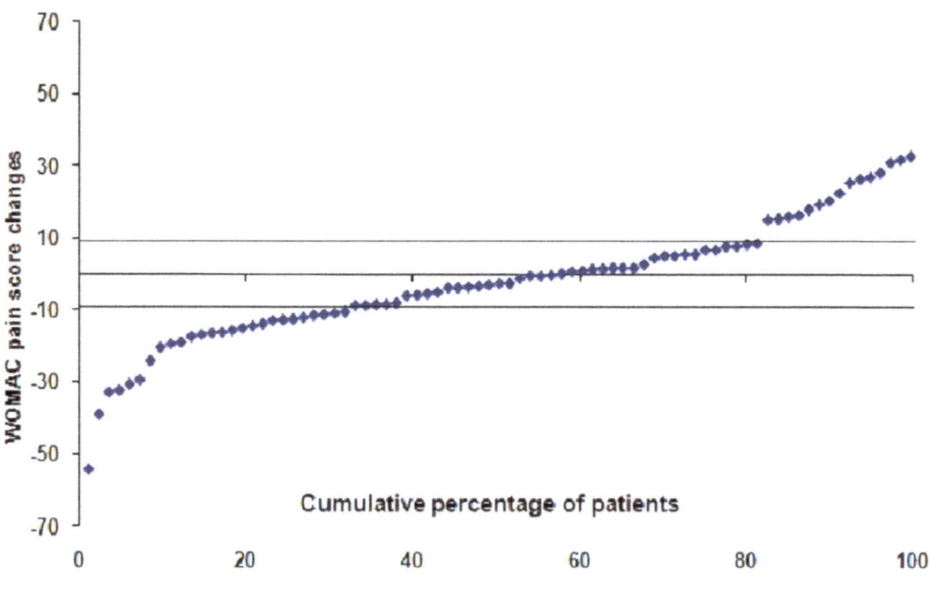

Figure 1a.

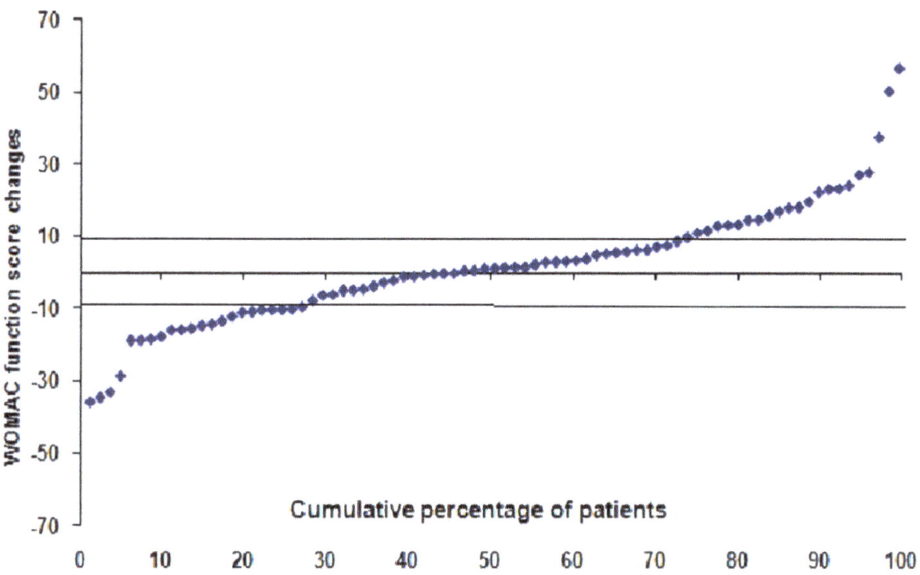

Figure 1. Cumulative probability plot of Western Ontario and McMaster Universities (WOMAC) scores change of patients without prosthesis during follow-up (n = 81) for WOMAC pain scores change (above) and WOMAC function scores change (below). The horizontal line above is the line set at minimal perceptible clinical improvement (MPCI) score which is used as the cut-off to define progression and the horizontal line below is the line set to define good prognosis.

Discussion

To our knowledge, the present study is the first which investigated determinants of clinical progression of knee and hip together. Clinical outcome is chosen because it is essential to patients. Clinical progression was present in 53% of patients; 33% by receiving joint prosthesis and 20% by deteriorating of self-reported pain or function.

Self-reported pain improved over 6 years in patients who received prostheses. Self-reported function did not change over 6 years regardless of joint replacement. The combination of WOMAC function changes in 1 year, limited tROM, and JSN scores provided the best explanation of variation in clinical progression of lower limb OA. Worsening WOMAC pain and function in 1 year were negatively associated with good prognosis. Patients in the highest tertile of worsening in WOMAC pain and WOMAC function in 1-year had 90% less chance to have good prognosis of their lower limb OA compared to patients with pain and function change in the lowest tertile.

The proportion of the study sample showing clinical progression in our study is comparable to results from the Bristol 'OA 500 study'. In that descriptive study, where the majority of the study population was also female, clinical change was reported by the patients as: better, same, and worse. They found that 63% and 54% of the patients reported worsening in overall condition for the knee and hip respectively, after 8 years follow-up.[9] In

Table 3. Determinants for clinical progression over 6 years of lower limb osteoarthritis.

Determinant	*Number of patients*		*Risk ratio (95% CI)* [1]	*Risk ratio (95% CI)* [2]
	Pro-gression (%)	*No pro-gression (%)*		
Age>60 years	59 (50)	50 (43)	1.0 (0.9 to 1.1)	na
Female sex	48 (41)	50 (43)	0.6 (0.3 to 1.0)	na
Body mass index (kg/m^2)				
<25.5	19 (16)	20 (17)	1	na
25.5 to 29.1	16 (14)	21 (18)	0.9 (0.5 to 1.2)	
>29.1	27 (23)	14 (12)	1.3 (0.9 to 1.7)	
WOMAC pain scores				
0 to 23.2	21 (18)	18 (15)	1	na
23.2 to 45.9	20 (17)	18 (15)	0.9 (0.5 to 1.3)	
>45.9	21 (18)	19 (16)	1.1 (0.7 to 1.4)	
WOMAC function scores				
0 to 18.0	20 (17)	20 (17)	1	na
18.0 to 40.9	22 (19)	16 (14)	1.2 (0.7 to 1.6)	
>40.9	20 (17)	19 (16)	1.1 (0.7 to 1.5)	
Change in WOMAC pain score in 1 year				
<−3.3	10 (9)	16 (14)	1	na
−3.3 to 10.1	15 (13)	11 (9)	1.6 (0.8 to 2.2)	
>10.1	17 (15)	9 (8)	1.9 (1.2 to 2.3)‡	
Change in WOMAC function score in 1 year				
<−1.4	9 (8)	17 (15)	1	1
−1.4 to 6.7	13 (11)	14 (12)	1.5 (0.9 to 2.7)	1.9 (0.9 to 2.6)
>6.7	20 (17)	5 (4)	2.4 (1.7 to 2.7)‡	2.3 (1.2 to 2.8)‡
Pain on physical examination	44 (38)	13 (11)	1.2 (1.0 to 1.5)‡	1.2 (0.8 to 1.2)
Total range of motion (°)				
>554	14 (12)	25 (21)	1	1
522 to 554	25 (21)	14 (12)	1.4 (1.01 to 1.7)	1.2 (0.9 to 1.2)
<522	23 (20)	16 (14)	1.4 (1.1 to 1.6)‡	1.2 (1.03 to 1.3)‡
Osteophyte scores				
1	19 (16)	28 (24)	1	na
2 to 4	19 (16)	10 (9)	1.4 (1.0 to 3.8)‡	
>4	11 (9)	8 (7)	1.5 (1.0 to 1.8)‡	
JSN scores				
1	19 (16)	32 (27)	1	1
2 to 4	16 (14)	12 (10)	1.5 (0.9 to 2.1)	1.6 (0.7 to 2.4)
>4	14 (12)	2 (2)	2.3 (1.5 to 2.6)‡	2.4 (1.9 to 2.7)‡

[1]except for determinants age, sex and BMI themselves, adjustment was made for age, sex and BMI.
[2]multivariate model using a backward selection (R^2 = 48.6%). The independent variables with univariate associations with a p-value ≤0.10 were included.
Both models are calculated using approximation formula of Zhang.[19].
‡: statistically significant.
Abbreviations: WOMAC: Western Ontario and McMaster Universities, JSN: joint space narrowing, na: not applicable.

the present study, self-reported pain and function for the whole group did not change in 6 years. This can be explained by the variation in progression between individuals as depicted in the cumulative probability plots (Figure 1a and 1b). Although some patients remained stable and even reported improvement, a considerable proportion of patients reported more pain and worse function. As a result the mean change is small. As expected in the sub-group of patients receiving joint prosthesis during follow-up, self-reported pain improved over 6 years, however, self-reported function did not. These results are consistent with the notion that joint replacement is an effective treatment for pain in lower limb OA. However, it seems that joint replacement cannot replace the function of the natural joint. Our results showed some parallels with a recent study by Nilsdotter et al.[20] They showed that patients had high preoperative expectations concerning reduction of pain and function but one year after knee replacement only the expectation regarding reduction of pain was fulfilled.

Table 4. Determinants of good prognosis of lower limb osteoarthritis over 6 years.

Determinant	*Number of patients*		*Risk ratio (95% CI)* [1]	*Risk ratio (95% CI)* [2]
	Good prognosis (%)	*Without good prognosis (%)*		
Age>60 years	28 (24)	3 (3)	1.0 (0.7 to 1.0)	na
Female sex	29 (25)	68 (58)	2.8 (0.8 to 6.3)	na
Body mass index (kg/m^2)				
<25.5	14 (12)	25 (21)	1	na
25.5 to 29.1	12 (10)	25 (21)	0.9 (0.4 to 1.6)	
>29.1	5 (4)	35 (30)	0.3 (0.1 to 0.9)	
WOMAC pain scores				
0 to 18.0	4 (4)	34 (29)	1	na
18.0 to 45.9	14 (12)	24 (20)	2.7 (0.7 to 3.6)	
>40.9	13 (11)	27 (23)	2.2 (0.7 to 3.8)	
WOMAC function scores				
0 to 18.0	6 (5)	34 (29)	1	na
18.0 to 40.9	13 (11)	24 (20)	2.5 (0.1 to 4.5)	
>40.9	12 (10)	27 (23)	1.9 (0.7 to 3.8)	
Change in WOMAC pain score in 1 year				
<−3.3	14 (12)	12 (10)	1	na
−3.3 to 10.1	5 (4)	21 (18)	0.3 (0.1 to 0.6)‡	0.6 (0.1 to 1.3)
>10.1	3 (3)	23 (20)	0.1 (0.1 to 0.8)‡	0.5 (0.1 to 1.1)
Change in WOMAC function score in 1 year				
<−1.4	15 (13)	11 (9)	1	1
−1.4 to 6.7	5 (4)	22 (19)	0.3 (0.1 to 0.7)‡	0.3 (0.1 to 0.8)‡
>6.7	2 (2)	23 (18)	0.1 (0.1 to 0.7)‡	0.2 (0.1 to 0.8)‡
Pain on physical examination	20 (17)	11 (9)	0.9 (0.6 to 1.1)	na
Total range of motion (°)				
>554	12 (10)	27 (23)	1	na
522 to 554	10 (9)	28 (24)	0.8 (0.3 to 1.7)	
<522	9 (8)	30 (26)	0.9 (0.4 to 1.8)	
Osteophyte scores				
1	17 (15)	30 (26)	1	na
2 to 4	6 (5)	23 (20)	0.6 (0.2 to 1.2)	
>4	4 (3)	15 (13)	0.5 (0.2 to 1.3)	
JSN scores				
1	18 (15)	33 (28)	1	na
2 to 4	7 (6)	21 (18)	0.7 (0.3 to 1.4)	
>4	2 (2)	14 (12)	0.4 (0.1 to 1.4)	

[1]except for determinants age, sex and BMI themselves, adjustment was made for age, sex and BMI.
[2]multivariate model using a backward selection ($R^2 = 43.3\%$). The independent variables with univariate associations with a p-value ≤0.10 were included.
Both models are calculated using approximation formula of Zhang.[19].
‡: statistically significant.
Abbreviations: WOMAC: Western Ontario and McMaster Universities, JSN: joint space narrowing, na: not applicable.

While self-reported pain at baseline was not associated with clinical progression, rapid deterioration in self-reported pain and function in the first year (even after correction for WOMAC scores at baseline that could confound the association) was associated with higher risk of progression over 6 years. This has not been studied before in OA, but it is in accordance with studies in rheumatoid arthritis (RA): worsening in self-reported disability measured with the health assessment questionnaire was a predictor for severe RA outcomes on the long term.[21] Interestingly, worsening in WOMAC pain and function score in 1-year were negatively associated with good prognosis. The consequence of these findings is that by following lower limb OA patients for 1 year, doctors can inform the patients about the progression of the OA in the long term. Therefore, it might advisable that doctors see their patients again 1-year after the first visit. It will be also interesting to investigate in a clinical trial whether modification of self reported pain or function one year after the presentation by means of physical therapy or better pain medication could stop the clinical progression of OA.

Pain on physical examination at baseline was associated with clinical progression. It was also the only pain variable that deteriorated over time. This observation reflects that pain as reported by the patient differs from pain on passive movement as found during physical examination as shown previously.[22]

Limited tROM (RR 1.4, 95%CI 1.1 to 1.6) and presence of pain on physical examination at baseline (RR 1.2, 95%CI 1.0 to 1.5) probably reflected the structural damage and might be used as a surrogate for osteophyte and JSN scores. In a recent EULAR recommendation for the diagnosis of knee OA, limited movement was indeed proposed as one of the clinical signs needed to make the diagnosis, probably because it was associated with radiological OA.[23]

Osteophytes and JSN scores were also identified as determinants of lower limb OA progression. Our findings support the findings of Lane and colleague, that osteophyte, JSN together with subchondral bone sclerosis were associated with hip OA progression.[4]

We showed that the WOMAC function changes in 1 year, limited tROM and higher JSN scores were independently significant determinants of clinical progression of lower limb OA. Although the main aim of this paper was to identify the determinants that were associated with clinical progression and not to build a prognostic model, we tried to get an impression on how good these determinants in predicting clinical progression when they were present together. We also tested the discriminative ability of this model to get an indication on how good the presence of these determinants predicts the clinical progression of lower OA. Their cumulative presence provided a very good explanation of variation in clinical progression, as shown with R^2 of 48.6%. The AUCs of the ROC curves of 0.80 also indicates a reasonable discriminative ability. This means that performing assessment on these three determinants in clinical practice will help clinician much in predicting the progression of lower limb OA and therefore give better patient information.

Roos et al showed that female sex was associated with worsening in self-reported pain and function and that older age and higher BMI were associated with worsening in function assessed on physical examination. On the other hand, we found no associations between demographic determinants and clinical progression.[5] Determinants for incidence are often failed to be identified as determinant of progression. The failure in finding determinants for progression is a common phenomenon that might be caused by methodological problem in studies restricted to subjects with existing disease.[24] Unfortunately, no method is yet available to overcome this problem. Another possible explanation in the difference in our results and results from Roos et al is the difference in patient population. The population in the study of Roos was a mix of knee OA patients and participants who underwent menisectomy in the past.

Our study sample that consists of selected sib-pairs with OA at multiple sites has strengths and limitations. Since generalized OA (GOA) population is associated with rapid OA progression [25], our study population is suitable to investigate OA progression within a relatively short period. However, the generalizability of our results in other population settings, especially to general practice clinics is arguably limited and we could not investigate GOA as determinant for progression. Yet, if we compare the 'severity of OA' by taking the incidence of joint prosthesis, we did not see much difference in the incidence of joint prosthesis in our study sample and in a hospital based OA population which was not selected for GOA, for a comparable follow-up time.[9] It supports the observations in other patient populations that generalized OA is also common and it is important to bear in mind that OA is often present at multiple sites while only the most symptomatic sites draw attention.[9], [25] To leave out the familial effect, we have performed a correction for familial factors in analysis.

The choice of the composite outcome that is a combination of two outcomes: joint prosthesis and increase in WOMAC pain or function scores above MPCI rewards comments. The two outcomes might be different; increase in WOMAC scores above MPCI might not always results in joint prosthesis. Also, the use of MPCI in defining progression is arbitrary. It was originally created to indicate clinical improvement in trials.[8] However, since no clinical outcome regarding clinical progression of knee or hip or lower limb OA is available at this moment, our choice of outcome could be considered to be used in observational studies.

It should be noted that our study population consists mainly of female. OA is known to be more common in female. The phenomenon that female tend to be overrepresented in OA studies is well known, such as in the large Bristol 'OA 500 study' mentioned above.[9] In the present study, effort has been taken to adjust for this possible confounder.

In summary, over a period of 6 years, more than half of the patients showed progression of lower limb OA, based on total joint replacement or change in self-reported pain or function above the MPCI. Performing combination of clinical and radiological assessment in clinical practice could evaluate the sub-group of patients with progression of lower limb OA. These findings would help doctors in patient information regarding progression of lower limb OA.

Acknowledgments

The authors would like to thank Dr. Naghmeh Riyazi and Dr. Stella Botha-Scheepers for performing clinical assessments. The authors would also like to acknowledge support of the cooperating hospitals (Bronovo Hospital, The Hague: Dr. ML Westedt; Jan van Breemen Instituut, Amsterdam: Dr. D van Schaardenburg; Leyenburg Hospital, The Hague: Dr. HK Ronday and Dr. LN Coene; Reinier de Graaf Gasthuis, Delft: Dr. AJ Peeters; Rijnland Hospital, Leiderdorp: Dr. EJ van Langelaan) and referring rheumatologists, orthopedic surgeons, and general practitioners.

Author Contributions

Conceived and designed the experiments: EY JB MK. Performed the experiments: EY JB HK MK. Analyzed the data: EY JB MK. Contributed reagents/materials/analysis tools: EY JB MK FR TH. Wrote the paper: EY JB MK. Drafted the article: EY JB MK Revised the article for important intellectual content: PS HK FR TH.

References

1. Lawrence RC, Helmick CG, Arnett FC, Deyo RA, Felson DT, et al. (1998) Estimates of the prevalence of arthritis and selected musculoskeletal disorders in the United States. Arthritis Rheum 41: 778–799.
2. Felson DT (2009) Developments in the clinical understanding of osteoarthritis. Arthritis Res Ther 11: 203.
3. Cooper C, Snow S, McAlindon TE, Kellingray S, Stuart B, et al. (2000) Risk factors for the incidence and progression of radiographic knee osteoarthritis. Arthritis Rheum 43: 995–1000.
4. Lane NE, Nevitt MC, Hochberg MC, Hung YY, Palermo L (2004) Progression of radiographic hip osteoarthritis over eight years in a community sample of elderly white women. Arthritis Rheum 50: 1477–1486.
5. Roos EM, Bremander AB, Englund M, Lohmander LS (2008) Change in self-reported outcomes and objective physical function over 7 years in middle-aged subjects with or at high risk of knee osteoarthritis. Ann Rheum Dis 67: 505–510.
6. O'Reilly SC, Muir KR, Doherty M (2000) Occupation and knee pain: a community study. Osteoarthritis Cartilage 8: 78–81.

7. Lacey RJ, Thomas E, Duncan RC, Peat G (2008) Gender difference in symptomatic radiographic knee osteoarthritis in the Knee Clinical Assessment–CAS(K): a prospective study in the general population. BMC Musculoskelet Disord 9: 82.
8. Ehrich EW, Davies GM, Watson DJ, Bolognese JA, Seidenberg BC, et al. (2000) Minimal perceptible clinical improvement with the Western Ontario and McMaster Universities osteoarthritis index questionnaire and global assessments in patients with osteoarthritis. J Rheumatol 27: 2635–2641.
9. Dieppe P, Cushnaghan J, Tucker M, Browning S, Shepstone L (2000) The Bristol 'OA500 study': progression and impact of the disease after 8 years. Osteoarthritis Cartilage 8: 63–68.
10. Belo JN, Berger MY, Reijman M, Koes BW, Bierma-Zeinstra SM (2007) Prognostic factors of progression of osteoarthritis of the knee: a systematic review of observational studies. Arthritis Rheum 57: 13–26.
11. Wright AA, Cook C, Abbott JH (2009) Variables associated with the progression of hip osteoarthritis: a systematic review. Arthritis Rheum 61: 925–936.
12. Riyazi N, Meulenbelt I, Kroon HM, Ronday KH, Hellio le Graverand MP, et al. (2005) Evidence for familial aggregation of hand, hip, and spine but not knee osteoarthritis in siblings with multiple joint involvement: the GARP study. Ann Rheum Dis 64: 438–443.
13. Altman R, Asch E, Bloch D, Bole G, Borenstein D, et al. (1986) Development of criteria for the classification and reporting of osteoarthritis. Classification of osteoarthritis of the knee. Diagnostic and Therapeutic Criteria Committee of the American Rheumatism Association. Arthritis Rheum 29: 1039–1049.
14. Altman R, Alarcon G, Appelrouth D, Bloch D, Borenstein D, et al. (1991) The American College of Rheumatology criteria for the classification and reporting of osteoarthritis of the hip. Arthritis Rheum 34: 505–514.
15. Ware JE, Jr., Sherbourne CD (1992) The MOS 36-item short-form health survey (SF-36). I. Conceptual framework and item selection. Med Care 30: 473–483.
16. Aaronson NK, Muller M, Cohen PD, Essink-Bot ML, Fekkes M, et al. (1998) Translation, validation, and norming of the Dutch language version of the SF-36 Health Survey in community and chronic disease populations. J Clin Epidemiol 51: 1055–1068.
17. Doyle DV, Dieppe PA, Scott J, Huskisson EC (1981) An articular index for the assessment of osteoarthritis. Ann Rheum Dis 40: 75–78.
18. Altman RD, Gold GE (2007) Atlas of individual radiographic features in osteoarthritis, revised. Osteoarthritis Cartilage 15 Suppl A: A1–56.
19. Zhang J, Yu KF (1998) What's the relative risk? A method of correcting the odds ratio in cohort studies of common outcomes. JAMA 280: 1690–1691.
20. Nilsdotter AK, Toksvig-Larsen S, Roos EM (2009) Knee arthroplasty: are patients' expectations fulfilled? A prospective study of pain and function in 102 patients with 5-year follow-up. Acta Orthop 80: 55–61.
21. Bykerk V (2009) Anti-cyclic citrullinated peptide antibody versus HAQ/MDHAQ: comparing apples and oranges? J Rheumatol 36: 1565–1567.
22. Bijsterbosch J, Wassenaar MJ, le Cessie S, Slagboom PE, Rosendaal FR, et al. (2010) Doyle Index is a valuable additional pain measure in osteoarthritis. Osteoarthritis Cartilage 18: 1046–50.
23. Zhang W, Doherty M, Peat G, Bierma-Zeinstra MA, Arden NK, et al. (2010) EULAR evidence-based recommendations for the diagnosis of knee osteoarthritis. Ann Rheum Dis 69: 483–489.
24. Zhang Y, Niu J, Felson DT, Choi HK, Nevitt M, et al. (2010) Methodologic challenges in studying risk factors for progression of knee osteoarthritis. Arthritis Care Res (Hoboken) 62: 1527–1532.
25. Ledingham J, Regan M, Jones A, Doherty M (1995) Factors affecting radiographic progression of knee osteoarthritis. Ann Rheum Dis 54: 53–58.

23

Polymorphisms in the Inflammatory Genes *CIITA*, *CLEC16A* and *IFNG* Influence BMD, Bone Loss and Fracture in Elderly Women

Maria Swanberg[1,2], Fiona E. McGuigan[1], Kaisa K. Ivaska[3], Paul Gerdhem[4,5], Kristina Åkesson[1,6]*

1 Clinical and Molecular Osteoporosis Research Unit, Department of Clinical Sciences, Lund University, Sweden, **2** Neurodegeneration and Inflammation Genetics Unit, Department of Experimental Medical Science, Lund University, Sweden, **3** Department of Cell Biology and Anatomy, Institute of Biomedicine, University of Turku, Turku, Finland, **4** Department of Clinical Science, Intervention and Technology, Karolinska Institute, Stockholm, Sweden, **5** Department of Orthopaedics, Karolinska University Hospital, Stockholm, Sweden, **6** Department of Orthopaedics, Skåne University Hospital, Malmö, Sweden

Abstract

Osteoclast activity and the fine balance between bone formation and resorption is affected by inflammatory factors such as cytokines and T lymphocyte activity, mediated by major histocompatibility complex (MHC) molecules, in turn regulated by the MHC class II transactivator (MHC2TA). We investigated the effect of functional polymorphisms in the MHC2TA gene (*CIITA*), and two additional genes; C-type lectin domain 16A (*CLEC16A)*, in linkage disequilibrium with *CIITA* and Interferon-γ (*IFNG*), an inducer of *CIITA;* on bone density, bone resorption markers, bone loss and fracture risk in 75 year-old women followed for up to 10 years (OPRA n = 1003) and in young adult women (PEAK-25 n = 999). *CIITA* was associated with BMD at age 75 (lumbar spine p = 0.011; femoral neck (FN) p = 0.049) and age 80 (total body p = 0.015; total hip p = 0.042; FN p = 0.028). Carriers of the *CIITA* rs3087456(G) allele had 1.8–3.4% higher BMD and displayed increased rate of bone loss between age 75 and 80 (FN p = 0.013; total hip p = 0.030; total body p = 3.8E^{-5}). Despite increasing bone loss, the rs3087456(G) allele was protective against incident fracture overall (p = 0.002), osteoporotic fracture and hip fracture. Carriers of *CLEC16A* and *IFNG* variant alleles had lower BMD ($p<0.05$) and ultrasound parameters and a lower risk of incident fracture (*CLEC16A*, p = 0.011). In 25-year old women, none of the genes were associated with BMD. In conclusion, variation in inflammatory genes *CIITA*, *CLEC-16A* and *INFG* appear to contribute to bone phenotypes in elderly women and suggest a role for low-grade inflammation and MHC class II expression for osteoporosis pathogenesis.

Editor: Stacey Cherny, University of Hong Kong, Hong Kong

Funding: This work was supported by grants from the Swedish Research Council www.vr.se (K2009-53X-14691-07-3, K2010-77PK-21362-01-2), FAS www.fas.se (Grant 2007–2125), Greta and Johan Kock Foundation www.kockskastiftelsen.se, A. Påhlsson Foundation, A. Osterlund Foundation, Knut and Alice Wallenberg Foundation www.wallenberg.com/kaw, the H Järnhardt foundation, King Gustav V and Queen Victoria Foundation, Åke Wiberg Foundation, Thelma Zoegas Foundation, Malmö University Hospital Research Foundation, Research and Development Council of Region Skåne, Sweden, the Swedish Medical Society www.slf.se. The funders had no role in study design, data collection and analysis, decision to publish, or preparation of the manuscript.

Competing Interests: The authors have declared that no competing interests exist.

* E-mail: Kristina.Akesson@med.lu.se

Introduction

Osteoporosis is a common disease in our ageing society and affects one in three women during the course of their lifetime. The disease is characterized by quantitative and qualitative changes to bone tissue and results in increased risk of fractures [1]. The etiology of osteoporosis is complex and contains both genetic and environmental risk factors, as well as interactions between them. As much as 80% of the population variance in bone mineral density (BMD) is genetically determined and results from many common alleles conferring small risk increments [2]. Genes may be phenotype specific or pleiotropic within the context of osteoporosis or shared with other complex diseases [2,3].

The role of the immune system is well established in conditions that are primarily inflammatory such as rheumatoid arthritis (RA), systemic lupus erythematosus (SLE) and multiple sclerosis (MS), however, systemic inflammatory processes are involved in other complex diseases such as obesity, diabetes and cardiovascular disease, and possibly also osteoporosis [4–6]. These diseases are generally more prevalent with increasing age and shared common risk factors have been identified [5,6]. While patients with some chronic inflammatory disorders are more likely to develop osteopenia, osteoimmunological interplay also constitutes part of normal physiological processes in bone.

The interplay between the immune system and bone metabolism includes molecular and cellular interactions between haematopoietic cells, lymphocytes, osteoblasts and osteoclasts, which are derived from the monocyte-macrophage lineage [2,3]. These interactions involve major histocompatibility complex (MHC) molecules and cytokines that have dual roles in bone homeostasis [3,7,8]. Antigen presentation on MHC molecules and the resulting activating patterns are crucial to the degree and type of immune response. Macrophage lineage cells are thus capable of both eliciting and modulating the inflammatory response by presenting MHCII molecules and activating T lymphocytes. The MHCII transactivator (MHC2TA) assembles transcription factors at promoter sites and is the master regulator of MHCII expression [9]. Expression of MHC2TA is crucial for proper antigen presentation [10] and is in turn induced by the cytokine interferon-γ (IFNγ).

Allelic variation in MHCII molecules contributes to several diseases including MS [11], RA [12,13] and osteoarthritis [14,15] while Genome-wide association studies (GWAS) of bone density and fracture have identified the human leukocyte antigen (HLA) region on chromosome 6p21, which encodes many immune-related genes including MHCII [16,17]. In the HLA region, the common rs3130340(T) allele was found to be associated with reduced BMD at the spine and increased risk of low trauma fractures [17]. Combining GWAS and gene expression data, Farber performed weighted gene co-expression network analysis (WGCNA) and identified a co-expression module highly enriched for genes involved in immune processes [18]. In addition, association studies have identified the pro-inflammatory interleukin 6 (IL6) gene as a determinant for low BMD [19–22], while in a previous study of the pro-inflammatory cytokine macrophage migration inhibitory factor (*MIF*) gene we reported association of *MIF* polymorphisms with bone loss and increased levels of bone resorption markers in elderly women [23].

A more pro-inflammatory profile characterized by increased levels of IFNγ and changes in cytokine regulation is evident in perimenopausal women and may induce bone loss. For example, activated T lymphocytes produce tumor necrosis factor-α (TNFα), an instrumental cytokine contributing to increased osteoclast activity and subsequent loss of bone density [24]. Studies in mice report a key role for MHC2TA in ovariectomy-induced bone loss, where the increased production of IFNγ increased MHC2TA expression, leading to lymphocyte activation and production of TNFα [25]. Based on the link between bone and inflammation, we hypothesize that polymorphisms of genes in the IFNγ-MHC2TA-MHCII pathway have implications for susceptibility to postmenopausal and senile osteoporosis. To date, this has not been explored as a determinant of bone loss and fracture with advancing age or at the time of maximal bone mass. In this study, we therefore analyzed polymorphisms in three genes encoding proteins regulating adaptive immune responses; MHC2TA (*CIITA*; 16p13), C-type lectin domain 16A (*CLEC16A*; 16p13) and IFNγ (*IFNG*; 12q14).

The rational for selecting these genes for analysis is based on considerable evidence. For example, null mutations in *CIITA* cause severe immunodeficiency [10] while common functional polymorphisms in the gene affect MHCII expression levels and susceptibility to inflammatory and complex diseases [26–33]. *CLEC16A* is located adjacent to and in linkage disequilibrium (LD) with *CIITA*, motivating analysis of this gene in conjunction with *CIITA*. Furthermore, CLECs play important roles in adaptive immunity by shaping the cytokine profile [34] and associations between *CLEC16A*, both in conjunction and independent of *CIITA* have been reported in several inflammatory conditions [31,35–38]. IFNγ induces MHCII expression through *CIITA* and polymorphisms in *IFNG* are associated with differential gene expression and disease susceptibility [39]. In postmenopausal women, the production of pro-inflammatory cytokines such as IFNγ is increased [40] and studies in ovariectomized mice have shown increased production of IFNγ, enhanced activation of T lymphocytes through MHC2TA and increased bone loss [25].

To address the genetic impact of polymorphisms in genes with possible effects on osteoimmunological interactions involving MHCII, T-lymphocytes and osteoclast activation, we studied both young and elderly women; 1003 75-year old women followed for up to 10 years and 999 25-year old women in order to capture age-related differences on BMD, bone loss and incident fracture risk.

Methods

Study Subjects

The Malmö Osteoporotic Prospective Risk Assessment (OPRA) cohort is a longitudinal population-based cohort of Caucasian women aged 75 years who were randomly selected from the Malmö city files between 1995 and 1999. No exclusion criteria were applied. A total of 1604 women were invited, 1044 (65%) attended at baseline and 715 women completed the 5 year follow-up visit.

In this study, BMD was measured at baseline and 5 years, with additional measurements available in 371 women at 10 years for hip and total body. Bone resorption markers were measured in serum at baseline and at the 1-, 3-, and 5-year follow-up visits. Information on medication, smoking and illness was collected by a questionnaire. Of the 1044 women at baseline, 145 (14%) were smokers, 208 (20%) were former smokers, 69 had diabetes, 48 were using hormone replacement therapy (HRT) or bisphosphonates at baseline (119 were using one or both of these medications at baseline or sometime during the 5 year follow-up period). Full details of this cohort have been reported previously [41].

The PEAK-25 cohort is a population-based cohort of Caucasian women aged 25 years living in Malmö. Initially, 2394 women randomly selected from the city files between 1999 and 2004 were invited, 1059 (44%) attended the full investigation. The exclusion criteria used were pregnancy or recent childbirth (n = 102, 7.6% of non-participants). Of those who participated, 56% were non-smokers 26% were current smokers and 18% were previous smokers. Full details of this cohort have been reported previously [42].

All participants gave written informed consent and the Lund University Ethics Committee approved the study. This study was performed according to the principles of the Helsinki declaration.

The data reported in this analysis is based on women for whom genotype and phenotype data was available, corresponding to 1003 women from the OPRA cohort at baseline and 999 women from the PEAK-25 cohort. Clinical characteristics of the women attending the baseline visit are shown in Table 1.

Marker Selection

Polymorphisms in *CIITA*, *CLEC16A* and *INFG* were selected based on previously reported associations with inflammatory disorders, other diseases or differential gene expression [29–31,33,35–37,39,43,44]. The SNPs have not previously been identified in GWAS of osteoporosis related traits. Marker details and criteria for selection are shown in Table 2.

Genotyping

Total genomic DNA was isolated from blood using the QIAamp 96 DNA blood kit (Qiagen, Valencia, CA, USA) according to the manufacturer's instructions.

Genotyping of *CLEC16A* (rs6498169) and *INFG* polymorphisms rs2069705 and rs2069727 was performed using Taqman SNP genotyping Assay (Applied Biosystems, Foster City, CA, USA). PCR was conducted in a Dual 384-well GeneAmp PCR system 9700 (Applied Biosystems), with an endpoint plate read on ABI 7900HT (Appied Biosystems) using the SDS 2.2.2 software. Polymorphisms for *CIITA* (rs3087456 and rs4774), *CLEC16A* (rs2903692 and rs725613) and *INFG* (rs2069718) were genotyped by Sequenom's iPlex Gold system (Sequenom, San Diego, CA). The overall success rate for both methods was >98 for all polymorphisms. Approximately 3% of the samples from each cohort were genotyped in duplicate with 100 percent concordance.

Table 1. Baseline clinical characteristics of the OPRA and PEAK-25 cohorts.

	OPRA (n = 1003)			PEAK-25 (n = 999)		
Variable	**Mean**	**±SD**	**(Range)**	**Mean**	**±SD**	**(Range)**
Age (years)	75.2	0.1	(75.0–75.9)	25.5	0.2	(25.0–25.9)
Weight (kg)	67.8	11.5	(41–110)	64.6	11.1	(40–135)
Height[a] (cm)	164.1	5.5	(145–180)	167.6	6.1	(150–187)
BMD (g/cm²)[b]						
Total body	1.007	0.097	(0.718–1.422)	1.174	0.073	(0.969–1.478)
Femoral neck	0.748	0.130	(0.153–1.230)	1.055	0.124	(0.746–1.604)
Total hip	0.849	0.149	(0.498–1.416)			
Lumbar spine	0.993	0.195	(0.518–1.855)	1.217	0.129	(0.824–1.868)
Ultrasound[c]						
BUA	102	10	(56–136)	118	11	(59–149)
SoS	1523	27	(1425–1643)	1575	32	(1498–1706)
Stiffness	72	13	(31–112)	99	15	(42–150)

[a]Height at age 20 (OPRA), Height at baseline visit, age 25 (PEAK25).
[b]BMD n = 904–946 (OPRA), n = 996–999 (PEAK-25).
[c]QUS n = 853 (OPRA), n = 853 (PEAK-25).

All polymorphisms conformed to Hardy-Weinberg equilibrium. Allele and genotype frequencies are reported in Supplementary Table S1.

Bone Density

The areal BMD was measured with dual-energy x-ray absorptiometry (DXA) by Lunar DPX-L for OPRA and Lunar Prodigy for PEAK-25 (Lunar Corporation WI, USA and GE Health Lunar Densitometry, WI, USA) at all sites (total body (TB), femoral neck (FN), total hip (TH) and lumbar spine L2–L4 (LS)). Analyses of OPRA scans were made with software versions 1.33 and 1.35 at baseline, 4.7b at five years and 4.7e at 10 years. The total hip scans were all analyzed with version 4.7b. There was no drift in phantom measurement results during the study period. Analyses of PEAK-25 scans were made with software versions 2.05, 2.15, 3.60, 5.70 and 7.70. DXA calibrations were performed daily using a manufacturer supplied phantom and the precision error (coefficient of variation) was total body; 0.94, LS; 1.45 and FN; 4.01 [45].

The rate of bone loss (RBL) between age 75 and 80 represents the annual change in BMD between the scan at baseline (BMD_{BL}) and the 5-year follow-up (BMD_{5Y}). It was calculated as $[(BMD_{5Y}\text{-}BMD_{BL})/BMD_{BL}/\text{years between scans}*100]$. The LS BMD at age 80 and LS RBL are not reported since previously we showed that LS BMD increased likely due to the presence of osteophytes, degenerative changes and compressive fractures common in women of this age [46]. Weight and BMD at age 75, 80 and 85 along with RBL is presented in Supplementary Table S3.

Quantitative Ultrasound

Quantitative ultrasound measurement speed of sound (SoS), broadband ultrasound attenuation (BUA) and stiffness index (SI, derived from of BUA and SoS) were assessed in both cohorts using a Lunar Achilles® system (Lunar Corporation, Madison, WI, USA). The right calcaneus was measured unless precluded by a previous history of injury or fracture. Precision was 1.5 for BUA and SOS [47] and calibrations were performed daily.

Fracture

Fractures in the OPRA cohort were self-reported for adult fractures (age 20–75) at the time of inclusion in the study and were verified from radiological files as previously reported [48]. In addition, incident fractures during the follow-up period (until November 2006) were recorded and verified by reviewing the related medical records [49]. The majority of fractures sustained (>99%) were attributable to low energy trauma. Fractures were classified as being osteoporotic if affecting the hip, distal radius, spine or proximal humerus.

Table 2. Markers used in the study and allele frequency in the OPRA cohort.

SNP ID	Location Chr (bp)	Common allele (frequency)	Minor allele (frequency)	Selection criteria
CIITA				
rs3087456	16 (10970902)	A (0.765)	G (0.235)	Association with inflammatory disease and differential gene expression. [29,30,33]
rs4774	16 (11000848)	G (0.689)	C (0.311)	
CLEC16A				
rs725613	16 (11169683)	T (0.660)	G (0.340)	Associated with type 1 diabetes and multiple sclerosis. [31,35,73–75]
rs2903692	16 (11238783)	G (0.678)	A (0.322)	
rs6498169	16 (11249329)	A (0.604)	G (0.396)	Associated with multiple sclerosis and rheumatoid arthritis [31,36,76]
IFNG				
rs2069727	12 (68548223)	T (0.532)	C (0.468)	Located 3′ near gene
rs2069718	12 (68550162)	C (0.582)	T (0.418)	Association with SLE. Located in intron 3 [39]
rs2069705	12 (68555011)	T (0.626)	C (0.374)	Association with SLE. Located 5′ upstream of gene [39]

Biochemistry

The serum bone markers C-terminal cross-linking telopeptide of type I collagen (S-CTX) and serum tartrate-resistant acid phosphatase 5b (S-TRACP5b) were analyzed in the OPRA cohort. S-TRACP5b was determined with BoneTRAP® assay (SBA Sciences/Immunodiagnostic Systems IDS Inc., Bolton, UK) and S-CTX was determined with Elecsys β-CrossLaps immunoassay (Roche Diagnostics, Indianapolis, IN). Details of the assays have been reported previously [46].

Longitudinal measures of bone resorption markers at baseline, 1-, 3-, and 5-years (age 80) were used. Among the 1003 women included in this study, data for all time points was available from 614 subjects for S-TRACP5b and from 606 subjects for S-CTX. Subgroups were created according to whether women had constantly low or constantly or high levels of S-CTX or S-TRACP5b over 5 years, as described previously. Those in the lowest or highest tertiles at three or more time points were considered to have constantly low or high levels, respectively, over the 5-year period. All others were classified into the intermediate group [50]. Among the 1003 women included in this study, 93 were constantly high and 108 constantly low for S-TRACP5b and 121 constantly high and 117 constantly low for S-CTX. Women using potent estrogen or bisphosphonates were excluded from the analyses (S-TRACP5b n = 76, S-CTX n = 77) since these medications have been shown to decrease S-CTX levels [51,52].

Routine biochemistry measured C-reactive protein (CRP, mg/L) in plasma, erythrocyte sedimentation rate (ESR, mm/h) in blood and leukocytes (BLC 10^9/L) in blood at 10-year follow-up.

Statistics

Deviation from Hardy-Weinberg equilibrium was calculated by the chi-square test. Linkage disequilibrium (LD) was evaluated within each gene and between *CIITA* and *CLEC-16A* using the Haploview program (http://www.broad.mit.edu/mpg/haploview/) and taking into consideration both D and r^2. Haplotypes were constructed for *CLEC16A* and *IFNG* using PHASE version 2.02 [53], and estimated haplotypes with a frequency >0.10 and a >0.8 probability of correct assignment were used for analysis.

ANOVA was used to determine associations between genotypes, bone density and rate of bone loss.

Bone resorption marker values were log-transformed prior to analysis due to non-normal distribution. The t-test was used for comparing mean S-CTX and S-TRACP5b values, and the Pearson Chi-Square test was used for analyzing consistently high and low levels of markers and association of polymorphisms with fracture incidence.

Linear regression was used to identify confounding factors for BMD, RBL and ultrasound and where indicated, multinomial logistic regression was used to adjust for total body BMD and weight at baseline in fracture analyses. Age was not included for adjustment since all the women within each cohort were of the same age.

The following covariates were used in the analyses of the OPRA cohort. BMD at baseline: weight (baseline), diabetes, current use of bisphosphonates (BPs) or potent estrogen (E) and smoking exposure (cigarettes per day*years smoking); BMD at 5-year follow-up: weight (5-year follow-up) and smoking exposure; BMD at 10-year follow-up: weight (10-year follow-up); RBL: use of E and/or BPs at baseline or during follow-up; QUS: weight (baseline), current use of BPs or E and smoking exposure. Exclusion of estrogen or bisphosphonate users from the analysis (n = 82) did not appreciably alter the results overall.

When indicated, weight change between baseline and 5-year follow-up visit was also used as covariate for RBL. Covariates used in the PEAK-25 cohort were height, weight and smoking for BMD; weight and smoking for ultrasound phenotypes.

Interaction between polymorphisms may contribute to opposite or synergistic effects on the phenotype of interest. To this end we performed pairwise interactions between SNPs to explore the effect on differences in BMD and QUS. Using general linear model-ANOVA (GLM-ANOVA), the model included an interaction term, covariates and assumed a co-dominant genetic model. In the results, p-values are reported for the interaction overall while in the tables mean BMD values defined by SNP_1-SNP_2 carriers compared to SNP_1-SNP_2 non-carriers are presented.

A priori power analyses indicated that the sample size of our studies allowed a >80% power to detect a difference in BMD of 0.1 standard deviations among genotype groups, while maintaining a type I error at 5%. This is based on the assumption of a SD of 0.13 g/cm^2 in BMD, which allows detection of a 0.065 g/cm^2 difference between genotype groups assuming a minor allele frequency of 0.21 or greater. Similarly, the OPRA study had >80% power to detect relative risks for fracture of at least 1.2.

All statistical analyses were performed using SPSS for Windows 18.0 (SPSS Inc., Chicago, IL) and associations with a p-value of <0.05 were considered nominally significant. The phenotypes and several of the markers studied are not independent (i.e. are correlated or in LD), therefore applying a Bonferroni correction would be over-stringent. We therefore report the uncorrected p-values and acknowledge the fact that multiple tests were performed.

Results

CIITA

The 2 SNPs in *CIITA* were not in strong LD with each other (D'<0.36, r^2<0.02) or with the 3 SNPs in the adjacent *CLEC16A* gene (D'<0.45, r^2<0.04). Haplotype estimates predicted 3 common (>10%) haplotypes (Supplementary Table S2). Haplotype analysis for *CIITA* did not add appreciably to the overall information obtained from genotype analyses (data not shown).

Bone Density and Bone Loss

In the OPRA cohort of elderly women, there was a moderate association between *CIITA* and BMD. Carriers of the rare rs3087456(G) allele displayed higher FN BMD at age 75 (baseline) and interaction between variant alleles rs3087456(G) and rs4774(C) was observed, resulting in higher LS BMD. At age 80 (5-year follow-up), FN BMD and TB BMD were also higher in rs3087456(G) carriers and an interaction between rs3087456(G) and rs4774(C) was associated with higher BMD at all sites (Table 3). At 10-year follow-up (n = 376), interaction between rs3087456(G) and rs4774(C) variant alleles was observed, with higher BMD at the FN (p = 0.019) TH (p = 0.027) and TB (p = 0.004) compared to common homozygotes (rs3087456(G): FN +0.4%, TH +1.7%, TB +1.8%; rs4774(C): FN +1.9%, TH +2.5%, TB +1.5%), data not shown.

The QUS results were in line with those for BMD with rs3087456(G) carriers having higher mean values for stiffness (72.9/70.6; p = 0.030) and BUA (102.6/101.1; p = 0.045).

Homozygotes for the rare *CIITA* allele rs3087456(G) had higher annual rates of bone loss (RBL) at the FN (p = 0.013), TH (p = 0.030) and TB (p = 0.00016). TB RBL was also higher for rs4774(C) homozygotes (p = 3.8E-5). This association was independent of weight change for FN and TB, but not for TH

Table 3. Associations between BMD and *CIITA*, *CLEC16A* and *IFNG* in the OPRA cohort.

Gene	SNP (rare allele)/haplotype	Site	Age	BMD mean[1] (g/cm²)	P-value*
CIITA	rs3087456(G)	FN	75	0.740/0.761	0.049
	rs3087456(G)*rs4774(C)	LS	75	0.967/0.992	0.011[2]
	rs3087456(G)	FN	80	0.702/0.726	0.041
	rs3087456(G)*rs4774(C)	FN	80	0.692/0.717	0.020[3]
	rs3087456(G)*rs4774(C)	TH	80	0.784/0.803	0.042
	rs3087456(G)	TB	80	0.989/1.009	0.015
	rs3087456(G)*rs4774(C)	TB	80	0.981/1.005	0.027
CLEC16A	Haplotype 1[4]	LS	75	1.002/0.983	0.037
	Haplotype 1[4]	FN	80	0.716/0.706	0.035
	Haplotype 1[4]	TH	80	0.802/0.794	0.039
	rs6498169	TB	80	0.997/1.002/0.985	0.037
IFNG	Haplotype 4[5]	TH	75	0.854/0.846	0.035
	rs2069727*rs2069705	LS	75	0.973/1.007/0.989 0.993/1.002/0.962	0.027

*Only associations where p<0.05 are reported.
[1]BMD values are reported as follows: For single SNP analysis (non-carrriers/carriers or common homozygotes/heterozygotes/variant homozygotes); For haplotypes (non-carriers/carriers); For interactions in allelic models (non-carriers of both variant alleles/carriers of both variant alleles); For interactions in genotypic models, values are given for each marker as common homozygotes/heterozygotes/variant homozygotes since no individuals were carriers of both variant alleles.
[2]For rs3087456 * rs4774 genotypic model, p = 0.011.
[3]For rs3087456 * rs4774 genotypic model, p = 0.028.
[4]CLEC16A haplotype 1: rs725613(T)/rs2903692(G)/rs6498169(A).
[5]IFNG haplotype 4: rs2069727(T)/rs2069718(T)/rs2069705(C).

(Table 4). In addition, there was interaction between SNPs rs3087456*rs4774 for TB RBL (p = 8.7E-5, adjusted 0.002).

CIITA was not associated with body weight at baseline, but to weight change between age 75 and 80 (rs3087456, p = 0.016, genotypic model). Women with the rs3087456(G/G) genotype had a mean weight loss of 2.8 kg compared to 1.4 kg for women with the rs3087456(A/A) genotype.

Bone resorption markers were not associated with *CIITA* genotype, neither was blood biochemistry (CRP, ESR) or blood leukocyte count.

Fracture

Among the OPRA participants, 51% (n = 507) had suffered at least one fracture between age 20 and 75, with no significant difference between the *CIITA* genotype groups. Incident fracture after age 75 was confirmed for 350 women (35%), resulting predominantly (99%) from low energy trauma. One or more osteoporotic fractures (at the hip, vertebra, distal radius or proximal humerus) occurred in 282 individuals (28%), of whom 110 (11%) had hip fracture.

The rs3087456(G) allele was protective against incident fracture overall, osteoporotic fractures and hip fracture (Table 5). The protective effect was significant even after correction for BMD and body weight at age 75 (Table 5).

Table 4. *CIITA* association with rate of bone loss between age 75 and 80.

Site	Marker	Mean BMD (g/cm²)[1]	P-value[2]	Adjusted P-value[3]
Femoral neck	rs3087456	−1.398/−1.498/−2.096	0.013	0.036
Total Hip	rs3087456	−1.123/−1.333/−1.599	0.030	NS
Total Body	rs3087456	−0.299/−0.250/−0.356	0.00016	0.0011
Total Body	rs4774	−0.286/−0.266/−0.348	0.000038	0.00069

[1]CC/CV/VV (c = common, v = variant allele).
[2]Genotypic model.
[3]Adjusted for weight change between age 75 and 80.

CLEC16A

LD between the *CLEC16A* SNPs was stronger between rs725613 and rs2903692 (D' = 0.95, $r^2 = 0.84$) than with rs6498169 (D'≥0.90, $r^2 \geq 0.27$). Three common (>10%) haplotypes were predicted (Supplementary Table S2).

Bone Density and Bone Loss

Carriers of *CLEC16A* haplotype 1 (rs725613(T)/rs2903692(G)/rs6498169(A)) had lower LS BMD at baseline (−2%) and lower BMD at the 5 year follow-up at the FN (−1.3%) and TH (−1.5%) (Table 3). Women with genotype rs6498169(G/G) displayed lower TB BMD at 5-year follow-up (0.98 vs 1.00, p = 0.037) compared to the rs6498169(A/A) or (A/G) genotypes. For bone loss between age 75 and 80, women with the rs2903692(A/A) genotype displayed reduced TB RBL (−1.30 vs −1.51, p = 0.033).

The rs2903692 marker was also associated with QUS parameters, as carriers of the rare (A) allele had lower stiffness values (71.2 vs 72.0; p = 0.040) while BUA was lowest in the (G/A) heterozygotes (GG: 101.9, GA: 101.5, AA: 101.9; p = 0.045).

Carriers of *CLEC16A* haplotype 1 had higher blood leucocyte counts at 10 years compared to non-carriers (BLC 7.0 vs 6.3×10^9/L, p = 0.002), while bone markers were not significantly associated.

Table 5. Association of *CIITA and CLEC16* polymorphisms with incident fractures between age 75 and 80 in the OPRA cohort.

Polymorphism	Genotype	Women without fracture (%)	Women with fracture (%)	p-value (adjusted)[1]	Odds Ratio (95% confidence interval)
Any fracture					
*CIITA*_ rs3087456	AA	349 (61)	223 (39)	0.002	
	AG/GG	294 (71)	122 (29)	(0.005)	0.657 (0.491–0.879)
CLEC16A_rs725613	TT	264 (61)	171 (39)	0.011	
	TG/GG	380 (69)	175 (32)	(0.013)	0.699 (0.526–0.928)
Hip fracture					
CIITA_ rs3087456	AA	498 (87)	74 (13)	0.025	
	AG/GG	381 (92)	35(8)	(0.038)	0.626 (0.402–0.975)
CLEC16A_rs725613	TT	392 (90)	43 (10)	NS	
	TG/GG	489 (88)	66 (12)	(NS)	
Osteoporotic fracture[2]					
CIITA_ rs3087456	AA	395 (69)	177 (31)	0.021	
	AG/GG	315 (76)	101 (24)	(0.047)	0.732 (0.538–0.996)
CLEC16A_rs725613	TT	297 (68)	138 (32)	0.027	
	TG/GG	415 (75)	140 (25)	(0.022)	0.705 (0.522–0.951)

[1]P-values calculated by χ^2; adjusted for variables weight and TB BMD at 75y (Any fracture, Osteoporotic fracture) or weight and FN BMD at 75y (Hip fracture).
[2]Osteoporotic fracture sites include hip, vertebrae, distal radius, proximal humerus.

Fracture

Carriage of the rare *CLEC16A* rs725613(G) allele or *CLEC16A* haplotype 7 (rs725613(G)/rs2903692(A)/rs6498169(A)) was similarly protective against incident fracture overall, including after correction for TB BMD and body weight. The rs725613(G) allele was also protective of osteoporotic fractures, but not hip fracture specifically (Table 5).

IFNG

The three markers in *IFNG* were in LD ($D' = 0.99$, $r^2 > 0.45$) and 3 common haplotypes were predicted (Supplementary Table S2).

Bone Density and Bone Loss

None of the individual genotypes were associated with BMD at baseline or follow-up; however carriers of haplotype 4 (rs2069727(T)/rs2069718(T)/rs2069705(C)) had 1% lower baseline BMD at the hip. Interaction between rs2069727*rs2069705 was also observed at the lumbar spine (Table 3).

For the QUS phenotypes, there were small but significant differences in mean values. The variant alleles for all 3 *IFNG* SNPs, but not their derived haplotypes, were associated with increased BUA, the most significant being rs2069727(C) ($p = 0.00003$). Carriers of rs2069705(G) and *IFNG* haplotype 4 had lower SoS values ($p = 0.003$). The rs2069727(C) and rs2069718(C/T) genotypes were associated with slightly higher stiffness values with both a single-marker and interactive model ($p = 0.033$-0.05). There was no association between polymorphisms in the *IFNG* gene and bone loss, fracture, bone markers or blood biochemistry.

Young Adult Women – the PEAK-25 Cohort

In young adult women representing peak bone mass, there was no association between *CIITA, CLEC16A or IFNG* SNPs and BMD. Small differences (<0.4%) between the genotype groups were observed between *CIITA* rs4774 and the QUS phenotype SoS ($p = 0.031$).

Discussion

This study suggests that inflammatory genes play a role in regulating bone mass and bone loss and influence the risk of incident fractures in elderly women. Specifically, we report association between polymorphisms in the inflammatory genes *CIITA, CLEC16A* and *IFNG* with BMD, ultrasound parameters, annual rate of bone loss and incident fractures in 75-year old women followed for 10 years. These results support inflammation and, specifically, MHCII expression as key components in postmenopausal or senile osteoporosis.

The reported association of *CIITA* and *IFNG* polymorphisms to BMD in elderly women is contrasted by the absence of association in young adult women, which suggests differential effects of these genes across the life span. It also supports our hypothesis that low-grade systemic inflammatory processes are elements of normal ageing in women, possibly due to the link between estrogen and cytokine levels. Estrogen receptors are expressed on both lymphocytes and mononuclear cells [54], making them responsive to changes in estrogen levels. Estrogen deficiency leads to increased immune activation mediated by antigen presenting cells (APCs) and cytokines (IFNγ, IL-7 and transforming growth factor-β), resulting in increased TNFα production from activated T lymphocytes [24]. By increasing both the production and sensitivity to RANKL, TNFα has potent effects on osteoclasts [24]. Polymorphisms affecting immune activation processes could therefore have an impact during periods with generally higher pro-inflammatory profile, such as old age and illness. We interpret the discrepant results between the elderly and young adult women as a reflection of differences in duration of exposure to low-grade systemic inflammation. The potentially deleterious effects of inflammation should be more pronounced if the systemic inflammatory processes have continued for years. This could also explain why, despite numerous GWAS of osteoporosis related phenotypes [16–18,55–71], these SNPs have not previously been identified; GWAS are not able to identify gene-environment interactions while the top 15 SNPs associated with BMD account for <3% of the variance of BMD [16].

Our observed results in elderly women - an association between functional polymorphisms in *CIITA*, BMD and fracture- is supported by previous reports evaluating the impact of the MHC2TA protein on molecular interactions and pathways. MHC2TA regulation of osteoclasts has been described in murine cells where it negatively regulated NFATc1 (nuclear factor of activated T-cells, cytoplasmic 1) and OSCAR by sequestering CBP/p300 from their promoter regions [72]. Decreased expression of *CIITA* would in this context lead to increased formation of osteoclasts. However, alternative mechanisms are also suggested since transgenic mice overexpressing *CIITA* display a hyper-osteoclastogenic phenotype and increased activation of signaling downstream of RANK (*E. Benasciutti and S. Cenci, personal communication).*

Based on our observations in this study and from earlier results from us and co-workers on expression levels [33], we postulate that the studied *CIITA* polymorphisms have osteoclast-stimulating effects that override the direct, inhibitory effect of IFNγ on osteoclasts [25]. Mechanistically this may be explained by estrogen deficiency after menopause, leading to increased production of IFNγ [24,25] and an induction of *CIITA* expression in cells of the monocyte/macrophage lineage. The resulting MHC2TA protein acts as a transcriptional transactivator at MHCII promoters, and induces expression of MHCII molecules on antigen presenting cells [9]. The T cell pool then increases due to inhibited T cell apoptosis by the increased amount of IFNγ and more T cells become activated by binding MHCII molecules. The activated T cells produce TNF, which could stimulate osteoclast activity through induction of RANKL, and increase osteoclast number through stimulating cytokines. The increase in osteoclast activity could then lead to decreased BMD and increased risk of fracture. The observed protective effect from the *CIITA* rs3087456(G) allele is associated with lower expression of *CIITA* and MHCII [33], which could slow down the process of T cell- and osteoclast stimulation and result in higher BMD and reduced fracture risk.

In the present study, the inverse effect of *CIITA* variant alleles on rate of bone loss compared to BMD and fracture is however somewhat contradictory. Individuals carrying *CIITA* variant alleles (mainly *CIITA* rs3087456(G)) lost more bone mineral density between age 75 and 80, but had higher BMD at age 75, 80 and 85 and, importantly, were protected from incident fracture during this time. *CIITA* variant alleles thus had a net positive effect on bone density and bone strength in elderly women at all time-points, despite also being associated with a higher rate of bone loss. Gene effects on bone turnover were not reflected by the bone resorption markers S-CTX and S-TRACP5b, however, the low numbers with consistently high or low turnover may have masked such effects. Furthermore, markers indicate turnover (and the potential effect of inflammatory processes on it) only at the time of sample collection and may not be able to capture the long-term effects of inflammation.

In addition to *CIITA*, *CLEC16A* and to a lesser extent *INFG* were associated with bone mass phenotypes. However, the contribution to fracture risk is less clear; *CLEC16A* was associated with a significantly reduced fracture risk, although less than *CIITA*, while *INFG* was not. A potential explanation would be that the *CLEC16A* marker most strongly associated with fracture (rs725613), is located closest to, and is in weak LD with *CIITA*.

The strengths of the study include the comprehensive and extended evaluation of the women in the OPRA-cohort, including detailed fracture information and bone turnover markers. We also have the possibility to make direct comparisons of ageing effects through the large cohort of young adult women in the PEAK-25 cohort. In this study, the reported association with bone phenotypes and overall fracture risk in the elderly women support the relevance of inflammatory genes affecting MCHCII expression in the pathogenesis of osteoporosis.

The study has some limitations, notably the large number of tests performed. Taking this into consideration and applying a conservative Bonferroni correction, the results can be considered to fall short of $p<0.05$. Performing adjustment at least for the 8 markers tested, association with BMD is non-significant, whereas association of CIITA with total body RBL, fracture and hip fracture is still significant. Importantly however the direction of effect of the SNPs within each gene is consistent indicating biological plausibility for the observations and importantly, both cohorts are of sufficient size to be confident of detecting true genotype related differences in the phenotypes analysed.

Replication studies are needed in order to fully evaluate the effect of the studied SNPs on osteoporosis-related phenotypes. Thus, replication in a similarly aged cohort to OPRA is necessary to corroborate the findings. Secondly, routine biochemistry including leukocyte count, CRP and ESR as clinical indicators of inflammation was only available on all OPRA participants at age 85. The finding that *CLEC16A* haplotypes were associated with higher counts of blood leukocytes with a similar trend for single markers, suggests that it would have been interesting to have complete longitudinal data. Thirdly, longitudinal data for the young adult women would be potentially interesting (including follow-up extending into the perimenopausal years) in order to facilitate evaluation of the natural course of inflammatory influence with normal ageing and transition to an estrogen deplete state. In a study comparing levels of IFNγ in young, perimenopausal and elderly women, the levels of IFNγ increased at menopause compared to young women, but fell to even lower levels in the elderly [40]. These results strongly argue for testing the studied *CIITA* and *IFNG* polymorphisms in cohorts of perimenopausal women for comparison.

We conclude that expression-related polymorphisms in the inflammatory genes *CIITA* and *CLEC16A* are associated with BMD and fracture in elderly women. These findings illustrate the importance of inflammation and MHCII expression in particular in the pathogenesis of reduced bone strength in the elderly.

Supporting Information

Table S1 Allele and genotype frequencies for *CIITA*, *CLEC16A* and *IFNG* in the OPRA and PEAK25 cohorts.

Table S2 *CIITA*, *CLEC16A* and *IFNG* haplotype frequencies in the OPRA and PEAK25 cohorts.

Table S3 Weight and BMD at age 75, 80 and 85 years (y) in the OPRA cohort (n = 1003) and rate of bone loss (RBL) between 75 and 80 y.

Acknowledgments

Thanks are extended to Lisa Jansson for genotyping support, to the research nurses at the Clinical and Molecular Osteoporosis Research Unit, Malmö and to all the women who kindly participated in the study.

Author Contributions

Conceived and designed the experiments: MS KÅ. Performed the experiments: MS. Analyzed the data: MS. Wrote the paper: MS FEM KVI PG KÅ. Conduct of study: MS. Data collection: PG KÅ. Data interpretation: MS FEM KÅ.

References

1. Cummings SR, Melton LJ (2002) Epidemiology and outcomes of osteoporotic fractures. Lancet 359: 1761–1767.
2. Ferrari S (2008) Human genetics of osteoporosis. Best Pract Res Clin Endocrinol Metab 22: 723–735.
3. Takayanagi H (2007) Osteoimmunology: shared mechanisms and crosstalk between the immune and bone systems. Nat Rev Immunol 7: 292–304.
4. Hofbauer LC, Brueck CC, Shanahan CM, Schoppet M, Dobnig H (2007) Vascular calcification and osteoporosis–from clinical observation towards molecular understanding. Osteoporos Int 18: 251–259.
5. Holmberg AH, Johnell O, Nilsson PM, Nilsson J, Berglund G, et al. (2006) Risk factors for fragility fracture in middle age. A prospective population-based study of 33,000 men and women. Osteoporos Int 17: 1065–1077.
6. Sennerby U, Farahmand B, Ahlbom A, Ljunghall S, Michaelsson K (2007) Cardiovascular diseases and future risk of hip fracture in women. Osteoporos Int 18: 1355–1362.
7. Dewhirst FE, Stashenko PP, Mole JE, Tsurumachi T (1985) Purification and partial sequence of human osteoclast-activating factor: identity with interleukin 1 beta. J Immunol 135: 2562–2568.
8. Takayanagi H, Ogasawara K, Hida S, Chiba T, Murata S, et al. (2000) T-cell-mediated regulation of osteoclastogenesis by signalling cross-talk between RANKL and IFN-gamma. Nature 408: 600–605.
9. Nagarajan UM, Bushey A, Boss JM (2002) Modulation of gene expression by the MHC class II transactivator. J Immunol 169: 5078–5088.
10. Steimle V, Otten LA, Zufferey M, Mach B (1993) Complementation cloning of an MHC class II transactivator mutated in hereditary MHC class II deficiency (or bare lymphocyte syndrome). Cell 75: 135–146.
11. Allen M, Sandberg-Wollheim M, Sjogren K, Erlich HA, Petterson U, et al. (1994) Association of susceptibility to multiple sclerosis in Sweden with HLA class II DRB1 and DQB1 alleles. Hum Immunol 39: 41–48.
12. Stastny P (1976) Mixed lymphocyte cultures in rheumatoid arthritis. J Clin Invest 57: 1148–1157.
13. Zanelli E, Breedveld FC, de Vries RR (2000) HLA class II association with rheumatoid arthritis: facts and interpretations. Hum Immunol 61: 1254–1261.
14. Pattrick M, Manhire A, Ward AM, Doherty M (1989) HLA-A, B antigens and alpha 1-antitrypsin phenotypes in nodal generalised osteoarthritis and erosive osteoarthritis. Ann Rheum Dis 48: 470–475.
15. Nakajima M, Takahashi A, Kou I, Rodriguez-Fontenla C, Gomez-Reino JJ, et al. (2010) New sequence variants in HLA class II/III region associated with susceptibility to knee osteoarthritis identified by genome-wide association study. PLoS One 5: e9723.
16. Rivadeneira F, Styrkarsdottir U, Estrada K, Halldorsson BV, Hsu YH, et al. (2009) Twenty bone-mineral-density loci identified by large-scale meta-analysis of genome-wide association studies. Nat Genet 41: 1199–1206.
17. Styrkarsdottir U, Halldorsson BV, Gretarsdottir S, Gudbjartsson DF, Walters GB, et al. (2008) Multiple genetic loci for bone mineral density and fractures. N Engl J Med 358: 2355–2365.
18. Farber CR (2010) Identification of a gene module associated with BMD through the integration of network analysis and genome-wide association data. J Bone Miner Res 25: 2359–2367.
19. Chung HW, Seo JS, Hur SE, Kim HL, Kim JY, et al. (2003) Association of interleukin-6 promoter variant with bone mineral density in pre-menopausal women. J Hum Genet 48: 243–248.
20. Ferrari SL, Ahn-Luong L, Garnero P, Humphries SE, Greenspan SL (2003) Two promoter polymorphisms regulating interleukin-6 gene expression are associated with circulating levels of C-reactive protein and markers of bone resorption in postmenopausal women. J Clin Endocrinol Metab 88: 255–259.
21. Ferrari SL, Garnero P, Emond S, Montgomery H, Humphries SE, et al. (2001) A functional polymorphic variant in the interleukin-6 gene promoter associated with low bone resorption in postmenopausal women. Arthritis Rheum 44: 196–201.
22. Murray RE, McGuigan F, Grant SF, Reid DM, Ralston SH (1997) Polymorphisms of the interleukin-6 gene are associated with bone mineral density. Bone 21: 89–92.
23. Swanberg M, McGuigan F, Ivaska KK, Gerdhem P, Lerner UH, et al. (2010) Polymorphisms in the macrophage migration inhibitory factor gene and bone loss in postmenopausal women. Bone 47: 424–429.
24. Weitzmann MN, Pacifici R (2006) Estrogen regulation of immune cell bone interactions. Ann N Y Acad Sci 1068: 256–274.
25. Cenci S, Toraldo G, Weitzmann MN, Roggia C, Gao Y, et al. (2003) Estrogen deficiency induces bone loss by increasing T cell proliferation and lifespan through IFN-gamma-induced class II transactivator. Proc Natl Acad Sci U S A 100: 10405–10410.
26. Bronson PG, Caillier S, Ramsay PP, McCauley JL, Zuvich RL, et al. (2010) CIITA variation in the presence of HLA-DRB1*1501 increases risk for multiple sclerosis. Hum Mol Genet 19: 2331–2340.
27. Bronson PG, Goldstein BA, Ramsay PP, Beckman KB, Noble JA, et al. (2011) The rs4774 CIITA missense variant is associated with risk of systemic lupus erythematosus. Genes Immun.
28. Grunewald J, Idali F, Kockum I, Seddighzadeh M, Nisell M, et al. (2010) Major histocompatibility complex class II transactivator gene polymorphism: associations with Lofgren's syndrome. Tissue Antigens 76: 96–101.
29. Lindholm E, Melander O, Almgren P, Berglund G, Agardh CD, et al. (2006) Polymorphism in the MHC2TA gene is associated with features of the metabolic syndrome and cardiovascular mortality. PLoS One 1: e64.
30. Martinez A, Alvarez-Lafuente R, Mas A, Bartolome M, Garcia-Montojo M, et al. (2007) Environment-gene interaction in multiple sclerosis: human herpesvirus 6 and MHC2TA. Hum Immunol 68: 685–689.
31. Martinez A, Perdigones N, Cenit MC, Espino L, Varade J, et al. (2010) Chromosomal region 16p13: further evidence of increased predisposition to immune diseases. Ann Rheum Dis 69: 309–311.
32. Skinningsrud B, Husebye ES, Pearce SH, McDonald DO, Brandal K, et al. (2008) Polymorphisms in CLEC16A and CIITA at 16p13 are associated with primary adrenal insufficiency. J Clin Endocrinol Metab 93: 3310–3317.
33. Swanberg M, Lidman O, Padyukov L, Eriksson P, Akesson E, et al. (2005) MHC2TA is associated with differential MHC molecule expression and susceptibility to rheumatoid arthritis, multiple sclerosis and myocardial infarction. Nat Genet 37: 486–494.
34. Geijtenbeek TB, Gringhuis SI (2009) Signalling through C-type lectin receptors: shaping immune responses. Nat Rev Immunol 9: 465–479.
35. Hakonarson H, Grant SF, Bradfield JP, Marchand L, Kim CE, et al. (2007) A genome-wide association study identifies KIAA0350 as a type 1 diabetes gene. Nature 448: 591–594.
36. Hafler DA, Compston A, Sawcer S, Lander ES, Daly MJ, et al. (2007) Risk alleles for multiple sclerosis identified by a genomewide study. N Engl J Med 357: 851–862.
37. Marquez A, Varade J, Robledo G, Martinez A, Mendoza JL, et al. (2009) Specific association of a CLEC16A/KIAA0350 polymorphism with NOD2/CARD15(–) Crohn's disease patients. Eur J Hum Genet 17: 1304–1308.
38. Zuvich RL, Bush WS, McCauley JL, Beecham AH, De Jager PL, et al. (2011) Interrogating the complex role of chromosome 16p13.13 in multiple sclerosis susceptibility: independent genetic signals in the CIITA-CLEC16A-SOCS1 gene complex. Hum Mol Genet.
39. Kim K, Cho SK, Sestak A, Namjou B, Kang C, et al. (2010) Interferon-gamma gene polymorphisms associated with susceptibility to systemic lupus erythematosus. Ann Rheum Dis 69: 1247–1250.
40. Deguchi K, Kamada M, Irahara M, Maegawa M, Yamamoto S, et al. (2001) Postmenopausal changes in production of type 1 and type 2 cytokines and the effects of hormone replacement therapy. Menopause 8: 266–273.
41. Gerdhem P, Brandstrom H, Stiger F, Obrant K, Melhus H, et al. (2004) Association of the collagen type 1 (COL1A 1) Sp1 binding site polymorphism to femoral neck bone mineral density and wrist fracture in 1044 elderly Swedish women. Calcif Tissue Int 74: 264–269.
42. McGuigan FE, Larzenius E, Callreus M, Gerdhem P, Luthman H, et al. (2007) Variation in the BMP2 gene: bone mineral density and ultrasound in young adult and elderly women. Calcif Tissue Int 81: 254–262.
43. Pravica V, Perrey C, Stevens A, Lee JH, Hutchinson IV (2000) A single nucleotide polymorphism in the first intron of the human IFN-gamma gene: absolute correlation with a polymorphic CA microsatellite marker of high IFN-gamma production. Hum Immunol 61: 863–866.
44. Morrison BA, Ucisik-Akkaya E, Flores H, Alaez C, Gorodezky C, et al. (2010) Multiple sclerosis risk markers in HLA-DRA, HLA-C, and IFNG genes are associated with sex-specific childhood leukemia risk. Autoimmunity 43: 690–697.
45. Lenora J, Akesson K, Gerdhem P (2010) Effect of precision on longitudinal follow-up of bone mineral density measurements in elderly women and men. J Clin Densitom 13: 407–412.
46. Lenora J, Ivaska KK, Obrant KJ, Gerdhem P (2007) Prediction of bone loss using biochemical markers of bone turnover. Osteoporos Int 18: 1297–1305.
47. Karlsson MK, Obrant KJ, Nilsson BE, Johnell O (1998) Bone mineral density assessed by quantitative ultrasound and dual energy X-ray absorptiometry. Normative data in Malmo, Sweden. Acta Orthop Scand 69: 189–193.
48. Gerdhem P, Akesson K (2007) Rates of fracture in participants and non-participants in the Osteoporosis Prospective Risk Assessment study. J Bone Joint Surg Br 89: 1627–1631.

49. Ivaska KK, Gerdhem P, Vaananen HK, Akesson K, Obrant KJ (2010) Bone turnover markers and prediction of fracture: a prospective follow-up study of 1040 elderly women for a mean of 9 years. J Bone Miner Res 25: 393–403.
50. Ivaska KK, Lenora J, Gerdhem P, Akesson K, Vaananen HK, et al. (2008) Serial assessment of serum bone metabolism markers identifies women with the highest rate of bone loss and osteoporosis risk. J Clin Endocrinol Metab 93: 2622–2632.
51. Okabe R, Nakatsuka K, Inaba M, Miki T, Naka H, et al. (2001) Clinical evaluation of the Elecsys beta-CrossLaps serum assay, a new assay for degradation products of type I collagen C-tlopeptides. Clin Chem 47: 1410–1414.
52. Seibel MJ (2006) Biochemical Markers of Bone Turnover Part II: Clinical Applications in the Management of Osteoporosis. Clin Biochem Rev 27: 123–138.
53. Stephens M, Smith NJ, Donnelly P (2001) A new statistical method for haplotype reconstruction from population data. Am J Hum Genet 68: 978–989.
54. Weusten JJ, Blankenstein MA, Gmelig-Meyling FH, Schuurman HJ, Kater L, et al. (1986) Presence of oestrogen receptors in human blood mononuclear cells and thymocytes. Acta Endocrinol (Copenh) 112: 409–414.
55. Cho YS, Go MJ, Kim YJ, Heo JY, Oh JH, et al. (2009) A large-scale genome-wide association study of Asian populations uncovers genetic factors influencing eight quantitative traits. Nat Genet 41: 527–534.
56. Duncan EL, Danoy P, Kemp JP, Leo PJ, McCloskey E, et al. (2011) Genome-wide association study using extreme truncate selection identifies novel genes affecting bone mineral density and fracture risk. PLoS Genet 7: e1001372.
57. Guo Y, Tan LJ, Lei SF, Yang TL, Chen XD, et al. (2010) Genome-wide association study identifies ALDH7A1 as a novel susceptibility gene for osteoporosis. PLoS Genet 6: e1000806.
58. Guo Y, Zhang LS, Yang TL, Tian Q, Xiong DH, et al. (2010) IL21R and PTH may underlie variation of femoral neck bone mineral density as revealed by a genome-wide association study. J Bone Miner Res 25: 1042–1048.
59. Hsu YH, Zillikens MC, Wilson SG, Farber CR, Demissie S, et al. (2010) An integration of genome-wide association study and gene expression profiling to prioritize the discovery of novel susceptibility Loci for osteoporosis-related traits. PLoS Genet 6: e1000977.
60. Karasik D, Hsu YH, Zhou Y, Cupples LA, Kiel DP, et al. (2010) Genome-wide pleiotropy of osteoporosis-related phenotypes: the Framingham Study. J Bone Miner Res 25: 1555–1563.
61. Koller DL, Ichikawa S, Lai D, Padgett LR, Doheny KF, et al. (2010) Genome-wide association study of bone mineral density in premenopausal European-American women and replication in African-American women. J Clin Endocrinol Metab 95: 1802–1809.
62. Kung AW, Xiao SM, Cherny S, Li GH, Gao Y, et al. (2010) Association of JAG1 with bone mineral density and osteoporotic fractures: a genome-wide association study and follow-up replication studies. Am J Hum Genet 86: 229–239.
63. Paternoster L, Lorentzon M, Vandenput L, Karlsson MK, Ljunggren O, et al. (2010) Genome-wide association meta-analysis of cortical bone mineral density unravels allelic heterogeneity at the RANKL locus and potential pleiotropic effects on bone. PLoS Genet 6: e1001217.
64. Styrkarsdottir U, Halldorsson BV, Gretarsdottir S, Gudbjartsson DF, Walters GB, et al. (2009) New sequence variants associated with bone mineral density. Nat Genet 41: 15–17.
65. Timpson NJ, Tobias JH, Richards JB, Soranzo N, Duncan EL, et al. (2009) Common variants in the region around Osterix are associated with bone mineral density and growth in childhood. Hum Mol Genet 18: 1510–1517.
66. Xiong DH, Liu XG, Guo YF, Tan LJ, Wang L, et al. (2009) Genome-wide association and follow-up replication studies identified ADAMTS18 and TGFBR3 as bone mass candidate genes in different ethnic groups. Am J Hum Genet 84: 388–398.
67. Kiel DP, Demissie S, Dupuis J, Lunetta KL, Murabito JM, et al. (2007) Genome-wide association with bone mass and geometry in the Framingham Heart Study. BMC Med Genet 8 Suppl 1: S14.
68. Kou I, Takahashi A, Urano T, Fukui N, Ito H, et al. (2011) Common variants in a novel gene, FONG on chromosome 2q33.1 confer risk of osteoporosis in Japanese. PLoS One 6: e19641.
69. Liu YZ, Pei YF, Liu JF, Yang F, Guo Y, et al. (2009) Powerful bivariate genome-wide association analyses suggest the SOX6 gene influencing both obesity and osteoporosis phenotypes in males. PLoS One 4: e6827.
70. Richards JB, Rivadeneira F, Inouye M, Pastinen TM, Soranzo N, et al. (2008) Bone mineral density, osteoporosis, and osteoporotic fractures: a genome-wide association study. Lancet 371: 1505–1512.
71. Zhao LJ, Liu XG, Liu YZ, Liu YJ, Papasian CJ, et al. (2010) Genome-wide association study for femoral neck bone geometry. J Bone Miner Res 25: 320–329.
72. Kim JH, Kim K, Youn BU, Jin HM, Kim N (2010) MHC class II transactivator negatively regulates RANKL-mediated osteoclast differentiation by downregulating NFATc1 and OSCAR. Cell Signal 22: 1341–1349.
73. Awata T, Kawasaki E, Tanaka S, Ikegami H, Maruyama T, et al. (2009) Association of type 1 diabetes with two Loci on 12q13 and 16p13 and the influence coexisting thyroid autoimmunity in Japanese. J Clin Endocrinol Metab 94: 231–235.
74. Wu X, Zhu X, Wang X, Ma J, Zhu S, et al. (2009) Intron polymorphism in the KIAA0350 gene is reproducibly associated with susceptibility to type 1 diabetes (T1D) in the Han Chinese population. Clin Endocrinol (Oxf) 71: 46–49.
75. Zoledziewska M, Costa G, Pitzalis M, Cocco E, Melis C, et al. (2009) Variation within the CLEC16A gene shows consistent disease association with both multiple sclerosis and type 1 diabetes in Sardinia. Genes Immun 10: 15–17.
76. Rubio JP, Stankovich J, Field J, Tubridy N, Marriott M, et al. (2008) Replication of KIAA0350, IL2RA, RPL5 and CD58 as multiple sclerosis susceptibility genes in Australians. Genes Immun 9: 624–630.

24

Herniation Pits in Human Mummies: A CT Investigation in the Capuchin Catacombs of Palermo, Sicily

Stephanie Panzer[1]*, Dario Piombino-Mascali[2], Albert R. Zink[2]

1 Department of Radiology, Trauma Center Murnau, Murnau, Germany, **2** EURAC - Institute for Mummies and the Iceman, Bolzano, Italy

Abstract

Herniation pits (HPs) of the femoral neck were first described in a radiological publication in 1982 as round to oval radiolucencies in the proximal superior quadrant of the femoral neck on anteroposterior radiographs of adults. In following early clinical publications, HPs were generally recognized as an incidental finding. In contrast, in current clinical literature they are mentioned in the context of femoroacetabular impingement (FAI) of the hip joint, which is known to cause osteoarthritis (OA). The significance of HPs in chronic skeletal disorders such as OA is still unclear, but they are discussed as a possible radiological indicator for FAI in a large part of clinical studies. In this paleoradiological study we examined a sample of mummies from the Capuchin Catacombs of Palermo, Sicily, by a mobile computed tomography (CT) scanner. Evaluation of the CT examinations revealed HPs in six out of 16 (37.5%) adult male mummies. The first aim of this study was to compare the characteristics of HPs shown in our mummy collection to the findings described in clinical literature. Thereby CT evaluation revealed that their osseous imaging characteristics are in accordance, consisting of round to oval subcortical lesions at the anterior femoral neck, clearly demarcated by a sclerotic margin. The second aim was to introduce HPs to the paleoradiological and paleopathological methodology as an entity that underwent a renaissance from an incidental finding to a possible radiological indicator of FAI in the clinical situation. As FAI plays an important role in the development of OA of the hip, which is a very common finding in human skeletal remains, HPs should always be considered in paleoradiological evaluation of hip joint diseases.

Editor: Erik L. Ritman, Mayo Clinic College of Medicine, United States of America

Funding: This study was supported by Dr. Dariusch Rafiy, 3W Production, Munich, Germany (http://www.3w-production.com) and the Foundation Südtiroler Sparkasse (http://www.stiftungsparkasse.it/). The funders had no role in study design, data collection and analysis, decision to publish, or preparation of the manuscript.

Competing Interests: Dr. Dariusch Rafiy, 3W Production, Munich, Germany made available the portable CT scanner for this study.

* E-mail: stephanie.panzer@bgu-murnau.de

Introduction

Paleopathology is the study of diseases and related conditions in skeletal and mummified remains that include the application of different methods and techniques and the use of various sources [1–3]. Since the first X-ray study of human and animal mummies, performed by König as early as 1896 [4], paleopathology has benefitted from the use of radiological methods and technical innovations in radiology, such as computed tomography (CT) and magnetic resonance imaging (MRI) by enhancing the possibility in diagnosing pathological conditions in ancient skeletons and mummies. Collaboration between anthropologists and musculoskeletal radiologists may facilitate solving diagnostic problems arising during analysis of ancient human remains, and radiological textbooks have become an important source in paleopathological studies [5]. Thereby, the contribution of musculoskeletal radiologists is not only to assist with diagnosis, but also to provide information on the clinical setting and relevance of diseases [6].

One of the most common described pathologies in ancient human remains is osteoarthritis (OA), or degenerative joint disease [7]. In studies of skeletal remains, OA of the hip is usually diagnosed by the presence of at least one of the following criteria: periarticular bone formation, subchondral bone resorption, and eburnation [2,8]. While eburnation is a clear indicator of advanced OA, in both clinical and paleopathological studies other surface modifications, such as pitting or porosity, have been proposed to be directly related to OA [9,10].

In paleoepidemiological studies, OA scores are widely used in order to reconstruct lifestyle, mobility and activity patterns in ancient populations with special emphasis on the biocultural context [11–15]. These studies are based on the assumption that activity, such as repetitive mechanical loading on muscles and joints, is the primary contributing factor [16]. This approach allows scholars to use osteoarthritic prevalence and severity in order to evaluate physical stress and specific activities in historic populations [12]. Nevertheless, most authors are aware of the complex etiopathogenesis of OA. Several other factors, such as sex, weight, nutrition, endocrine status and genetic influences may in fact contribute to the development of OA. Moreover, it has also been noted that anatomical variation can affect joints differently and influence the onset of OA. As an example, Reijmann and colleagues [17] showed that patients with acetabular dysplasia have a higher risk of hip OA.

Another condition associated with hip osteoarthritis is femoroacetabular impingement (FAI). In FAI, morphologic abnormalities of the proximal femur, acetabulum or both cause abnormal contact between the femur and acetabulum during motion, especially during flexion and internal rotation. This contact causes abnormal stress on the acetabular labrum and articular cartilage. The resulting degeneration, tearing of the labrum and damage to the adjacent acetabular cartilage can lead to OA of the hip joint [18,19]. In the current clinical literature, minor osseous changes located in the femoral neck, or the so-called herniation pits (HPs), were mentioned in the context of FAI.

Herniation pits were first described by Pitt and colleagues in 1982 [20]. On anteroposterior (AP) radiographs of adult femoral necks, the authors identified well-delineated, round to oval radiolucencies in the proximal superior quadrant of the femoral neck, projected 5–15 mm below the superior neck margin, directly beneath the anterior cortex, bordered by a thin, organized sclerotic margin. Pitt and co-workers [20] generally recognized HPs as benign and incidental and believed that HPs, although sharing a common teleologic mechanism of soft-tissue herniation characteristic of some ganglia, are a different, unique entity.

Since this first definition of HPs, a number of case reports and reviews in clinical literature were published, describing especially the radiological findings in CT, MRI, micro-CT and bone scanning, the macro-pathology and histology, as well as the location and the prevalence of HPs [21–31]. In contrast to the early publications, in which HPs were generally described as an incidental finding [20,22], more recent clinical studies regard them as a possible radiographic indicator for FAI [e.g., 32–38].

In this study, we focus on the paleoradiological investigation of HPs in a sample of human mummies from the Capuchin Catacombs in Palermo, Sicily. Until now, HPs and FAI have not been widely taken into consideration in paleopathological or paleoradiological studies. Chhem and Brothwell [6] describe HPs, but classify them as normal variants, while Villotte and Knüsel [39] discuss the role of FAI with regard to osseous non-metric traits of the femoral neck. Therefore, the goal of our study was to introduce HPs to the paleoradiological and paleopathological methodology as a possible indicator of FAI.

As FAI plays an important role in the development of hip OA, which is a very common finding in human skeletal remains, we believe that HPs should be taken into account in future paleopathological studies.

Materials and Methods

In December of 2010 we had the opportunity to examine a sample group of 26 mummies, including 16 adult males and 10 immature individuals preserved in the Capuchin Catacombs of Palermo. At the end of the 16th century, the Catacombs were constructed as a burial site for deceased friars. Over the course of time, extensive subterranean corridors were carved out of massive deposit of tuff that underlies the Capuchin Church and Convent. The first mummified bodies were placed there in 1599, and the last ones in the early 20th century [40,41]. Today the Catacombs form an impressive site where over twelve hundred bodies, many of which still retain soft tissue, are displayed along the sides of the corridors (Figure 1). The Catacomb mummies of Sicily are mainly the result of a spontaneous-enhanced preservation mechanism. Shortly after death, bodies were taken to special preparation rooms, and laid on terracotta racks designed to allow draining of the body fluids and promote spontaneous desiccation of the cadavers. The rooms were then sealed for approximately one year, after which time the corpses were exposed to the air, washed with vinegar and dressed. Some bodies were also preserved with anthropogenic methods, such as briefly immersing the bodies in lime or by means of arterially injecting specific chemicals [40–43].

For the present study, only the adult sample group, consisting of 16 males dating from the late 18th to the late 19th centuries AD, was considered. The sample selection was mainly based on the accessibility and preservation state of the bodies. Furthermore, the short time availability of the mobile CT scanner only allowed a small number of mummies to be studied. Any available information on these subjects, such as age, identity, occupation and time of death was either determined through observation of the artifacts associated with the bodies and the coffins, the embalming technique employed, or gleaned from the death records present in the Archives of the Capuchin Convent and in the Municipal Archives of Palermo. At least six bodies from the sample group underwent a process of anthropogenic mummification.

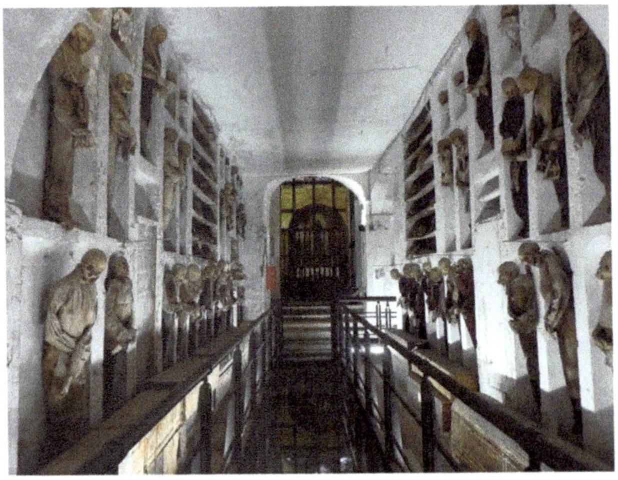

Figure 1. Image of one of the corridors of the Catacombs. Over eighteen hundred bodies, many of which still retain soft tissue, are displayed along the sides of the different corridors. Many of them are stored in wall niches or upon shelves while others lie in wooden coffins. Over time, bodies were grouped according to sex, age and occupation. Almost all mummies are clothed and wear hats, shoes or even gloves.

The mummies were examined by a mobile 4-section CT scanner (Alliance Medical, Warwick, UK; LightSpeed Plus, GE Healthcare, Milwaukee, Wisconsin, USA) which was positioned in front of the Capuchin Church next to the entrance of the Catacombs. All examinations were obtained as whole body CT in helical technique with slice thickness of 1.25 mm, interval of 1.25 mm and pitch of 0.75 with 120 kV in a standard algorithm. Paleoradiological evaluation as well as performance of multiplanar reconstructions (MPR) was carried out at the Picture Archiving and Communicating System (ImpaxEE, Agfa HealthCare, Bonn, Germany) in the Department of Radiology by the first author who is also experienced in paleoradiology and musculoskeletal radiology.

HPs at the femoral neck were characterized by size, shape, margin, cortical breaks and Hounsfield Unit (HU) representing the density values in CT examinations. In case of mummies with HPs, MPRs of the respective hip joint were generated. The location of each HP was classified in the parasagittal plane in which the anterior, almost semicircular half of the femoral neck was divided into a superior and inferior portion and the transition zone between the two [37].

To determine the femoral head-neck junction, the angle α introduced by Nötzli et al. [44] was measured on a plane parallel to the axis of the femoral neck passing through the centre of the femoral head. The angle α was defined by two lines: the first line between the centre of the femoral head and the anterior point

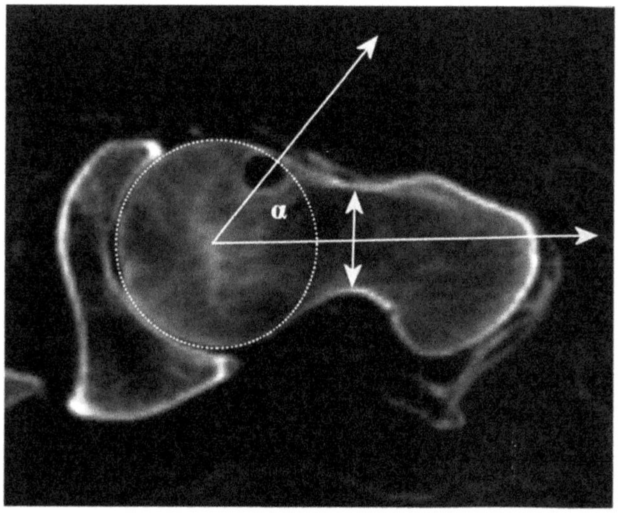

Figure 2. Measurement of the angle α. Paraaxial (parallel to the axis of the femoral neck) reformation CT image in case 3. The angle α was defined by a line between the centre of the femoral head and the anterior point, where the distance of the centre of the femoral head exceeds the radius of the surface of the femoral head and a second line between the centre of the femoral head and the centre of the femoral neck at its narrowest point.

where the distance of the centre of the femoral head exceeds the radius of the surface of the femoral head and the second line between the centre of the femoral head and the centre of the femoral neck at its narrowest point (Figure 2).

Degenerative disease of the hip joints containing HPs was evaluated by the assessment of osteophytes, subchondral cysts and eburnation. The criterion of joint space narrowing, which is used in the clinical situation, is not applicable to paleoradiology as soft tissues and joint alignment in mummies are known to change as a result of dehydration [6].

Results

All investigated mummies showed very good preservation status of the skeletal structures, allowing precise assessment of morphological changes. In some mummies, preserved parts of the joint capsule and labrum were visible (Figure 3).

CT examination revealed a total of 11 HPs in six out of the 16 investigated adult male mummies (Table 1), while no HPs were detected in the child mummies. According to the death records, one person died at the age of 56 years and another one at the age of 73 years. The remaining four cases were estimated to an age range of about 40 to 70 years based on the radiological appearance. Two mummies showed bilateral HPs as well as multiplicity in one femur of each case (Figure 3). Two mummies had a single HP in the left femur, and two had a single HP in the right femur. The femur of case 6 was disarticulated postmortem (Figure 4). The maximum diameter of the 11 HPs ranged from 3 to 13 mm with a mean of 7.4 mm. They were round or round to oval in shape and in three cases they were slightly lobulated. All HPs were demarcated by a complete sclerotic margin (Figure 3, Figure 4, Figure 5B, D). Cortical breaks were discernible in six HPs (Figure 3D). HU values measured within the HPs ranged from −763 to −980 with a mean of −908.8. All HPs were located below the growth plate of the femoral head, five in the superior portion of the femoral neck (Figure 5B) and six in the transition zone between the superior and inferior portion (Figure 5D). The angle α ranged from 33° to 68° with a mean of 42.4° (Table 2).

Evaluation of OA of the hip joints with HPs (Table 2) revealed slight osteophytes of the lateral acetabular roof in cases 1, 3, 5 and 6 with additional slight osteophytes of the femoral head in case 6. Case 4 showed moderate osteophytes and small subchondral cysts of the acetabular roof as well as slight osteophytes of the femoral head. At the anterior border of the right acetabulum of case 2 and of case 5 respectively, one round to oval lesion with a well-defined sclerotic margin and a diameter of 4 to 5 mm was found subcortically/subchondrally, both representing small cysts (Figure 3A). The lesion in case 2 showed a cortical break. Eburnation was not found in any case.

As additional findings which did not affect the hip joint directly, case 1 showed a subcortical lobulated lesion with well-defined sclerotic margins and osseous septa in the ventrolateral aspect of the right acetabulum. The maximum diameter was 2.7 cm. The lesion revealed a cortical break. In case 3, a lobulated lesion with well-defined sclerotic margins and a thin peripheral osseous septum was detectable subcortically/subchondrally in the ventrolateral part of the acetabular roof. The maximum diameter was 2 cm and a cortical break was visible. In both mummies the described lesions were monostotic. Both lesions represent benign tumors or tumor-like lesions, e.g., simple bone cysts or fibrous dysplasia.

Discussion

We found HPs in six out of 16 (37.5%) adult male mummies respectively in eight out of 32 (25%) femora. Prevalence of HPs in clinical studies ranged from 2.6% (four out of 152 patients) [26] to 42.5% (85 out of 200 patients) [37], respectively 4.6% (one out of 22 femora) [45] to 35.4% [35] if referring to the single femora. Thereby the investigated collectives differed mainly between normal adults [20,22], incidental collectives [24,37] and clinically symptomatic patients with FAI [35,45–48]. Collectives with normal adults and incidental collectives ranged from 4.2% [22] to 42.5% [37] referring to patients. In clinical literature, the age of patients ranged from 22 to 62 years in case reports on HPs [21,23,25–30], and from 14 to 96 years in studies on FAI mentioning HPs (37,45).

In this study, we were only able to investigate a small collection of exclusively male adult mummies, making a comparison with clinical studies difficult. Nevertheless, the prevalence and age we found in the mummies of the Capuchin Catacombs lies inside the range of published data from the clinical literature. Bilateral HPs and multiplicity of HPs in a femur as shown in two of our investigated mummies are also known findings [37].

The size of HPs in our collection, with a mean diameter of 7.4 mm, was comparable to the average size given in clinical publications. According to Pitt et al. [20] the maximum diameter of HPs is usually less than 10 mm. Studies based on high case numbers report an average diameter of 5 mm (range 3–15 mm) on x-rays [47] and 5.3 mm (range 2–11 mm) in CT examinations [37].

The usual appearance of HPs in clinical CT examinations is a round to oval, sometimes lobulated, subcortical lesion containing connective tissue and fat, surrounded by a sclerotic margin. Cortical perforations or breaks are frequently discernible [20,23,28,37]. The CT appearance of the HPs detected in our mummies was in full accordance with the described osseous characteristics. The density measured inside the HPs (HU values ranging from −763 to −980) was significantly lower than that generally measured in studies on living patients, in which density

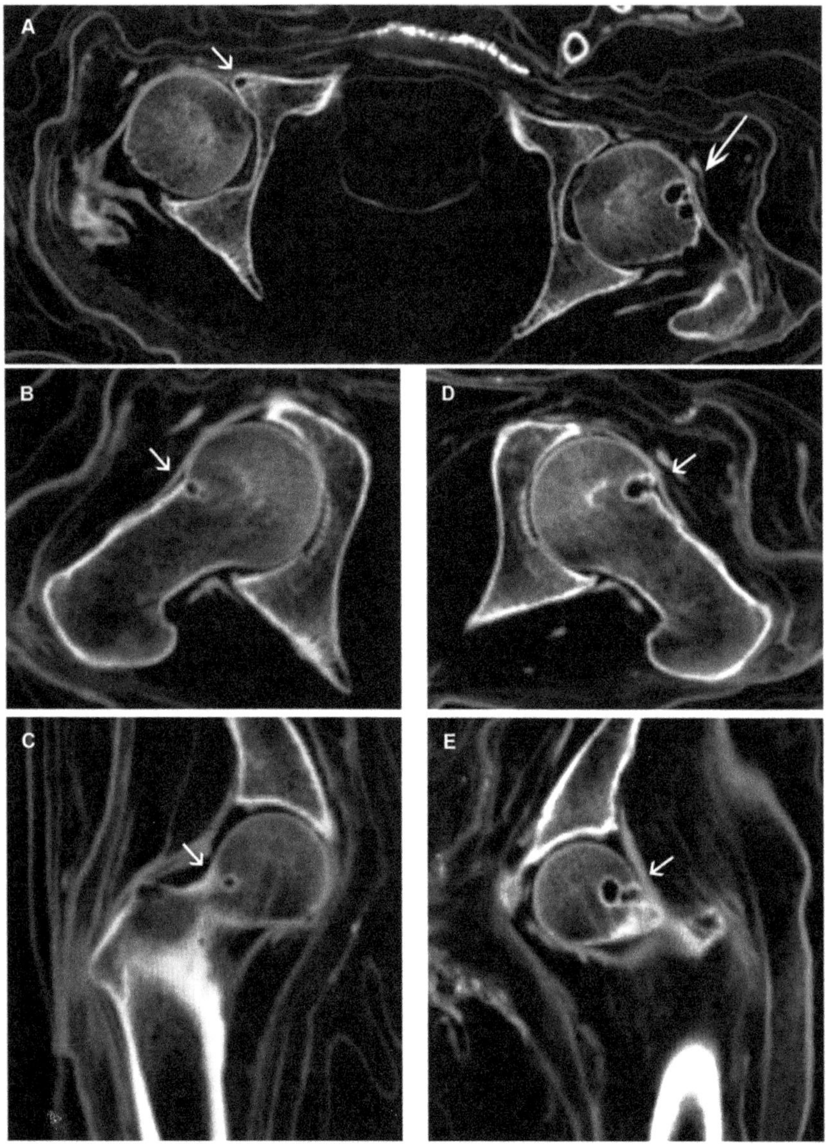

Figure 3. CT examination of case 2 with bilateral and multifocal HPs. (**A**) Axial CT slice illustrating a small subcortical/subchondral cyst inside the anterior border of the right acetabulum (short arrow) and multifocal HPs in the left anterior femur (long arrow). (**B**) Paraxial and (**C**) paracoronar CT reformation images of the right femur showing a small round HP with sclerotic margin (arrow). (**D**) Paraxial CT reformation image of the left femur demonstrating a HP with clearly visible cortical break (arrow). Note partial preservation of the joint capsule including labral structures. (**E**) Paracoronar CT reformation image of the left femur showing one round to oval HP medially and one round to oval lobulated HP laterally (arrow).

(HU) values were ranging from −79 to 380, as described by Panzer et al. [37] in a large-scale study. This can be explained by the fact that the HPs in the studied mummies are mainly filled with air as at least most of the fat and connective tissue inside the HPs has degraded over time.

The typical location of HPs is the superior portion of the anterior femoral neck [20], while in some cases HPs are located in the inferior anterior femoral neck [28,37] or at the transition zone between the superior to inferior anterior portion [37]. In the mummy sample group HPs were found in the superior portion of the femoral neck as well as in the transition zone.

Pitt et al. [20] showed that HPs are formed by herniation of soft tissues through erosions or perforations, which result from abrasive action of the overlying hip capsule. They believed that the HP is a unique entity. In recent publications, it is postulated that HPs are intraosseous ganglia [31,47]. Furthermore, the results of the study of Leunig et al. [47] indicated that there is a close spatial relationship between HPs and the site of FAI, favoring the theory that flexion-induced pressure causes the production of HPs.

In differential diagnosis, HPs must be differentiated from subchondral cysts that occur in OA. The latter are usually located in the central area of the joint surface where the stress of weight bearing has the highest impact [49]. In contrast to subchondral cysts, HPs are predominantly localized at the peripheral side of the anterior femoral neck. Further differential diagnoses that should be taken into account are osteoid osteomas [20,22,25,28,30,47], malignant diseases such as atypical osseous metastasis [22,29,30,47] and lymphoma [47], inflammatory disease such as Brodie's abscess [20,22,25,29,30] or iliopsoas tendinitis, -bursitis [30] as well as focal avascular necrosis [22,30], focal osteoporosis,

Table 1. CT-characteristics and location of HPs.

Case	**1**	**2**			**3**				**4**	**5**	**6**
Femur	**right**	**right**	**left**	**left**	**right**	**right**	**right**	**left**	**left**	**right**	**left**
Size (mm)	12	5	9	8	7	4	3	13	3	10	7
Shape	round-oval, lobul.	round	round-oval	round-oval, lobul.	round-oval	round	oval	round-oval	round-oval	round-oval	round-oval, lobul.
Margin	sclerotic	sclerotic	sclerotic	sclerotic	sclerotic	sclerotic	sclerotic	sclerotic	sclerotic	sclerotic	sclerotic
Cortical Breaks	-	-	1	1	-	1	-	1	1	1	-
HU	−873	−888	−958	−960	−948	−949	−893	−980	−763	−935	−850
Location	trans.	superior	superior medial	superior lateral	trans. medial	trans. middle	trans. lateral	trans.	superior	superior	trans.

HU Hounsfield Units.
lobul. lobulated.
trans. transition zone.

unspecific trabecular restructuring and degenerative changes [31]. Nevertheless, HPs should be clearly differentiable from these by means of their typical CT appearance as round to oval subcortical/subchondral lesions with encircling sclerotic margin and their typical location at the anterior femoral neck.

In early clinical publications, HPs were generally reported as an incidental finding [20,22], whereas in current radiological and orthopedic literature they are mentioned within the context of FAI and OA of the hip [38]. The etiology of OA of the hip has long been considered primary (presuming some underlying abnormality of the articular cartilage) or secondary (e.g. due to congenital or developmental deformities). Recent findings support a hypothesis that the so-called primary OA has also to be regarded as secondary OA due to tenuous developmental abnormalities in which the underlying mechanism is FAI [19]. Four decades ago, Murray [50] proposed the term "tilt deformity of the femoral head" in order to describe an abnormal relationship of the femoral head to the femoral neck as a slight anatomical variation. Anteroposterior radiographs suggested a mild degree of the deformity commonly occurring after a minimal slipped capital femoral epiphysis [19]. Stulberg et al. [51] introduced the term "pistol-grip deformity" for a femoral head and neck configuration, consisting of a flattening of the usually concave surface of the lateral femoral neck and a bump on the anterolateral surface of the femoral neck visible on AP radiographs. Two different types of FAI have been described. Cam-type FAI, which is more prevalent in young male patients, is caused by an offset pathomorphology between the head and neck of the femur that leads to an outside-in delamination of the acetabulum. Pincer-type FAI, which is more prevalent in middle-aged women, is caused by a more linear impact between a local (retroversion of the acetabulum) or general overcoverage (coxa profunda/protrusion) of the acetabulum. Most hips however show a mixed FAI pattern with cam predominance [19,52].

In the numerous ongoing studies on FAI, a tendency towards the association of HPs to cam-type became apparent [19,53–55]. The use of CT and MRI allowed the introduction of new measurements for FAI in any desired plane and even for three-dimensional analysis [55]. A relatively simple measurement for the assessment of pathomorphological changes in the femoral head and neck in CT and MRI examinations is the determination of the angle α [44]. In this study, we have chosen this measurement of the anterior position of the femoral head-neck junction as it represents, together with the anterosuperior position, the most frequent location for FAI [19,56].

In the mummy samples, one out of a total of 8 femora with the presence of HPs showed an angle α larger than 50° (case 6, angle α

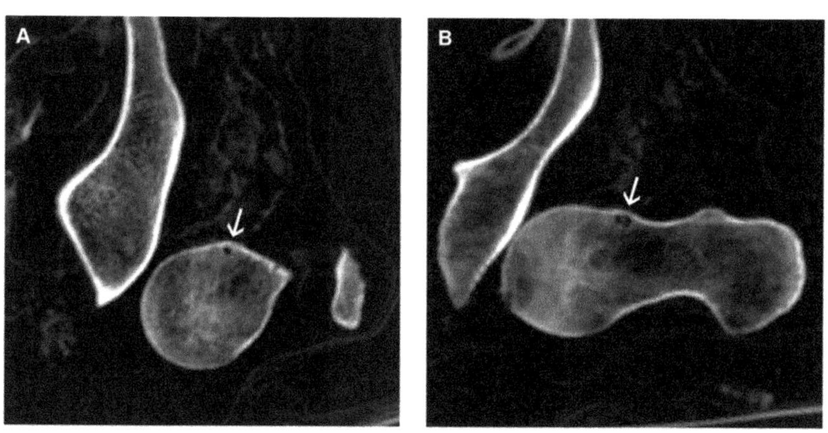

Figure 4. CT examination of case 6 with HP and a prominent anterior femoral head neck junction. Disarticulated left femur. (**A**) Axial CT slice illustrating a small round to oval HP (arrow). (**B**) Paraxial CT reformation image demonstrating the prominent anterior femoral head neck junction and the HP at the femoral neck (arrow).

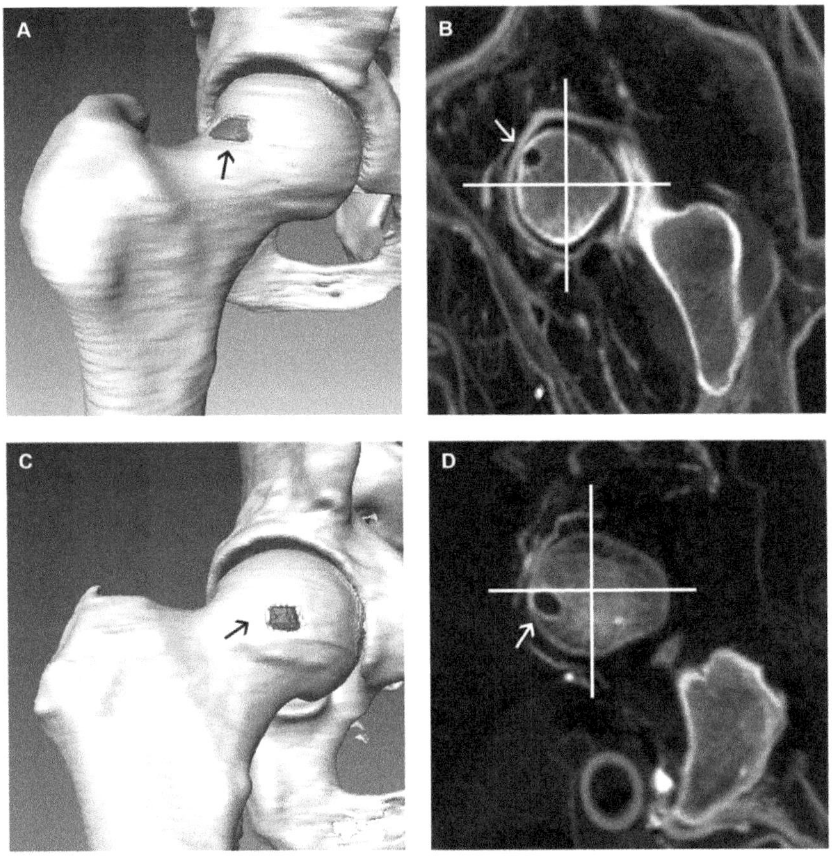

Figure 5. Location of HPs. Typical location of HPs in the superior portion of the anterior femoral neck (**A, B**) and less common location in the transition zone between the superior and inferior portion of the anterior femoral neck (**C, D**). (**A, C**) Modified three-dimensional CT reconstructions of living patients with HPs. (**B, D**) Parasagittal (perpendicular to the femoral neck axis) CT reformation images of case 2 and 3 with division into a superior (between 9 and 12 o'clock) and inferior (between 6 and 9 o'clock) portion.

68°, see Table 2), which is the cut-off angle in the description of [44]. In another femur (case 3) an angle α of exactly 50° was measured. We can thus provide evidence for one femur showing the typical pathomorphology of the head neck junction indicating cam-type FAI and another one that has to be regarded as a borderline case. The remaining 6 femora did not show any abnormal anatomy of the head neck junction based on the measurement of the angle α.

Slight degenerative changes of the hip joint were found in four cases, including the two femora with an angle α of 50° respectively 68°. In these two cases, the prominent head neck junction could have led to FAI resulting in mild degenerative disease. One case with moderate degenerative changes had a normal angle α of 38°. In this case the development of OA cannot be directly linked to a pathological anatomy of the proximal femur, despite the presence of a HP.

In paleopathology, OA or degenerative joint disease is a very common and well-described disease [3,49,57]. It is widely used in paleoepidemiological studies as a main indicator for mechanical stress and activity in ancient populations [12–14]. Although the complexity of the pathogenesis of OA has been noted by some authors [58–60], little attention has drawn to the role of morphological alterations in the etiology of OA of the hip and OA in general [7]. It is important to note, that in the clinical literature, OA of the hip is mainly linked to morphological deformities, such as developmental dysplasia of the hip [61]. In more recent work, FAI was brought out as an important mechanism for the development of hip OA [19,35]. Therefore, more focus should be placed on abnormal hip morphology as a cause for OA in paleopathological studies. In radiological but also morphological examinations of human remains, the above described angle α could be easily determined as an indicator for FAI. As HPs can apparently be linked to FAI and OA of the hip, they should be recognized and documented as a finding in the paleoradiological evaluation of hip joint diseases, in addition to the well-established criteria of degenerative disease like eburnation, osteophytes and subchondral cysts. In skeletons or mummies, it is rarely possible to assess labral or chondral structures, but as shown in case 2 and 5 of our study, the small subcortical/subchondral cysts in the peripheral part of the anterior acetabulum can serve as indicators for chondral and labral tears. In particular, chondral abnormalities situated peripherally at the labral-chondral transition zone lead to changes in the adjacent subchondral bone including the development of subchondral cysts [18,48,62]. Labral tears predispose toward extraosseous ganglia formation with splitting of the labrum and acetabular cartilage. This allows synovial fluid to penetrate into the subchondral bone, leading to a subchondral cyst formation [33]. The acetabular findings in case 1 and 3, representing benign tumors or tumor-like lesions, are most probably not associated with pathologies of the hip joint.

As far as possible, CT should be favored over conventional X-ray for the investigation of HPs in paleoradiological studies. CT

Table 2. Angle α of the femurs with HPs and signs of OA of the respective hip joint.

Case	1	2		3		4	5	6
Femur	**right**	**right**	**left**	**right**	**left**	**left**	**right**	**left**
Angle α	45°	33°	38°	38°	50°	38°	42°	68°
Osteo-phytes	slight acetabular	-	-	slight acetabular	sligth acetabular	moderate acetabular, slight femoral	slight acetabular	slight acetabular
Cysts	-	anterior acetabular border	-	-	-	acetabular roof	anterior acetabular border	-

scans allow a much better imaging of skeletal structures without any superimposition and are independent of the positioning during the examination. As an example, in our own previous study one of the mummies (case 1) was examined by means of digital X-ray [42]. The HP inside the right femur of this case was not detectable, despite a recent re-evaluation of the X-ray images.

The CT investigation of the mummy collection in this study showed that HPs could clearly be diagnosed in mummies and that the osseous imaging characteristics were comparable to those described in clinical literature. HPs can be identified in CT scans as round to oval subcortical/subchondral lesions at the anterior femoral neck, which is clearly demarcated by an encircling sclerotic margin. In the course of the last 30 years, the perception of HPs underwent a renaissance in clinical, radiological and orthopedic literature from an incidental finding to a possible radiological indicator for FAI, which is known to cause OA of the hip joint. OA of the hip joint is a very common observation in paleopathology and the discussed clinical relevance of HPs should also be addressed in paleoradiology. We believe that HPs should be detected and documented in paleoradiological diagnosis of hip joint disease and even subtle morphological changes of the hip joint, indicating FAI, should be taken into consideration as a cause for this condition.

Acknowledgments

We are most grateful to Gaetano Gullo, Superintendent to the Cultural and Environmental Heritage of Palermo, as well as to Father Vincenzo Marchese, Minister of the Order of the Capuchin Friars for the Province of Palermo, for advocating and supporting the project.

Author Contributions

Conceived and designed the experiments: SP DP AZ. Performed the experiments: SP DP AZ. Analyzed the data: SP. Contributed reagents/materials/analysis tools: SP DP AZ. Wrote the paper: SP AZ.

References

1. Roberts C, Manchester K (1995) The Archaeology of Disease. 2nd ed. Ithaca: Cornell University Press. pp 1–29.
2. Aufderheide AC, Rodríguez Martín C (1998) The Cambridge Encyclopedia of Human Paleopathology. Cambridge, England: Cambridge University Press. pp XV–XVI; 93–96.
3. Ortner DJ (2003) Identification of pathological conditions in human skeletal remains. San Diego, London: Academic Press. pp 545–558.
4. König W (1896) 14 Photographien von Röntgen-Strahlen aufgenommen im physikalischen Verein zu Frankfurt a. M. Leipzig: Johan Ambrosius Barth.
5. Resnick D, Niwayama G (1988) Diagnosis of bone and joint disorders. Philadelphia: WB Saunders.
6. Chhem RK, Brothwell DR (2008) Paleoradiology. Imaging mummies and fossils. Berlin, Heidelberg: Springer. pp 1–14.
7. Weiss E, Jurmain R (2007) Osteoarthritis revisited: a contemporary review of aetiology. Int J Osteoarchaeol 17: 437–450.
8. Buikstra JE, Ubelaker DH (1994) Standards for data collection from human skeletal remains. Fayetteville: Arkansas, Archaeological Survey Research Series No. 44. pp 122–123.
9. Woods RJ (1995) Biomechanics of osteoarthritis of the knee. PhD thesis, Ohio State University: Columbus OH.
10. Rothschild BM (1997) Porosity: a curiosity without diagnostic significance. Am J Phys Anthropol 104: 529–533.
11. Larsen CS, Ruff CB, Kelly RL (1995) Structural analysis of the Stillwater postcranial human remains: behavioral implications of articular joint pathology and long bone diaphysial morphology. In: Larsen CS, Kelly RL, eds. Bioarchaeology of the Stillwater Marsh: prehistoric human adaptation in the Western Great Basin. New York: American Museum of Natural History, Anthropological Papers no. 77. pp 107–133.
12. Larsen CS (1997) Bioarchaeology. Interpreting behavior from the human skeleton. Cambridge, England: Cambridge University Press. pp 160–194.
13. Walker PL, Holliman SE (1989) Changes in osteoarthritis associated with development of a maritime economy among southern Californian Indians. Int J Anthropol 4: 171–183.
14. Lieverse AR, Weber AW, Bazaliiskiy VI, Goriunova OI, Savel'ev NA (2007) Osteoarthritis in Siberia's Cis-Baikal: Skeletal indicators of hunter-gatherer adaptation and cultural change. Am J Phys Anthropol 132: 1–16.
15. Klaus HD, Spencer Larsen C, Tam ME (2009) Economic intensification and degenerative joint disease: life and labor on the postcontact north coast of Peru. Am J Phys Anthropol 139: 204–221.
16. Kellgren JH, Lawrence JS (1958) Osteo-arthrosis and disc degeneration in an urban population. Ann Rheum Dis 17: 388–397.
17. Reijman M, Hazes JMW, Pols HAP, Koes BW, Bierma-Zeinstra SMA (2005) Acetabular dysplasia predicts incident osteoarthritis of the hip. Arthritis and Rheumatism 52: 787–793.
18. Filigenzi JM, Bredella MA (2008) MR imaging of femoroacetabular impingement. Appl Radiol 37: 12–19.
19. Ganz R, Leunig M, Leunig-Ganz K, Harris WH (2008) The etiology of osteoarthritis of the hip. An integrated mechanical concept. Clin Orthop Relat Res 466: 264–272.
20. Pitt MJ, Graham AR, Shipman JH, Birkby W (1982) Herniation pit of the femoral neck. AJR 138: 1115–1121.
21. Thomason CB, Silverman ED, Walter RD, Olshaker R (1983) Focal bone tracer uptake associated with a herniation pit of the femoral neck. Clin Nucl Med 8: 304–305.
22. Nokes SR, Vogler JB, Spritzer CE, Martinez S, Herfkens RJ (1989) Herniation pits of the femoral neck: appearance at MR imaging. Radiology 172: 231–234.
23. Crabbe JP, Martel W, Matthews LS (1992) Rapid growth of femoral herniation pit. AJR 159: 1038–1040.
24. Hedvabny Z, Zidkova H, Kofranek I (1993) Herniation pit. Acta Chir Orthop Traumatol Cech 60: 351–353.
25. Polger M, Aliabadi P (1993) Radiologic vignette: the radiographic findings are typical of herniation pit of the femoral neck. Arthritis Rheum 36: 572–574.
26. Schedel H, Wicht L, Mäurer J (1994) Differential diagnosis in variants or abnormalities of the hip on MRI. Bildgebung 61: 20–24.
27. Lerais JM, Jacob D, Thibaud JC, Fourrer C, Cercueil JP, et al. (1995) Disparition spontanée d'une lacune sous-corticale du col fémoral. J Radiol 76: 593–595.
28. Daenen B, Preidler KW, Padmanabhan S, Brossmann J, Tyson R, et al. (1997) Symptomatic herniation pits of the femoral neck: anatomic and clinical study. AJR 168: 149–153.
29. Lee L, Manolios N, De Costa R, Howe G, Spencer G (2000) Herniation pit of the femoral neck. J Rheumatol 27: 2278–2280.

30. Borody C (2005) Symptomatic herniation pit of the femoral neck: a case report. J Manipulative and Physiological Therapeutics 28: 449–451.
31. Panzer S, Esch U, Abdulazim AN, Augat P (2010) Herniation pits and cystic-appearing lesions at the anterior femoral neck: an anatomical study by MSCT and μCT. Skeletal Radiol 39: 645–654.
32. Ganz R, Parvizi J, Beck M (2003) Femoroacetabular impingement. A cause for osteoarthritis of the hip. Clin Orthop Relat Res 417: 112–120.
33. Bredella M, Stoller DW (2005) MR Imaging of FAI. Magn Reson Imaging Clin N Am 13: 653–664.
34. James SLJ, Connell DA, O'Donnell P, Saifuddin A (2007) Femoroacetabular impingement: bone marrow edema associated with fibrocystic change of the femoral head and neck junction. Clin Radiology 62: 472–478.
35. Tannast M, Kubiak-Langer M, Langlotz F, Puls M, Murphy SB, et al. (2007) Noninvasive three-dimensional assessment of femoroacetabular impingement. J Orthop Res 25: 122–131.
36. Tannast M, Siebenrock KA, Anderson SE (2007) Femoroacetabular impingement: radiographic diagnosis-what the radiologist should know. AJR 188: 1540–1552.
37. Panzer S, Augat P, Esch U (2008) CT assessment of herniation pits: prevalence, characteristics, and potential association with morphological predictors of femoroacetabular impingement. Eur Radiol 18: 1869–1875.
38. Panzer S, Augat P, Scheidler J (2010) Hernation pits und ihre Renaissance im Zusammenhang mit femoroazetabulärem Impingement. Fortschr Röntgenstr 182: 565–572.
39. Villotte S, Knüsel CJ (2009) Some remarks about femoroacetabular impingement and osseous non-metric variations of the proximal femur. Bulletins et Mémoires de la Société d'Anthropologie de Paris, n.s 21(1–2): 93–96.
40. Piombino-Mascali D, Aufderheide AC, Panzer S, Zink AR (2010) Mummies from Palermo. In: Wieczorek A, Rosendahl W, eds. Mummies of the World. Munich, London, New York: Prestel. pp 357–361.
41. Aufderheide AC (2003) The scientific study of mummies. Cambridge, England: Cambridge University Press. pp 195–197.
42. Panzer S, Zink AR, Piombino-Mascali D (2010) Radiologic evidence of anthropogenic mummification in the Capuchin Catacombs of Palermo, Sicily. Radio Graphics 30: 1123–1132.
43. Piombino-Mascali D (2009) Il Maestro del Sonno Eterno. Palermo: La Zisa.
44. Nötzli HP, Wyss TF, Stoecklin CH, Schmid MR, Treiber K, et al. (2002) The contour of the femoral head-neck junction as a predictor for the risk of anterior impingement. J Bone Joint Surg Br 84: 556–560.
45. Jäger M, Wild A, Westhoff B, Krauspe R (2004) Femoroacetabular impingement caused by a femoral osseous head-neck bump deformity: clinical, radiological, and experimental results. J Orthop Sci 9: 256–263.
46. Kassarjian A (2006) Hip MR arthrography and femoroacetabular impingement. Sem Muskuloskelet Radiol 10: 208–209.
47. Leunig M, Beck M, Kalhor M, Kim YJ, Werlen S, et al. (2005) Fibrocystic changes at anterosuperior femoral neck: prevalence in hips with femoroacetabular impingement. Radiology 236: 237–246.
48. James SLJ, Ali K, Malara F, Young D, O'Donell J, et al. (2006) MRI findings of femoroacetabular impingement. AJR 187: 1412–1419.
49. Steinbock RT (1976) Paleopathological diagnosis and interpretation: Bone diseases in ancient human populations. Springfield: Charles C. Thomas. pp 277–286.
50. Murray RO (1965) The aetiology of primary osteoarthritis of the hip. Br J Radiol 38: 810–824.
51. Stulberg SD, Cordell LD, Harris WH, Ramsey PL, MacEwen GD (1975) Unrecognized childhood hip disease: a major cause of idiopathic osteoarthritis of the hip. In: The hip, Proceedings of the third open scientific meeting of The Hip Society. Mosby: St. Louis. pp 212–228.
52. Leunig M, Beaulé PE, Ganz R (2009) The concept of femoroacetabular impingement. Current status and future perspectives. Clin Orthop Relat Res 467: 616–622.
53. Anderson LA, Peters CL, Park BB, Stoddard GJ, Erickson JA, Crim JR (2009) Acetabular cartilage delamination in femoroacetabular impingement. Risk factors and magnetic resonance imaging diagnosis. J Bone Joint Surg Am 91: 305–313.
54. Fadul DA, Carrino JA (2009) Imaging of femoroacetabular impingement. J Bone Joint Surg Am 91: 38–143.
55. Kavanagh EC, Read P, Carty F, Zoga AC, Parvizi J, Morrison WB (2011) Three-dimensional magnetic resonance imaging analysis of hip morphology in the assessment of femoral acetabular impingement. Clin Radiol 66: 742–747.
56. Pfirrmann CW, Mengiardi B, Dora C, Kalberer F, Zanetti M, et al. (2006) Cam and pincer femoroacetabular impingement: Characteristic MR Arthrographic findings in 50 patients. Radiology 240: 778–785.
57. Wells C (1963) Hip disease in ancient man. Report of three cases. J Bone Joint Surg Br 45: 790–791.
58. Jurmain R (1977) Stress and etiology of osteoarthritis. Am J Phys Anthropol 46: 353–366.
59. Jurmain R (1999) Stories from the skeleton: behavioral reconstruction in human osteology. Amsterdam: Gordon and Breach.
60. Waldron T (2009) Paleopathology. Cambridge, England: Cambridge University Press. pp 26–40.
61. Harris WH (1986) Etiology of osteoarthritis of the hip. Clin Orthop Relat Res 213: 20–33.
62. Beall DP, Sweet CF, Martin HD, Lastine CL, Grayson DE, et al. (2005) Imaging findings of femoroacetabular impingement syndrome. Skeletal Radiol 34: 691–701.

Use of Alendronate Sodium (Fosamax) to Ameliorate Osteoporosis in Renal Transplant Patients: A Case-Control Study

Wen-Hung Huang[1,2], Shen-Yang Lee[1,2], Cheng-Hao Weng[1,2], Ping-Chin Lai[1,2]*

1 Department of Nephrology, Chang Gung Memorial Hospital, Linkou, Taiwan, Republic of China, **2** Chang Gung University College of Medicine, Taoyuan, Taiwan, Republic of China

Abstract

Background: Renal transplant patients often have severe bone and mineral deficiencies. While the clinical effects of immunosuppressive agents like calcineurin inhibitors (CIs) and sirolimus on bone turnover are unclear, bisphosphonates are effective in bone recovery in these patients. Gender is significantly associated with osteoporosis and affects bone turnover, which is different in women and men. The effective gender-related site of action of bisphosphonates is unknown.

Methods: Initially, we enrolled 84 kidney recipients who had received their transplants at least 5 months ago; of these, 8 were excluded and 76 were finally included in the study. First bone mineral density (BMD) at the lumbar spine, hip, and femoral neck was determined using dual-energy X-ray absorptiometry (DXA) between September 2008 and March 2009. These 76 patients underwent a repeat procedure after a mean period 14 months. Immunosuppressive agents, bisphosphonates, patients' characteristics, and biochemical factors were analyzed on the basis of the BMD determined using DXA.

Results: After the 14-month period, the BMD of lumbar spine increased significantly (from 0.9 g/cm^2 to 0.92 g/cm^2, $p<0.001$), whereas that of the hip and femoral neck did not. Ordinal logistic regression analysis was used to show that Fosamax improved bone condition, as defined by WHO ($p = 0.007$). The use of immunosuppressive agents did not affect bone turnover ($p>0.05$). Moreover, in subgroup analysis, Fosamax increased the BMD at the lumbar spine and the hipbone in males ($p = 0.028$ and 0.03, respectively) but only at the lumbar spine in females ($p = 0.022$).

Conclusion: After a long periods after renal transplantation, the detrimental effects of steroid and immunosuppressive agents on bone condition diminished. Short-term Fosamax administration effectively improves BMD in these patients. The efficacy of Fosamax differed between male and female renal transplant patients.

Editor: Bin He, Baylor College of Medicine, United States of America

Funding: The authors have no support or funding to report.

Competing Interests: The authors have declared that no competing interests exist.

* E-mail: williammaxima@gmail.com

Introduction

Patients maintained on dialysis for end-stage renal disease exhibit severe mineral and bone deficiencies. While renal transplantation restores defective kidney function in patients with chronic renal disease, the associated steroid and other immunosuppressive therapies continuously damage the bones [1,2]; the expected correction of established bone lesions does not occur. Although transplantation can resolve many biochemical imbalances, such as hyperparathyroidism, associated with chronic renal failure, progressive loss of BMD in the trabecular bone often occurs early after renal transplantation [3]. Investigators have not agreed on the risk factors that are most strongly associated with reduced BMD [4,5] after renal transplantation, except on an accumulated dose of steroid. At present, the use of biochemical markers of bone turnover in the serum or urine is not recommended for diagnosis [6]. The World Health Organization (WHO) defines osteoporosis as a condition in which the difference between the mean BMDs for the lumbar spine (LS), femoral neck (FN), or hip (H) of the patients and healthy young adults is more than 2.5 standard deviations (SDs), as measured by dual energy X-ray absorptiometry (DXA). Further, osteopenia is defined as a condition in which the difference between the mean BMDs of the patients and healthy young adults is between 1 and 2.5 SDs [6]. Several studies have shown the beneficial effects of bisphosphonates on post-transplantation osteoporosis [7–9]. Other studies have shown that calcineurin inhibitors (CIs) have deleterious effects on bone mineral metabolism in rats [10–12], and that at least one cyclosporine has a protective effect on bone [13]. Other immune-modifying drugs, such as azathioprine, mycophenolate mofetil, and sirolimus, which are used in conjunction with glucocorticoids and CIs, have not been shown to promote bone loss, neither experimentally nor clinically [14,15]. Osteoporosis caused by portosystemic shunting [16], or by steroid or CIs through receptor activator of nuclear factor kappa-B ligand

(RANKL)-dependent pathways, may be partially ameliorated using sirolimus [17]. Moreover, the physiology of bone turnover differs according to gender, particularly in menopausal women [18–21], and the efficacy of alendronate in the treatment of postmenopausal osteoporosis has been well established [22]. To our knowledge, the gender-related efficacy of alendronate in renal transplant subjects has rarely been reported. The aim of this randomized case-control study was to assess the impact of immunosuppressive agents and alendronate on BMD, as estimated by DXA, and to determine whether the response to alendronate in renal transplant subjects is gender-dependent.

Materials and Methods

This case-control study complied with the guidelines of the Declaration of Helsinki and approved by the Medical Ethics Committee of Chang Gung Memorial Hospital, a tertiary referral center located in the northern part of Taiwan. Since this study involved retrospective review of existing data, the Institutional Review Board approval was obtained, but without specific informed consent from patients. In addition, all individual information was securely protected (by delinking identifying information from main data set) and available to investigators only. Furthermore, all the data were analyzed anonymously. On the other hand, if this study involved retrospective review of existing data plus retrospective analysis of remaining biological samples, both Institutional Review Board approval and specific informed consent must be obtained from all patients. The Institutional Review Board of Chang Gung Memorial Hospital has specifically waived the need for consent. Finally, all primary data were collected according to strengthening the reporting of observational studies in epidemiology guidelines. The form described above was referenced from the Liu et al.'s publication [23].

Study population

We randomly enrolled 84 kidney recipients (40 men and 44 women) who had undergone transplantation at least 5 months ago. We used DXA to obtain BMD measurements of the lumbar spine (LS), left hip (H), and femoral neck (FN) between September 2008 and March 2009 [24]. Bone condition was defined on the basis of the WHO criteria: a BMD value >2.5 standard deviations (SD, T score) below the young adult mean indicated osteoporosis and that between 1.0 and 2.5 SDs below the mean indicated osteopenia. The immunosuppressive agents that the patients had received included prednisolone (5 mg/tablet), cyclosporine (25 mg/tablet and 100 mg/tablet), tacrolimus (0.5 mg/tablet and 1 mg/tablet), sirolimus (1 mg/tablet), and mycophenolate (250 mg/tablet). Fosamax (alendronate sodium; 70 mg/tablet, 70 mg per week) was administered to the patients who were initially diagnosed with osteoporosis. Fasting blood levels of serum creatinine (Cr), blood urea nitrogen (BUN), calcium, inorganic phosphate, and uric acid were obtained. The patients' medical records were studied for the history of diabetes mellitus (DM), smoking frequency, alcohol intake, and hepatitis B (HBV), hepatitis C (HCV), and cytomegalovirus (CMV) infections. All the doses of immunosuppressive agents administered between the 2 BMD measurements were considered as the accumulated dose. After 14±1.6 months of follow-up, the 76 remaining patients (8 of the 84 patients were excluded—2 subjects had died, 2 had graft failure, and the initial BMD measurements of 4 patients was lost) received a second measurement of BMD and fasting blood tests.

Precautions and contraindications for the use of Fosamax

The first DXA report was obtained between September 2008 and March 2009. Fosamax (70 mg per week) was administered to the patients diagnosed with osteoporosis based on this DXA report unless 1 or more of the following conditions was present: bisphosphonate allergy; blood calcium levels <8 mg/dL; active stomach problems (e.g., esophagitis, gastritis, or ulcers); renal insufficiency (estimated glomerular filtration rate [eGFR] <30 mL/[min·1.73 m^2] or serum Cr level >3 mg/dL); difficulty swallowing or the inability to stand/sit upright for at least 30 min, and pregnancy and breastfeeding. The patients did not receive Fosamax prior to obtainment of the first DXA data. Furthermore, the patients were informed that they should take the drug only upon rising for the day with 3 to 4 swallows of water and that they should stand, walk, or sit and fast for 30–45 min afterwards, and then eat breakfast. Lying down or reclining after taking the drug is prohibited. At least 30 min should pass after the intake of alendronate before taking supplements or other drugs.

Immunosuppressive protocol

In our hospital, we mainly use a CI-based immunosuppressive regimen in the initial months of transplantation. Most of our patients also receive mycophenolic acid plus prednisolone during this stage. Immediately after transplantation, the targeted cyclosporine concentration at 2 h post-dose (C_2) is approximately 1300–1100 ng/mL and the tacrolimus trough level is maintained at approximately 12–10 ng/mL. These concentrations are tapered gradually in the first year. In patients that have been transplanted for more than 12 months, the cyclosporine C_2 level is maintained at approximately 500–600 ng/mL and tacrolimus level at 3–4 ng/mL. Prednisolone is maintained at 1.25–10 mg per day, according to patient's condition. An mTOR inhibitor is added to the regimen if the patient's condition is suitable (proteinuria <800 mg/day and eGFR >40 mL/[min·1.73 m^2]). The trough level of the mTOR inhibitor is maintained at approximately 3–8 ng/mL. Once the mTOR inhibitor has been added, the CI and mycophenolic acid dose are cut by 50% overnight, while prednisolone is maintained at the same dosage. Subsequently, the CI dose is tapered as much as possible. Most of the patients in this study received only 25 mg cyclosporine or 0.5 mg tacrolimus per day if an mTOR inhibitor was used.

Statistical analysis

The data, given as median and interquartile ranges in non-normal distribution variables, are expressed as mean ± SD in normal distribution variables. The paired *t* test and the Wilcoxon signed-rank test were used to compare data of the patients at presentation and follow-up. The Kruskal–Wallis test and one-way analysis of variance (ANOVA) were performed to compare data of the different bone conditions defined by the WHO criteria. Comparisons among groups were performed using the Mann–Whitney test and Student's *t* test. We used multivariate ordinal logistic regression to test the expected value between clinical variables and the change of bone condition (grade 1: change to better, grade 2: no change, and grade 3: deterioration; change to better: from osteoporosis to osteopenia or normal, or from osteopenia to normal; no change: no change in bone condition at start and follow-up; deterioration: from normal to osteopenia or osteoporosis, or from osteopenia to osteoporosis), as defined by WHO. The Chi-square test was used to determine the correlation between the 2 binary variables; a p value <0.05 was considered statistically significant. All statistical analyses were performed using the Statistical Package for the Social Sciences (SPSS) Version 12.0 for Windows (SPSS Inc., Chicago, IL, USA).

Results

Characteristics of the study population

After a follow-up period of 14±1.6 months, 76 subjects received a second BMD measurement. Among these patients, 12 had a medical history of DM; 10 were infected with HBV, 15 with HCV, and 13 with CMV; 10 men were habitual tobacco users, and 8 men and 1 woman regularly consumed alcohol. Thirty-four patients received Fosamax, 57, prednisolone; 55, mycohenolate; 30, tacrolimus; 26, cyclosporine; and 34, sirolimus. Eight patients (11%) received a single immunosuppressive agent, 21 patients (28%) received 2 immunosuppressive agents, 36 (47%) received 3, and 11 (14%) received 4.

Bone mineral density (BMD) at baseline and at follow-up

Table 1 shows the changes in BMD and blood biochemistry after 14±1.6 months of follow-up. In the 76 patients, calcium level decreased from 9.45±0.51 mg/dL to 9.29±0.52 mg/dL ($p<0.001$) and albumin from 4.42±0.29 g/L to 4.34±0.4 g/L ($p=0.009$), both levels were still within the normal range. However, BMD of the lumbar spine increased from 0.9 to 0.92 g/cm^2, ($p<0.001$). No correlation between the use of Fosamax and that of the immunosuppressive agents could be demonstrated, as determined by the Chi-square test ($p>0.05$). No patient who received Fosamax exhibited a deterioration in the condition of his bone structure, as defined by WHO criteria. Thirty patients showed no change in their bone condition, but 4 showed improvement. In patients who had not received Fosamax, 6 (14%) showed deterioration and 1 (2%) showed improvement.

BMD in patients with osteoporosis and without

In 41 patients with and 35 without osteoporosis at baseline, the lumbar spine bone density increased (from 0.83 to 0.86 g/cm^2 [$p<0.001$] and from 0.99 to 1.0 g/cm^2 [$p=0.02$]; respectively) after the mean 14-month follow-up period, but hip and femoral neck densities did not (Table 2). In order to detect any difference in BMD due to the use of immunosuppressive agents in different conditions of the bone, the patients were divided into 3 groups: normal, osteopenia, and osteoporosis, on the basis of the initial DXA findings. The osteoporosis group received a greater cumulative steroid dose than the osteopenia group (1326.5 mg vs. 724.5 mg; $p=0.005$; Figure 1A), and the increase in the lumbar spine BMD was greater in the osteoporosis group (0.033 g/cm^2 vs. 0.009 g/cm^2; $p=0.028$; Figure 1B). Otherwise, the cumulative dose of immunosuppressive agents among the 3 groups did not differ significantly ($p>0.05$; Figure 1A). Interestingly, of our 41 osteoporosis patients, 7 did not receive Fosamax due to their intolerance of the side effects. Among those 41 patients, those administered Fosamax showed a greater increase in BMD (0.035 g/cm^2 vs. 0.003 g/cm^2) but not significant ($p>0.05$).

Factors associated with bone turnover

To deepen our investigation of the influence of clinical features on bone condition, we used a univariate binary logistic regression to evaluate the association between bone condition (osteoporotic and not osteoporotic at follow-up) and the clinical variables in 76 patients. The use of both prednisolone (odds ratio [OR], 5.18; 95% confidence interval [CI], 1.6–16.4; $p=0.005$) and Fosamax (OR, 18.75; 95% CI, 5.42–64.76; $p<0.001$) showed an association in patients with osteoporosis (Figure 2A). In an ordinal logistic regression with multivariate analysis of the change in bone condition (grade 1, improvement; grade 2, no change; and grade 3, deterioration; as defined by WHO criteria) and the clinical variables, after adjusting for age, sex, status of diabetes, smoking, alcohol consumption, time since transplantation, age at transplant, and use of prednisolone, the use of Fosamax (OR, −3.115; 95% CI, −5.364; −0.866; $p=0.007$) was found to be associated with a positive prognosis (Figure 2B).

Table 1. Data reported at baseline and at follow-up, n = 76.

	Baseline	follow-up	P value
LS-BMD (g/cm^2)	0.90±0.14	0.92±0.14	<0.001
H-BMD (g/cm^2)	0.81±0.14	0.81±0.14	NS
FN-BMD (g/cm^2)	0.68±0.12	0.69±0.13	NS
LS T	−1.53±1.24	−1.32±1.26	<0.001
H T	−1.76±0.97	−1.68±1.07	NS
FN T	−2.45±0.96	−2.42±1.02	NS
Smoking	10/76		
Alcohol	9/76		
DM	12/76		
HBV	10/76		
HCV	15/76		
CMV	13/76		
BUN (mg/dL)	19.7±10.0	19.8±10.9	NS
Cr (mg/dL)	1.18±0.54	1.20±0.54	NS
Ca (mg/dL)	9.45±0.51	9.29±0.52	<0.001
P (mg/dL)	3.21±0.54	3.23±0.59	NS
Uric acid (mg/dL)	6.24±1.68	6.45±1.70	NS
Albumin (g/L)	4.42±0.29	4.34±0.40	0.009
TC (mg/dL)	201±44	190±46	NS
TG (mg/dL)	147±82	148±113	NS
Normal	5/76	5/76	
Osteopenia	30/76	29/76	
Osteoporosis	41/76	42/76	

At follow-up, LS-BMD was significantly greater than its initial value. The albumin and calcium levels also had decreased significantly, but they remained within normal range.

Abbreviations: LS-BMD, lumbar spine bone mineral density; H-BMD, hip bone mineral density; FN-BMD, femoral neck bone mineral density; T, number of standard deviations (SD) above or below the mean value of a sex-matched, young adult mean of BMD. DM, diabetes mellitus; BUN, blood urea nitrogen; Cr, blood creatinine; Ca, serum calcium; P, serum inorganic phosphate; TC, serum total cholesterol; TG, serum triglyceride; HBV, hepatitis B virus infection; HCV, hepatitis C virus infection; CMV, cytomegalovirus infection; NS, no significance, $p>0.05$.

Gender differences in the effect of Fosamax on bones

In our study, we found no gender-related differences in bone turnover of renal transplant patients during the mean 14-month follow-up period. Seeking a gender-related difference in the physiology of bone turnover, we examined the bone response to Fosamax in the 2 sexes. We found no differences in bone turnover with respect to age, time since transplant, or the changes in blood values for creatinine, albumin, or calcium, and neither was the change in BMD or the cumulative immunosuppressive agents different in the 2 sexes. However, when we compared BMD before and after Fosamax treatment within the male and female groups, we found Fosamax to be more effective in men than in women. Among the patients who received Fosamax, BMD in the lumbar spine and the hip ($p=0.028$ and $p=0.03$, respectively) increased in 14 men; however, the increase in the BMD was observed only

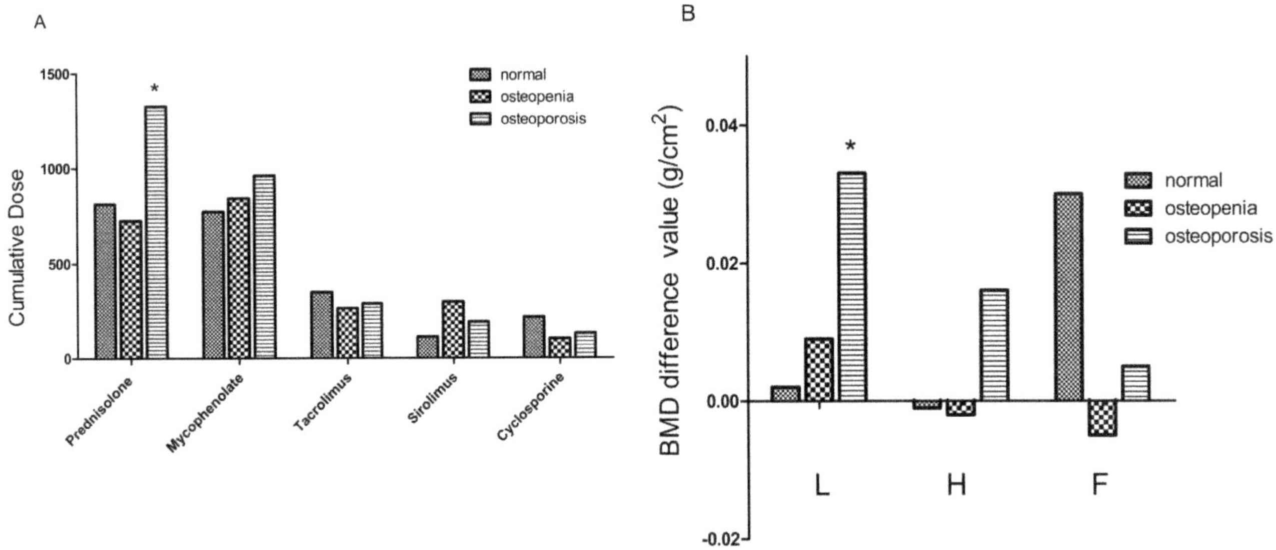

Figure 1. Cumulative dose of immunosuppressive agents and bone mineral density change between three bone conditions by WHO. The patients were divided, according to their baseline DXA, into normal (n = 5), osteopenia (n = 30), and osteoporosis (n = 41) groups. The osteoporosis group received a significantly greater cumulative prednisolone dose than did the osteopenia group (1326.5 mg vs. 724.5 mg; p = 0.005; Figure 1A), and the increase in lumbar spine bone mineral density was also significantly greater in the osteoporosis group (0.033 g/cm^2 vs. 0.009 g/cm^2; p = 0.028; Figure 1B). The drugs included in the analysis of cummulative immunosuppresive therapy were prednisolone, 5 mg; mycophenolate, 250 mg; tacrolimus, 0.5 mg; sirolimus, 1 mg; and cyclosporine, 100 mg. Abbreviations: L, lumbar spine; H, hipbone; F, femoral neck. *Statistical significance at p<0.05.

in the lumbar spine (p = 0.022; Table 3) in 20 women. Among the above-mentioned men and women who used Fosamax, the BMD difference values were not different (p>0.05). Thus, we find that the sites of action of Fosamax differ across the 2 sexes.

Discussion

In this study, we have shown that short-term weekly use of Fosamax can improve both BMD and bone condition, in accordance with the WHO criteria, regardless of effect of immunosuppressive agents after a long period after renal transplantation. In renal transplant subjects with osteoporosis, Fosamax improved the BMD of the lumbar spine. Although the bone condition after renal transplantation did not vary according to gender, the bone regions in which Fosamax was effective did vary.

An increase in bone mass loss is multifactorial and is affected by age [21], sex [19–21], renal function, and duration of time for which the patient was on dialysis before transplantation [20]. A major influencing and well-known factor causing increased loss of bone mass is high-dose steroid therapy during the early period after transplantation and continuous long-term steroid administration [2]. CIs such as cyclosporine and tacrolimus also are known to have serious effects and cause rapid and severe bone losses in both animal models and humans. The role of T-lymphocyte action via RANKL seems to be of essence in triggering bone loss [14]. Other immune-modifying drugs such as azathioprine, mycophenolate mofetil, and sirolimus, which are used in conjunction with glucocorticoids and CIs, have—neither experimentally nor clinically—been shown to promote bone loss. Recent studies [17,25] suggest that sirolimus could promote an osteoclastic balance between the effects of steroid and of calcineurine inhibitors. Moreover, under sirolimus-based maintenance immunosuppression [26] after bone surgery, no radiologic advantage or disadvantage to bone healing was noted. Therefore, in our clinical estimation, a bias may exist between the biochemical markers and DXA–WHO criteria in osteoporosis to evaluate bone condition.

Interestingly, the lumbar spine BMD in our 35 non-osteoporotic patients increased slightly. As was true with the steroids, the cumulative dose of immunosuppressive agents in the non-osteoporosis and osteoporosis groups did not differ. In the past decade, the use of corticosteroids in the peritransplantation period has been dramatically reduced and replaced by CIs and other adjunctive agents. To our knowledge, the first 3 to 6 months after transplantation is the critical period for the loss in bone mass [4,27,28]. In a long-term study, the ongoing accelerated lumbar bone mass loss was 1.7±2.8% per year [29], but in the 12 months following cardiac transplantation, the LS BMD value was restored to that at the time of transplant [30]. Twenty-four months after transplantation, the yearly loss of absolute BMD was parallel to the age-dependent physiological decline in absolute BMD [5]. In our study, the time since transplant of non-osteoporotic subjects was 78±60 months. From the studies cited above and from our observations during the long post-transplantation period, we can explain the slightly increased BMD of lumbar spine in our patients who did not receive Fosamax. Otherwise, as the use of immunosuppressive agents changes in the long period of renal transplantation, the effective power of steroid on bone turnover may be increasingly minor.

In this study, when we analyzed the subgroups of the subjects with osteoporosis, we observed that Fosamax was not equally effective in men and women in the different bone regions. Several previous studies have shown that bisphosphonates continued to improved bone mineral density after renal transplantation [7–9,31,32] and most of them showed the effect on both lumbar spine and femoral neck BMD. In a meta-analysis review of 1209 patients [33], treatment with bisphosphonates increased BMD in lumbar spine and femoral neck. No measurable change in the BMD of the hip area was observed. In another population-based longitudinal study [18], both the bone turnover and the sites of bone loss

Table 2. Comparison of patients with (41) and without (35) osteoporosis at presentation and follow-up.

	Non-osteoporosis patients (35)			Osteoporosis patients (41)			P value
	Baseline	**1st follow up**	**P value**	**Baseline**	**1st follow up**	**P value**	
LS-BMD(g/cm²)	0.99±0.12	1.00±0.13	0.02	0.83±0.11	0.86±0.12	<0.001	
H-BMD(g/cm²)	0.91±0.12	0.90±0.13	NS	0.72±0.11	0.73±0.10	NS	
FN-BMD (g/cm²)	0.78±0.09	0.78±0.11	NS	0.605±0.058	0.607±0.066	NS	
LS T score	−1.0 [−1.6,−0.2]	−0.9 [−1.5,0.3]	0.047	−2.15±1.02	−1.9±1.07	<0.001	
H T score	−1.06±0.65	−1.01±0.89	NS	−2.35±0.79	−2.25±0.86	NS	
FN T score	−1.59±0.68	−1.68±0.78	NS	−3.14±0.47	−3.09±0.54	NS	
Gender (F/M)		16/19			24/17		
Smoking		5/35			5/41		
Alcohol		5/35			4/41		
DM		7/35			5/41		
BUN (mg/dL)	17.7±7.6	17.7±6.3	NS	21.27±11.77	21.55±13.46	NS	NS*
Cr (mg/dL)	1.09±0.45	1.15±0.41	0.043	1.24±0.6	1.28±0.62	NS	NS*
Ca (mg/dL)	9.52±0.49	9.33±0.56	0.002	9.4±0.53	9.24±0.49	0.007	NS*
P (mg/dL)	3.22±0.58	3.22±0.57	NS	3.2±0.52	3.25±0.62	NS	NS*
Uric acid (mg/dL)	6.0±1.7	6.6±1.9	NS	6.44±1.73	6.26±1.59	NS	NS*
Albumin (g/L)	4.48±0.31	4.39±0.43	0.035	4.38±0.27	4.31±0.41	NS	NS*
TC (mg/dL)	198.1±40.2	190.5±44.3	NS	203.67±47.5	187.78±49.4	NS	NS*
TG (mg/dL)	159.9±85.5	152.5±106.3	NS	137.77±79.35	146.03±129.37	NS	NS*
Normal	5	5		0	0		
Osteopenia	30	25		0	4		
Osteoporosis	0	5		41	37		
Cumulative dose of immunosuppressant agent							
Prednisolone (mg)		872±730			1326.5±961		p = 0.003
Mycophenolate (tablets)		833.6±823.8			962.2±812.5		NS*
Tacrolimus (tablets/1 mg)		275.0±393.6			288.1±447.1		NS*
Sirolimus (tablets)		270.8±302.0			191.5±301.1		NS*
Cyclosporine (100 mg tablets)		119.20±210.85			131.12±177.79		NS*
Increase in BMD							
LS-BMD (g/cm²)		0.011±0.027			0.030±0.028		p = 0.005
H-BMD (g/cm²)		−0.005±0.03			0.007±0.036		NS*
FN-BMD (g/cm²)		0.003 ±0.052			0.002±0.031		NS*

The mean follow-up period was 14 months. In both the non-osteoporosis and the osteoporosis group, the LS-BMD significantly increased. At the end of the period, the cumulative dose of prednisolone and the LS-BMD differential were greater in the osteoporosis group.
NS*: $p>0.05$ between the osteoporosis and non-osteoporosis group.
Abbreviations: LS-BMD, lumbar spine bone mineral density; H-BMD, hip bone mineral density; FN-BMD, femoral neck bone mineral density; T score, number of standard deviations (SD) different from the mean value of the corresponding gender-matched young adult mean BMD. DM, diabetes mellitus; BUN, blood urea nitrogen; Cr, blood creatinine; Ca, serum calcium concentration; P, serum inorganic phosphate level; TC, serum total cholesterol level; TG, serum triglyceride level; NS: not significant, $p>0.05$.

differed according to gender. In a 2-year double-blind trial of men with osteoporosis (mean age, 63 years), alendronate significantly increased bone mass of spine and hipbone and helped prevent vertebral fractures [34]. Iwamoto et al. [35] have suggested that although alendronate treatment in men effectively increased lumbar BMD from baseline, its efficacy appeared to be no greater than that in postmenopausal women with osteoporosis. Studies on the comparative effects in a renal transplant population of bisphosphonates according to gender and bone site are limited. In our study on men and women who presented no significant differences in the increase in their BMD with Fosamax, the 14 osteoporotic men showed improved BMD at the hip and lumbar spine and the 20 osteoporotic females responded well only at the lumbar spine.

Fosamax is absorbed and partitioned rapidly, with approximately 50% binding to the exposed bone surface and the remainder being excreted unchanged by the kidneys [36]. Therefore, Fosamax should be used carefully in patients with renal insufficiency or in anuric patients because of concerns regarding drug accumulation. The major side effect of Fosamax is ulceration of the esophagus, which may require hospitalization and intensive treatment. Gastric and duodenal ulceration may also

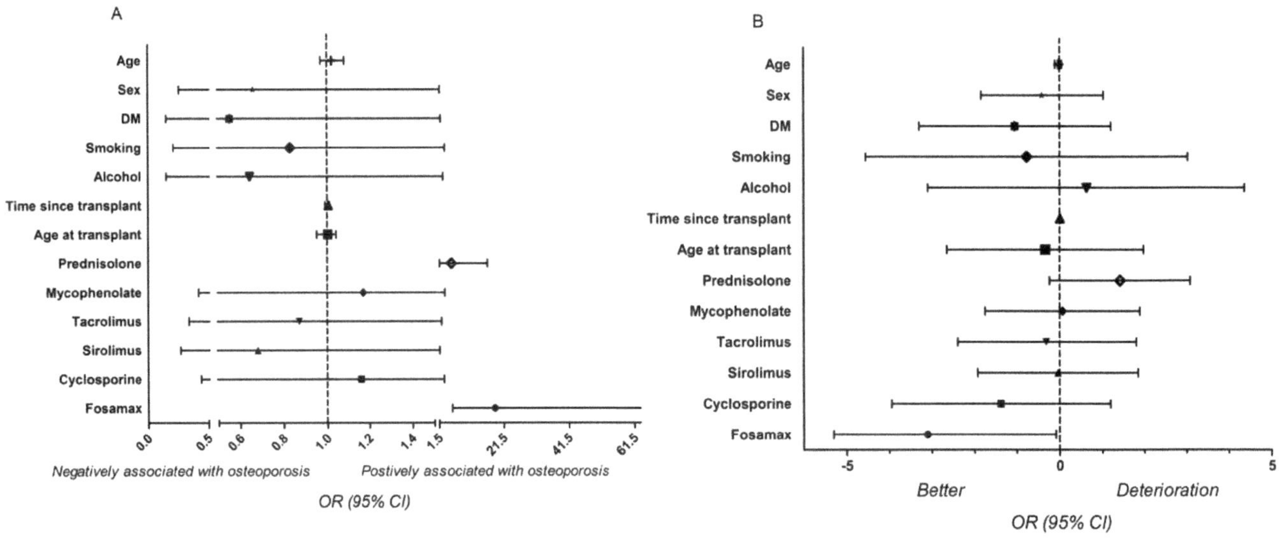

Figure 2. Clinical variables associated with bone condition change. A binary (non-osteoporosis and osteoporosis in follow-up) logistic regression analysis was performed to identify the variables associated with osteoporosis. The dependent variable was non-osteoporosis or osteoporosis. The independent variables were age, sex, DM, smoking, alcohol consumption, age at transplantation, time since transplant, use of immunosuppressive agents and use of Fosamax. Both the use of prednisolone (odds ratio [OR], 5.18; 95% confidence interval [CI], 1.6–16.4; $p = 0.005$) and the use of Fosamax (OR, 18.75; 95% CI, 5.42–64.76; $p < 0.001$) were associated with the symptoms of osteoporosis (Figure 2A). In an ordinal logistic regression with multivariate analysis of the change of bone condition (grade 1, changed to the better; grade 2, no change; and grade 3, deterioration, as defined by WHO criteria and clinical variables), after adjusting for age, sex, status of diabetes (DM), smoking, alcohol consumption, time since transplant, age at transplant, and use of prednisolone, the use of Fosamax (OR, −3.115; 95% CI, −5.364 to −0.866; $p = 0.007$) was found to be associated with a positive prognosis (Figure 2B).

Table 3. Comparison of the use and non-use of Fosamax in men and women.

	Male patients (36)			**Female patients (40)**			**P value**
	Non-Fosamax (22)	**Fosamax (14)**	**P value**	**Non-Fosamax (20)**	**Fosamax (20)**	**P value**	
Age (years)	48±10.4	51.9±9.0	NS	49.7±7.6	53.3±8.8	NS	NS*
Time since transplant (months)	92±68.1	103.7±59.4	NS	61.4±39.6	97.6±72.9	NS	NS*
Creatinine difference value (mg/dL)	0 (−0.072, 0.122)	0.04 (−0.09, 0.21)	NS	0.05 (−0.035, 0.225)	0.01 (−0.075, 0.16)	NS	NS*
Albumin difference value (g/L)	−0.06 (−0.21, 0.08)	0.01 (−0.33, 0.18)	NS	−0.02 (−0.26, 0.047)	−0.1 (−0.21, 0.15)	NS	NS*
Calcium difference value (mg/dL)	−0.3 (−0.4, 0)	−0.2 (−0.4, 0.025)	NS	−0.15 (−0.27, 0)	−0.1 (−0.5, 0.17)	NS	NS*
BMD difference value							
LS-BMD difference value (g/cm^2)	0.018 (−0.002, 0.036)	0.039 (0.02, 0.056)	0.028	0.004 (−0.004, 0.033)	0.032 (0.01, 0.051)	0.022	NS*
H-BMD difference value (g/cm^2)	−0.0085 (−0.025, 0.015)	0.015 (−0.0035, 0.029)	0.03	0.003 (−0.015, 0.019)	0.023 (−0.043, 0.039)	NS	NS*
FN-BMD difference value (g/cm^2)	0.004 (−0.021, 0.030)	0.0095 (−0.0065, 0.03)	NS	−0.0015 (−0.024, 0.017)	−0.0035 (−0.024, 0.016)	NS	NS*
Cumulative dose of Immunosuppressive agents							
Prednisolone (mg)	1054±700	1477±1072	NS	434 (0, 616)	1295 (751, 2151)	<0.001	NS*
Mycophenolate (tablets)	971±933	1079±902	NS	613±487	994±856	NS	NS*
Tacrolimus (tablets/1 mg)	0 (0, 178)	0 (0, 677)	NS	0 (0,705)	147 (0, 770)	NS	NS*
Sirolimus (tablets)	350 (0, 556)	0 (0, 425)	NS	0 (0, 383)	0 (0, 385)	NS	NS*
Cyclosporine (tablets/100 mg)	0 (0,402)	0 (0, 404)	NS	0 (0, 192)	0 (0, 253)	NS	NS*

Under similar conditions (characteristics, BMD differences, and cumulative use of immunosuppressive agents) the use of Fosamax in male patients increased the BMD of both lumbar spine and hip bone, but in female patients it increased the BMD only of lumbar spine.
NS*: $p > 0.05$ between male and female patients.
Abbreviations: LS-BMD, lumbar spine bone mineral density; H-BMD, hip bone mineral density; FN-BMD, femoral neck bone mineral density;
NS, no significance, $p > 0.05$.

occur [37,38]. The co-administration of Fosamax and calcium, antacids, or oral medications containing multivalent cations interferes with the absorption of alendronate [38]. The short-term use of a low dose of Fosamax (40 mg per week) was safe in hemodialysis patients [39]. Alendronate treatment safely and effectively increased BMD and decreased fractures in women with normal to severely impaired renal function [40], and no differences in adverse events were observed in these women according to their renal function. The use of Fosamax for a mean of 14 months did not deteriorate renal function in male and female renal transplant patients (Table 3). To our knowledge, studies on the interaction between Fosamax and immunosuppressant agents are limited. The studies cited above and our own observations suggest that the interaction between these agents is subtle.

Although the limitations of our study with regard to its retrospective design and small sample size are evident, to our knowledge, these are the first data reporting the differences between men and women with regard to the sites at which Fosamax is effective in renal transplant patients; these findings refer to short-term treatment after a long post-renal transplantation period.

Conclusions

In conclusion, this randomized case-control study has shown that short-term use of Fosamax increased BMD and that the effect of concomitant steroid was not significantly correlated with bone turnover. Moreover, Fosamax increased the BMD of the lumbar spine and hip significantly in men, but only in the lumbar spine in women. Immunosuppressive agents such as CIs, sirolimus, and mycohenolate were not correlated with any change in BMD.

Acknowledgments

We thank the members of the Immune Transplant Center in Chang Gung Memorial Hospital for their invaluable and dedicated assistance.

Author Contributions

Conceived and designed the experiments: WHH PCL. Performed the experiments: WHH SYL CHW. Analyzed the data: WHH SYL PCL. Contributed reagents/materials/analysis tools: WHH CHW. Wrote the paper: WHH.

References

1. Parker CR, Freemont AJ, Blackwell PJ, Grainge MJ, Hosking DJ (1999)Cross-sectional analysis of renal transplantation osteoporosis. J Bone Miner Res 14(11):1943–1951.
2. Kodras K, Haas M (2006) Effect of kidney transplantation on bone. Eur J Clin Invest 36:Suppl-75.
3. Rodino MA, Shane E (1998) Osteoporosis after organ transplantation. Am J Med 104(5):459–469.
4. Julian BA, Laskow DA, Dubovsky J, Dubovsky EV, Curtis JJ, et al. (1991) Rapid loss of vertebral mineral density after renal transplantation. N Engl J Med 325(8):544–550.
5. Grotz WH, Mundinger FA, Rasenack J, Speidel L, Olschewski M, et al. (1995) Bone loss after kidney transplantation: a longitudinal study in 115 graft recipients. Nephrol Dial Transplant 10(11):2096–2100.
6. Sweet MG, Sweet JM, Jeremiah MP, Galazka SS (2009) Diagnosis and treatment of osteoporosis. Am Fam Physician 79(3):193–200.
7. Nayak B, Guleria S, Varma M, Tandon N, Aggarwal S, et al. (2007)Effect of bisphosphonates on bone mineral density after renal transplantation as assessed by bone mineral densitometry. Transplant Proc 39(3):750–752.
8. Palmer SC, McGregor DO, Strippoli GF (2007) Interventions for preventing bone disease in kidney transplant recipients. Update of Cochrane Database Syst Rev (3):CD005015
9. El-Agroudy AE, El-Husseini AA, El-Sayed M, Mohsen T, Ghoneim MA (2005) A prospective randomized study for prevention of postrenal transplantation bone loss. Kidney Int 67(5):2039–2045.
10. Buchinsky FJ, Ma Y, Mann GN, Rucinski B, Bryer HP, et al. (1996)T lymphocytes play a critical role in the development of cyclosporin A-induced osteopenia. Endocrinology 137(6):2278–2285.
11. Movsowitz C, Epstein S, Fallon M, Ismail F, Thomas S (1988) Cyclosporin-A in vivo produces severe osteopenia in the rat: effect of dose and duration of administration. Endocrinology 123(5):2571–2577.
12. Schlosberg M, Movsowitz C, Epstein S, Ismail F, Fallon MD, et al. (1989)The effect of cyclosporin A administration and its withdrawal on bone mineral metabolism in the rat. Endocrinology 124(5):2179–2184.
13. Carlini RG, Rojas E, Weisinger JR, Lopez M, Martinis R, et al. (2000) Bone disease in patients with long-term renal transplantation and normal renal function. Am J Kidney Dis 36(1):160–166.
14. Tamler R, Epstein S (2006) Nonsteroid immune modulators and bone disease. Ann N Y Acad Sci 1068:284–296.
15. Abdelhadi M, Ericzon BG, Hultenby K, Sjoden G, Reinholt FP, et al. (2002) Structural skeletal impairment induced by immunosuppressive therapy in rats: cyclosporine A vs tacrolimus. Transpl Int 15(4):180–187.
16. van der Merwe SW, Conradie MM, Bond R, Olivier BJ, Fritz E, et al. (2006) Effect of rapamycin on hepatic osteodystrophy in rats with portasystemic shunting. World J Gastroenterol 12(28):4504–4510.
17. Westenfeld R, Schlieper G, Woltje M, Gawlik A, Brandenburg V, et al. (2011) Impact of sirolimus, tacrolimus and mycophenolate mofetil on osteoclastogenesis-implications for post-transplantation bone disease. Nephrol Dial Transplant 26(12):4115–4123.
18. Dennison E, Eastell R, Fall CH, Kellingray S, Wood PJ, et al. (1999) Determinants of bone loss in elderly men and women: a prospective population-based study. Osteoporos Int 10(5):384–391.
19. Kokado Y, Takahara S, Ichimaru N, Toki K, Kyo M, et al. (2000) Factors influencing vertebral bone density after renal transplantation. Transpl Int 13:Suppl-5.
20. Aroldi A, Tarantino A, Montagnino G, Cesana B, Cocucci C, et al. (1997) Effects of three immunosuppressive regimens on vertebral bone density in renal transplant recipients: a prospective study. Transplantation 63(3):380–386.
21. Hung CJ, Lee PC, Song CM, Chang YT, Tsai MT, et al. (1996) Clinical implication of hormone treatment in postmenopausal kidney transplants. Transplant Proc 28(3):1548–1550.
22. Cranney A, Guyatt G, Griffith L, Wells G, Tugwell P, et al. (2002) Meta-analyses of therapies for postmenopausal osteoporosis. IX: Summary of meta-analyses of therapies for postmenopausal osteoporosis. Endocr Rev 23(4):570–578.
23. Liu SH, Lin JL, Weng CH, Yang HY, Hsu CW, et al.(2012) Heart rate-corrected QT interval helps predict mortality after intentional organophosphate poisoning. PLoS One 7(5):e36576.
24. Huang WH, Lai PC (2011)Age at transplant–one of the factors affecting bone mineral density in kidney recipients–a single-center retrospective study. Ren Fail 33(8):776–80.
25. Campistol JM, Holt DW, Epstein S, Gioud-Paquet M, Rutault K, et al. (2005) Bone metabolism in renal transplant patients treated with cyclosporine or sirolimus. Transpl Int 18(9):1028–1035.
26. Cavadas PC, Hernan I, Landin L, Thione A (2011) Bone healing after secondary surgery on hand allografts under sirolimus-based maintenance immunosuppression. Ann Plast Surg 66(6):667–669.
27. Horber FF, Casez JP, Steiger U, Czerniak A, Montandon A, et al. (1994) Changes in bone mass early after kidney transplantation. J Bone Miner Res 9(1):1–9.
28. Ezaitouni F, Westeel PF, Fardellone P, Mazouz H, Brazier M, et al. (1998) Long-term stability of bone mineral density in patients with renal transplant treated with cyclosporine and low doses of corticoids. Protective role of cyclosporine?. Presse Med 27(15):705–712.
29. Pichette V, Bonnardeaux A, Prudhomme L, Gagne M, Cardinal J, et al. (1996) Long-term bone loss in kidney transplant recipients: a cross-sectional and longitudinal study. Am J Kidney Dis 28(1):105–114.
30. Leidig-Bruckner G, Hosch S, Dodidou P, Ritschel D, Conradt C, et al. (2001) Frequency and predictors of osteoporotic fractures after cardiac or liver transplantation: a follow-up study. Lancet 357(9253):342–347.
31. Torregrosa JV, Fuster D, Pedroso S, Diekmann F, Campistol JM, et al. (2007)Weekly risedronate in kidney transplant patients with osteopenia. Transpl Int 20(8):708–711.
32. Giannini S, D'Angelo A, Carraro G, Nobile M, Rigotti P, et al. (2001) Alendronate prevents further bone loss in renal transplant recipients. J Bone Miner Res 16(11):2111–2117.
33. Palmer SC, Strippoli GF, McGregor DO (2005) Interventions for preventing bone disease in kidney transplant recipients: a systematic review of randomized controlled trials. Am J Kidney Dis 45(4):638–649.
34. Orwoll E, Ettinger M, Weiss S, Miller P, Kendler D, et al. (2000) Alendronate for the treatment of osteoporosis in men. N Engl J Med 343(9):604–610.
35. Iwamoto J, Takeda T, Sato Y, Uzawa M (2007) Comparison of the effect of alendronate on lumbar bone mineral density and bone turnover in men and postmenopausal women with osteoporosis. Clin Rheumatol 26(2):161–167

36. Shinkai I, Ohta Y (1996) New drugs–reports of new drugs recently approved by the FDA. Alendronate. Bioorg Med Chem 4(1):3–4.
37. de Groen PC, Lubbe DF, Hirsch LJ, Daifotis A, Stephenson W, et al. (1996) Esophagitis associated with the use of alendronate. N Engl J Med 335(14):1016–1021
38. Full prescribing information for FOSAMAX (2012) Merck Sharp & Dohme, June 2012.
39. Wetmore JB, Benet LZ, Kleinstuck D, Frassetto L (2005) Effects of short-term alendronate on bone mineral density in haemodialysis patients. Nephrology 10(4):393–399.
40. Jamal SA, Bauer DC, Ensrud KE, Cauley JA, Hochberg M, et al. (2007) Alendronate treatment in women with normal to severely impaired renal function: an analysis of the fracture intervention trial. J Bone Miner Res 22(4):503–508.

26

Epidemiological Evidence for Work Load as a Risk Factor for Osteoarthritis of the Hip

Sandra I. Sulsky[1]*, Laura Carlton[1], Frank Bochmann[2], Rolf Ellegast[2], Ulrich Glitsch[2], Bernd Hartmann[3], Dirk Pallapies[4], D. Seidel[3], Yi Sun[2]

1 ENVIRON International Corporation, Amherst, Massachusetts, United States of America, **2** Institut für Arbeitsschutz der Deutschen Gesetzlichen Unfallversicherung (IFA), Sankt Augustin, Germany, **3** Berufsgenossenschaft der Bauwirtschaft (BG BAU), Arbeitsmedizinisch-Sicherheitstechnischer Dienst, Berlin, Germany, **4** Institut für Prävention und Arbeitsmedizin der Deutschen Gesetzlichen Unfallversicherung (IPA), Bochum, Germany

Abstract

Objective: Osteoarthritis of the hip (OA) is a common degenerative disorder of the joint cartilage that presents a major public health problem worldwide. While intrinsic risk factors (e.g, body mass and morphology) have been identified, external risk factors are not well understood. In this systematic review, the evidence for workload as a risk factor for hip OA is summarized and used to derive recommendations for prevention and further research.

Methods: Epidemiological studies on workload or occupation and osteoarthritis of the hip were identified through database and bibliography searches. Using pre-defined quality criteria, 30 studies were selected for critical evaluation; six of these provided quantitative exposure data.

Results: Study results were too heterogeneous to develop pooled risk estimates by specific work activities. The weight of evidence favors a graded association between long-term exposure to heavy lifting and risk of hip OA. Long-term exposure to standing at work might also increase the risk of hip OA.

Conclusions: It is not possible to estimate a quantitative dose-response relationship between workload and hip OA using existing data, but there is enough evidence available to identify job-related heavy lifting and standing as hazards, and thus to begin developing recommendations for preventing hip OA by limiting the amount and duration of these activities. Future research to identify specific risk factors for work-related hip OA should focus on implementing rigorous study methods with quantitative exposure measures and objective diagnostic criteria.

Editor: Nick Harvey, University of Southampton, United Kingdom

Funding: The authors have no support or funding to report.

Competing Interests: SS and LC are employees of ENVIRON International Corporation. There are no patents, products in development or marketed products to declare. No other authors have any conflicts to declare.

* E-mail: ssulsky@environcorp.com

Introduction

Osteoarthritis or osteoarthrosis of the hip (hip OA) is a degenerative disorder of the joint cartilage and its underlying bone that can affect one or both hip joints [1]. It is a common joint disease in the elderly, is recognized as a major cause of pain, disability, and social expenditure, and presents a major public health problem throughout the world [2–5].

The diagnosis of hip OA is based on clinical criteria consisting of hip pain and impaired inner rotation in combination with radiographically confirmed joint degeneration [6]. Hip pain alone is not a sufficient indicator for OA because the majority of people with hip complaints do not show clinical or radiological evidence of osteoarthrosis, and not all people with radiographically confirmed hip OA experience pain [7]. Several systems for scoring morphological changes in hip joints have been developed and used over time, and they are more or less comparable. However, there is no gold standard method of scoring the radiographic evidence of hip OA. The first standardized system was proposed by Kellgren and Lawrence (K&L-score) in 1957 [8]. Their criteria were later accepted as a diagnostic method by the World Health Organization [9]. Revisions have attempted to address questions about the validity of the original scoring system, mainly related to the relative importance of the presence of osteophytes for defining OA (K&L-score grade 2 and above). Some believe that osteophytes are a natural phenomenon of age-related bone and joint remodeling, and thus should not contribute to the diagnosis of pathology [10]. Others suggest that the presence of osteophytes is the most specific criterion leading to OA diagnosis, and are as sensitive a criterion as joint space narrowing, especially for hip OA [11]. At least 10 other radiographic scoring systems for hip OA have been developed since the early 1980s [12]. These systems address nearly the same radiographic features, but weight their relative importance differently. Because the majority of persons with radiographic evidence of hip OA are symptom-free, alternative case definitions have been proposed. For example, epidemiological studies may identify OA cases on the basis of radiological findings, symptoms, or both. The primary consideration should be to develop consistent and reproducible methods for identifying cases.

Clinical and epidemiological studies of hip OA have investigated factors that correlated with the occurrence of symmetric OA including genetic predisposition [13,14];arthritis of knee and finger joints, particularly in women [14–16]; malformations of hip, hip dysplasia or femoracetabular impingements [17]; demographic factors, such as race or gender [14,18]; systemic factors, such as obesity or metabolic disorders [14,18]; participation in certain sports, such as long distance running [19]; and occupational factors such as farming or heavy physical work load [18]. The peak incidence of hip OA is typically between ages 70 and 79 years [14]. Among women, the incidence rate per 100,000 person-years increases from approximately 50 in those aged 50–59 to approximately 600 in those aged 70–79; in men, incidence increases from approximately 30 in those aged 50–59 to approximately 430 per 100,000 person-years in those aged 70–79 [14]. Incidence and prevalence rates of hip OA vary across the world, but are generally high, and expected to increase due to demographic changes, in Western countries. The age standardized incidence rate for hip OA has been estimated as 53.3 per 100,000 for women and 38.1 per 100,000 for men in the defined WHO region EURO A of 26 European countries [20]. Prevalence rates for the same region were estimated at 577 per 100,000 for women and 413 per 100,000 for men. In Germany, about 8% of all orthopedic treatments and 2% of all early retirements were due to hip OA in 2002 [21].

The association between hip OA and heavy physical work load has reported consistently in the scientific literature, but the size of the effect estimates and the specific occupational activities reported to increase risk vary between studies. Eleven systematic reviews published between January 1999 and March 2010 evaluated the association between occupational activities and/or work load and the risk of hip OA (Tables S1 and S2). The evidence for an effect of long-term physical work load or strain on the risk of hip OA was generally characterized as moderate or strong [22–28], or described as showing a positive or consistent association [29–31]. However, D'Souza found the methodological limitations of the underlying studies substantial enough to characterize the relationship with work load as only "suggestive" [32]. Lifting was identified as a specific risk factor for hip OA by several authors, with a few also characterizing risk associated by weight and frequency [24–26,28,31]. Other occupational activities considered to be among the characteristics of physically demanding work that increase the risk of hip OA included stair climbing, kneeling, and walking [25,26,30]. Two authors, however, judged the evidence for these associations with hip OA to be weak, inconsistent, and/or inadequate to reach a conclusion [23,24,28]. The lack of quantitative exposure data and/or reliance on cross-sectional or case-control study designs were consistently identified as weaknesses in the existing literature. Additionally, the variability across studies in methods and results has made developing specific preventive measures difficult, because of the uncertainty about key risk factors.

In all literature reviews and syntheses, quality differences between the underlying studies may play an important role in determining the size of the estimated effect. For example, the author of at least one review noted that studies with low quality scores tended to report higher effect estimates than studies with higher quality scores [25]. Most previous reviews have been qualitative, focusing on the authors' judgment regarding the association between physical work load and hip OA, rather than providing quantitative exposure-response relationships. As a result, the findings of these reviews provide only limited guidance for the development of preventive measures to reduce the incidence of work-related hip OA. The current review was undertaken with the goal of identifying valid, quantitative estimates of exposure to occupational activities that might increase the risk of hip OA, in order to develop specific work-place recommendations to prevent future cases. The analysis emphasizes studies with high quality designs and quantitative exposure data. Based on this analysis, we assessed the extent to which the current body of literature can inform the development of preventive measures for hip OA and occupational exposures. Possible prevention measures are discussed, along with recommendations on aspects of exposure assessment, diagnostic criteria and specific needs for future research.

Methods

The authors identified studies from their personal libraries, and MEDLINE and EMBASE were searched to identify other studies of occupational work load and hip OA following previously recommended search strategies [33,34]. Additional searches for literature reviews were done in MEDLINE, EMBASE and the Cochrane Occupational Health Field [35]. The bibliographies of key articles and the reviews were also checked for pertinent references not identified previously. An example of the multipart search strategy implemented in MEDLINE is as follows:

a) Search (occupational diseases) OR (occupational risk)
b) Search lifting OR carrying
c) Search (hip joint endoprosthesis) OR (hip endoprosthesis) OR (hip joint prosthesis) OR (hip prosthesis) OR ("osteoarthritis, hip"[MeSH Terms] OR ("osteoarthritis"[All Fields] AND "hip"[All Fields]) OR "hip osteoarthritis"[All Fields] OR "coxarthroses"[All Fields])
d) Search ("osteoarthritis, hip"[MeSH Terms] OR ("osteoarthritis"[All Fields] AND "hip"[All fields"] OR "hip osteoarthritis"[All Fields] OR "coxarthrosis"[All Fields]) OR ("osteoarthritis, hip"[MeSH Terms] OR ("osteoarthritis"[All Fields] AND "hip"[All Fields]) OR "hip osteoarthritis"[All Fields] OR "coxarthroses"[All Fields])

combine b OR c OR d = e
combine e AND a
Limits: Humans

After excluding duplicates, 262 original studies were screened to identify: 1, primary research; 2, studies that used radiographic evidence or total hip replacement surgery to diagnosis hip OA; and 3, studies that provided quantitative occupational exposure estimates. Studies that used quantitative exposure estimates but less rigorous case definitions, semi-quantitative exposure characterization (e.g., low, medium and high), or qualitative estimates of exposure intensity (e.g., "much" standing) were considered lesser quality, but included for their potential to contribute to the weight of evidence (Figure 1).

The majority of the initial screening and categorization of studies was performed by one staff person. One epidemiologist (LC) reviewed a random, 10% sample of all articles identified through database searches and other sources to assess the accuracy of the initial quality assessment, and a further 10% of the articles excluded at initial screening or classified in one of the "questionable quality" categories were re-screened. Among all articles rescreened for quality assurance, only one was found to have been excluded instead of classified as "questionable quality"; this study was later excluded for focusing on prognosis instead of incidence of hip OA.

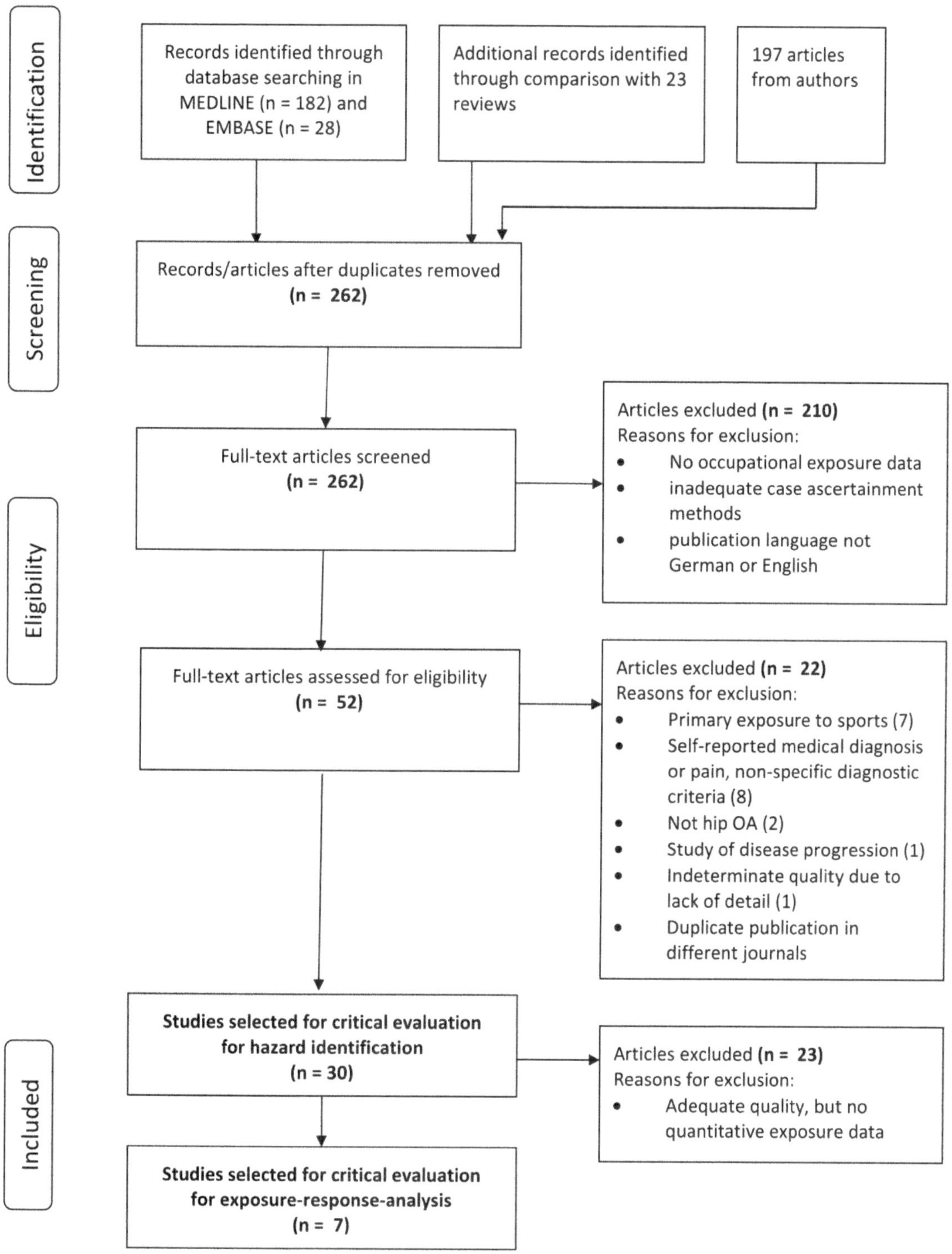

Figure 1. Flow diagram on identification of literature for critical evaluation.

Results

Fifty-two of the 262 studies met preliminary inclusion criteria (Figure 1). After full text review by two epidemiologists (SS and LC), we implemented the following additional exclusions:

- Exposures were related to recreational or professional sports activity [19,36–41];
- Cases were ascertained by self-reported prior hip OA diagnosis [42–45] or self-reported hip pain [46];
- Outcome was rheumatoid arthritis [47] or hand osteoarthritis [15], not hip OA;
- Outcome was progression from mild to severe hip OA, not development of hip OA [48];
- The data were duplicated in another publication [49–51];

- Joint spaces were measured, but criteria for diagnosing hip OA were not specified [52–54]; and
- Inadequate information was provided in the publication to allow a fair quality assessment [55].

We rated each of the 30 studies remaining for quality of their case ascertainment (Table 1) and exposure assessment methods (Table 2). Quality criteria and weighting of quality characteristics were developed and agreed upon prior to commencing the review (Table 3). The studies were divided between two epidemiologists (SS and LC) for quality assessment; a sample of studies was cross-reviewed to ensure agreement in quality assessments. Any discrepancies or questions were discussed until agreement was reached. The study attributes contributing the most weight to the quality assessments were: study design and methodology, likelihood of bias, and control for confounding (i.e., methodological threats to the validity of the reported findings). Characteristics most indicative of high quality study design included timing of exposure assessment (information gathered prior to onset of disease was considered more reliable); source and comparability of case and reference populations; and type of study, where cohort, case-control and cross-sectional designs were considered strongest to weakest, respectively. We judged the likelihood of selection bias, recall bias, and misclassification based on the description of the study methods, with special attention to the data collection methods and the sources and participation rates of case or exposed and reference populations. We looked specifically for information on the following potential confounders: age, gender, some measure of weight (e.g., body mass index, obesity), smoking, and non-occupational exposures. The clarity of the text describing study methods and results also factored in to our quality assessment, such that studies whose methods were unclear or that did not provide specific results received lower quality scores.

Summary quality assessments for all 30 studies are provided in Table S3. Details, including key elements of study design and specific results, are provided in Table S4 and discussed in the Appendix S1. After considering the exposure and outcome ascertainment scores and the study quality, six of the 30 studies were found to include quantitative exposure data. Of the 24 studies that could not be used for an exposure-response analysis:

- Four employed quantitative occupational exposure assessments, but used less rigorous case identification methods, were assessed as prohibitively low quality, or expressed exposures in non-generalizable (farming-specific) metrics;
- Seven employed semi-quantitative or qualitative estimates of exposure intensity with varying adequacy of case definition; and
- Thirteen employed only qualitative occupational exposure assessments with varying adequacy of case definition.

Results from these 24 studies nevertheless contribute to the weight of evidence regarding the presence/absence of an association between occupational physical demands and risk of hip OA. Nearly all of the studies reported higher prevalence of hip OA among the groups identified as exposed to higher levels of occupational physical activity or workload compared to others. Exceptions were Cvijectic et al. [56], Jacobsen et al. [53], and van Dijk et al. [57]. These authors did not detect statistically significant associations between risk of radiographically or clinically determined hip OA and either occupational work load or duration of exposure to work load categorized by level of intensity. Each of these studies was hampered by methodological problems, however, including potential information bias and misclassification of exposure and outcome. If in operation, any or all of these limitations would have reduced the magnitude of any true association between work load and hip OA, if one existed. Jacobsen et al. [53] was additionally difficult to interpret due to the authors' failure to report specific study results. Study details are provided in the Appendix S1 and Tables S3 and S4.

Cohort studies are generally considered the study design least prone to bias. Each of the five cohort studies included in this review [58–62] are briefly described, below, with more details provided in the Appendix S1 and Table S3 and S4. All five studies were limited by the authors' use of qualitative or semi-quantitative exposure metrics.

Flugsrud et al. (case ascertainment score: 3; exposure assessment score: 2) [58] matched exposure data from a large prospective cohort study with outcome data from a national THR registry to examine risk factors for hip OA in Norway. A total of 50,034 participants were eventually enrolled, including 672 participants who underwent a first THR for primary hip OA (cases). By using THR surgery to define cases, some participants with hip OA who had not undergone THR may be misclassified as non cases, potentially biasing risk estimates towards the null.

At baseline, participants classified their work during the past year as sedentary or requiring moderate, intermediate, or intensive physical activity. There were 6–12 years between baseline assessments and start of follow-up, and the average duration of follow-up was nine years. Analyses were performed using Cox proportional hazards regression, adjusting for age at screening, body mass index, sex, body weight, marital status, smoking status, and physical activity during leisure time. Compared to those with self-rated sedentary jobs, risk of THR for hip OA was higher for those in higher categories self-rated work intensity among both men and women. After adjusting for all variables described above,

Table 1. Definition of level of evidence for diagnostic evaluation of studies on osteoarthritis of the hip.

Diagnosis Criteria	Score*: Case ascertainment
Medical history/questionnaire: hip pain without clinical check	1
Hip pain and clinical reduction of movement without radiographic features or Radiographic features without clinical examination without THR	2
Hip pain with clinical reduction of movement and clearly defined radiographic features (joint space narrowing or K&L-score grade 2 and above or comparable criteria) or Diagnostic with indication for total hip replacement (THR)	3

*Score 1 = low quality; score 3 = high quality.

Table 2. Definition of quality for exposure assessment of studies on osteoarthritis of the hip (score 1–5).

Exposure Assessment	Score*: Exposure assessment
Profession, job title, classification of occupation	1
Qualitative specification of exposure in different work activities (lifting, climbing stairs, sitting)	2
Quantitative specification of exposure in different work activities/physical strains with information on intensity (e.g. load weight steps) and duration	3
Quantitative specification of exposure (as above) with additional plausibility check (e.g. information on daily work output or special controls through video analysis)	4
Direct measurement or biomechanical model calculation of hip joint strain	5

*Score 1 = low quality; score 5 = high quality.

the hazard ratio (HR) for men was 1.5 (95% CI: 1.0, 2.2) for moderate work, 1.7 (95% CI: 1.1, 2.4) for intermediate work, and 2.1 (95% CI: 1.5, 3.0) for intensive work compared to sedentary work. Compared to sedentary workers, women had HRs of 1.1 (95% 0.8, 1.6) for work in the moderate category, 1.4 (95% CI: 0.9, 2.0) for work in the intermediate category, and 2.1 (95% CI: 1.3, 3.3) for intensive work activity compared to sedentary work. Tests for trend were statistically significant for men ($p<0.0001$) and women ($p<0.0003$). In contrast, after controlling for all other variables, risk was not associated with higher categories of intensity of leisure activity for either men or women.

Jarvholm et al. (case ascertainment score: 3; exposure assessment score: 1) [59] collected data at multiple time points and recorded information on potential confounders (smoking habits, body weight and height), but categorized exposure only on the basis of job title from the first examination and did not report the results of any analyses that assessed or controlled for confounding. The cohort comprised Swedish men who received physical examinations every three to five years between 1971 and 1992. Hip OA incidence from 1987 to 1998 was determined through record linkage with the Swedish Hospital Discharge Register. Cases were defined as workers receiving surgical treatment for primary OA in the hip, with traumatic, secondary OA, or secondary hip replacement cases excluded. Relative risks for construction workers compared to white collar workers were estimated by Mantel-Haenszel statistics. After all exclusions were applied, the analytic cohort included 204,741 men, of whom 9,136 were considered to be white-collar workers. A total of 1,260 cases of hip OA were identified during the follow-up period. Relative risk estimates for hip OA by construction job title ranged from 0.77 to 1.58 when compared to white-collar workers, with none statistically significant. As with the Flugsrud et al. study, the use of THR surgery to define cases would bias risk estimates towards the null if the comparison group included men with hip OA that had not yet been surgically treated.

Table 3. Study attributes and their contribution to assessment of quality.

Study Attribute	Quality criteria
Study objectives	Clearly stated Relevant to research questions
Study methods	Adequately described Appropriate for objectives Minimize selection and information bias Reasonable statistical power
Outcome measurement	Well-defined, reasonably specific Accurate measurement or diagnosis Proper time frame for risk of outcome
Exposure measurement	Individual level, not group level data Direct quantitative measurements Accounts for changes over time
Control of confounding	Known risk factors considered and measured Reasonable analysis method(s) used (stratification, multivariate statistical models)

Between 1978 and 1980, Juhakoski et al. (case ascertainment score: 2; exposure assessment score: 2) [60] invited a representative sample of 8,000 Finns ages 30 and over, identified from population registers, to participate in the Mini-Finland Health Examination Survey. Ninety percent (7,217 subjects) completed baseline questionnaires, interviews, and laboratory and joint function tests. Those who reported experiencing hip pain leading to difficulty walking, squatting or climbing stairs were asked to attend a clinical examination. Study physicians diagnosed hip OA based on history of diagnoses and on clinical evidence. Between 2000 and 2001, subjects from the original sample were identified and invited to a follow-up examination (n = 1,286). Of the 909 agreeing to participate, 69 were excluded for having a hip OA diagnosis at baseline or withdrawing from the workforce, leaving a final study population of 840. This represents only 11.6% of the original 7,217 participants, an extremely low follow-up rate. Non-participants, including those not invited and those declining participation, were older, had fewer years of education, higher BMI, and were less likely to be in a sedentary occupation and to have reported regular leisure-time physical exercise at baseline compared to members of the final study population. All of these factors are potentially related to hip OA, and the differences by participation status indicate that selection bias may have affected the results. If so, the results could be biased in either direction.

Hip OA was diagnosed at the follow-up examination using the same clinical criteria as were used at baseline. Occupational exposures, self-reported at baseline, were classified into 6 groups: Group 1, light sedentary work; Group 2, other sedentary work but involving fairly heavy objects; Group 3, light standing work or light work involving movement; Group 4, fairly light or medium heavy work involving movement; Group 5, heavy manual work; and Group 6, very heavy manual work. Logistic regression was used to compare odds of definite or probable hip OA among exposure groups, adjusted for age, sex, years of education, BMI, smoking status, alcohol intake, leisure time physical activity, and history of injury. Compared to those with light sedentary work, odds of hip OA was statistically significantly higher in Group 4 workers (OR = 3.1, 95% CI: 1.2, 8.0) and Group 5 workers (OR = 6.7, 95% CI: 2.3, 19.5). Only 12 people were classified in

Group 6, and no hip OA cases were observed among them. Group 4 occupations were described as involving "a great deal of moving about and a fair amount of stooping down or carrying light objects, walking up and down the stairs or fairly rapid motion over rather long distances," and group 5 work involves "either mostly standing work involving much lifting of light objects or lifting and carrying heavy objects, drilling excavating, hammering, etc., but with some sitting or standing." Note that the categories combine multiple activities and do not offer any quantitative descriptions of weights lifted, distances walked, etc.

Thelin et al. (case ascertainment score: 2; exposure assessment score: 1) [61]) followed a cohort of 1,220 Swedish farmers, 1,130 non-farmer, but occupationally active, rural referents, and 1,087 urban referents from 1990 to 2003. Hip OA cases were determined through the Swedish national register of hospital care using ICD-9 and -10 diagnosis codes. Exposure information, apart from occupational category, was not collected. Hazard ratios for hip OA in farmers compared to both referent groups were calculated using Cox regression, with adjustment only for age. Farmers had three times the risk of hip OA (HR = 3.0, 95% CI: 1.7, 5.3) compared with the urban referent group; risks among the rural, non-farming group were similar to the urban referents (HR = 1.2, 95% CI: 0.8, 1.6).

Tuchsen et al. (case ascertainment score: 2; exposure assessment score: 1) [62]) used Danish national population and hospital registers to identify all employed men aged 20–59 years in 1981, 1986, 1991 and 1994. The men were followed for four years to identify first hospital admissions for hip OA, and standardized hospitalization rates (SHR) were calculated in a manner analogous to standardized mortality rates, using data for all employed men in Denmark. The SHR for hip OA was generally about twice as high as expected for farmers compared to the general population of Danish men, with some variability in the point estimates depending upon which occupational code was used to identify farmers. The lowest reported SHR was 114 (95% CI: 89, 147) for men "employed in agriculture and horticulture" in 1981–1985, and the highest was 286 (95% CI: 262 to 313) for "self employed farmers" in 1994–1999. The only exposure metric used in this study was occupational title, and no potential confounders were measured or assessed.

Thus, although these five cohort studies would be considered high quality based only on their design, they were each methodologically weak due to their choice of exposure metrics (job title or semi-quantitative categories) and/or the lack of control for confounding.

Two of the six studies that provided quantitative exposure data and met outcome ascertainment requirements were determined to be of low quality based on high likelihood for bias and confounding [63,64], and one study was internally inconsistent in its exposure estimation methods [65]. All three were, therefore, excluded from the quantitative exposure-response analysis; study details are provided in the Appendix S1, and in Tables S1 and S2. The remaining three studies were judged to be of reasonable epidemiological quality and met our *a priori* requirements for characterization of exposure and outcome; they are described in detail, below:

Croft 1992b (Case ascertainment score: 2; Exposure assessment score: 3) [66]

Croft, Cooper et al. performed a case-control study among men ages 60–75, identified from hospital x-ray registers as having undergone an outpatient urogram between 1982 and 1987, most often for prostate symptoms. Men who had a THR for hip OA or had JS ≤2.5 mm were identified as cases. A subset of "severe" cases included those with a THR for hip OA or JS ≤1.5 mm in at least one hip. Controls were those men identified by urogram review of having a JS ≥3.5 mm in both hips and no other radiographic indication of hip OA. The proportion of the cases identified by THR, and the JSN information for these cases, is not reported. While it seems unlikely that a THR for hip OA would occur without severe joint space narrowing, it is not clear from the methods whether cases identified by THR also met the minimal joint space criteria.

Lifetime occupational histories were determined through blinded interview, and then coded according to the 1970 Office of Population Censuses and Survey classification. Exposure levels were determined by length of time spent in specific work activities. Cases and controls had similar participation rates (69% and 68%, respectively), and a total of 245 (53 severe) cases and 294 controls completed interviews.

Associations between hip OA and duration of exposure to various work activities were examined using logistic regression, adjusting for age group and hospital. Height and weight, although measured at the time of interview, were not controlled in the analyses. Risk of severe hip OA in this study was found to be higher for those with the highest BMI, but the association was not statistically significant (OR for hip OA comparing highest vs. lowest tertiles of BMI was 1.6, 95% CI: 0.7, 3.4). Nevertheless, an analysis of the potential for confounding by height and weight was warranted, and the omission of control for these variables may affect the magnitude of the reported risk estimates.

Hip OA was evaluated for its association with each of the following occupational activities: sitting, standing, or bending for >2 hours/day; kneeling or squatting for >30 minutes/day; walking or walking over rough ground for >2 miles/day; running for >1 hour/day; climbing ladders; climbing >30 flights of stairs/day; manually lifting or moving weights >56 lbs; and driving for >4 hours/day. In analyses including all cases (JS ≤2.5 mm), no clear patterns emerged with any occupational activities and the only statistically significant association with hip OA was among men with 20 or more years' exposure to jobs requiring standing for >2 hrs per day, among whom odds of hip OA were nearly doubled compared to men not required to stand at work. A positive association was also reported between odds of severe hip OA (JS ≤1.5 mm) and the number of years in a job requiring standing for >2 hours/day. Compared to those with <20 years of standing >2 hours/day, the OR for severe hip OA was 1.5 (95% CI: 0.5, 4.8) for those with 20–39 years of exposure and 2.7 (95% CI: 1.0, 7.3) for those with 40+ years exposure.

Time spent in jobs requiring manual lifting or moving weights >56 lbs was also positively associated with odds of hip OA: compared to those with <1 year of exposure, odds were higher for men with 1–19 years (OR = 1.2, 95% CI: 0.5, 2.9) and ≥20 years (OR = 2.5, 95% CI: 1.1, 5.7) of this type of work. Other activities were generally associated with higher odds of severe hip OA comparing those with longer vs. shorter duration of exposure, but the trends were not consistent, results were not statistically significant and the magnitude of the associations was small, with ORs not exceeding 2. After adjustment for combined exposure to standing, walking, walking over rough ground, heavy lifting, participation in sports activities and BMI, the odds of severe hip OA was doubled (OR = 2.1, 95% CI: 0.7, 6.6) and odds were 60% higher (OR = 1.6, 95% CI: 0.5, 5.1) among men with more than 20 years' exposure to heavy lifting and more than 40 years' exposure to standing >2 hrs/day, compared to men <20 years exposure to heavy lifting and <50 years exposure to standing >2 hrs/day, respectively.

The main strength of this study was its use of urograms from local hospital registries to identify cases and controls, minimizing misclassification and ensuring that subjects were drawn from the same population pool. The similar participation rates for cases and controls also suggested that selection bias was unlikely. However, the extent and type of illness in the controls is not described, beyond the statement that most urograms were performed due to prostate symptoms. This study is considered to be of good methodological quality, and it provides data that potentially could be useful for a quantitative exposure-response analysis.

Roach 1994 (Case ascertainment score: 3; Exposure assessment score: 3) [67]

In a case-control study of US Military Veterans attending a Veteran's outpatient clinic to obtain hip radiographs for diagnosis of hip pain or as follow up for THR, Roach et al. identified 212 cases of hip OA based on either Kellgren or Croft grade 3 or 4. Four hundred eighty-one men from the same clinic with outpatient IV pyelogram x-ray films on file that allowed for visualization of the hip joint were identified as controls, if measured JS>1.5 mm. All participants responded to self-administered questionnaires to identify those with >15 years employment in jobs with activities requiring heavy or light lifting, defined on the basis of specific work activities whose forces on the hip joint were estimated in mathematical models. Compression forces of more than twice body weight were considered "heavy", and compression forces of less than body weight were considered "light". All others were classified as "intermediate", and excluded from analysis. After adjusting for prior cancer diagnosis (mostly bladder and prostate), obesity at age 40 and history of running for exercise, men who had been exposed to heavy work for at least 15 years had 2.5 times higher odds of hip OA than men with light work (95% CI: 1.5, 5.0), and this association was statistically significant.

This study was considered to be of good quality. Its strengths included internal validity stemming from the objective identification of both cases and controls from the same patient population; the methods used to estimate work load were substantiated from prior research; and the questionnaire was carefully designed to identify the critical elements of work history needed for the estimation of work load. The main limitations of this study were as follows:

- Its reliance on long-term recall of work history may have introduced recall bias, if the cases with hip OA were more likely to accurately report or to over-report the work load they experienced in the past. If recall bias played a role in this study, the association between prior work load and hip OA would have been exaggerated.
- Some of the men with heavy work load may have been misclassified as having had intermediate exposures. Because the intermediate exposure group was excluded, the only effect would have been to reduce the statistical power of the analysis to detect differences between groups.
- The study sample design led to its inability to assess tobacco smoking as a potential modifier of the effect of work load. Although data on smoking history were collected, the study was designed such that controls were more likely to have had a cancer diagnosis than cases. Because smoking is a risk factor for the types of cancer most commonly diagnosed among the controls, the controls were also more likely to have been smokers than the cases. Statistical control for confounding by both factors was thus necessary.

The authors categorized work load using different, incompatible mathematical models to estimate the compression forces conferred by various activities. They did not distinguish between quasi-static (average force) and dynamic peak forces.

Vingard 1997b (Case ascertainment score: 3; Exposure assessment score: 3) [68]

This is a high-quality case-control study of women aged 50–70 years, residing in one of 5 counties in Sweden between 1991 and 1994. Cases of primary hip OA (n = 242) were identified from the Swedish national THR register, with diagnosis performed according to a standardized protocol including clinical and radiographic examinations. Women with other forms of arthritis and/or a history of leg injury, thought to be a risk factor for development of hip OA, were excluded. Controls (n = 298) were recruited from population registers covering the same regions in which the cases resided, and were matched on age (within one year) at the time of the survey. Surgery had taken place an average of 4.5 years (range: 0, 13) prior to participation. Potential controls with hip disorders were excluded.

Structured, in-person interviews were conducted with each woman to determine health and medication status and history, number of children, height and weight, and occupational and non-occupational physical activity history from age 16 until age 50. Categories of activities including hours spent sitting and standing, numbers of flights of stairs climbed, number of jumps, and number of heavy lifts were divided into categories of low (i.e., lowest 25%), medium (i.e., 25% to 75%) and high (75% to 100%) based on the distribution observed among controls. Information was collected and categorized separately on sports activities.

After adjustment for age, body mass index, use of cigarettes, past sports activities, number of children, and hormone therapy, high exposure to each of the work activities except for number of hours per day spent sitting was associated with higher odds of hip OA, with ORs between 1.5 and 2.1. High exposure to non-occupational physical activity was associated with a two-fold higher odds of hip OA (OR = 2.3, 95% CI: 1.5, 3.6), and sports activity increased the odds of hip OA when cross-classified by levels of occupational activity.

Strengths of this study included: its focus on exposures occurring prior to the surgery for cases (i.e., attention to temporal ordering of exposure and outcome); careful questionnaire design to identify activities contributing to physical load on the hip during periods of similar activity intensity; separate ascertainment of work and non-work activities; assessment and control of confounding, including tobacco use, hormone therapy, and BMI at age 40; and use of an enumerated population to develop the study population, minimizing selection bias and allowing for risk estimation. Selection bias is also minimized by the high and relatively similar participation rates reported for the cases (90%) and controls (82%).

The primary limitations of the study stem from its reliance on exposures recalled from the distant past (30–40 years prior) and the resulting possibility of potentially differential misclassification due to recall bias. For example, recall of recent activity levels may contaminate recall of activities from years ago. If this occurred, women with hip OA may have under-reported their past activity levels, because they would be less likely to have remained physically active compared to women without arthritis or knee problems. If this occurred, the magnitude of the observed associations would be attenuated.

When we compared exposure metrics across the three studies, we found that the use of biomechanical models and exposure measures differed so greatly that the data could not be combined. The individual quantitative results of the three studies are

Table 4. Standing, Sitting and Stair Climbing results from three studies eligible for exposure response analysis.

Author, year	Odds ratio (95% confidence interval)	Exposure categories
Published results		
Standing		
Vingard, 1997b	1.0 (referent)	<22,792 hours
	1.4 (0.8, 2.2)	22,793–51,546 hours
	1.6 (0.9, 2.8)	51,547–67,760 hours
Croft, 1992	1.0 (referent)	<20 years
	1.5 (0.5, 4.8)	20–39 years
	2.7 (1.0, 7.3)	≥40 years
Roach, 1994	1.0 (referent)	<15 years (mean 2.2 years)
	2.2	15–24 years (mean 19.8 years)
	3.0	25–34 years (mean 28.9 years)
	2.2	>34 years (mean 41.2 years)
Sitting		
Vingard, 1997b	1.0 (referent)	<13,563 hours
	0.8 (0.5, 1.2)	13,564–35,816 hours
	0.8 (0.4, 1.3)	35,817–65,384 hours
Croft, 1992	1.0 (referent)	<1 year
	1.0 (0.4, 2.2)	1–19 years
	0.8 (0.3, 1.7)	≥20 years

Table 5. Heavy lifting results from three studies eligible for exposure response analysis.

Heavy lifts		
Vingard, 1997b	1.0 (referent)	<20,328 lifts
	1.1 (0.7, 1.7)	20,329–44,088 lifts
	1.5 (0.9, 2.5)	44,089–95,040 lifts
Croft, 1992	1.0 (referent)	<1 year
	1.2 (0.5, 2.9)	1–19 years
	2.5 (1.1, 5.7)*	≥20 years
Roach, 1994	1.0 (referent)	<15 years (mean 2.2 years)
	2.2	15–24 years (mean 19.8 years)
	3.0	25–34 years (mean 28.9 years)
	2.2	>34 years (mean 41.2 years)
Stair climbing		
Vingard, 1997b	1.0 (referent)	<64,680 flights
	1.3 (0.8, 2.0)	64,681–564,960 flights
	2.1 (1.2, 3.6)*	564,961–3,353,400 flights
Croft, 1992	1.0 (referent)	<1 year
	1.2 (0.6, 2.5)	≥1 year

*Results are statistically significant at alpha level of 0.05.

summarized in Tables 4 and 5. Overall, the data suggest risk of hip OA may increase with long term exposures to standing and heavy lifting at work, but the risk is not high and there is a large amount of variability in the results. There is some indication that long term occupational exposure to stair climbing may increase risk of hip OA, but results are inconsistent. Sitting at work does not appear to be associated with risk of hip OA based on these data.

Discussion

The objective of this review was to determine whether the existing body of literature on work load and hip OA is sufficient for developing preventive exposure guidelines. Studies were first evaluated on exposure characterization, outcome definition, and methodological quality, and only studies meeting requirements for exposure and outcome definitions and determined to be of adequate epidemiological quality were compared on results and conclusions.

An assessment of study quality depends on the authors including a detailed description of methods. If the methods were not sufficiently described in an article selected for review, a study that might otherwise have been considered high quality would have been excluded. It should be noted that the evaluation of the studies in this review was performed with the objective of providing valid evidence in guiding the development of measures to prevent work-related hip OA, and this objective influenced our quality assessments.

Six studies were identified as meeting exposure characterization, outcome definition, and three of the six were of good epidemiological quality. Despite differences in study design and methods, and potential for biases and heterogeneity, the six studies were consistent in their results suggesting increasing exposure-response trends with increasing duration [63,66] or intensity [64,67,68] of heavy lifting or heavy work load. The majority of the published reviews addressing the association between heavy work load and risk of hip OA also concluded there is positive and consistent evidence for a causal association [22–31]. Several reviews attempted to characterize the exposure-response relationship between heavy lifting and hip OA, and concluded that long-term, frequent lifting of 10–25 kg loads increased risk [24,25,28]. Results were mixed for other frequently evaluated occupational risk factors for work load and hip OA, especially sitting, standing, stair climbing and walking.

Potential biases

Studies in the English or German languages were selected for review, which may have introduced some bias if high quality, quantitative data that failed to show an association between work load and risk of hip OA were available in other languages, but inappropriately excluded. Eight studies in languages other than German or English (specifically: Dutch, Italian, French, Swedish and Danish) were identified in preliminary searches, but not included in this review.

Any literature review is subject to publication bias. We did not attempt to identify or obtain unpublished data, as peer review was a preliminary and *a priori* criterion for inclusion. Several of the papers discussed in this review reported null findings, however, suggesting that bias towards publishing only positive findings was at least not universal.

All of the six key studies with quantitative exposure data used the case-control design, which is more susceptible than prospective studies to recall and selection biases. Specifically, several may have misclassified participants' exposures or outcomes, and we identified those with the potential for uncontrolled confounding in the preceding summaries and the Appendix S1. Although the five available cohort studies were less prone to bias due to their design, these studies also were limited by methodological weaknesses including selection and information biases, misclassification of exposure or outcome, and use of non-quantitative exposure measures.

Exposures based on self-reported work history through questionnaire or interview can be strongly affected by recall ability, especially when data are collected on exposures experienced over decades of work [69–71]. For example, Coggon (1998) included people up to 91 years of age and characterized physical work load experienced anywhere from 24 to 70 years prior to the interview [63]. Depending on the wording of interview or questionnaire items, it can be extremely difficult for respondents to provide reliable and complete quantitative information on timing, duration, frequency and intensity of specific work activities. In addition, those diagnosed with a condition suspected of being related to physically demanding work may more accurately remember or over-estimate historical work activity compared to individuals without such conditions, as they may have actively reflected on potential causes after learning of their diagnosis or beginning to experience symptoms. Such recall bias was likely in several of the included studies in which participants were asked to characterize occupational exposures from a time years to decades prior to the interview [63,64,66–68].

Because radiographically confirmed hip OA does not always produce symptoms, misclassification of outcome may have occurred in studies that failed to verify that the nominal control group was free from hip OA. In addition, the studies that identified hip OA cases from THR registries or waiting lists may have excluded mild or moderate hip OA cases [63,64,68,72]. Misclassification of outcome could artificially reduce the risk estimates either if non-cases were mis-categorized as cases or if cases were mis-categorized as non-cases, but would not introduce bias if it occurred more or less equally across exposure groups.

Selection bias was minimized in several studies by appropriately selecting cases and controls from same source population [66–68]. However, differential participation rates by cases and controls in one study (Coggon 1998) [63] indicated selection bias was likely to have occurred. Selection bias and uncontrolled confounding may affect the results of a study in either direction.

All of the key studies controlled for potential confounding by age and sex, either through restriction of the study population, matching, or statistical adjustment. Other risk factors identified in studies of hip OA include BMI or obesity [25], smoking [73], and leisure-time activity [27]. Previous joint trauma, joint deformity, and certain disorders, such as dysplasia, may increase risk of OA in the affected joint [18]. Participation in certain sports may also increase risk of hip OA [18]. Four of the six studies with quantitative exposure data controlled for BMI or obesity [63,65,67,68], while the remaining two studies investigated differences in BMI, but did not control for it in their analyses [64,66]. Five studies controlled for or considered some measure of non-occupational physical activity or sports participation [64–68], and two controlled for smoking [65,68]. All studies excluded or adjusted for some combination of previous joint trauma, malformations, or history of a disorder that may increase risk of OA [63–68].

Heterogeneity

Common sources of heterogeneity between research studies, in general, include differences in study methods, distribution of risks in the source populations, and inclusion and exclusion criteria. Heterogeneity was prevalent in the studies included in this review. Some evaluated very specific populations, such as farmers [61,74], construction workers [59] or ballet dancers [57], while others included mixed populations. The ages included also varied considerably (e.g. 20 to 59 years [62], 20 to 80 years [75] or 65 to 75 years [66]), and this contributed to lack of comparability across study results. Use of different case definitions, exposure classification methods, and time periods of exposure relative to diagnosis also may have affected the comparability of results across studies:

- When cases are identified from THR registries or waiting lists [63–65,68], disease may be more severe than when cases are identified radiologically [66,67]. Eligibility criteria for THR may differ by location, so heterogeneity may be present even when studies identify cases from the same types of sources. Participants with less severe hip OA may be misclassified as non-cases, potentially reducing the magnitude of associations.
- All six studies with quantitative exposure data relied on self-reported occupational history to determine exposure status, but they used different methods to classify exposures. For example, Croft [66] coded lifetime occupational history to a standard classification system, while Coggon [63] recorded work history only for jobs held longer than one year. The time period of exposure relative to the onset of hip OA varied across studies. Coggon [63] collected work history only up to age 30 or up to 10 years prior to study entry, while relevant occupational history for women participating in Vingard [68] covered time intervals anywhere from 0–20 years prior to study entry.

Diagnostic criteria, methods

The diagnostic criteria described in this body of literature included versions with and without radiological imaging data, and some investigators identified cases based on pending or performed joint replacement therapy (THR), clinical findings or previous medical diagnosis. In a series of 227 Dutch patients, Bierma-Zeinstra et al. [76] found that agreement was poor between methods using only clinical findings and those combining clinical and radiological diagnostic methods (kappa 0,11), but high between two sets of criteria that both included radiological assessment (either smallest joint spaces or Kellgren scores). Regardless, a valid diagnosis considering the level of morphological damage can only be expected if radiological criteria were part of case ascertainment. All six of the studies with quantitative exposure data also used objective imaging criteria for diagnosing cases, and all except Roach [67] identified potential cases from THR registries. Nevertheless, there may be subtle differences in the severity of the cases included in each study, because the indication for THR may not be consistently defined or applied.

Exposure assessment

In spite of the consistent, positive association between risk of hip OA and heavy lifting, variability across studies in exposure assessment methods and data collected contributed uncertainty to the conclusions that can be drawn from this literature review, as well as uncertainty in developing preventive measures. For example, exposures were assessed using simple yes/no questions [75], job titles (e.g., job at first medical examination) [59], longest held occupation [75], and comprehensive interviews on physical loads [63]) as well as combinations of these methods. Only six of 30 studies reviewed provided quantitative exposure data, and only three studies provided quantitative estimates of lifted weights that were similar enough to be combined. Unfortunately, the data required substantial manipulation and application of assumptions before they were similar enough to be combined; although we provide quantitative exposure-response estimates, these should be considered rough indicators of the risk of hip OA associated with lifting. No other exposure was reported in quantitative terms that could be combined, so it should not be assumed that lifting is the only occupational risk factor associated with a graded risk of hip OA.

The following sections provide a more specific evaluation of the various exposure assessment methods encountered in this body of literature, and discusses their utility for developing preventive guidelines.

Simple exposure parameters – levels 1 and 2. Studies that used qualitative or semi-quantitative exposure assessments (levels 1 and 2), i.e., job titles and time in those jobs (e. g. Lindberg and Danielsson 1984, Thelin 1990, Chitnavis 2000, Rossignol et al. 2003, Thelin and Holmberg 2007, Jarvholm et al. 2008 [2,59,61,77–79]) do not provide sufficient information to support development of recommendations for preventive measures. This is because of variability in the actual exposures associated with any given job title or profession: each includes a range of different jobs and tasks, so conclusions about the specific work activities that increase risk cannot be reached.

Complex exposure parameters – level 3. The assessment of frequency and duration of specific work activities can be used to develop preventive guidelines, if they can be linked to a quantitative estimate of physical strain. Simple identification of job tasks, not modified by intensity levels (e.g., walking, standing or sitting) allows a rough quantitative estimate of exposure that depends only on duration. More detailed estimates of risk can be developed by including the time spent in specific work activities and repetitiveness of tasks per time unit during the work day or week. More complex jobs, like lifting and carrying of loads, require more detailed data to adequately assess risk. Ideally, exposure assessments should include, for example, the weight of the load, the distance carried and/or the height lifted, and the frequency and intensity of exposure to the task.

Although six studies captured quantitative exposure data in at least some detail, variability and uncertainty in the estimated exposures remains. For example, Jacobsen et al. [53] assigned daily lifting operations of 50×20 kg and 20×50 kg as equivalent, assuming that intensity and frequency confer equal stress on hip joints; hence a reduction of the weight per load only reduces stress if the frequency of loads does not in turn increase. Other authors also used categories that considered both weight and frequency [63,64,66,80]. While quantitative exposure assessments such as these are more useful than qualitative or semi-quantitative exposure metrics, it is still necessary to be cautious in comparing and interpreting exposures across studies. Specifically, when authors report quantitative exposure estimates as cumulative exposure time, there is a high likelihood of misclassification due to grouping study participants with long duration, low exposure and short duration, high intensity exposure. This will lower the chances of identifying an association between work tasks and risk of hip OA, if one exists. Exposure metrics that account for both intensity and frequency of effort are better, but are still subject to misclassification if grouped into categories that are too wide for either frequency or intensity, or if any of the categories are open-ended. Finally, no individual-level exposure measurements were completed for these studies, nor would individual measurements be practical for large-scale epidemiological assessments of work load. Thus, even the most apparently objective exposure metrics only provide graded estimates of exposure. If such metrics are used to estimate an average intensity or frequency of exposure in a given time frame, it is necessary to apply stringent assumptions that might not be valid.

Self-reported exposures are more practical for epidemiological studies, and they may be at least partially validated by conducting plausibility checks, for example, by comparing recalled exposures to daily work output diaries or quantitative exposure databases. Overall, there is a need for objective assessment of specific occupational exposures that are not subject to recall and reporting issues [81], that are accurate and detailed, and that are capable of characterizing hip joint strain from load-bearing activities. Besides the demand for objective exposure assessment, identified occupational risk factors for hip OA should be examined for their biological plausibility, i.e. it should be determined whether or not there is an identifiable mechanism for hip joint damage associated with each job task that appears to increase the risk of hip OA. An exposure-response analysis that fulfils these validation and plausibility requirements can provide the evidence needed to develop specific prevention strategies that include occupational exposure limits.

Hazard, exposure-response characterization. Profound differences in the procedures for assessment and quantification of exposures in the best currently available studies make it impossible to pool data across studies, or to clearly characterize the type and levels of work load that increase risk for development of hip OA. The pattern of increasing risk of hip OA associated with heavy lifting is consistent with the conclusions summarized in the other systematic reviews, several of which attempted to quantify the exposure-response relationship between heavy lifting and hip OA. These concluded that long-term, frequent lifting of 10–25 kg loads was sufficient to increase risk [24,25,28]. Only one review has individually considered exposure to stair climbing and risk of hip OA; it concluded there was insufficient evidence for a causal association [24,28]. No reviews concluded there is a specific risk of hip OA associated with standing or sitting exposures.

In summary, the only type of physical work load that has been quantified and for which there is adequate and consistent evidence of an association with osteoarthritis of the hip is heavy lifting over a long time period. While it seems to be unlikely that weights below 10 kg have any relevant effect on hip OA, it remains to be established the level at which cumulative long-term heavy lifting exposure does indeed lead to an increased risk. We concur with the conclusions presented in previous systematic reviews: the lack of quantitative exposure data and/or reliance on cross-sectional or case-control study designs is a weakness of the existing evidence base. The studies reviewed here generally are limited by a lack of objective exposure assessment.

Conclusions

This review attempted to identify occupational risk factors for hip OA, which are generally difficult to measure and usually have no gold standard for assessment. Despite variability across studies in their methods, populations, exposure and outcome definitions and measures, there is consistent evidence that extended exposure to heavy physical work load can increase the risk for osteoarthritis of the hip. The studies that provided quantitative exposure data consistently reported positive, graded associations between development of hip OA and occupational tasks or jobs requiring lifting and possibly standing. The association between hip OA and stair climbing or jumping was not clear, and there appeared to be no association between hip OA and sitting or walking on the job. Even taking into account clear problems in exposure assessment as discussed above, the consistent 2 to 3 fold increased risk for osteoarthritis of the hip in those participant groups with the highest physical work load suggests some association which cannot be fully explained by bias or confounding. Thus, we would conclude that very high physical work load is likely to be an independent risk factor for osteoarthritis of the hip, although the available data do not allow this to be defined. There is some indication of an exposure-response relationship, but quantification of this relationship is not possible based on the current body of literature.

Options for prevention

The inability to determine a threshold value for physical work load limits the development of specific preventive approaches. General recommendations for guidelines to help prevent hip OA can be developed from these data, as follows:

- Job activities with high physical work load should be minimized to the extent possible.
- Training and guidelines for appropriate ergonomic approaches to materials handling and other work activities should be made available and implemented.
- In workplaces where jobs require exposure to high work load, companies should promote preventive health measures for workers. Programs should focus on limiting exposure to extended standing etc. as well as providing physical training to prevent musculoskeletal diseases.
- Better work organisation may reduce unnecessary physical work load.
- Older employees and employees with hip disorders, hip deformity, former injuries or known intrinsic risks for THR should not be exposed to high physical work load.
- Tasks related to agricultural work should be specifically evaluated to identify the components that increase stresses on the hip joint.

Recommendations for further research

Several gaps in the existing body of literature on occupational work load and hip OA have been identified that limit the ability of current research to inform detailed preventive measures. Future research could improve upon aspects of exposure assessment, diagnosis definition, and study design as follows:

Exposure assessment

- To facilitate objective assessment of physical work load exposures, industry-specific job-exposure-matrices should be developed based on objective measurements, homogenous exposure groups, and biomechanical models that are valid and reproducible. The matrices could be established using measurement data from work shift monitoring in combination with laboratory studies on task specific hip joint loading.
- Studies on occupational physical work load (e.g. lifting and carrying) should measure not only the level of exposure but also the frequency and duration of the exposure, with attention paid to heterogeneous activity demands within and between job titles.
- If questionnaires are used to collect exposure information, data should be obtained by a trained interviewer. Measures of plausibility should be introduced to detect under- and overestimations of exposure, and to assess the probability of recall bias. Questionnaire data should validated, to the extent possible, against objective measurements [82] or exposure databases.
- If physical work loads are expressed in terms of compressive joint forces or joint moments, static (-mean) levels and dynamic peaks must be distinguished.
- High occupational physical work load does not necessarily implicate high physical loading of the hip joint. Thus, consistent biomechanical models for assessing the loads on the hip joints with respect to the different occupational tasks have to be developed and applied.

Diagnosis

- The diagnosis of hip OA should always include clearly defined radiological features (osteophytes, joint space narrowing or K&L-score grade 2 and above). Consideration of alternative diagnostic criteria, e.g., those described by Altmann 1991 [6], is also recommended.
- Different clinical patterns of hip OA (unilateral, bilateral or generalized form with multi-joint involvement) and their relationship with physical work load should be clarified.

Study design. Hip OA is a chronic, insidious disease that tends to develop slowly over an extended period of time. The precise timing of disease onset is often unknown, and incidence can be difficult to accurately measure. These characteristics present challenges in designing epidemiological studies to study risk factors for hip OA, and are especially prohibitive for prospective cohort studies. To balance cost-effectiveness and study quality, use of the nested case-control design is recommended for future studies, in which cases and controls can be identified within a well-documented baseline population (such as a medical insurance population). In addition to work related exposures, the data on additional risk factors for OA should be collected and evaluated: age; sex; body mass index or weight; previous joint diseases (including congenital diseases like hip dysplasia or femoracetabular impingements) and injuries; OA of other joint groups; and sport and other non-occupational activities that may increase risk of hip OA.

Supporting Information

Table S1 Main conclusions of systematic reviews of hip OA and occupational factors, and supporting studies.

Table S2 Studies considered highest quality in reviews that also characterized heavy lifting exposures.

Table S3 Summary of quality assessment: Thirty occupational epidemiological papers discussing osteoarthritis of the hip, with best quality papers indicated in bold face type.

Table S4 Study Details.

Appendix S1 Studies contributing to hazard identification.

Author Contributions

Conceived and designed the experiments: SS LC FB RE UG BH DP DS YS. Performed the experiments: SS LC FB RE UG BH DP DS YS. Analyzed the data: SS LC FB RE UG BH DP DS YS. Contributed reagents/materials/analysis tools: SS LC FB RE UG BH DP DS YS. Wrote the paper: SS LC FB RE UG BH DP DS YS.

References

1. Sun Y, Brenner H, Sauerland S, Gunther KP, Puhl W, et al. (2000) Serum uric acid and patterns of radiographic osteoarthritis–the Ulm Osteoarthritis Study. Scand J Rheumatol 29: 380–386.
2. Rossignol M, Leclerc A, Hilliquin P, Allaert FA, Rozenberg S, et al. (2003) Primary osteoarthritis and occupations: a national cross sectional survey of 10 412 symptomatic patients. Occup Environ Med 60: 882–886.
3. Badley EM (1995) The effect of osteoarthritis on disability and health care use in Canada. J Rheumatol 22: 19–22.
4. Felson DT (1988) Epidemiology of hip and knee osteoarthritis. Epidemiol Rev 10: 1–28.
5. Sun Y, Sturmer T, Gunther KP, Brenner H (1997) Incidence and prevalence of cox- and gonarthrosis in the general population. Z Orthop Ihre Grenzgeb 135: 184–192.
6. Altman R, Alarcon G, Appelrouth D, Bloch D, Borenstein D, et al. (1991) The American College of Rheumatology criteria for the classification and reporting of osteoarthritis of the hip. Arthritis Rheum 34: 505–514.
7. Odding E, Valkenburg HA, Algra D, Vandenouweland FA, Grobbee DE, et al. (1998) Associations of radiological osteoarthritis of the hip and knee with locomotor disability in the Rotterdam Study. Ann Rheum Dis 57: 203–208.
8. Kellgren JH, Lawrence JS (1957) Radiological assessment of osteo-arthrosis. Ann Rheum Dis 16: 494–502.
9. WHO (1993) The epidemiology of chronic rheumatism, Atlas of standard radiographs of arthritis. Oxford: Blackwell Scientific.
10. Spector TD, Hochberg MC (1994) Methodological problems in the epidemiological study of osteoarthritis. Ann Rheum Dis 53: 143–146.
11. Croft P, Cooper C, Coggon D (1994) Case definition of hip osteoarthritis in epidemiologic studies. J Rheumatol 21: 591–592.
12. Sun Y, Gunther KP, Brenner H (1997) Reliability of radiographic grading of osteoarthritis of the hip and knee. Scand J Rheumatol 26: 155–165.
13. Riyazi N, Rosendaal FR, Slagboom E, Kroon HM, Breedveld FC, et al. (2008) Risk factors in familial osteoarthritis: the GARP sibling study. Osteoarthritis and Cartilage 16: 654–659. doi: DOI: 10.1016/j.joca.2007.10.012.
14. Zhang Y, Jordan JM (2008) Epidemiology of osteoarthritis. Rheum Dis Clin North Am 34: 515–529.
15. Dahaghin S, Bierma-Zeinstra SM, Reijman M, Pols HA, Hazes JM, et al. (2005) Does hand osteoarthritis predict future hip or knee osteoarthritis? Arthritis Rheum 52: 3520–3527.
16. Gunther KP, Sturmer T, Sauerland S, Zeissig I, Sun Y, et al. (1998) Prevalence of generalised osteoarthritis in patients with advanced hip and knee osteoarthritis: the Ulm Osteoarthritis Study. Ann Rheum Dis 57: 717–723.
17. Heliovaara M, Makela M, Impivaara O, Knekt P, Aromaa A, Sievers K (1993) Association of overweight, trauma and workload with coxarthrosis. A health survey of 7,217 persons. Acta Orthop Scand 64: 513–518.
18. Felson DT, Lawrence RC, Dieppe PA, Hirsch R, Helmick CG, et al. (2000) Osteoarthritis: new insights. Part 1: the disease and its risk factors. Ann Intern Med 133: 635–646. 200010170-00016 [pii].
19. Kujala UM, Kaprio J, Sarna S (1994) Osteoarthritis of weight beraring jointsof lower limbs in former elite male athletes. BMJ 308: 308–234; 819.
20. Symmons D, Mathers C, Pfleger B (2006) Global Burden of Osteoarthritis in the Year 2000. In: Global Burden of Diseases 2000 WHO.
21. Merx H, Dreinhofer KE, Gunther KP (2007) [Socioeconomic relevance of osteoarthritis in Germany]. Z Orthop Unfall 145: 421–429.
22. Bierma-Zeinstra SM, Koes BW (2007) Risk factors and prognostic factors of hip and knee osteoarthritis. Nat Clin Pract Rheumatol 3: 78–85.
23. da Costa BR, Vieira ER (2010) Risk factors for work-related musculoskeletal disorders: A systematic review of recent longitudinal studies. Am J Ind Med 53: 285–323.
24. Jensen LK (2008) Hip osteoarthritis: influence of work with heavy lifting, climbing stairs or ladders, or combining kneeling/squatting with heavy lifting. Occup Environ Med 65: 6–19.
25. Lievense A, Bierma-Zeinstra S, Verhagen A, Verhaar J, Koes B (2001) Influence of work on the development of osteoarthritis of the hip: a systematic review. J Rheumatol 28: 2520–2528.
26. Aluoch MA, Wao HO (2009) Risk factors for occupational osteoarthritis: a literature review. AAOHN J 57: 283–290.
27. Vignon E, Valat JP, Rossignol M, Avouac B, Rozenberg S, et al. (2006) Osteoarthritis of the knee and hip and activity: a systematic international review and synthesis (OASIS). Joint Bone Spine 73: 442–455.
28. Jensen LK (2006) Osteoarthritis in the hip and knee. Influence of work with heavy lifting, climbing stairs or ladders, or combining kneeling/squatting with heavy lifting. pp 1–83.
29. Maetzel A, Makela M, Hawker G, Bombardier C (1997) Osteoarthritis of the hip and knee and mechanical occupational exposure–a systematic overview of the evidence. J Rheumatol 24: 1599–1607.
30. Schouten JS, de Bie RA, Swaen G (2002) An update on the relationship between occupational factors and osteoarthritis of the hip and knee. Curr Opin Rheumatol 14: 89–92.
31. Bolm-Audorff U (2000) Zusammenhang zwischen beruflichen Einwirkungen und Coxarthrose- ein Uberlick. Arbeitsmed Sozialmed Umweltmed 35: 471–475.
32. D'Souza JC, Franzblau A, Werner RA (2005) Review of epidemiologic studies on occupational factors and lower extremity musculoskeletal and vascular disorders and symptoms. J Occup Rehabil 15: 129–165.
33. PEROSH Working Group (2011) Clearinghouse of Systematic Reviews on Occupational Safety and Health. PEROSH Website. Available: http://www.perosh.eu/p/clearinghouse. Accessed 2011 Jul 26.
34. Euler U (2010) Recommended search strategies for systematic reviews on "Does physical work load lead to hip osteoarthritis?" in *Search documentation form* of the Clearinghouse of Systematic Reviews on Occupational Safety and Health. PEROSH Website. Available: http://www.perosh.eu/p/8C4GZT. Accessed 2011 Jul 26.
35. Cochrane OSH (2011) Occupational Safety and Health Review Group. OSH Website. Available: http://osh.cochrane.org/. Accessed 2011 Jul 26.
36. Cooper C, Inskip H, Croft P, Campbell L, Smith G, et al. (1998) Individual risk factors for hip osteoarthritis: Obesity, hip injury, and physical activity. Am J Epidemiol 147: 516–522.
37. Vingard E, Alfredsson L, Goldie I, Hogstedt C (1993) Sports and osteoarthrosis of the hip. An epidemiologic study. Am J Sports Med 21: 195–200.
38. Vingard E, Alfredsson L, Malchau H (1998) Osteoarthrosis of the hip in women and its relationship to physical load from sports activities. Am J Sports Med 26: 78–82.
39. Schmitt H, Rohs C, Schneider S, Clarius M (2006) Is competitive running associated with osteoarthritis of the hip or the knee?. Orthopade 35: 1087–1092.
40. Schmitt H, Brocai DR, Lukoschek M (2004) High prevalence of hip arthrosis in former elite javelin throwers and high jumpers: 41 athletes examined more than 10 years after retirement from competitive sports. Acta Orthop Scand 75: 34–39.
41. Marti B, Knobloch M, Tschopp A, Jucker A, Howald H (1989) Is excessive running predictive of degenerative hip disease? Controlled study of former elite athletes. BMJ 299: 91–93.
42. Sandmark H (2000) Musculoskeletal dysfunction in physical education teachers. Occup Environ Med 57: 673–677.
43. Shepard GJ, Banks AJ, Ryan WG (2003) Ex-professional association footballers have an increased prevalence of osteoarthritis of the hip compared with age matched controls despite not having sustained notable hip injuries. Br J Sports Med 37: 80–81.
44. Drawer S, Fuller CW (2001) Propensity for osteoarthritis and lower limb joint pain in retired professional soccer players. Br J Sports Med 35: 402–408.
45. Kettunen JA, Kujala UM, Kaprio J, Koskenvuo M, Sarna S (2001) Lower-limb function among former elite male athletes. Am J Sports Med 29: 2–8.
46. Pope DP, Hunt IM, Birrell FN, Silman AJ, Macfarlane GJ (2003) Hip pain onset in relation to cumulative workplace and leisure time mechanical load: a population based case-control study. Ann Rheum Dis 62: 322–326.
47. Lawrence JS, Molyneux MK, ngwall-Fordyce I (1966) Rheumatism in foundry workers. Br J Ind Med 23: 42–52.
48. Reijman M, Hazes JM, Pols HA, Bernsen RM, Koes BW, et al. (2005) Role of radiography in predicting progression of osteoarthritis of the hip: prospective cohort study. BMJ 330: 1183.
49. Lau E, Lam T, Chan NH (2007) Risk factors for primary osteoarthritis of the hip and knee in the Hong Kong Chinese population. Hong Kong Med J 13: S9–14.
50. Jacobsen S, Sonne-Holm S (2005) Hip dysplasia: a significant risk factor for the development of hip osteoarthritis. A cross-sectional survey. Rheumatology 44: 211–218.
51. Olsen O, Vingard E, Koster M, Alfredsson L (1994) Etiologic fractions for physical work load, sports and overweight in the occurrence of coxarthrosis. Scand J Work Environ Health 20: 184–188.
52. Elsner G, Nienhaus A, Beck W (1995) Coxarthrosis and occupational work load. J Public Health 3: 131–144.
53. Jacobsen S, Sonne-Holm S, S°balle K, Gebuhr P, Lund B (2004) Factors influencing hip joint space in asymptomatic subjects: A survey of 4151 subjects of the Copenhagen City Heart Study: The Osteoarthritis Substudy. Osteoarthritis and Cartilage 12: 698–703. doi: DOI: 10.1016/j.joca.2004.06.002.
54. Teitz CC, Kilcoyne RF (1998) Premature osteoarthrosis in professional dancers. Clin J Sport Med 8: 255–259.
55. Cunningham RJ (1992) Farmer's hip. BMJ 305: 118–119.
56. Cvijetic S, Kanic-Ozegovic D, Campbell L, Cooper C, Potocki K (1999) Occupational physical demands and hip osteoarthritis. Arh Hig Rada Toksikol 50: 371–379.
57. van Dijk CN, Lim LS, Poortman A, Strubbe EH, Marti RK (1995) Degenerative joint disease in female ballet dancers. Am J Sports Med 23: 295–300.
58. Flugsrud GB, Nordsletten L, Espehaug B, Havelin LI, Meyer HE (2002) Risk factors for total hip replacement due to primary osteoarthritis: a cohort study in 50,034 persons. Arthritis Rheum 46: 675–682.
59. Jarvholm B, From C, Lewold S, Malchau H, Vingard E (2008) Incidence of surgically treated osteoarthritis in the hip and knee in male construction workers. Occup Environ Med 65: 275–278.
60. Juhakoski R, Heliovaara M, Impivaara O, Kroger H, Knekt P, et al. (2009) Risk factors for the development of hip osteoarthritis: a population-based prospective study. Rheumatology 48: 83–87.
61. Thelin A, Holmberg S (2007) Hip osteoarthritis in a rural male population: A prospective population-based register study. Am J Ind Med 50: 604–607.

62. Tuchsen F, Hannerz H, Jensen MV, Krause N (2003) Socioeconomic status, occupation, and risk of hospitalisation due to coxarthrosis in Denmark 1981–99. Ann Rheum Dis 62: 1100–1105.
63. Coggon D, Kellingray S, Inskip H, Croft P, Campbell L, et al. (1998) Osteoarthritis of the hip and occupational lifting. Am J Epidemiol 147: 523–528.
64. Yoshimura N, Sasaki S, Iwasaki K, Danjoh S, Kinoshita H, et al. (2000) Occupational lifting is associated with hip osteoarthritis: a Japanese case-control study. J Rheumatol 27: 434–440.
65. Vingard E, Hogstedt C, Alfredsson L, Fellenius E, Goldie I, et al. (1991) Coxarthrosis and physical work load. Scandinavian Journal of Work and Environmental Health 17: 104–109.
66. Croft P, Cooper C, Wickham C, Coggon D (1992) Osteoarthritis of the hip and occupational activity. Scand J Work Environ Health 18: 59–63.
67. Roach KE, Persky V, Miles T, Budiman-Mak E (1994) Biomechanical aspects of occupation and osteoarthritis of the hip: a case-control study. J Rheumatol 21: 2334–2340.
68. Vingard E, Alfredsson L, Malchau H (1997) Osteoarthrosis of the hip in women and its relation to physical load at work and in the home. Ann Rheum Dis 56: 293–298.
69. Barrero LH, Katz JN, Dennerlein JT (2009) Validity of self-reported mechanical demands for occupational epidemiologic research of musculoskeletal disorders. Scand J Work Environ Health 35: 245–260.
70. Lissner L, Potischman N, Troiano R, Bengtsson C (2004) Recall of physical activity in the distant past: the 32-year follow-up of the Prospective Population Study of Women in Goteborg, Sweden. Am J Epidemiol 159: 304–307.
71. Wiktorin C, Karlqvist L, Winkel J (1993) Validity of self-reported exposures to work postures and manual materials handling. Stockholm MUSIC I Study Group. Scand J Work Environ Health 19: 208–214.
72. Vingard E, Alfredsson L, Goldie I, Hogstedt C (1991) Occupation and osteoarthrosis of the hip and knee: a register-based cohort study. Int J Epidemiol 20: 1025–1031.
73. Vingard E, Alfredsson L, Malchau H (1997) Lifestyle factors and hip arthrosis. A case referent study of body mass index, smoking and hormone therapy in 503 Swedish women. Acta Orthop Scand 68: 216–220.
74. Thelin A, Vingard E, Holmberg S (2004) Osteoarthritis of the hip joint and farm work. Am J Ind Med 45: 202–209.
75. Rossignol M, Leclerc A, Allaert FA, Rozenberg S, Valat JP, et al. (2005) Primary osteoarthritis of hip, knee, and hand in relation to occupational exposure. Occup Environ Med 62: 772–777.
76. Bierma-Zeinstra S, Ginai A, Prins A, Verhaar J (1999) Validity of American College of Rheumatology criteria for diagnosing hip osteoarthritis in primary care research. J Rheumatol 26: 1129–1133.
77. Lindberg H, Danielsson LG (1984) The relation between labor and coxarthrosis. Clin Orthop Relat Res. pp 159–161.
78. Thelin A (1990) Hip joint arthrosis: an occupational disorder among farmers. Am J Ind Med 18: 339–343.
79. Chitnavis J, Sinsheimer JS, Suchard MA, Clipsham K, Carr AJ (2000) End-stage coxarthrosis and gonarthrosis. Aetiology, clinical patterns and radiological features of idiopathic osteoarthritis. Rheumatology (Oxford) 39: 612–619.
80. Lau EC, Cooper C, Lam D, Chan VNH, Tsang KK, et al. (2000) Factors Associated with Osteoarthritis of the Hip and Knee in Hong Kong Chinese: Obesity, Joint Injury, and Occupational Activities. Am J Epidemiol 152: 855–862.
81. Okunribido O (2009) Lower Limb MSD - Scoping work to help inform advice and research planning. HSL RR706: 1–84.
82. Benke G, Sim M, Fritschi L, Aldred G (2000) Beyond the job exposure matrix (JEM): the task exposure matrix (TEM). Ann Occup Hyg 44: 475–482.

Cost-Effectiveness of Total Hip and Knee Replacements for the Australian Population with Osteoarthritis: Discrete-Event Simulation Model

Hideki Higashi*, Jan J. Barendregt

School of Population Health, The University of Queensland, Herston, Queensland, Australia

Abstract

Background: Osteoarthritis constitutes a major musculoskeletal burden for the aged Australians. Hip and knee replacement surgeries are effective interventions once all conservative therapies to manage the symptoms have been exhausted. This study aims to evaluate the cost-effectiveness of hip and knee replacements in Australia. To our best knowledge, the study is the first attempt to account for the dual nature of hip and knee osteoarthritis in modelling the severities of right and left joints separately.

Methodology/Principal Findings: We developed a discrete-event simulation model that follows up the individuals with osteoarthritis over their lifetimes. The model defines separate attributes for right and left joints and accounts for several repeat replacements. The Australian population with osteoarthritis who were 40 years of age or older in 2003 were followed up until extinct. Intervention effects were modelled by means of disability-adjusted life-years (DALYs) averted. Both hip and knee replacements are highly cost effective (AUD 5,000 per DALY and AUD 12,000 per DALY respectively) under an AUD 50,000/DALY threshold level. The exclusion of cost offsets, and inclusion of future unrelated health care costs in extended years of life, did not change the findings that the interventions are cost-effective (AUD 17,000 per DALY and AUD 26,000 per DALY respectively). However, there was a substantial difference between hip and knee replacements where surgeries administered for hips were more cost-effective than for knees.

Conclusions/Significance: Both hip and knee replacements are cost-effective interventions to improve the quality of life of people with osteoarthritis. It was also shown that the dual nature of hip and knee OA should be taken into account to provide more accurate estimation on the cost-effectiveness of hip and knee replacements.

Editor: Pieter H. M. van Baal, Erasmus University Rotterdam, The Netherlands

Funding: Financial support for this study was provided by a grant from the Australian National Health and Medical Research Council (Health Services Research grant no. 351558). The funder had no role in study design, data collection and analysis, decision to publish, or preparation of the manuscript.

Competing Interests: The authors have declared that no competing interests exist.

* E-mail: h.higashi@ uqconnect.edu.au

Introduction

Musculoskeletal conditions constitute a major burden to the Australian population. Over 6.1 million people (of a population of 20 million) were estimated to suffer from a musculoskeletal condition in 2004 [1]. Musculoskeletal conditions are among the most frequently managed diseases by general practitioners accounting for 17% of consultations in 2003–2004 [2]. In 2002, musculoskeletal conditions were selected as the 7th National Health Priority Area [3]. Amongst the various conditions, osteoarthritis (OA) is the most common type. According to the Australian Burden of Disease and Injury study 2003 [4], OA accounted for 34,578 disability-adjusted life-years (DALYs) and was the largest contributor to musculoskeletal disease burden. The health expenditure associated with OA was AUD 1.1 billion in 2000-2001, or 25% of all musculoskeletal conditions that was the third largest component of the total health expenditure accounting for 9.4% [3]. One of the characteristics of OA is that the prevalence is higher amongst lower socio-economic quintiles, but not necessarily among the Indigenous population [5].

Currently there are limited measures to prevent OA, and there is no absolute cure [3]. However, various non-surgical and surgical procedures have become available to manage the symptoms associated with OA and improve physical mobility and quality of life of the affected population. Guidelines for non-surgical therapies and surgical referrals have been developed for general practitioners in Australia [2,6]. Whilst several options are available for surgical interventions, joint arthroplasty for hips and knees have been shown to be particularly efficacious to improve the quality of life of people with OA [7]. Studies from Australia and other countries have demonstrated hip and knee replacements to be a cost-effective option [8,9,10,11]. However, we are not aware of an analysis which accounted for the fact that people have two hips and two knees, and that within each pair joints are likely to have different severities of OA. Evaluations that take only a single joint into account may overestimate the benefit of surgical intervention because a sizable proportion of patients have OA in both joints, and pain relief will therefore be limited.

The aim of this study is to evaluate the cost-effectiveness of total hip and knee replacements for OA patients in Australia by accounting for two joints of the individuals. It was conducted as part of a large project which compares the cost-effectiveness of over 150 preventive and curative health interventions in Australia [12]. Therefore, this study complies with the economic protocol of the project in order to enable comparisons with all other interventions. This included the use of disability-adjusted life year (DALY) as the health outcome measure, which had a major implication on the methods to model the intervention effects.

Methods

The economic protocol of the parent project of this study guided the choice of methods for this study. The following sections provide the details of methods employed for the cost-effectiveness analysis. Further details are provided in Text S1 that is available online.

Perspective

A health system perspective was employed for this study. Although guidelines for economic evaluations often advocate a societal perspective, the broadest among various alternatives [13], the most appropriate perspective varies with each study depending on the target audiences and decision-making contexts. The parent project of this study aimed to assist policy makers and health services managers in making practical decisions about what services to provide within the available resources in the health sector. Given the aim, a health system perspective was deemed most appropriate for the project and was adopted in the economic protocol to which this study mostly adheres.

Discrete-event simulation model

The analysis employed a discrete-event simulation (DES) model. This type of model has over 50 years of history as a major tool for operational research [14]. Originally developed in the steel industry [15], DES models expanded over various sectors particularly in manufacturing, industry and service sectors [16]. Although the application to the health sector has been less extensive [14], experts lists healthcare as one of growing priority areas for DES model application [17]. This is reflected in the annual number of publications using DES in the healthcare domain which has nearly doubled since 2004 [18]. Application in the healthcare setting has been typically in modeling situations where populations of patients interact with healthcare delivery system, (e.g. elective surgery, operation room management, transplantable organ-allocation, patient-flow forecasting), interaction of individuals (e.g. infectious diseases), resource planning, and economic evaluation [19,20,21].

In economic evaluations, DES model has the flexibility to accommodate a richer structure without making it unmanageable in size [20]. Our study models OA stage progression, decision for joint replacement, durability and time of repetitive revisions for each joint separately, which requires a large number of attributes and events that likely exceeds the manageable size of a Markov model. Further, the time to event (e.g. decision for replacement, revision) depends on the time the joints have spent in the previous attribute. Such "memories" can be attached to the individuals in a DES model, which is difficult to achieve with a cohort Markov approach [20]. In a DES model, individual life histories are created by drawing randomly from distributions that describe the time to the occurrence of particular events. The individuals from the study population would move from one attribute to another, driven by events, by means of time to progression of OA severity, time to decision for surgery, probability of surgical success and death, survival time of implants to revisions, and time to death. We accounted for the right and left joints for each individual, with in the baseline analysis the assumption that the attributes of hip or knee joints are independent of each other (this assumption was examined in a sensitivity analysis (see Text S1 Section 3.3).

Figure 1 provides the schematic depiction of the model. An individual aged 40 or over in 2003 enters the model if the person has at least one joint with moderate OA (grade 2 with symptoms or grade 3–4 without symptoms) or worse. The other joint may or may not have OA, but both joints are at risk for progression of OA severity (or incidence) for some time. Following the assumption set for the Burden of Disease Study [4], the background mortality rate for these people was assumed to be higher with a relative risk of 1.1 compared to the rest of population without OA. The person with OA will receive non-surgical therapies, such as simple analgesia, non-steroidal anti-inflammatory drugs, land-based exercise and others, until the OA reaches a severity level that becomes too difficult to manage. Once the decision for a joint replacement is made, the person will receive the surgery which may either be successful (the DW of the joint will improve by the estimated effect size, either with complications or without) or unsuccessful (surgical death). After a successful replacement of a joint, the implant will function for a certain time until an event prompts a revision (e.g. dislocation, loosening etc.). The process of surgery and implant failure will repeat for each OA affected joint for life.

In modelling such events for each individual, we have drawn parameters from various sources. The information on the progression of OA severities was obtained from the Bristol OA 500 study [22] which followed-up patients with OA for eight years. The time to decision of surgery was modelled from the annual surgical rate among severe OA patients, which was calculated as the proportion of surgeries reported in the National Joint Replacement Registry [23] for 2003 and the number of OA patients at grade 3–4 (symptomatic) from the Burden of Disease study. The time to revision of implants was modelled by distinguishing short- and long-term causes. The information on the time to failure of implants due to short-term causes was obtained from the revision rates over seven years reported in the National Joint Replacement Registry [24]. The information on long-term causes was obtained from follow-up studies in international literature. We assumed separate Weibull distributions for short- and long-term causes for implant failures. The probability density curves for implant failures from the two Weibull distributions were then combined to a mixture distribution, normalized (i.e. the surface under the mixture distributions equals unity) and adjusted to fit the observed values by means of the Solver function in MS-Excel. Figure 2 provides an example of the combined distribution curve of time to revision of hip implants (see Text S1 Section 1.9 for further details of methods and outputs).

In simulating the progression of OA severity, time to decision of surgery and time to implant failure for each individual, we converted each estimated parameter to a continuous survival curve from which random draws determined the time to the next events. Other events, such as death from surgery, were determined by assessing the outcome of a Bernoulli trial based on the probabilities of such events obtained from literature (see Text S1 Section 1.6). The model was implemented in MS-Excel, using the Ersatz add-in [25] to perform the simulation. Table 1 provides the sources of information from which the input parameters were obtained.

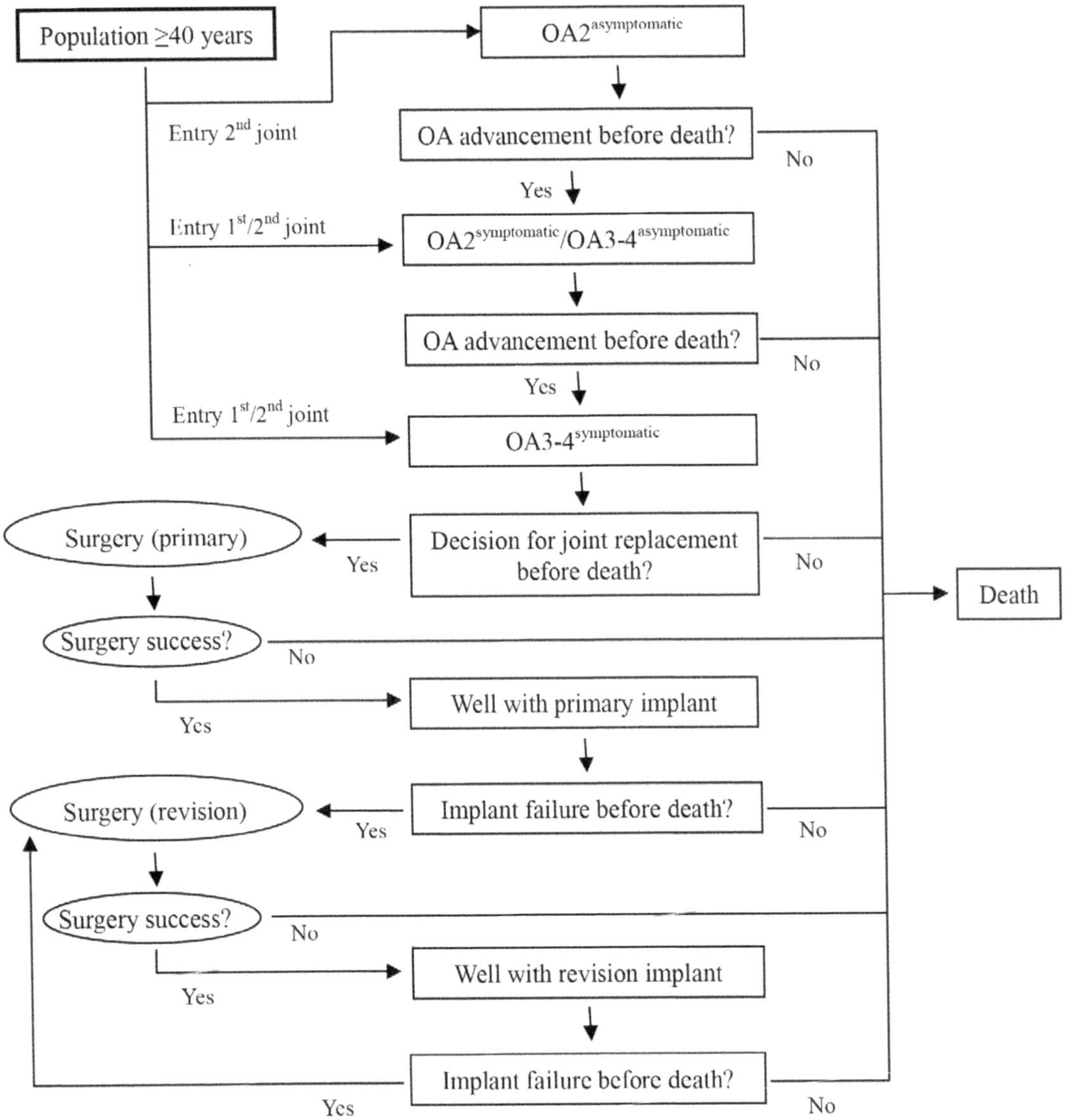

Figure 1. Event pathway of people with osteoarthritis in the discrete-event simulation model.

Study Population

The study population comprised of Australians with OA who were 40 years of age or older in 2003 as was estimated in the Australian Burden of Disease and Injury study. In the Burden of Disease study, OA was divided into four grades with different disability weights (DWs) assigned (see Table 2 and Text S1 Section 1.8) [4,66]. We limited the inclusion to males and females who had at least one hip or knee with grade 2 symptomatic OA or higher. The number of individuals for each sex/age-group was obtained from the Burden of Disease study. The study did not distinguish people with hip and knee OA. We therefore assumed that the proportion of hip and knee OA was the same as the age-group specific proportions of hip and knee replacement surgeries conducted in Australia in 2003 [23]. 68,908 individuals (30,347 males and 38,561 females) with hip OA and 100,657 individuals (42,930 males and 57,727 females) with knee OA entered the analysis and were followed-up until extinct.

Interventions

The interventions are total replacement of hips and knees. Whilst alternative methods are available for primary surgeries (i.e. hip resurfacing, uni-compartmental knee arthroplasty etc.), only primary conventional total hip replacements and primary total knee replacements, as defined in the National Joint Replacement Registry [23], including their subsequent revisions, were considered in this analysis as they constitute the majority of surgeries in Australia (91% of OA primary hip, 86% of OA primary knee) [24], and the evidence on efficacy of other types of implants has yet to be well established. All patients were assumed to have received a series of non-surgical treatments until these become insufficient prior to the decision to undergo surgery. The comparator for both hip and knee replacements is 'doing nothing' (continued non-surgical therapies without joint replacements).

OA is a chronic non-fatal disease which significantly affects the well-being of patients. Surgical intervention primarily aims to

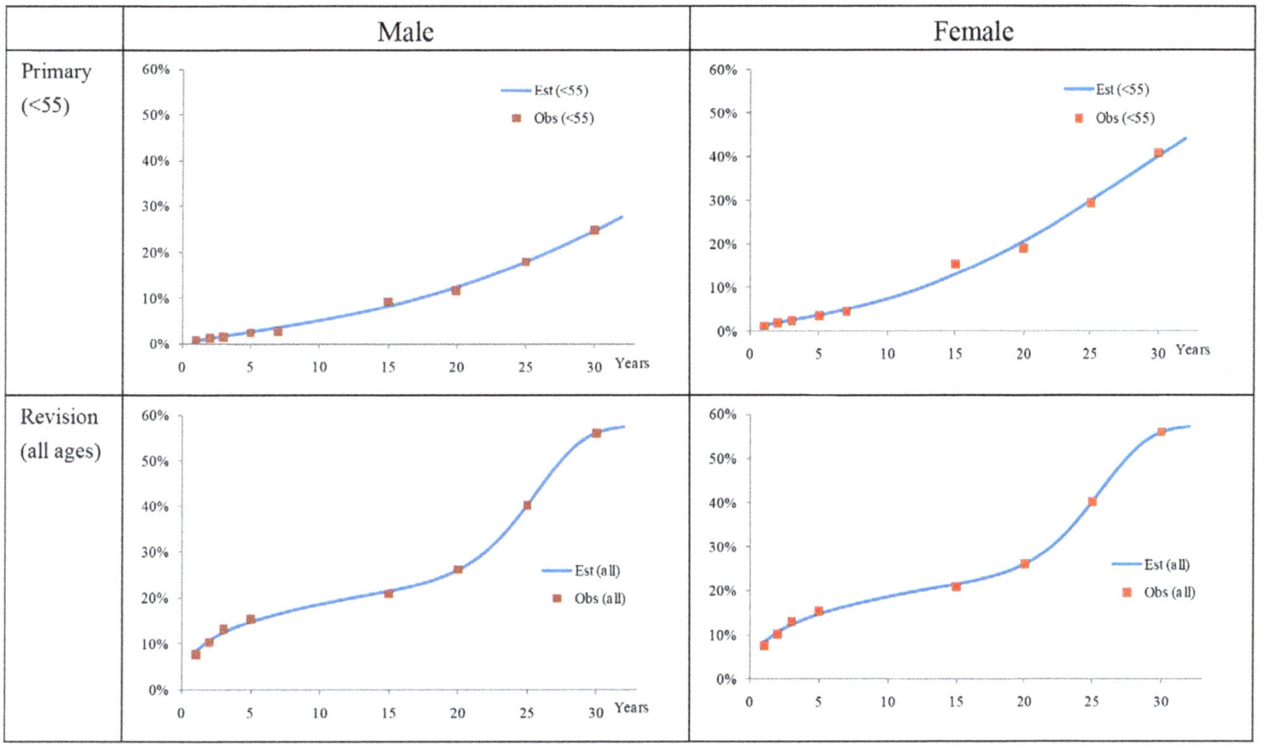

Figure 2. Cumulative distribution curve of time to revision with observed values (hip implants).

improve the quality of life of people with OA. The efficacies of hip and knee replacement surgeries have been evaluated by various instruments in the literature. Such instruments can range from generic (e.g. SF-36: Medical Outcomes Study Short-Form 36; HAQ: Health Assessment Questionnaire) [67,68], arthritic-specific (e.g. WOMAC: Western Ontario and McMaster University Osteoarthritis Index) [69], or utility (e.g. EQ-5D: EuroQol 5-dimensions [70]). As mentioned, we used the DALY disability weight (DW) from the Burden of Disease study to quantify the impact of OA on the quality-of-life faced by OA patients. However, we were not able to identify any literature utilizing this instrument to measure the effect of hip and knee replacement. Therefore, we estimated the effect size on the DW from literature utilizing other instruments in the following manner:

$$Effect = \left(1 - Score_{post}\right) / \left(1 - Score_{pre}\right) \quad (1)$$

$$DW_{post} = DW_{pre} * Effect \quad (2)$$

where *Effect* denotes the effect size of an intervention, $Score_{post}$ the single index of post-surgery scores from other instruments, $Score_{pre}$ the single index of pre-surgery score of other instruments, DW_{post} the DW at post-surgery, and DW_{pre} the DW at pre-surgery. For instruments that do not use scores that fall between 0 and 1, we adjusted the scores to fall within this range (e.g. HAQ uses scores between 0 and 3, so we divided the scores by 3). The underlying assumptions for this novel approach were two. First, although the scores used in other instruments are fundamentally different and are not comparable to each other, the ratios between pre- and post-intervention scores in each instrument reflect the same relative health improvements from the intervention. Second, the effect sizes calculated as per the above equation are comparable between instruments and serve as proxies for the effects on the DWs. In order to test for the plausibility of this technique, a sensitivity analysis was performed to compare the cost-effectiveness results between DALY and EQ-5D as health outcome measures for hip replacements where both results proved fairly comparable (see Text S1 Section 3.3).

We used different approaches to calculate $Score_{pre}$ and $Score_{post}$ for hip and knee replacements depending on the available data. To calculate the scores for hip replacements, we used the regression model from Briggs et al. [46] which they employed to estimate the pre- and post-surgical quality of life scores of hip replacements using EQ-5D. We assumed normal distributions to each regression coefficient and calculated the pre- and post-surgical quality of life scores, which were then assigned to Expressions 1 and 2 to extrapolate the post-surgical DW.

On the other hand, we were not able to identify an appropriate source for knee replacement providing a regression model like this. Therefore, we used the literature included in a systematic review [7] reporting the pre-and post-surgical scores of knee replacements in EQ-5D, HAQ, and SF-36. We performed a non-parametric bootstrap on Expression 1 with 5,000 iterations by assigning the scores reported in 13 primary studies with 16 indexes (i.e. one EQ-5D, one HAQ, and fourteen SF-36 indexes) to derive the mean effect sizes and confidence intervals [47,48,49,50,51,52,53,54,55,56,57,58,71]. In order to derive a single score from studies using SF-36, we referred to the transfer to utility (TTU) technique, a tool developed by Segal et al. [8] to convert the multiple sub-scales of SF-36 to a single utility score for OA and subsequently applied to stroke [72]. In recognition of the critique raised by Viney et al. [73] regarding the TTU due to the fundamental differences between the concepts underlying health-related quality of life-scores and utilities, our aim was to estimate the effect size of the intervention under the assumptions set out above rather than to

Table 1. Data sources.

Parameters	Sources of information
Population and demographic	
Population	Burden of Disease 2003 [4]
Mortality rate	Burden of Disease 2003
Prevalent years lived with disability	Burden of Disease 2003
OA	
Prevalence (all)	National health survey 2001 [1]
Prevalence (grade 2 symptomatic+)	Burden of Disease 2003
Proportion of number of people in each grade	Burden of Disease 2003, literature [26,27]
Mortality relative risk (OA)	Burden of Disease 2003
Progression of OA severity	Literature[22], Burden of Disease 2003
Proportion of bilateral OA	Literature [28,29,30,31,32,33,34,35,36]
DW	Burden of Disease 2003
Intervention (hip and knee replacement)	
Proportion of OA as primary diagnosis	Joint replacement registry 2007 [37]
Number of operations	Joint replacement registry 2004 [23]
Surgical death rate	CIHI 2007 [38], Joint replacement registry 2007
Revision rate (short term)	Joint replacement registry 2008 [24]
Revision rate (long term)	Literature [39,40,41,42,43,44,45]
Effect	Literature [7,46,47,48,49,50,51,52,53,54,55,56,57,58]
Cost	
Hip and knee replacement surgery	Australian hospital statistics (2003-04), National hospital cost data collection (2003–2004) [59,60]
Health expenditure for OA and all other health conditions	Disease costing and impact study (2000-01) [61]
Patient's out of pocket payment	Literature [62]
Patient's time cost	Average weekly earnings [63], Labour Force Statistics 2003 [64]
Price deflator	Health expenditure in Australia (2003-04) [65]

OA: osteoarthritis; CIHI: Canadian Institute for Health Information.

estimate the utility score itself. In light of the purpose of this study to compare the cost-effectiveness of disparate interventions, and in the absence of evidence on the effect size of hip and knee replacements on DWs, we regarded the TTU technique as an acceptable tool. Table 3 shows the estimated effect sizes on DWs (refer to Text S1 Section 1.8 for further details).

The health gains from the interventions were expressed as DALYs averted which were calculated using the following equation:

$$DALYs\ averted = \sum\left[(1\text{-}PYLD_a) * (1\text{-}DW1_{post}) * (1\text{-}DW2_{post})\right] - \sum\left[(1\text{-}PYLD_a) * (1\text{-}DW1_{pre}) * (1\text{-}DW2_{pre})\right] \quad (3)$$

where $PYLD_a$ denotes the prevalent years lived with disabilities (excluding those due to OA) of a person at age a since the time of primary joint replacement (for the intervention arm) or the time

Table 2. Case definition and sequelae.

OA sequelae	Definition
Grade 2 (radiological)	Definite osteophytes in hip or knee
Grade 2 (symptomatic)	Grade 2 and pain for at least 1 month in last 12
Grade 3-4 (asymptomatic)	Osteophytes and joint space narrowing in hip or knee, deformity also present for Grade 4
Grade 3-4 (symptomatic)	Grade 3+ and pain for at least 1 month in last 12

OA: osteoarthritis.
Source: The burden of disease and injury in Australia 2003 [4].

Table 3. Effect size of hip and knee replacements on disability-weights.

Joint	Type	Sex	Mean	SD	LCI 95%	HCI 95%
Hip	Primary	Male	0.3358	0.0454	0.2548	0.4319
		Female	0.3479	0.0376	0.2793	0.4260
	Revision	Male	0.5339	0.0830	0.3883	0.7115
		Female	0.5527	0.0709	0.4256	0.7018
Knee	Primary	Male	0.5202	0.0697	0.3888	0.6606
		Female	0.5205	0.0687	0.3891	0.6580
	Revision	Male	0.6610	0.0492	0.5642	0.7573
		Female	0.6698	0.0474	0.5772	0.7621

SD: standard deviation; LCI: lower confidence interval limit; HCI: higher confidence interval limit.

since the person was eligible for primary replacement should the person were to receive it (for the comparator arm), and $DW1_{post/pre}$ and $DW2_{post/pre}$ the disability experienced by the first and second joints for the person with and without joint replacements.

Intervention Cost and Cost Offset

Given the health system perspective employed for this study, all costs that fall on the health sector with the interventions were included in the analysis, both in the government and private sectors. The private sector costs included those born by the patients such as co-payment, travel costs and time costs. Health sector costs that can be saved due to the interventions are also included in the analysis.

Costs for surgeries were derived from the average cost per diagnosis-related group in 2003 [59,60] and the disease costing and impact study 2000-2001 [61]. We distinguished the surgical costs between primary replacements and revisions, and with and without complications. The probability of having complications for primary replacements and revisions were extrapolated from the proportion of complications in 2003, which were estimated from the reports of National Joint Replacement Registry and cost per diagnosis-related group. A random value from the Bernoulli trial determined the presence or absence of complications for the individuals in the simulation (see Text S1 Section 2.1).

Patient's out of pocket costs related to surgery were obtained from March et al. [62] assuming that the personal spending which accrue three months pre- and post surgery is part of the intervention costs. Patient's time costs were defined as those directly involved in receiving surgery-related services including travelling, waiting, pre-surgical visits, operation and recuperation. Unit costs associated with patient's time were obtained from the average weekly earnings in 2003 [63]. Future costs which are to be offset as the result of interventions were calculated from the annual OA expenditure obtained from disease costing and impact study 2000-2001 [61]. Unrelated health care costs, which would accumulate in the future due to extended life years of OA patients after joint replacements, were also obtained from the same source. Further details of the estimation of different costs are provided in Text S1 Section 2. The full data sources and estimated intervention costs are summarized in Tables 1 and 4. The exchange rate for Australian dollar (AUD) in 2003 was 1 AUD = 0. 67 USD (07/01/2003) [74]. The costs obtained from different years were all adjusted to the AUD 2003 value by means of price deflator [65].

Accounting for Uncertainties

Uncertainty distributions were provided for input parameters where appropriate in order to account for sampling uncertainties. The model underwent Monte Carlo simulation (often also known as probabilistic sensitivity analysis) by re-sampling the values of parameters 2,000 times from the given distributions. The distributions provided for each parameter are shown in Table 5.

The model was implemented in Microsoft Excel 2007, with the Ersatz add-in [25] for uncertainty analysis. We conducted the simulation under different scenarios based on the inclusion or exclusion of cost offset and patient's time cost. Future costs and health gains were discounted at an annual rate of 3% to account for time preference. The internal consistency of model was tested by comparing the proportions of total joint replacements occurring in each sex/age-group for a given year between the joint registry [23] and our simulation.

Results

Among those who have undergone successful hip and knee replacement surgeries at least once, 49% of males and 42% of females with hip OA had their second joints replaced along their course of life. The proportions of bilateral replacements for people with knee OA were 57% and 52% for males and females respectively. The test for internal consistency provided reasonably comparable outputs between the joint registry and our simulation (see Text S1 Section 3.4). Tables 6, 7, and 8 provide the costs, health gains, and incremental cost-effectiveness ratios (ICERs) and 95% uncertainty intervals (UIs) (sex-specific results provided in Text S1 Section 3.1). The results are reported at the population-level due to the aim of this study to inform policy makers at the national-level. While the protocol of the parent project of this study excluded the unrelated health care costs that would accumulate in the future due to prolonged life-years of patients [12], we report the results with the inclusion of such costs as an additional scenario (Table 9). Both hip and knee replacements were cost-effective compared to the pre-defined threshold level of AUD 50,000 per DALY averted by the overarching project of this study [12]. Although the ICERs become less favourable if we excluded the cost offset, or included the future unrelated health care costs, they are consistently below the threshold level. The scatter plots of hip and knee replacements are provided in Figure 3.

Discussion

This study has found favourable cost-effectiveness for hip and knee replacement in Australia. Given the sizable burden of OA in Australia, the interventions contribute substantially to the improvement of people's quality of life at reasonable costs. However, there were substantial differences in the cost-effective-

Table 4. Intervention cost (per surgery).

Cost item	Cost per surgery (AUD)
Government cost	
Hip replacement surgery (primary–Cscc)	13,648
Hip replacement surgery (primary+Cscc & revision–Cscc)	16,744
Hip replacement surgery (revision+Cscc)	30,648
Knee replacement surgery (primary–Cscc)	13,640
Knee replacement surgery (primary+Cscc & revision–Cscc)	19,620
Knee replacement surgery (revision+Cscc)	35,912
Other costs related to surgery (non-admitted visits etc.)	2,254
Patient out of pocket cost	
Out of pocket cost pre- and post-surgery (hip)	839
Out of pocket cost pre- and post-surgery (knee)	1,019
Time cost	
Pre-surgical visits (hip)	168
Surgery & recuperation (hip, male, primary–Cscc)	2,227
Surgery & recuperation (hip, male, primary+Cscc & revision–Cscc)	3,781
Surgery & recuperation (hip, male, revision+Cscc)	5,629
Surgery & recuperation (hip, female, primary–Cscc)	1,576
Surgery & recuperation (hip, female, primary+Cscc & revision–Cscc)	2,677
Surgery & recuperation (hip, female, revision+Cscc)	3,985
Pre-surgical visits (knee)	171
Surgery & recuperation (knee, male, primary–Cscc)	2,096
Surgery & recuperation (knee, male, primary+Cscc & revision–Cscc)	4,197
Surgery & recuperation (knee, male, revision+Cscc)	6,246
Surgery & recuperation (knee, female, primary–Cscc)	1,484
Surgery & recuperation (knee, female, primary+Cscc & revision–Cscc)	2,970
Surgery & recuperation (knee, female, revision+Cscc)	4,422

Cscc: catastrophic or severe complications and comorbidities.

Table 5. Distributions assumed for each parameter.

Parameters	Distributions
Time to primary replacement of hip and knee joints*	Empirical
Time to death*	Empirical
Time to revision of hip and knee implants*	Weibull†
Intervention effect (regression coefficients for hip replacement)	Normal‡
Intervention effect (knee replacement)	Beta‡
Intervention cost (hip and knee surgeries)	Gamma§
Patient's out of pocket payment pre/post-surgeries	Gamma§, Triangular**
Patient's time cost for surgeries	Gamma§, Triangular**
Average length of stay for hip and knee surgeries and recuperations	Gamma§

*These parameters accounted for the first-order uncertainties (individual level), and others the second-order uncertainties (population level).
†Time to failure due to short-run and long-run causes were distinguished. We assumed separate Weibull distributions for each cause, and modelled the time to revision as the normalized sum of these two. The Weibull parameters are provided in Text S1 Section 1.9.
‡The values are provided in Text S1 Section 1.8.
§The parameters of Gamma distributions consist of Alpha = unit cost, Beta = 1.
**Triangular distribution was used to model the uncertainty of unit costs (±20%), and Gamma distribution for the time spent in hospital.

Table 6. Health gains.

	Hip (DALY averted)		Knee (DALY averted)	
	Mean	**95%UI**	**Mean**	**95%UI**
DALY averted	115,000	98,800 - 129,000	113,000	93,200 - 133,000
DALY averted (per person)*	1.7 per person		1.1 per person	

DALY: disability-adjusted life-years; UI: uncertainty interval.
NB: The values are discounted by 3%, and rounded to the three digits of significance.
* Mean value divided by the number of people (68,908 for hip, 100,657 for knee).

ness between hip and knee replacements. Hip replacements were substantially more cost-effective than knee replacements. The ICER for knee replacements without cost offsets was AUD 21,000, or AUD 26,000 including unrelated health care costs, per DALY averted with time costs, and was about half that for hip replacements (AUD 12,000, or AUD 15,000 including unrelated health care costs, per DALY). The difference became slightly more prominent if we included the cost offsets in the analysis (ICER for knee: AUD 12,000, or AUD 17,000 including unrelated health care costs, per DALY with time costs; ICER for hip: AUD 5,000, or AUD 8,600 including unrelated health care costs, per DALY). There are a number of reasons for the more favourable results of hip replacements. First, the post-surgery health outcomes for hip replacements consistently surpass that for knee replacements in the literature [7]. This was reflected in our result where the cumulative health benefits was similar for hip and knee replacements despite the smaller number of people included in the hip replacement analysis (see Table 6). Second, more revisions were required for knee replacements (see Text S1 Section 1.10). Since a hip replacement provides better health outcome at lower costs compared to a knee replacement, it is more cost-effective. Although females have slightly more favourable ICERs for both hip and knee replacements, the UIs largely overlap with those of males. On the other hand, the ICERs can substantially vary between age-groups. Age-group specific results are provided in Text S1 Section 3.2 which shows less favourable ICERs for elderly patients, yet mostly within the threshold level.

An earlier study in Australia by Segal et al. [8] also reported favourable cost-effectiveness for joint replacements (AUD 4,535 – 6,953 per QALY for hip replacement and AUD 7,671 – 11,671 for knee replacement) although the findings are noticeably more favourable than ours (AUD 9,000 – 12,000 per DALY for hip replacement and AUD 16,000 – 23,000 per DALY for knee replacement, without cost offset, time cost, and unrelated health care cost) and not directly comparable due to methodological differences. Studies from other countries suggest the cost-effectiveness of hip replacement ranges between cost-saving and AUD 10,900 per QALY, and between AUD 9,000 and 24,400 per QALY for knee replacement [9,10,11]. In order to make the results from our study more comparable to the other ones, we conducted a sensitivity analysis by restricting one joint of all individuals to be free from OA for life (unilateral OA for both hips and knees), and by replacing the health outcome measure from DALY to QALY (EQ-5D) for hip replacement (this was difficult for knee replacement since the employed effect size was a pooled product from multiple studies using different instruments). The results from the analysis where one joint was always free from OA were AUD 6,900 per DALY and AUD 11,000 per DALY for hip and knee replacements, respectively (Text S1 Section 3.3). Further, replacing the health outcome measure for hip replacement to QALY and restrict one hip to be free from OA provided a cost-effectiveness ratio of AUD 6,500 per QALY (Text S1 Section 3.3). Interestingly all these results fell within the range of the ones from Segal et al., which support the hypothesis that accounting for only

Table 7. Costs under different scenarios.

Scenario	Hip (AUD Millions)		Knee (AUD Millions)	
	Mean	**95%UI**	**Mean**	**95%UI**
With cost offset				
Without time cost	420	400 - 440	1,100	1,100 - 1,200
With time costs	580	520 - 670	1,400	1,300 - 1,500
Without cost offset				
Without time cost	1,200	1,100 - 1,200	2,100	2,100 - 2,200
With time costs	1,300	1,300 - 1,400	2,400	2,300 - 2,500
*Cost per person**				
With cost offset (without time costs)	6,100 per person		11,000 per person	
Without cost offset (without time cost)	17,000 per person		21,000 per person	

AUD: Australian Dollar; UI: uncertainty interval.
NB: The values are discounted by 3%, and rounded to the two digits of significance.
*Mean value without time cost (unit: AUD) divided by the number of people in the model.

Table 8. Incremental cost-effectiveness ratio.

Scenario	Hip (AUD per DALY averted)		Knee (AUD per DALY averted)	
	Mean	95%UI	Mean	95%UI
With cost offset				
Without time cost	3,600	3,200 - 4,200	10,000	8,400 - 12,000
With time costs	5,000	4,200 - 6,200	12,000	10,000 - 15,000
Without cost offset				
Without time cost	10,000	9,000 - 12,000	19,000	16,000 - 23,000
With time costs	12,000	10,000 - 13,000	21,000	18,000 - 26,000

AUD: Australian Dollar; DALY: disability-adjusted life-years; UI: uncertainty interval.
NB: The values are discounted by 3%, and rounded to the two digits of significance.

one joint in the analysis yields too favourable cost-effectiveness ratios for hip and knee replacement surgeries.

Our analysis made a number of assumptions and has some limitations which are worth noting. First the quantification of the intervention effects was problematic. Whilst the change in the DALY DW plays a key role in measuring the intervention effects, we were not able to identify studies utilizing this instrument to measure the effects of hip and knee replacements. Therefore we extrapolated the effects from other instruments with assumptions which potentially could have under- or over-estimated the true DW post-interventions. However, the extrapolations were in line with the findings from a systematic review that the post-replacement indexes are consistently better than pre-surgery, and hip replacements have consistently better health outcomes than knee replacements. Further, as mentioned above, the sensitivity analysis comparing the results between DALY and EQ-5D as health outcome measures suggested the plausibility of these assumptions.

Another limitation was that the durability of hip and knee implants were modelled from historical data, which may be under estimating the current survivorship of implants given the technological advancement over decades. This issue has potentially resulted in a less favourable cost-effectiveness, since an improved durability of implants would reduce the number of revisions. Further, the revision rates of hip implants obtained from the National Joint Replacement Registry included replacement cases due to fractured neck of femur which are known to have a shorter lifespan than from other causes and were not included in our study population. This may have potentially caused an underestimation of the true survivorship of implants. However, the proportion of replacements due to fractures is small (2.8% between 1999 and 2004) [75], and so is not likely to have affected the estimation substantially.

The independence of OA progression and time to revision of implants assumed for the right and left joints warrants due attention. Whilst some correlation may exist between the two joints, the actual degrees are unknown. Therefore we performed a sensitivity analysis by assuming an extreme correlation between the two joints; i.e. ±0.99. The analysis did not provide significant deviations from our original results (see Text S1 Section 3.3), and so our findings are robust with respect to this assumption.

On the other hand, the study has its own strength. The nature of the intervention, which may or may not require repeated revisions at varying intervals for one or two joints, favoured the employment of a DES model. The model has the potential to account for variations at both (or either) individual levels (first order) and population levels (second order). This is one of the advantages of this study which would reflect the variations at the population level more accurately. Another strength was that the model was able to account for two hips or knees for each individual with OA. Modelling two joints separately for a person would have been difficult with other approaches. As discussed above, modelling just one joint overestimates health benefits since a sizable proportion of OA patients suffer from bilateral problems and hence replacement of one joint will leave the problem on the other joint. In this regard, a further study that account for OA problems in multiple sites of a patient (i.e. both hip and knee joints) may be warranted as more epidemiological data on OA become available.

In conclusion, the findings suggest that both hip and knee replacements are highly cost-effective with ICERs significantly lower than the AUD 50,000 per DALY threshold level. The interventions substantially contribute to the improvement of quality of life of population suffering from OA. Despite the limitations of the study, the overall conclusions from the analysis

Table 9. Incremental cost-effectiveness ratio including future unrelated health care costs.

Scenario	Hip (AUD per DALY averted)		Knee (AUD per DALY averted)	
	Without time cost	With time cost	Without time cost	With time cost
With cost offset	7,100	8,600	15,000	17,000
Without cost offset	13,000	15,000	24,000	26,000

AUD: Australian Dollar; DALY: disability-adjusted life-years.
NB: The values are discounted by 3%, and rounded to the two digits of significance.

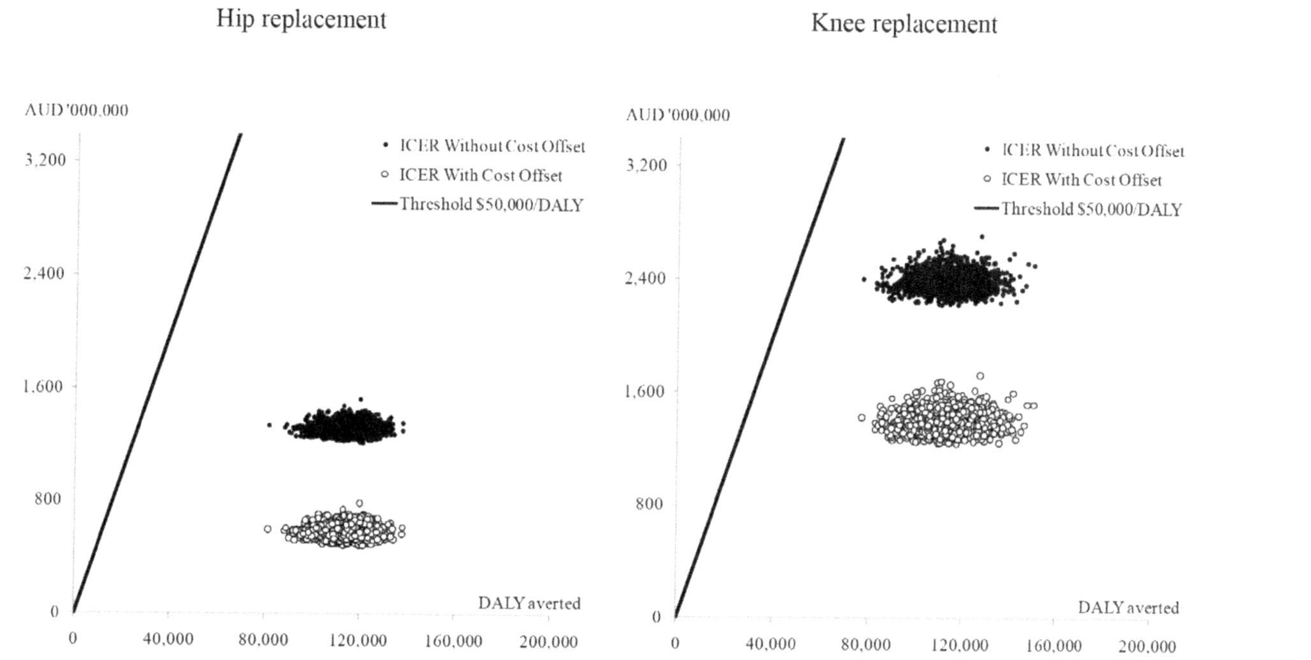

Figure 3. Cost-effectiveness of hip and knee replacements illustrated on a cost-effectiveness plane with AUD 50,000 per DALY threshold line (without time cost). The graphs represent population total rather than per patient outcomes (hip replacement: 68,908 individuals; knee replaceement: 100,657 individuals).

are not likely to be affected. It was also shown that we should take the dual nature of hip and knee OA into account to provide more accurate estimation on the cost-effectiveness of hip and knee replacements.

Supporting Information

Text S1 Details of methods, input data and additional results.

Acknowledgments

The authors greatly acknowledge Dr. Scott Crawford, Director of Orthopaedic Surgery, Prince Charles Hospital, for his technical advice on joint replacement surgeries, and Professor Robert Carter, Deakin University, for his advice on the costing part of the analysis.

Author Contributions

Analyzed the data: HH JJB. Contributed reagents/materials/analysis tools: HH JJB. Wrote the paper: HH JJB.

References

1. Australian Bureau of Statistics (2006) National health survey: summary of results, 2004-05. Canberra: Australian Bureau of Statistics.
2. The Royal Australian College of General Practitioners (2009) Guideline for the non-surgical management of hip and knee osteoarthritis. Melbourne: The Royal Australian College of General Practitioners.
3. Australian Institute of Health and Welfare (2005) Arthritis and musculoskeletal conditions in Australia, 2005. Canberra: Australian Institute of Health and Welfare.
4. Begg S, Vos T, Barker B, Stevenson C, Stanley L, et al. (2007) The burden of disease and injury in Australia 2003. Canberra: Australian Institute of Health and Welfare.
5. National Arthritis and Musculoskeletal Conditions Advisory Group (2005) A national action plan for osteoarthritis, rheumatoid arthritis and osteoporosis: a national health priority area. Canberra: Australian Government Department fo Health and Ageing.
6. The Royal Australian College of General Practitioners (2007) Referral for joint replacement: a management guide for health providers. Melbourne: Joint Replacement Waiting List Working Group, The Royal Australian College of General Practitioners.
7. Ethgen O, Bruyere O, Richy F, Dardennes C, Reginster JY (2004) Health-related quality of life in total hip and total knee arthroplasty. A qualitative and systematic review of the literature. J Bone Joint Surg Am 86-A: 963–974.
8. Segal L, Day S, Chapman A, Osborne R (2004) Priority setting in osteoarthritis. Melbourne: Centre for Health Economics, Monash University.
9. Lavernia C, Guzman J, Gachupin-Garcia A (1997) Cost effectiveness and quality of life in knee arthroplasty. Clin Orthop 1: 134–139.
10. Chang RW, Pellisier JM, Hazen GB (1996) A cost-effectiveness analysis of total hip arthroplasty for osteoarthritis of the hip. Journal of the American Medical Association 275: 858–865.
11. Rissanen P, Aro S, Sintonen H, Asikainen K, Slätis P, et al. (1997) Costs and cost-effectiveness in hip and knee replacements: a prospective study. Int J Technol Assess Health Care 13: 574–588.
12. Vos T, Carter R, Barendregt J, Mihalopoulos C, Veerman L, et al. (2010) Assessing cost-effectiveness in prevention (ACE-Prevention): Final report. Brisbane and Melbourne: University of Queensland, Deakin University.
13. Drummond MF, Jefferson TO (1996) Guidelines for authors and peer reviewers of economic submissions to the BMJ. BMJ 313: 275–283.
14. Taylor SJE, Eldabi T, Riley G, Paul RJ, Pidd M (2009) Simulation modelling is 50! Do we need a reality check? J Oper Res Soc 60: S69–S82.
15. Hollocks BW (2006) Forty Years of Discrete-Event Simulation: A Personal Reflection. The Journal of the Operational Research Society 57: 1383–1399.
16. Cao X, Day S, Shah S, McGee S (2006) Discrete event simulation in pharmaceutical research-a package line model. In: Robinson S, Taylor S, Brailsford S, Garnett J, eds. Birmingham. pp 1123–1130.
17. Taylor SJE, Robinson S (2006) So where to next? A survey of the future for discrete-event simulation. Journal of Simulation 1: 1–6.
18. Guenal MM, Pidd M (2010) Discrete event simulation for performance modelling in health care: a review of the literature. Journal of Simulation 4: 42–51.
19. Weinstein MC (2006) Recent Developments in Decision-Analytic Modelling for Economic Evaluation. Pharmacoeconomics 24: 1043–1053.
20. Barton P, Bryan S, Robinson S (2004) Modelling in the economic evaluation of health care: selecting the appropriate approach. J Health Serv Res Policy 9: 110–118.
21. Comas M (2008) Application of discrete-event simulation to health services research: analysis of needs and demand for elective surgery. Barcelona: Universitat Politècnica de Catalunya.

22. Dieppe P, Cushnaghan J, Tucker M, Browning S, Shepstone L (2000) The Bristol 'OA500 study': progression and impact of the disease after 8 years. Osteoarthritis Cartilage 8: 63–68.
23. Australian Orthopaedic Association National Joint Replacement Registry (2004) Annual report. Adelaide: Australian Orthopaedic Association.
24. Australian Orthopaedic Association National Joint Replacement Registry (2008) Annual report. Adelaide: Australian Orthopaedic Association.
25. Epigear (2010) Ersatz 1.1. Brisbane: Epigear International PTY LTD.
26. Guccione A, Felson D, Anderson J (1990) Defining arthritis and measuring functional status in elders: methodological issues in the study of disease and physical disability. Am Public Health Assoc. pp 945–949.
27. Felson D (1990) The epidemiology of knee osteoarthritis: results from the Framingham Osteoarthritis Study. Semin Arthritis Rheum 20: 42–50.
28. Dawson J, Linsell L, Zondervan K, Rose P, Randall T, et al. (2004) Epidemiology of hip and knee pain and its impact on overall health status in older adults. Rheumatology 43: 497–504.
29. Tepper S, Hochberg MC (1993) Factors associated with hip osteoarthritis: data from the first national health and nutrition examination survey (NHANES-1). Am J Epidemiol 137: 1081–1088.
30. Hochberg M, Lethbridge-Cejku M, Scott W, Reichle R, Plato C, et al. (1995) The association of body weight, body fatness and body fat distribution with osteoarthritis of the knee: data from the Baltimore Longitudinal Study of Aging. J Rheumatol 22: 488–493.
31. Mannoni A, Briganti MP, Di Bari M, Ferrucci L, Costanzo S, et al. (2003) Epidemiological profile of symptomatic osteoarthritis in older adults: a population based study in Dicomano, Italy. Ann Rheum Dis 62: 576–578.
32. Ingvarsson T, Hagglund G, Lohmander LS (1999) Prevalence of hip osteoarthritis in Iceland. Ann Rheum Dis 58: 201–207.
33. Davis MA, Ettinger WH, Neuhaus JM (1990) Obesity and osteoarthritis of the knee: evidence from the national health and nutrition examination survey (NHANES I). Semin Arthritis Rheum 20: 34–41.
34. Zhang Y, Xu L, Nevitt MC, Aliabadi P, Yu W, et al. (2001) Comparison of the prevalence of knee osteoarthritis between the elderly Chinese population in Beijing and whites in the United States: The Beijing osteoarthritis study. Arthritis & Rheumatism 44: 2065–2071.
35. Ledingham J, Regan M, Jones A, Doherty M (1995) Factors affecting radiographic progression of knee osteoarthritis. Ann Rheum Dis 54: 53–58.
36. Lacey R, Thomas E, Duncan R, Peat G (2008) Gender difference in symptomatic radiographic knee osteoarthritis in the Knee Clinical Assessment - CAS(K): a prospective study in the general population. BMC Musculoskeletal Disorders 9: 82.
37. Australian Orthopaedic Association National Joint Replacement Registry (2007) Annual report. Adelaide: Australian Orthopaedic Association.
38. Canadian Institute for Health Information (2007) Canadian joint replacement registry report: total hip and total knee replacements in Canada. Ottawa: Canadian Institute for Health Information.
39. Schulte KR, Callaghan JJ, Kelley SS, Johnston RC (1993) The outcome of Charnley total hip arthroplasty with cement after a minimum twenty-year follow-up. The results of one surgeon. J Bone Joint Surg Am 75: 961–975.
40. Callaghan JJ, Albright JC, Goetz DD, Olejniczak JP, Johnston RC (2000) Charnley total hip arthroplasty with cement: minimum twenty-five-year follow-up. J Bone Joint Surg Am 82: 487–497.
41. Callaghan JJ, Templeton JE, Liu SS, Pedersen DR, Goetz DD, et al. (2004) Results of Charnley total hip arthroplasty at a minimum of thirty years. A concise follow-up of a previous report. J Bone Joint Surg Am 86: 690–695.
42. Madey SM, Callaghan JJ, Olejniczak JP, Goetz DD, Johnston RC (1997) Charnley total hip arthroplasty with use of improved techniques of cementing. The results after a minimum of fifteen years of follow-up. J Bone Joint Surg Am 79: 53–64.
43. Schreurs BW, Bolder SBT, Gardeniers JWM, Verdonschot N, Slooff TJJH, et al. (2004) Acetabular revision with impacted morsellised cancellous bone grafting and a cemented cup: A 15- to 20-year follow-up. J Bone Joint Surg Br 86-B: 492–497.
44. Rand JA, Trousdale RT, Ilstrup DM, Harmsen WS (2003) Factors affecting the durability of primary total knee prostheses. J Bone Joint Surg Am 85-A: 259–265.
45. Rand J, Ilstrup D (1991) Survivorship analysis of total knee arthroplasty. Cumulative rates of survival of 9200 total knee arthroplasties. J Bone Joint Surg Am 73: 397–409.
46. Briggs A, Sculpher M, Dawson J, Fitzgerald R, Murray D, et al. (2003) Modelling the cost-effectiveness of primary hip replacement: how cost-effective is the Spectron compared to the Charnley prosthesis? York: Centre for Health Economics, The University of York.
47. Brazier JE, Harper R, Munro J, Walters SJ, Snaith ML (1999) Generic and condition-specific outcome measures for people with osteoarthritis of the knee. Rheumatology 38: 870–877.
48. Van Essen GJ, Chipchase LS, O'Connor D, Krishnan J (1998) Primary total knee replacement: short-term outcomes in an Australian population. J Qual Clin Pract 18: 135–142.
49. Bennett K, Torrance G, Moran L, Smith F, Goldsmith C (1997) Health state utilities in knee replacement surgery: the development and evaluation of McKnee. J Rheumatol 24: 1796–1805.
50. Dawson J, Fitzpatrick R, Murray D, Carr A (1998) Questionnaire on the perceptions of patients about total knee replacement. J Bone Joint Surg Br 80: 63–69.
51. Heck D, Robinson R, Partridge C, Lubitz R, Freund D (1998) Patient outcomes after knee replacement. Clin Orthop 356: 93–110.
52. Kiebzak G, Campbell M, Mauerhan D (2002) The SF-36 general health status survey documents the burden of osteoarthritis and the benefits of total joint arthroplasty: but why should we use it. Am J Manag Care 8: 463–474.
53. Kiebzak G, Vain P, Gregory A, Mokris J, Mauerhan D (1997) SF-36 general health status survey to determine patient satisfaction at short-term follow-up after total hip and knee arthroplasty. J South Orthop Assoc 6: 169–172.
54. Shields R, Enloe L, Leo K (1999) Health related quality of life in patients with total hip or knee replacement. Arch Phys Med Rehabil 80: 572–579.
55. Jones C, Voaklander D, Johnston D, Suarez-Almazor M (2001) The effect of age on pain, function, and quality of life after total hip and knee arthroplasty. Arch Intern Med 161: 454–460.
56. Jones C, Voaklander D, Johnston D, Suarez-Almazor M (2000) Health related quality of life outcomes after total hip and knee arthroplasties in a community based population. J Rheumatol 27: 1745–1752.
57. Bachmeier CJ, March LM, Cross MJ, Lapsley HM, Tribe KL, et al. (2001) A comparison of outcomes in osteoarthritis patients undergoing total hip and knee replacement surgery. Osteoarthritis Cartilage 9: 137–146.
58. Hozack W, Rothman R, Albert T, Balderston R, Eng K (1997) Relationship of total hip arthroplasty outcomes to other orthopaedic procedures. Clin Orthop 344: 88–93.
59. Australian Institute of Health and Welfare (2005) Australian hospital statistics 2003-04. Canberra: Australian Institute of Health and Welfare.
60. Australian Government Department of Health and Ageing (2005) National hospital cost data collection: cost report round 08 (2003-2004) AR-DRGv4.2. Canberra: Australian Government Department of Health and Ageing.
61. Australian Institute of Health and Welfare (2001) Disease costs and impact study 2000-01. Canberra: Australian Institute of Health and Welfare.
62. March L, Cross M, Tribe K, Lapsley H, Courtenay B, et al. (2002) Cost of joint replacement surgery for osteoarthritis: the patients' perspective. J Rheumatol 29: 1006–1014.
63. Australian Bureau of Statistics (2004) Average weekly earnings: November 2003. Camberra: Australian Bureau of Ststistics.
64. Australian Bureau of Statistics;Persons not in the labour force. Camberra: Australian Bureau of Ststistics.
65. Australian Institute of Health and Welfare (2005) Health expenditure Australia 2003-04. Canberra: Australian Institute of Health and Welfare.
66. Stouthard MEA, Essink-Bot ML, Bonsel GJ, Barendregt JJ, Kramers PGN, et al. (1997) Disability weights for diseases in the Netherlands. Rotterdam: Department of Public Health, Erasmus University.
67. Ware J, Sherbourne C (1992) The MOS 36-item short-form health survey (SF-36). I. Conceptual framework and item selection. Med Care 30: 473–483.
68. Fries JF, Spitz P, Kraines RG, Holman HR (1980) Measurement of patient outcome in arthritis. Arthritis & Rheumatism 23: 137–145.
69. Bellamy N, Buchanan W, Goldsmith C, Campbell J, Stitt L (1988) Validation study of WOMAC: a health status instrument for measuring clinically important patient relevant outcomes to antirheumatic drug therapy in patients with osteoarthritis of the hip or knee. J Rheumatol 15: 1833–1840.
70. EuroQol Group (1990) EuroQol - a new facility for the measurement of health-related quality of life. Health Policy 16: 199–208.
71. Bayley K, London M, Grunkemeier G, Lansky D (1995) Measuring the success of treatment in patient terms. Med Care.
72. Mortimer D, Segal L, Sturm J (2009) Can we derive an'exchange rate'between descriptive and preference-based outcome measures for stroke? Results from the transfer to utility (TTU) technique. Health and quality of life outcomes 7: 33.
73. Viney R, King M, Savage E, Hall J (2004) Use of the TTU is questionable. The Medical Journal of Australia 181: 338.
74. The United Nations (2003) Operational Rates of Exchange. New York: United Nations Treasury.
75. Australian Orthopaedic Association National Joint Replacement Registry (2005) Annual report supplementary. Adelaide: Australian Orthopaedic Association.

Permissions

All chapters in this book were first published in PLOS ONE, by The Public Library of Science; hereby published with permission under the Creative Commons Attribution License or equivalent. Every chapter published in this book has been scrutinized by our experts. Their significance has been extensively debated. The topics covered herein carry significant findings which will fuel the growth of the discipline. They may even be implemented as practical applications or may be referred to as a beginning point for another development.

The contributors of this book come from diverse backgrounds, making this book a truly international effort. This book will bring forth new frontiers with its revolutionizing research information and detailed analysis of the nascent developments around the world.

We would like to thank all the contributing authors for lending their expertise to make the book truly unique. They have played a crucial role in the development of this book. Without their invaluable contributions this book wouldn't have been possible. They have made vital efforts to compile up to date information on the varied aspects of this subject to make this book a valuable addition to the collection of many professionals and students.

This book was conceptualized with the vision of imparting up-to-date information and advanced data in this field. To ensure the same, a matchless editorial board was set up. Every individual on the board went through rigorous rounds of assessment to prove their worth. After which they invested a large part of their time researching and compiling the most relevant data for our readers.

The editorial board has been involved in producing this book since its inception. They have spent rigorous hours researching and exploring the diverse topics which have resulted in the successful publishing of this book. They have passed on their knowledge of decades through this book. To expedite this challenging task, the publisher supported the team at every step. A small team of assistant editors was also appointed to further simplify the editing procedure and attain best results for the readers.

Apart from the editorial board, the designing team has also invested a significant amount of their time in understanding the subject and creating the most relevant covers. They scrutinized every image to scout for the most suitable representation of the subject and create an appropriate cover for the book.

The publishing team has been an ardent support to the editorial, designing and production team. Their endless efforts to recruit the best for this project, has resulted in the accomplishment of this book. They are a veteran in the field of academics and their pool of knowledge is as vast as their experience in printing. Their expertise and guidance has proved useful at every step. Their uncompromising quality standards have made this book an exceptional effort. Their encouragement from time to time has been an inspiration for everyone.

The publisher and the editorial board hope that this book will prove to be a valuable piece of knowledge for researchers, students, practitioners and scholars across the globe.

List of Contributors

Hermien Janneke Schutte, Sofie Jansen, Nathalie van der Velde and Sophia E. J. A. de Rooij
Section of Geriatric Medicine, Department of Medicine, Academic Medical Center, Amsterdam, The Netherlands

Matthias U. Schafroth
Department of Orthopedic Surgery, Academic Medical Center, Amsterdam, The Netherlands

J. Carel Goslings
Trauma Unit, Department of Surgery, Academic Medical Center, Amsterdam, The Netherlands

François Genêt, Claire Jourdan and Alexis Schnitzler
Service de Médecine Physique et de Réadaptation, Hôpital Raymond Poincaré, Garches, France

Christine Lautridou, Thierry Judet and Philippe Denormandie
Service de Chirurgie Orthopédique et Traumatologique, Hôpital Raymond Poincaré, Garches, France

Didier Guillemot
Unité Fonctionnelle de Santé Publique, Hôpital Raymond Poincaré, Garches, France

Serge Poiraudeau
Service de Médecine Physique et de Réadaptation, Hôpital Cochin, Paris, France

Kerryl E. Piper, Marta Fernandez-Sampedro, Kathryn E. Steckelberg, Melissa J. Karau, James M. Steckelberg, Elie F. Berbari and Douglas R. Osmon
Division of Infectious Diseases, Department of Medicine, Mayo Clinic College of Medicine, Rochester, Minnesota, United States of America

Jayawant N. Mandrekar
Division of Biomedical Statistics and Informatics, Department of Health Sciences Research, Mayo Clinic College of Medicine, Rochester, Minnesota, United States of America

Robin Patel
Division of Infectious Diseases, Department of Medicine, Mayo Clinic College of Medicine, Rochester, Minnesota, United States of America
Division of Clinical Microbiology, Department of Laboratory Medicine and Pathology, Mayo Clinic College of Medicine, Rochester, Minnesota, United States of America

Arlen D. Hanssen, David G. Lewallen, Robert H. Cofield, John W. Sperling, Joaquin Sanchez-Sotelo and Paul M. Huddleston, Mark B. Dekutoski, Michael Yaszemski and Bradford Currier
Department of Orthopedic Surgery, Mayo Clinic College of Medicine, Rochester, Minnesota, United States of America

Thomas W. Lewis and Sarah C. Blott
Kennel Club Genetics Centre at the Animal Health Trust, Animal Health Trust, Newmarket, United Kingdom

John A. Woolliams
The Roslin Institute and Royal (Dick) School of Veterinary Studies, University of Edinburgh, Roslin, United Kingdom

Kelly L. Corbett, Akosua A. Nti and Julian J. Z. Prokopetz
Department of Orthopedic Surgery, Orthopedic and Arthritis Center for Outcomes Research, Brigham and Women's Hospital, Boston, Massachusetts, United States of America

Elena Losina
Department of Orthopedic Surgery, Orthopedic and Arthritis Center for Outcomes Research, Brigham and Women's Hospital, Boston, Massachusetts, United States of America
Division of Rheumatology, Immunology and Allergy, Brigham and Women's Hospital, Harvard Medical School, Boston, Massachusetts, United States of America
Department of Biostatistics, Boston University School of Public Health, Boston, Massachusetts, United States of America

Jeffrey N. Katz
Department of Orthopedic Surgery, Orthopedic and Arthritis Center for Outcomes Research, Brigham and Women's Hospital, Boston, Massachusetts, United States of America
Division of Rheumatology, Immunology and Allergy, Brigham and Women's Hospital, Harvard Medical School, Boston, Massachusetts, United States of America
Department of Epidemiology, Harvard School of Public Health, Boston, Massachusetts, United States of America

Caterina A. Lund, Ann M. Møller
Department of Anaesthesia and Intensive Care, Herlev University Hospital, Herlev, Denmark

Jørn Wetterslev and Lars H. Lundstrøm
Copenhagen Trial Unit, Centre for Clinical Intervention Research, Rigshospitalet, Copenhagen University Hospital, København, Denmark

Lars H. Lundstrøm
Department of Anaesthesia, Nordsjællands Hospital, Hillerød University Hospital, Hillerød, Denmark

Karl Michaëlsson and Liisa Byberg
Department of Surgical Sciences, Section of Orthopaedics, Uppsala University, Uppsala, Sweden
Uppsala Clinical Research Center, Uppsala University, Uppsala, Sweden

Håkan Melhus
Uppsala Clinical Research Center, Uppsala University, Uppsala, Sweden
Department of Medical Sciences, Section of Clinical Pharmacology, Uppsala University, Uppsala, Sweden

Anders Ahlbom and Bahman Y. Farahmand
The Institute of Environmental Medicine, Karolinska Institutet, Stockholm, Sweden

Zhengkui Zhou
College of Animal Science and Technology, Northwest A&F University, Yangling, China,
Institute of Animal Science, Chinese Academy of Agricultural Sciences, Beijing, China
Department of Clinical Sciences, College of Veterinary Medicine, Cornell University, Ithaca, New York, United States of America

Xihui Sheng
Institute of Animal Science, Chinese Academy of Agricultural Sciences, Beijing, China
Department of Clinical Sciences, College of Veterinary Medicine, Cornell University, Ithaca, New York, United States of America
Department of Animal Science and Technology, Beijing University of Agriculture, Beijing, China

Junya Li, Shangzhong Xu and Lixin Du
Institute of Animal Science, Chinese Academy of Agricultural Sciences, Beijing, China

Steve G. Friedenberg, Linda S. Hunter, Wendy S. Vandenberg-Foels, William E. Hornbuckle, Ursula Krotscheck, Elizabeth Corey, Nancy S. Moise, Nathan L. Dykes and Rory J. Todhunter
Department of Clinical Sciences, College of Veterinary Medicine, Cornell University, Ithaca, New York, United States of America

Zhiwu Zhang
Institute for Genomic Diversity, Cornell University, Ithaca, New York, United States of America

Keyan Zhao
Department of Computational Biology and Statistics, Cornell University, Ithaca, New York, United States of America

Lan Zhu
Department of Statistics, Oklahoma State University, Stillwater, Oklahoma, United States of America

Gang Guo and Yachun Wang
Department of Animal Science, China Agricultural University, Beijing, China

Jody Sandler
Guiding Eyes for the Blind, Yorktown Heights, New York, United States of America

Gregory M. Acland and George Lust
Baker Institute for Animal Health, Cornell University, Ithaca, New York, United States of America

Feng Zhang and Yin-Ping Zhang
The Key Laboratory of Environment and Genes Related to Diseases, Xi'an Jiaotong University College of Medicine, Ministry of Education, Xi'an, Shaanxi, People's Republic of China

Yao-Zhong Liu
Department of Biostatistics, Tulane University School of Public Health and Tropical Medicine, New Orleans, Louisiana, United States of America

Yan Guo, Xiao-Gang Liu, Xiang-Hong Xu, Yan-Fang Guo, Yuan Chen and Feng Pan
The Key Laboratory of Biomedical Information Engineering, Xi'an Jiaotong University School of Life Science and Technology, Ministry of Education and Institute of Molecular Genetics, Xi'an, Shaanxi, People's Republic of China

Xue-Zhen Zhu
University of Shanghai for Science and Technology, Shanghai, People's Republic of China

Hong-Wen Deng
Department of Biostatistics, Tulane University School of Public Health and Tropical Medicine, New Orleans, Louisiana, United States of America
The Key Laboratory of Biomedical Information Engineering, Xi'an Jiaotong University School of Life Science and Technology, Ministry of Education and Institute of Molecular Genetics, Xi'an, Shaanxi, People's Republic of China
University of Shanghai for Science and Technology, Shanghai, People's Republic of China

Yali Hou and Yachun Wang
College of Animal Science & Technology, China Agricultural University, Beijing, China

George Lust
Baker Institute for Animal Health, College of Veterinary Medicine, Cornell University, Ithaca, New York, United States of America

Lan Zhu
Department of Statistics, Oklahoma State University, Stillwater, Oklahoma, United States of America

Zhiwu Zhang
Institute for Genomic Diversity, Cornell University, Ithaca, New York, United States of America

Rory J. Todhunter
Department of Clinical Sciences, College of Veterinary Medicine, Cornell University, Ithaca, New York, United States of America

Yiqiong Zhao, Dong Fu, Kai Chen, Guodong Li, Zhengdong Cai, Yan Shi and Xiaobing Yin
The Tenth People's Hospital Affiliated with Tong Ji University Shanghai, China

Klaas A. Hartholt
Department of Internal Medicine - Section of Geriatric Medicine, Erasmus MC, University Medical Center Rotterdam, Rotterdam, The Netherlands
Department of Surgery-Traumatology, Erasmus MC, University Medical Center Rotterdam, Rotterdam, The Netherlands

Christian Oudshoorn and Tischa J. M. van der Cammen
Department of Internal Medicine - Section of Geriatric Medicine, Erasmus MC, University Medical Center Rotterdam, Rotterdam, The Netherlands

Stephanie M. Zielinski, Paul T. P. W. Burgers and Peter Patka
Department of Surgery-Traumatology, Erasmus MC, University Medical Center Rotterdam, Rotterdam, The Netherlands

Martien J. M. Panneman
Consumer and Safety Institute, Amsterdam, The Netherlands

Ed F. van Beeck
Department of Public Health, Erasmus MC, University Medical Center Rotterdam, Rotterdam, The Netherlands

Eric C. Sayre
Arthritis Research Centre of Canada, Vancouver, British Columbia, Canada
School of Population and Public Health, University of British Columbia, Vancouver, British Columbia, Canada
Department of Medicine, University of British Columbia, Vancouver, British Columbia, Canada

Jacek A. Kopec
Arthritis Research Centre of Canada, Vancouver, British Columbia, Canada
School of Population and Public Health, University of British Columbia, Vancouver, British Columbia, Canada

Linda C. Li
Arthritis Research Centre of Canada, Vancouver, British Columbia, Canada
Department of Physical Therapy, University of British Columbia, Vancouver, British Columbia, Canada

John M. Esdaile and Jolanda Cibere
Arthritis Research Centre of Canada, Vancouver, British Columbia, Canada
Division of Rheumatology, Department of Medicine, University of British Columbia, Vancouver, British Columbia, Canada

Sherry Bar
Primary Health Care, British Columbia Ministry of Health Services, Victoria, British Columbia, Canada

Norihide Sugisaki
Center for Environment, Health and Field Sciences, Chiba University, Kashiwa, Chiba, Japan
Waseda Institute for Sport Sciences, Waseda University, Tokorozawa, Saitama, Japan

Sadao Kurokawa
Center for Liberal Arts, Meiji Gakuin University, Yokohama, Kanagawa, Japan

Junichi Okada
Faculty of Sport Sciences, Waseda University, Tokorozawa, Saitama, Japan

Hiroaki Kanehisa
National Institute of Fitness and Sports in Kanoya, Kanoya, Kagoshima, Japan

Thomas W. Lewis and Sarah C. Blott
Kennel Club Genetics Centre at the Animal Health Trust, Animal Health Trust, Newmarket, United Kingdom

John A. Woolliams
The Roslin Institute and Royal (Dick) School of Veterinary Studies, University of Edinburgh, Roslin, United Kingdom

Agnes Dechartres, Isabelle Boutron, Carine Roy, Gabriel Baron and Philippe Ravaud
INSERM, U738, Paris, France
Université Paris 7, UFR de Médecine, Paris, France
AP-HP, Hôpital Bichat, Département d'Epidémiologie, Biostatistique et Recherche Clinique, Paris, France

Remy Nizard
Assistance Publique-Hôpitaux de Paris (AP-HP), Hôpital Lariboisie` re, Service d'Orthopé die, Paris, France
Université Paris VII, Paris, France

Serge Poiraudeau
Assistance Publique-Hôpitaux de Paris (AP-HP), Hôpital Cochin, Service de Médecine Physique et de Réadaptation, Paris, France
Université Paris V, Paris, France
Institut Fédé ratif de Recherche sur le Handicap, Paris, France

Jean-François Ravaud
INSERM, U750-CERMES, Paris, France
Institut Fédé ratif de Recherche sur le Handicap, Paris, France

François Genêt, Claire Jourdan, Clément Chehensse and Alexis Schnitzler
Service de Médecine Physique et de Réadaptation, CHU R.Poincaré, Garches, France

Christine Lautridou and Philippe Denormandie
Service de chirurgie Orthopédique, CHU R.Poincaré, Garches, France

Kambiz Minooee
Service de Rhumatologie et de Médecine Physique, CHU Erasme, Bruxelles, Belgique

Bethany J. Wilson, Frank W. Nicholas, John W. James, Claire M. Wade, Imke Tammen,
Herman W. Raadsma, Kao Castle and Peter C. Thomson
Faculty of Veterinary Science, The University of Sydney, Sydney, New South Wales, Australia

Claire Jourdan
AP-HP, Hôpital R. Poincaré , Service de Médecine Physique et Réadaptation, Garches, France
Institut National de la Santé et de la Recherche Médicale (INSERM) E 0738, Centre d'Epidémiologie Clinique, Université Paris Descartes, Paris, France

Stéphane Descamps, Stéphane Boisgard and Myriam Galvin
CHU Clermont-Ferrand, Hôpital Gabriel Montpied, Service d'Orthopé die, Traumatologie, Chirurgie plastique et reconstructive, Université Claude Monnet, Clermont-Ferrand, France

Rémy Nizard
AP-HP, Hôpital Lariboisiére, Service de Chirurgie Orthopédique et Traumatologique, Université Paris 7, Paris, France

Serge Poiraudeau, Moussa Hamadouche and Philippe Anract
AP-HP, Hôpital Cochin, Service d'Orthopédie, Université Paris Descartes, Paris, France

Philippe Ravaud
Institut National de la Santé et de la Recherche Médicale (INSERM) E 0738, Centre d'Epidémiologie Clinique, Université Paris Descartes, Paris, France

Jennifer Seida, Ben Vandermeer and Donna M. Dryden
Department of Pediatrics, Alberta Research Centre for Health Evidence, University of Alberta, Edmonton, Canada

Lisa Hartling
Department of Pediatrics, Alberta Research Centre for Health Evidence, University of Alberta, Edmonton, Canada
Department of Pediatrics, Cochrane Child Health Field, University of Alberta, Edmonton, Alberta, Canada

Ricardo M. Fernandes
Gulbenkian Programme for Advanced Medical Education; Departamento da Criança e da Família (Child and Family Department), Hospital de Santa Maria; Laboratório de Farmacologia Clínica e Terapêutica (Clinical Pharmacology and Therapeutics), Instituto de Medicina Molecular, Lisboa, Portugal

Lihong Fan, Xiaoqian Dang and Kunzheng Wang
Department of Orthopaedic Surgery, Second Affiliated Hospital, Medical School of Xi'an Jiaotong University, Xi'an, Shaanxi Province, People's Republic of China

Margreet Kloppenburg
Department of Rheumatology, Leiden University Medical Center, Leiden, The Netherlands,
Department of Clinical Epidemiology, Leiden University Medical Center, Leiden, The Netherlands

Erlangga Yusuf, Jessica Bijsterbosch and Tom W. J. Huizinga
Department of Rheumatology, Leiden University Medical Center, Leiden, The Netherlands

P. Eline Slagboom
Department of Molecular Epidemiology, Leiden University Medical Center, Leiden, The Netherlands

Herman M. Kroon
Department of Radiology, Leiden University Medical Center, Leiden, The Netherlands

Frits R. Rosendaal
Department of Clinical Epidemiology, Leiden University Medical Center, Leiden, The Netherlands

Fiona E. McGuigan
Clinical and Molecular Osteoporosis Research Unit, Department of Clinical Sciences, Lund University, Sweden

Maria Swanberg
Clinical and Molecular Osteoporosis Research Unit, Department of Clinical Sciences, Lund University, Sweden
Neurodegeneration and Inflammation Genetics Unit, Department of Experimental Medical Science, Lund University, Sweden

Kaisa K. Ivaska
Department of Cell Biology and Anatomy, Institute of Biomedicine, University of Turku, Turku, Finland

Paul Gerdhem
Department of Clinical Science, Intervention and Technology, Karolinska Institute, Stockholm, Sweden
Department of Orthopaedics, Karolinska University Hospital, Stockholm, Sweden,

Kristina Å kesson
Clinical and Molecular Osteoporosis Research Unit, Department of Clinical Sciences, Lund University, Sweden
Department of Orthopaedics, Skåne University Hospital, Malmö, Sweden

Stephanie Panzer
Department of Radiology, Trauma Center Murnau, Murnau, Germany

Dario Piombino-Mascali and Albert R. Zink
EURAC - Institute for Mummies and the Iceman, Bolzano, Italy

Wen-Hung Huang, Shen-Yang Lee, Cheng-Hao Weng and Ping-Chin Lai
Department of Nephrology, Chang Gung Memorial Hospital, Linkou, Taiwan, Republic of China
Chang Gung University College of Medicine, Taoyuan, Taiwan, Republic of China

Sandra I. Sulsky and Laura Carlton
ENVIRON International Corporation, Amherst, Massachusetts, United States of America

Frank Bochmann, Rolf Ellegast, Ulrich Glitsch and Yi Sun
Institut für Arbeitsschutz der Deutschen Gesetzlichen Unfallversicherung (IFA), Sankt Augustin, Germany

Bernd Hartmann and D. Seidel
Berufsgenossenschaft der Bauwirtschaft (BG BAU), Arbeitsmedizinisch-Sicherheitstechnischer Dienst, Berlin, Germany

Dirk Pallapies
Institut für Prävention und Arbeitsmedizin der Deutschen Gesetzlichen Unfallversicherung (IPA), Bochum, Germany

Hideki Higashi and Jan J. Barendregt
School of Population Health, The University of Queensland, Herston, Queensland, Australia

Index